Orthotic Intervention for the Hand and Upper Extremity

SPLINTING PRINCIPLES AND PROCESS

Second Edition

MaryLynn Jacobs, MS, OTR/L, CHT
Partner/Owner/Hand Therapist
Attain® Therapy + Fitness
Corporate Office
East Longmeadow, MA

Noelle M. Austin, MS, PT, CHT
Owner/Instructor
CJ Education and Consulting, LLC
Woodbridge, CT

Hand Therapist
The Orthopaedic Group
Hamden, CT

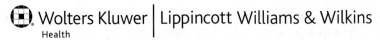
Wolters Kluwer | Lippincott Williams & Wilkins
Health
Philadelphia • Baltimore • New York • London
Buenos Aires • Hong Kong • Sydney • Tokyo

Acquisitions Editor: Michael Nobel
Product Manager: Paula C. Williams
Marketing Manager: Shauna Kelley
Production Project Manager: Marian Bellus
Designer: Teresa Mallon
Manufacturing Coordinator: Margie Orzech
Compositor: Absolute Service, Inc.

351 West Camden Street	Two Commerce Square
Baltimore, MD 21201	2001 Market Street
	Philadelphia, PA 19103

Printed in China

9 8 7 6 5 4 3 2 1

Library of Congress Cataloging-in-Publication Data

Splinting the hand and upper extremity.
  Orthotic intervention for the hand and upper extremity : splinting principles and process / [edited by] MaryLynn Jacobs, Noelle Austin. — Second Edition.
     p. ; cm.
  Preceded by: Splinting the hand and upper extremity : principles and process / [edited by] MaryLynn A. Jacobs, Noelle M. Austin. c2003.
  Includes bibliographical references and index.
  ISBN 978-1-4511-4530-4
  I. Jacobs, MaryLynn A., editor of compilation. II. Austin, Noelle M., editor of compilation. III. Title.
  [DNLM: 1. Hand. 2. Splints. 3. Arm Injuries—rehabilitation. 4. Arm. 5. Hand Injuries—rehabilitation. 6. Orthotic Devices. WE 26]
  RD559
  617.5'74044—dc23

                                                                                  2013021398

DISCLAIMER

Care has been taken to confirm the accuracy of the information present and to describe generally accepted practices. However, the authors, editors, and publisher are not responsible for errors or omissions or for any consequences from application of the information in this book and make no warranty, expressed or implied, with respect to the currency, completeness, or accuracy of the contents of the publication. Application of this information in a particular situation remains the professional responsibility of the practitioner; the clinical treatments described and recommended may not be considered absolute and universal recommendations.

The authors, editors, and publisher have exerted every effort to ensure that drug selection and dosage set forth in this text are in accordance with the current recommendations and practice at the time of publication. However, in view of ongoing research, changes in government regulations, and the constant flow of information relating to drug therapy and drug reactions, the reader is urged to check the package insert for each drug for any change in indications and dosage and for added warnings and precautions. This is particularly important when the recommended agent is a new or infrequently employed drug.

Some drugs and medical devices presented in this publication have Food and Drug Administration (FDA) clearance for limited use in restricted research settings. It is the responsibility of the health care provider to ascertain the FDA status of each drug or device planned for use in their clinical practice.

To purchase additional copies of this book, call our customer service department at **(800) 638-3030** or fax orders to **(301) 223-2320**. International customers should call **(301) 223-2300**.

Visit Lippincott Williams & Wilkins on the Internet: http://www.lww.com. Lippincott Williams & Wilkins customer service representatives are available from 8:30 am to 6:00 pm, EST.

RRS1306

This Book is Dedicated

To Our Families and all the patients we have treated throughout the years

Foreword

As a therapist who has written about and taught hand splinting (now accurately called orthotic fabrication) for many years, I commend MaryLynn Jacobs and Noelle Austin on giving you, the reader, this second edition of *Splinting the Hand and Upper Extremity: Principles and Process*, which now has the updated title of *Orthotic Intervention for the Hand and Upper Extremity: Splinting Principles and Process*.

This book is your doorway into the complex, skill-based, real world of orthotic intervention for the upper extremity. Therapists who want to specialize in treating upper extremity patients must have a wide range of knowledge and ability in orthotic intervention by developing an understanding of the underlying anatomical principles, how tissue heals and matures, how to apply mechanical principles to orthotic design, how to skillfully handle orthotic tools and materials, and how to evaluate and determine the need for and the appropriate design of an orthosis. Then they must be able to design, fabricate, fit, adjust, and describe for billing, as well as reevaluate the effectiveness of the orthotic intervention. This book delivers all of this information and more to the reader.

Why Should You Read This Book?

I have observed therapists in the clinic wanting a book, which will give them a pattern for an orthosis and how to construct it but nothing more. But an orthosis is only part of the treatment approach and cannot be separated from a comprehensive understanding of the pathology and how a therapist can influence the outcome. This book combines the "how to" with the "why" and directs you to resources, which can further your understanding. To appreciate the entire therapy process and not just the construction, an orthosis should be every therapist's goal.

A number of features of this book set it apart from others on this subject. Not all orthoses need to be made of low-temperature thermoplastics, and the authors' discussion of casting, taping, use of neoprene and prefabricated orthoses completes your armamentarium to address the wide range of specific patient needs. The real-life "Clinical Pearls" included throughout the book give you insight from experienced clinicians who have learned on-the-job tips and tricks to increase efficiency and patient comfort.

For therapists who are looking for a starting point, the section on "Orthotic Fabrication" gives you a step-by-step design and construction process, while concurrently the section on "Orthotic Intervention for Specific Diagnoses and Populations" provides deeper insight to the appropriate orthotic intervention for specific diagnostic problems. The case study accompanying each chapter in this latter section illustrates direct application to a specific situation.

Reading this book as well as some of the recommended references will take you a long way toward gaining orthotic skills. In our current busy clinic climate, time to practice and learn orthotic skills is scarce and we must find innovative methods and resources to build and maintain this skill set.

Why Was I Willing to Write This Foreword?

I wrote this because it matters that we, as therapists, develop and maintain a high level of orthotic intervention skills for our patients as part of our treatment spectrum. No one else can integrate the use of an orthosis into the treatment but us. My recommendation is to keep this book at your bedside as well as next to your treatment area. Read a few pearls each day and incorporate them into your clinical practice or make an unfamiliar orthosis on a coworker as self- training. You will build your skill and knowledge arsenal each day.

Who knows . . . perhaps you will contribute to the text on orthotic intervention for the next generation.

Judy C. Colditz, OTR/L, CHT, FAOTA
HandLab
Raleigh, NC
June 1, 2013

Preface

Orthotic Intervention for the Hand and Upper Extremity: Splinting Principles and Process, Second Edition, was inspired by clinicians and students who, in our teaching experience, were requesting one resource that would clarify all appropriate traditional orthosis fabrication /splinting, casting, and taping managements for upper extremity diagnoses. Although an upper extremity therapist tends to fabricate thermoplastic orthoses most of the time, there are many situations when casting, taping, neoprene, or even a prefabricated orthosis is a more appropriate choice. This book is unique in that it provides orthosis patterns for most upper extremity diagnoses as well as in-depth discussions and instructions for fabricating and choosing these other options. This feature truly distinguishes this book from all others currently on the market. We do not delve into the specifics of rehabilitation techniques and surgical interventions; instead, we provide overviews of the various diagnoses described to clarify a particular rationale specific to an orthosis design or protocol. Chapters on **Neoprene Orthoses**, **Peripheral Nerves Injuries**, **Adult Neurological Dysfunction**, **Tendon Injuries**, and **The Pediatric Patient** have been totally revised and expanded. A new chapter on **Hand and Upper Extremity Transplantation** has been added. The reference and suggested reading lists for each chapter are located online to guide the student to further study on a particular topic.

Organization Highlights and Features

This book is divided into four sections. **Section I** focuses on the fundamentals. Much of the mystery surrounding orthotic fabrication can be eliminated if the therapist has a good working knowledge of appropriate nomenclature (to interpret referrals), upper extremity anatomy, tissue healing guidelines, and a concrete understanding of mechanical principles. This section provides the foundation necessary to plan and create an orthosis. **Chapter 1** presents a modified version of the American Society of Hand Therapists (ASHT) orthosis nomenclature, which is used consistently throughout the book. **Chapter 2** systematically reviews the bony and neuromuscular anatomy, specifically as it relates to the application of orthoses. **Chapter 3** describes the stages of healing, factors that influence healing, and the relationship of specific stages of healing to orthosis selection and application. **Chapter 4** defines the fundamental mechanical terms and concepts pertinent to orthosis design and fabrication and discusses the clinical relevance and application of these basic principles using specific examples. **Chapter 5** surveys the proper equipment crucial to effective orthosis fabrication. **Chapter 6** outlines the entire process of creating an accurate orthosis design, from obtaining an appropriate referral to properly dispensing the device. It also introduces the PROCESS concept used in Section II.

Section II is the working section of the book and is organized into four chapters that cover immobilization (**Chapter 7**), mobilization (**Chapter 8**), restriction (**Chapter 9**), and nonarticular (**Chapter 10**) orthoses.

Each chapter includes pattern illustrations and accompanying photography of the orthosis described. Most of the pattern descriptions include **Clinical Pearls** and **Pattern Pearls** that apply to that particular orthosis. These pearls relate to our personal experience and the experience of our colleagues. They include fabrication and orthosis modification tips as well as insight for improving cost containment and maximizing time efficiency. Most orthosis patterns have alternative design options in the event that the therapist cannot fabricate a custom orthosis. Common diagnoses and general positioning are recommended. However, one must appreciate that the diagnoses appropriate for an orthosis and the recommended positioning can be varied and depend on many factors. The pattern designs illustrated are suggestions of the ones we have found simple to visualize and use. The Pattern Pearls give alternative pattern designs that we have used in our clinical practice. The therapist is encouraged to modify the pattern according to specific patient needs. Section II is meant as a guideline for orthosis construction—use your creativity to individualize each device. The Clinical Pearls are not always unique to a particular orthosis, and many apply to a variety of orthoses. A complete list of Clinical Pearls is provided at the front of the book to help the student locate specific points of interest.

Section III describes alternative interventions for immobilization, mobilization, or restriction of a body part. Because of time constraints, monetary issues, or perhaps lack of product availability, it is not always practical or appropriate to make an orthosis from thermoplastic materials. The chapters included in this section provide information on alternative means of orthotic fabrication. Chapter 11 outlines the considerations and options related to the use of prefabricated orthoses, including information on how to become an educated consumer on the availability, application, and modification of these devices. Chapter 11 also reviews some of the commonly used and currently available orthoses on the market. Chapter 12 describes casting as a treatment technique that has the ability to provide outcomes that no other orthotic intervention approach can offer. It familiarizes the clinician with the characteristics of casting products so he or she can choose the material that best meets the patient's needs. Chapter 13 provides a brief overview of three popular taping methods: traditional athletic taping, McConnell taping, and elastic therapeutic taping. Each technique is described with specific instructions and multiple clinical examples. Chapter 14 is a noteworthy chapter because neoprene is becoming increasingly popular. It reviews the basic information regarding the benefits of neoprene, qualities of neoprene materials, and a variety of thought provoking options and alternatives for orthotic management.

Each chapter in Section IV goes into depth regarding a specific diagnosis or patient population including stiffness, fractures, arthritis, tendon injuries, peripheral nerves injuries, the athlete, adult neurologic dysfunction, the pediatric patient, burns, the musician, and, lastly, the newly added chapter, the transplanted upper extremity. This chapter highlights emerging concepts on the postoperative management of this unique population.

After an overview of the topic, the chapters include common orthotic interventions and specific considerations. Many chapters include tables that clarify information and decrease redundancy within the text. Case Studies accompany each chapter and are meant to stimulate clinical reasoning and synthesize information reviewed in the text.

Appendix A, located on thePoint companion Web site, is a list of orthotic vendors/resources that offer equipment, materials, and prefabricated orthoses. Appendices B and C, on thePoint companion Web site, provides examples of forms used in a clinical setting. The Index allows the reader to access information about orthoses by their common names as well as by the ASHT terminology.

Features

- **Chapter Objectives:** At the beginning of each chapter, these guide both students and instructors to the material in the chapter and help prepare for the information provided.
- **Key Terms:** Appearing at the beginning of each chapter, these are defined in the glossary to emphasize basic terminology associated with orthotic fabrication.
- **Case Studies:** Located in the chapters and online, these foster critical thinking to apply concepts to clinical practice.
- **Clinical Pearls:** Appearing in Section II, these illustrate tips on ways to modify the design or alter the fabrication process to improve efficiency or maximize patient specificity.
- **Pattern Pearls:** Presented in Section II, these provide alternative pattern designs or other orthotic options.
- **ASHT Orthotics Nomenclature:** Nomenclature is described in detail for better understanding.

- **Chapter Review Questions:** Located at the end of each chapter, these help students review and retain the information they have encountered in each chapter.
- **Discussion Points:** At the end of Section II chapters, these questions challenge students to use critical thinking to recall concepts and theories learned in these chapters.
- Orthotic fabrication for a spectrum of diagnoses and special populations
- **Multiple Views of Orthoses:** These provide an overall full view of specific orthoses.
- **Glossary:** This provides a list of terms and definitions.

This book reviews numerous pattern designs and other options for orthotic management for the upper extremity. Although this endeavor documents a spectrum of orthotic management, the possibilities for different options extend far beyond a single text. New challenges face the clinician daily; and it is with each patient that we learn something new, building on our previous knowledge. This book is meant to stimulate clinical skills and clinician creativity, encouraging the integration of principles and process from which a clinician can create new orthoses.

ADDITIONAL RESOURCES

Orthotic Intervention for the Hand and Upper Extremity: Splinting Principles and Process includes additional resources for both instructors and students that are available on the book's companion Web site at http://thePoint.lww.com.

Instructor Resources

Approved adopting instructors will be given access to the following additional resources:
- Image bank
- PowerPoint Presentation as "Clinic in the Classroom"
- Sample Syllabi
- Lab Exercises
- Answers to Chapter Review Questions
- Answers to Discussion Points

Student Resources

Students who have purchased *Orthotic Intervention for the Hand and Upper Extremity: Splinting Principles and Process* have access to the following additional resources:
- Videos called *Video Pearls* showing the most common injuries and splints
- Interactive Quiz Bank
- Online Case Studies
- Checklist
- Anatomy Reference Tables
- Appendix A: Distributors of Orthotic Fabrication Products
- Appendix B: Occupational/Physical Therapy Examination
- Appendix C: Care and Use of Your Custom Orthosis
- References

In addition, purchasers of the book can access the searchable full text online by going to the *Orthotic Intervention for the Hand and Upper Extremity: Splinting Principles and Process* Web site at http://thePoint.lww.com. See the inside front cover of this book for more details, including the passcode you will need to gain access to the Web site.

Contributors

Gary P. Austin, PT, PhD
Associate Professor of Physical Therapy
Director, Orthopaedic Physical Therapy
  Residency Program
Director, Certificate Program in Advanced
  Orthopaedic Physical Therapy
Sacred Heart University
Fairfield, CT

Board Certified Orthopaedic Clinical
  Specialist
Fellow, American Academy of Orthopaedic
  Manual Physical Therapists
Fellow, Applied Functional Science
American Academy of Orthopaedic Manual
  Physical Therapists
Baton Rouge, LA

Physical Therapist
Sacred Heart University Sports Medicine
  and Rehabilitation Center
Fairfield, CT

Noelle M. Austin, MS, PT, CHT
Owner/Instructor
CJ Education and Consulting, LLC
Woodbridge, CT

Hand Therapist
The Orthopaedic Group
Hamden, CT

Guest Lecturer
Physical Therapy Program
Sacred Heart University
Fairfield, CT

Richard A. Bernstein, MD
Partner, The Orthopaedic Group
New Haven, CT

Assistant Clinical Professor, Department of
  Orthopaedics and Rehabilitation
Yale University School of Medicine
New Haven, CT

**Salvador Bondoc, OTD, OTR/L, BCPR,
CHT, FAOTA**
Associate Professor of Occupational Therapy
Quinnipiac University
Hamden, CT

Occupational Therapist
Griffin Hospital
Derby, CT

Sabrina Cassella, MEd, OTR/L, CHT
Senior Hand Therapist
Attain® Therapy + Fitness
Springfield, Belchertown & Wilbraham, MA

Guest Lecturer
Springfield College
Springfield Technical Community College
Springfield, MA

Nancy Chee, OTR/L, CHT
Hand Therapist
California Pacific Medical Center
San Francisco, CA

Adjunct Assistant Professor
MOT Program/Department of
  Occupational Therapy
Samuel Merritt University
Oakland, CA

Shrikant Chinchalkar, M.Th.O, B.Sc.OT, OTR, CHT, OT. Reg. (ONT)
Hand Therapist
Hand Therapy Division, Hand and Upper
  Limb Centre
St. Joseph's Hospital
London, Ontario, Canada

Instructor
Rehab Education, LLC
Tallman, NY

Jennifer Stephens Chisar, MS, PT, CHT
Supervisor of Hand Therapy
Rehabilitation Services
John Muir Health
Walnut Creek, CA

Evan D. Collins, MD
Chief, The Methodist Hand and Upper
  Extremity Center
The Methodist Hospital
Houston, TX

Faculty
Weill Cornell Medical College
New York, NY

Ruth Coopee, OTR/L, CHT, CLT, LMT
Owner, Therapist
Body Holistics
Pinellas Park, FL

Hand Therapist
Largo Medical Center
Largo, FL

Instructor
Klose Training & Consulting, LLC
Lafayette, CO

Jerry Coverdale, OTR/L, CHT
American Society of Hand Therapists
  (ASHT) Past President

Director, Hand Therapist
Broward Orthopedic Specialists
Fort Lauderdale, FL

Rebecca Harris, MS, OTR/L, CHT
Hand Therapist
2 Thumbs Up Hand Therapy, LLC
Plymouth and Norwell, MA

Hand Therapist
Quincy Medical Center
Quincy, MA

MaryLynn Jacobs, MS, OTR/L, CHT
Partner/Owner/Hand Therapist
Attain® Therapy + Fitness
Corporate Office
East Longmeadow, MA

Guest Lecturer
Physical & Occupational therapy
Springfield College
American International College
Springfield, MA

Colleen Lowe, MPH, OTR/L, CHT
Senior Therapist
Hand Therapy Outpatient Service,
  Occupational Therapy Department
Massachusetts General Hospital
Boston, MA

Alexandra MacKenzie, OTR/L, CHT
Section Manager, Department of
  Hand Therapy
Hospital for Special Surgery
New York, NY

Jonathan Niszczak, MS, OTR/L
Clinical Specialist
Bio Med Sciences, Inc.
Allentown, PA

Senior Burn Therapist
Temple University, Physical Medicine and
  Rehabilitation
Philadelphia, PA

Marie Pace, OTR/L, CHT
Senior Occupational Therapist
Centers for Rehab Services
University of Pittsburgh Medical Center
Pittsburgh, PA

Jill Peck-Murray, MOT, OTR/L, CHT
Occupational Therapist/Hand Therapist
Rady Children's Hospital
San Diego, CA

Instructor
Rehab Education, LLC
Tallman, NY

Joey Pipicelli, M.Sc.OT, CHT, OT Reg. (ONT)
Sessional Instructor
Faculty of Health Sciences, School of
 Occupational Therapy
Western University
London, Ontario, Canada

Hand Therapist
Division of Hand Therapy, Hand and Upper
 Limb Centre
St. Joseph's Health Care
London, Ontario, Canada

Director of Hand Therapy
Talbot Trails Physiotherapy and
 Musculoskeletal Centre
St. Thomas, Ontario, Canada

Reg Richard, MS, PT
Clinical Research Coordinator Burn
 Rehabilitation
U.S. Army Institute of Surgical Research
 Burn Center
Fort Sam Houston, TX

Jessica Griffin Scheff, MS, OTR/L
Hand Therapist
Attain® Therapy + Fitness
Springfield, MA

Karen Schultz, MS, OTR/L, FAOTA, CHT
Director, Hand Therapist
Rocky Mountain Hand Therapy
Edwards, CO

Adjunct Faculty
Rocky Mountain University of Health
 Professions
Provo, UT

Kimberly Goldie Staines, OTR, CHT
Hand Therapist
Michael E. DeBakey Veterans Affairs
 Medical Center
Houston, TX

Adjunct Faculty
Baylor College of Medicine
Plastic Hand Surgery Fellowship, Orthopedic
 Residency, Physical Medicine and
 Rehabilitation Residency
Houston, TX

Kimberly Zeske-Maguire, MS, OTR/L, CHT
Senior Occupational Therapist,
 Facility Director
Hand and Upper Extremity Rehab Clinic,
 Centers for Rehab Services
University of Pittsburgh Medical Center
Pittsburgh, PA

Guest Lecturer
Occupational Therapy Program
University of Pittsburgh
Pittsburgh, PA

Reviewers

Michael Borst, BA, MS, OTD
Assistant Professor Occupational Therapy
Concordia University Wisconsin
Mequon, WI

Marianne McKittrick Crary, OTR/L, CHT
Occupational Therapy Assistant
Bismarck, ND

Connie Danko, BA, BS, OT
Registered Occupational Therapist
Niskayuna, NY

Emily Eckel, MS, OTR/L, CHT
Assistant Professor
Master of Occupational Therapy Program
Chatham University
Pittsburgh, PA

Chris Eidson
Assistant Professor
Occupational Therapy Department
University of Alabama at Birmingham
Birmingham, AL

Wendy J. Holt, OTR, CHT
Occupational Therapy Department
University of Florida
Gainesville, FL

Pamela Kasyan-Itzkowitz, MS, OTR/L,
CHT
Nova Southeastern University
Fort Lauderdale, FL

Consuelo Kreider, MSH, OTR/L
Department of Occupational Therapy
University of Florida
Gainesville, FL

Linda M. Martin, PhD, OTR/L, FAOTA
Chair/Professor
Florida Gulf Coast University
Fort Myers, FL

Victoria Priganc, PhD, OTR, CHT, CLT
Occupational Therapist
Hand Therapist
Richmond, VT

Katherine Schofield, DHS, OTR, CHT
Assistant Professor
School of Occupational Therapy
University of Indianapolis
Glendale, AZ

Deborah Schwartz, BS, OTR/L, CHT
Physical Rehabilitation
Marlton, NJ

Elizabeth Spencer Steffa, BS, OTR/L,
CHT
Occupational Therapist
Tallman, NY

Acknowledgments

The undertaking of this second edition would not be possible if it were not for the patient and gentle approach Paula Williams, our product manager, provided for us. Sincere thanks to Doug Smock and Terry Mallon, our design coordinators, for assisting with updating the design and Jennifer Clements, our art director, for the overwhelming task of organizing the hundreds of additional photographs and illustrations we added to this updated book. We truly appreciate the hard work and patience provided by Harold Medina, Project Manager at Absolute Service, Inc., during this revision. He successfully conquered the daunting task of creating a user-friendly format to present the images and information.

No book is solely the work of its authors. We would like to thank all the patients who were so generous in allowing us to photograph their upper extremities and provide such a plethora of examples for our book. We would like to express our gratitude to the many therapists and physicians we have worked with over the years who contributed to our knowledge base, professional growth, and clinical skills. So many of you have urged and supported us to always dig deeper and be as creative as possible! Your trust in our expertise and appreciation for what we do has fueled the underlying passion for the writing of this book.

Many thanks to the following individuals, who have contributed their time and expertise in reviewing various chapters or giving us valuable information and/or feedback: Gary P. Austin, PT, PhD; Richard A. Bernstein, MD; Sabrina Cassella, MEd, OTR/L, CHT; Judy C. Colditz, OTR/L, CHT, FAOTA; Gail Garfield Dadio, MHSc, OTR/L, CHT, CLT; Dominic L. DeMello, MD; Barry R. Jacobs, MD; Julianne Lessard, OTR/L, CHT; Pat McKee, M.Sc.OT Reg. (Ont), OT(C); Pranay Parikh, MD; Erik Rosenthal, MD; Caryn Salwen, MEd, OTR/L; Jessica Griffin Scheff, MS, OTR/L; Joan Simmons, MS, OTR/L, PhD; and Steven Wenner, MD.

We would like to especially thank Patterson Medical, especially Paul England, Director of Marketing, Orthopedics for the generous support in supplying the majority of thermoplastic materials and components used in Section II for the photography. We have thoroughly enjoyed working with all your materials, especially TailorSplint. Thanks so much!

Finally, we would like to express our sincere thanks to our families who have been so patient and understanding during the first edition and didn't commit us when we undertook the project of this revision! Without their love, support, and ongoing patience, we would not have been able to tackle such a huge, detail-oriented task successfully.

Contents

SECTION I Fundamentals of Orthotic Fabrication

SECTION II   Orthotic Fabrication

by MaryLynn Jacobs, MS, OTR/L, CHT, and Noelle M. Austin, MS, PT, CHT

SECTION III   Optional Methods

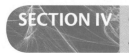 **SECTION IV**   **Orthotic Intervention for Specific Diagnoses and Populations**

Clinical Pearls

 CLINICAL PEARLS

CLINICAL PEARLS

 ADDITIONAL CLINICAL PEARLS

Fundamentals of Orthotic Fabrication

Concepts of Orthotic Fundamentals

MaryLynn Jacobs, MS, OTR/L, CHT
Jerry Coverdale, OTR/L, CHT

Chapter Objectives

After study of this chapter, the reader should be able to:

- Detect the proper nomenclature used to describe orthoses for communication to peers, payers, and referral sources.
- Understand the clinical reasoning process for selecting the most appropriate orthosis for a patient.

- Explain the specific differences and uses for the terms *static*, *dynamic*, *serial static*, and *static progressive* orthoses.
- List the objectives for intervention for immobilization, mobilization, and restrictive orthoses and be able to describe an example of each.

Key Terms

American Society of Hand Therapists
Articular
Centers for Medicare & Medicaid Services
Current Procedural Terminology
Custom fabricated
Durable Medical Equipment, Prosthetics, Orthotics, and Supplies
Dynamic orthoses
Healthcare Common Procedure Coding System Level II

Immobilization
Immobilization orthosis
L-Code
Medicare Administrative Contractors
Mobilization
Mobilization orthoses
Modified Orthosis Classification System
Modifier
National Supplier Clearinghouse
Nonarticular orthosis

Prefabricated orthosis
Provider Enrollment, Chain and Ownership System
Restriction
Restriction orthoses
Serial static orthoses
Splint Classification System
Static progressive orthoses
Static Orthoses

Introduction

Fabrication of upper extremity orthoses requires a unique combination of the therapist's creative abilities and a sound knowledge of anatomical, biomechanical, physiologic, and healing principles as they relate to injury, surgery, and disease. Orthosis fabrication can be one of the most challenging and most enjoyable aspects of being a therapist. Before delving into the fabrication of orthoses, one must not only understand proper nomenclature for universal communication but also develop a solid understanding of the clinical reasoning process for selecting the most appropriate orthosis for the patient. Owing to the growing recognition of specialists who treat the upper extremity and the increasing use of custom-fabricated orthoses, it has been necessary to develop a standard language that clearly and uniformly describes an orthosis to those who refer, fabricate, and/or pay for the devices. The **American Society of Hand Therapists (ASHT)** recognized the need to standardize, organize, and simplify terms and in 1992 developed the **Splint Classification System (SCS)** that grouped orthoses into progressively more refined categories (American Society of Hand Therapists [ASHT], 1992). The first edition of this book was based on a modified version of this classification. This second edition continues to support and integrate our historical nomenclature; however, the authors recognize that the current climate of hand therapists dispensing and fabricating orthoses has drastically changed. Occupational therapists (OTs) and physical therapists (PTs) who practice in this arena have found their rights and qualifications questioned. It has become imperative that adapting the language put forth by the **Centers for Medicare & Medicaid Services (CMS)** along with clinician documentation be very descriptive and streamlined. It is to this end that the authors of this chapter have taken the ASHT SCS and the current CMS **L-Codes** (a specific description of a custom or prefabricated orthosis) and developed a modified and simplified version to be used for the purpose of teaching in this book and is referred to as the **Modified Orthosis Classification System (MOCS)**. A comprehensive and detailed description of the expanded ASHT SCS can be found in the book *Rehabilitation of the Hand*, Sixth Edition (Fess, 2011).

The authors of this chapter and the editors of this book have combined these two systems for several reasons. The first reason is to simply link clinical documentation to orthosis billing. For example, in a clinical note, a therapist may describe an orthosis by using more traditional terminology; however, that clinician will be responsible for choosing the correct L-Code to bill for that orthosis (which is in CMS language). Second, the classification systems were combined to provide clear, consistent, and accurate communication with all payers, physicians, and peers regarding exactly what orthosis is being dispensed or fabricated. The CMS L-Code system is just not detailed enough to meet the second requirement; therefore, the historical nomenclature has been woven into this MOCS (Table 1–1 and Fig. 1–1).

Nomenclature: Orthosis versus Splint

The qualifications of licensed/registered OTs and PTs dispensing and fabricating orthotic devices have been questioned by CMS and state legislatures over the years. In 2000, Congress passed legislation that required CMS to develop a regulation, through a negotiated rulemaking process, to restrict payment for custom-fabricated orthoses and all prosthetics to only those that are provided by qualified practitioners and suppliers. OTs and PTs are included as qualified practitioners in the law through state licensure and certification examinations completed after receiving an entry-level degree at an accredited institution. OTs and PTs have the educational background, clinical exposure, and clinical assessment/reasoning skills to design, fabricate, fit, and educate a client safely and effectively with an orthotic device. This education includes, but is not limited to, orthosis training, knowledge of anatomy, biomechanics, kinesiology, disease/injury processes (including surgical procedures and wound healing physiology), and the psychosocial aspects of injury/disease. The CMS-negotiated rulemaking failed to reach consensus, and CMS has not issued a regulation to implement this legislation at the time of the printing of this

book (ASHT, 2009; Centers for Medicare & Medicaid Services [CMS], 2008; Healthcare Common Procedure Coding System [HCPCS], 2011; McKee & Rivard, 2011).

Because OT and PT qualifications to dispense and fabricate orthoses have been questioned by policymakers and payers, it is extremely important that clinicians use the proper language that has been adopted by CMS. This is especially important because many payers follow CMS guidelines. The term *splint* has been used in therapy professions for decades; however, CMS does not recognize these devices by that name. They designate the term *orthotic devices* (orthoses), as defined in the 2008 **Durable Medical Equipment, Prosthetics, Orthotics, and Supplies (DMEPOS Quality Standards)** manual as the reimbursable language (CMS, 2008). Therefore, it is imperative that clinicians make a shift in terminology in all of the following areas:

- Documentation
- Patient education
- Academic/student education
- Continuing education courses
- Publications/presentations
- Literature/research
- Communication with physicians, insurance carriers, and colleagues

TABLE 1–1

Relevant Terminology Definitions

CMS
Centers for Medicare & Medicaid Services is a federal agency within the U.S. Department of Health and Human Services that administers the Medicare program and works in partnership with state governments to administer Medicaid and other such programs.

CPT
Current Procedural Terminology
This refers to a number/code assigned to the majority of tasks and services a medical practitioner may provide to a patient. It is then linked to a determined amount of reimbursement by the insurer. Level II of the HCPCS is a standardized coding system that is used primarily to identify products, supplies, and other services *not* included in these CPT codes (such as orthoses). CPT codes are developed and published by the American Medical Association (AMA, 2011) and revised yearly.

DME
Durable Medical Equipment
This is a term used to describe any medical equipment used in the home to aid in an improved quality of life. Examples are walkers, wheelchairs, power scooters, hospital beds, and home oxygen equipment. Clinicians often refer to orthoses as DME equipment; however, the proper terminology is DMEPOS.

DMEPOS
Durable Medical Equipment, Prosthetics, Orthotics, and Supplies
Durable medical equipment is often referred to as DMEPOS because Medicare also covers prosthetics, orthotics, and certain supplies (POS). Prosthetics are devices that can replace a missing body part, such as a hand or leg. Orthotics are devices that help to immobilize, mobilize, or restrict a body part.

HCPCS
Healthcare Common Procedure Coding System
HCPCS is a comprehensive, standardized system that classifies similar products that are medical in nature into categories for the purpose of efficient claim processing and ensures uniformity. It is used primarily to identify products, supplies, and services *not* included in the CPT codes, such as durable medical equipment, prosthetics, orthotics, and supplies (DMEPOS) when used outside a physician's office. Because Medicare and other insurers cover a variety of services, supplies, and equipment that are *not* identified by CPT codes, the level II HCPCS codes were established for submitting claims for these items.

L-Code
L-Codes describe orthoses by identifying which body parts they are used for (**S**, shoulder; **E**, elbow; **W**, wrist; **H**, hand; and **F**, finger), followed by the letter **O** for orthosis. They are also described as static (without joint) or dynamic (nontorsion joint and elastic bands and turnbuckles) and specify whether an orthosis is custom or prefabricated. The L-Code is the number linked to the specific description of a custom or prefabricated orthosis for proper communication to the insurance carrier.

MAC
Medicare Administrative Contractors
L-Codes are not billed to CMS directly but rather through regional/jurisdiction MAC. There are currently four jurisdictions based on which region of the United States you are billing from.

Modifiers
A code added to the end of a CPT code to clarify the services and increase accuracy regarding what is being billed. Modifiers offer a way in which the service can be altered without changing the procedure code.

NPI
National Provider Identification number
This is a unique 10-digit identification number issued to health care providers in the United States by CMS. This number is a required identifier for Medicare services and is used by other payers, including commercial healthcare insurers. All healthcare providers and facilities must obtain an NPI number to use in all standard transactions. Therefore, a clinician and/or facility must have this number in order to bill for orthotic services.

NSC
National Supplier Clearinghouse
This organization processes the enrollment applications submitted by DMEPOS suppliers for their NSC (DMEPOS) number. This process is done online via PECOS enrollment.

PECOS
Provider Enrollment Chain Ownership System
Allows DME suppliers to initially enroll for an NSC (DMEPOS) number, make changes to an existing number, update information (such as adding a new provider), check on the status of an application or reenroll online. Anyone wishing to become a Medicare provider must apply through PECOS. In addition, as the supplier of the **DMEPOS**, you will be denied payment **if** your referral source is not enrolled in PECOS.

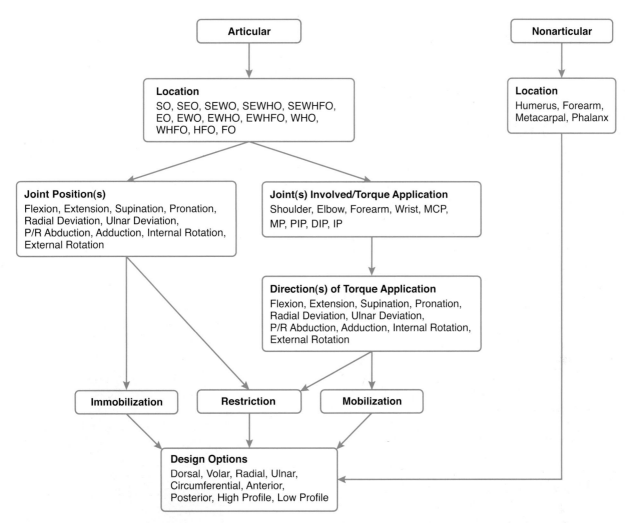

FIGURE 1–1 **The authors recommended Modified Orthosis Classification System (MOCS).** Note that the Centers for Medicare & Medicaid Services (CMS) does not recognize the thumb as a separate body part. The thumb is classified as F, the same distinction used for the index, middle, ring, and small digits.

Definition

Orthosis

An orthosis is a rigid and/or semirigid device used for the purpose of support, alignment, prevention or correction of deformity, or to improve function or restrict motion of a movable body part (CMS, 2008). Orthotic devices are described by the CMS using L-Codes that are found in the **Healthcare Common Procedure Coding System (HCPCS) Level II** manual.

What is the proper terminology to use?

- **Orthosis** is a noun and should be used in place of the word *splint.*
- **Orthoses** is a plural noun and should be used to replace the term for multiple splints.
- **Fabricating an orthosis** should be used in place of the verb *splinting.*

- **Orthotic** is an adjective and is used to describe a noun associated with the science of orthotics, such as orthotic device, orthotic treatment plan, orthotic intervention, orthotic fabrication, or orthotic coding.

The second edition of this book has adopted much of the terminology put forth by CMS while continuing to gently blend the historical nomenclature that so many physicians and therapists are accustomed to. The editors and authors of this publication strongly believe that unified terminology is paramount when referring to orthoses in every aspect of our professions. Threaded throughout this chapter, the reader will find occasional examples of CMS language (WHO, SO . . .) and in Figures 1–2 through 1–5 corresponding L-Codes for the orthosis described. The reader must note that the L-Codes described in this chapter are only discussed in this chapter as examples and are reflective of the time of this publication. L-Codes can be changed or altered by CMS at any time. It is important to keep current with individual insurance carrier changes (including CMS) and the associated reimbursements. It is the authors' intent to continually reinforce the important relationship between documentation and billing.

Overview of Orthosis Classification

It would be erroneous to have a book dedicated to orthoses and not discuss coding choices for reimbursement. This section is dedicated to assisting in proper L-Code selection and to promote unification of selection across our profession.

The codes used for reimbursement for orthoses are the L-Codes found in the HCPCS manual. Although it is CMS that uses the HCPCS coding system, many payers tend to follow CMS guidelines. However, not all insurance carriers may recognize all the L-Codes that CMS recognizes. Other carriers may cover all or just a few. In addition, they may not reimburse at the same rate that CMS does for the exact same product. Each clinic/organization must abide by the contract they have with the individual insurance carriers and accept the negotiated rates mutually agreed upon through the contract period. The reimbursement for orthoses will depend on how each clinic/organizations individual insurance contract is written, what is included within it, what L-Codes are covered, and what exactly is the rate for each. This may greatly differ from clinic to clinic, state to state, private practice to hospital setting, and so forth.

Easily identifying the reimbursement L-Codes is simple and rendered timeless by being based on the anatomical structure (joints) that the orthosis supports and/or crosses. Each joint is recognized with the first letter of that joint. For example, "SO" would represent shoulder orthosis; "EO," elbow orthosis; "WHO," wrist and hand orthosis; and so on. The combination of each letter will determine the structures that the orthosis crosses. The following coding examples include the anatomical headings and the CMS descriptions of the corresponding L-Code (Table 1–2). In the coding examples (Figs. 1–2 to 1–5), the actual numerical number associated with that L-Code description (e.g., L3908) has been recommended. Each provider (clinician/organization) is encouraged to communicate with their local insurance companies to determine acceptable L-Codes that they cover. This should be done yearly as well as staying informed on any bulletin a payer may put forth regarding this issue.

Coding examples:

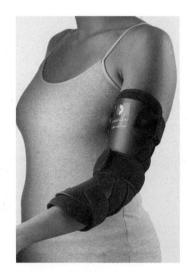

FIGURE 1–2 Immobilization prefabricated orthosis: (EO). L3762 Elbow orthosis, rigid, without joints, includes soft interface material, prefabricated, and includes fitting and adjustment. Photo courtesy of Corflex Inc. The Ventral Cubital Tunnel Splint.

TABLE 1–2	
Key to Anatomical Headings	
SEWHFO	shoulder, elbow, wrist, hand, finger/thumb orthosis
SEWHO	shoulder, elbow, wrist, hand orthosis
SEO	shoulder, elbow orthosis
EWHFO	elbow, wrist, hand, finger/thumb orthosis
EWHO	elbow, wrist, hand orthosis
WHFO	wrist, hand, finger/thumb orthosis
WHO	wrist, hand orthosis
HFO	hand, finger/thumb orthosis
SO	shoulder orthosis
EO	elbow orthosis
HO	hand orthosis
FO	finger/thumb orthosis

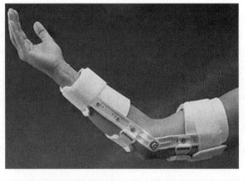

FIGURE 1–3 Mobilization prefabricated orthosis: (EO). L3760 Elbow orthosis, with adjustable position locking joint(s), prefabricated, includes fitting and adjustments, any type. Photo courtesy of Patterson Medical; The Rolyan® Pre-Formed Elbow Hinge Splint.

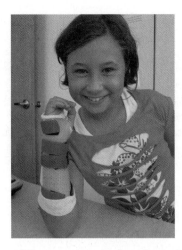

FIGURE 1–4   Immobilization custom-fabricated orthosis: (WHO). L3906 Wrist hand orthosis, without joints, may include soft interface, straps, custom fabricated, includes fitting and adjustment.

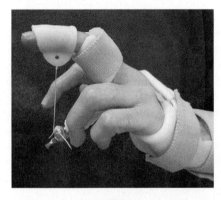

FIGURE 1–5   Mobilization custom-fabricated orthosis: (WHFO). L3806 Wrist-hand-finger orthosis, includes one of more nontorsion joint(s), turnbuckles, elastic bands/springs, may include soft interface material, straps, custom fabricated, includes fitting and adjustment.

Every L-Code has a detailed description. Each description explains whether or not that L-Code is **prefabricated** or **custom fabricated** and if it is an orthosis that is used to mobilize (dynamic, serial static, or static progressive) or immobilize (static) the anatomical structures. If the L-Code is for an immobilization orthosis, then the description will contain the words *without joint* to indicate no joints are mobilized. If the L-Code is for a mobilization orthosis, then the description will contain words such as "nontorsion joints, elastic bands, and turnbuckles," indicating there is at least one joint that the orthosis crosses which a torque is being applied via elastic bands, springs, or turnbuckles but may also include at least one joint which torque is **not** applied. This language primarily applies to the custom-fabricated orthoses. The prefabricated orthoses descriptors have not been altered by CMS and use words such as "rigid" to denote an immobilizing or restricting orthosis and "adjustable or locking joints" for a mobilizing orthosis (HCPCS, 2011).

The L-Code is generally inclusive of the evaluation, cost of base materials, fabrication, fitting, and adjustments to the orthosis. The **Current Procedural Terminology (CPT)** code 97760 (a time-dependent code) may be used in conjunction with the L-Code *only* if training goes above and beyond what is considered customary. The CPT code should not be used for basic and routine training for use and care. It is imperative that documentation must justify why the training time was lengthened and what that training entailed. An evaluation CPT code (97003 OT or 97001 PT) can only be charged at the time of orthotic fabrication/dispensing if the orthosis is part of a treatment plan and the patient will be seen for ongoing treatment. If bilateral orthoses are dispensed or fabricated, then a **modifier** is required on the billing form: "Rt" for right upper extremity and "Lt" for the left upper extremity.

For example, a therapist receives a referral for a patient with the diagnosis of bilateral distal radius fractures and the prescription is for bilateral wrist orthoses, evaluation, and treatment. At the time of this publication, the clinician can bill an evaluation CPT code as well as treatment CPT codes, which are billed directly to CMS. The L-Codes (L3906 in this example) are billed using modifiers Rt and Lt to denote that two orthoses were fabricated for the right and left upper extremities. The L-Codes are billed to the **National Supplier Clearinghouse (NSC)** via **Medicare Administrative Contractors (MACs)** instead of directly to CMS and require that the provider have an NSC number, also known as a DMEPOS number. Therapists apply for this DMEPOS number via the Internet through **Provider Enrollment, Chain and Ownership System (PECOS)**. Refer to Table 1–1 for greater detail. If the referral is *only* for bilateral wrist orthoses, then the therapist would not bill the evaluation CPT code but only the WHO (L3906) code using the right and left modifiers to the NSC.

Challenges in the Use of L-Codes

The clinician may be challenged to find the proper code to describe what has been fabricated. Because of the vast possibilities of designs, it is near impossible to have a code description for everything. If a code cannot be found to match up with the orthosis fabricated, then the code that *best* describes the orthosis should be chosen. Clear, proper, and meticulous documentation must justify this choice.

For example, there is no code that accounts for using an immobilization orthosis to function as a static progressive (mobilization) device that can be sequentially adjusted over several treatment sessions. The CPT code 97762 may be used when it is necessary to serially modify the immobilization orthosis in order to provide a mobilizing force. Remember that this code is considered a *timed code* based on 15-minute increments; therefore, this code should not be used for basic or quick modifications.

An additional challenge is the limited options for codes describing nonarticular orthoses, with the exception of hand

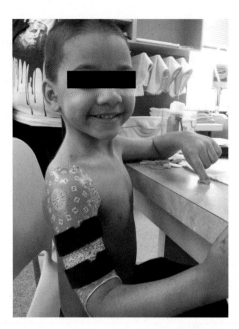

FIGURE 1–6 **Nonarticular humerus orthosis: (SO).** A humeral fracture brace used to stabilize and protect a healing midshaft humerus fracture. Although labeled as nonarticular, the orthosis partially crosses the shoulder joint. The most appropriate L-Code is L3671.

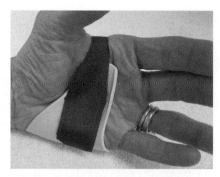

FIGURE 1–7 **Nonarticular hand orthosis: (HO).** A hand immobilization orthosis for treatment of a midshaft fifth metacarpal fracture; the pressure applied through the volar–dorsal nature of this device during fabrication minimizes the tendency for the bone fragments to shift.

orthosis (HO) that can be used for midshaft metacarpal fractures. Therefore, if a therapist fabricates a custom humeral orthosis to protect a midshaft humeral fracture, then the code chosen for billing would have to closely describe this orthosis. A choice could be a custom-fabricated immobilization orthosis or L3671 shoulder orthosis (SO); "shoulder joint design, without joints, may include soft interface, straps, custom fabricated, and includes fitting and adjustments" (HCPCS, 2011). Even though the description actually states it immobilizes the shoulder joint, it is the closest description offered (Fig. 1–6).

Summary of the Modified Orthosis Classification System

Articular and Nonarticular Orthoses

Orthoses are divided into one of two broad groups: **articular** and **nonarticular**. Articular orthoses are those that cross one or more joints. Nonarticular orthoses provide support and protection to a healing bone (e.g., humerus, metacarpal, or phalanx) or to a soft tissue structure (e.g., annular pulley or musculotendinous junction of the medial or lateral epicondyle). There are far fewer nonarticular orthoses than articular orthoses (Fig. 1–7).

When interpreting a referral, it is advantageous to distinguish between articular and nonarticular orthoses so that a joint is not unnecessarily immobilized. For example, if the word *nonarticular* does not precede the words *proximal forearm immobilization orthosis* on the referral, then the therapist may assume that the elbow or wrist needs to be

included in the design. By adding the word *nonarticular*, the description becomes far more specific. In Section II, the articular orthoses are separated from the nonarticular to aid in pattern location; the term *articular* does not need to appear in the description because the name of the orthosis (e.g., wrist immobilization orthosis or WHO) indicates whether a joint is included. However, the term *nonarticular* does need to appear in the descriptions (e.g., nonarticular humerus orthosis or SO L3671 and nonarticular metacarpal orthosis or HO L3919), so there is no ambiguity as in Figures 1–6 and 1–7. Note: for billing purposes, the CMS codes chosen here are the best choice (to this publication date) available to describe these devices for reimbursement.

Location

Location, the next level in the MOCS, refers to the joint, set of joints, or body part on which the orthosis acts according to its main intent. Therefore, in order to simplify naming, if there are several joints involved, as commonly seen after a severe crushing injury to the hand, MOCS groups the joints together. For example, if a crush injury involves all the metacarpophalangeal (MCP), proximal interphalangeal (PIP), and distal interphalangeal (DIP) joints, the proper name would be a hand and digit immobilization orthosis or HFO. If the crush injury involves the three joints of only the middle finger (MF), then the orthosis is described as a digit immobilization orthosis or FO.

Nonarticular orthoses are described in much the same way. For example, an orthosis used to immobilize a fifth metacarpal fracture is described as a nonarticular fifth metacarpal orthosis or HO (Fig. 1–7). Similarly, an orthosis used to protect a recently reconstructed annular pulley is described as a nonarticular proximal phalanx orthosis or FO (Fig. 1–8).

Joint(s) Involved/Torque Application

A mobilization orthosis may require immobilization support of adjacent joints or, occasionally, mobilization in more than one direction *within* the same orthosis. When noting the anatomical locations that the orthosis crosses, it is imperative to

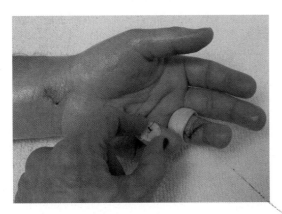

FIGURE 1–8 **Nonarticular proximal phalanx orthosis: (FO).** This circumferential designed orthosis provides protection to a recently reconstructed A2 annular pulley.

note which joint(s) are immobilized and which joint(s) have torque applied to them. An example may be managing metacarpal phalangeal (MP) joint extension contractures after a distal radius fracture. The wrist may require continued immobilization, whereas the MCPs would benefit from flexion mobilization, as shown in Figure 1–24. This orthosis would be noted for billing as a WHFO (L3806), and the written documentation would reflect a statement such as "wrist extension immobilization, MCP flexion mobilization orthosis." A mobilization orthosis may also require torque application to more than one joint and in different directions. An example may be managing a claw hand from a long-standing ulnar nerve injury where the patient exhibits MCP extension and interphalangeal (IP) flexion contractures. The joint torque in this case would be applied to the MPs in the direction of flexion and simultaneously to the IPs in the direction of extension. This orthosis would be noted for billing as an HFO (L3921) and for documentation as a small finger and ring finger (SF/RF) MCP flexion/IP extension mobilization orthosis.

Direction

The **direction** descriptor, the next level in the MOCS, refers to the position of the primary joint in an immobilization orthosis, the joint boundary of a restrictive orthosis, and the direction of torque in a mobilizing orthosis. The direction descriptor provides critical information necessary for accurately fabricating the orthosis. Prior to fabrication, the specific purpose of the orthosis must be known before the therapist can add the direction descriptor. Direction defines the position of the involved joints (immobilization orthosis), the desired direction of the mobilizing force (mobilization orthosis), or the direction in which motion is to be blocked (restriction orthosis). For example, by adding a direction term (e.g., RF PIP extension orthosis), the orthosis' intent is further clarified, in this case by indicating that the joint is to be extended. As noted in the next section—by then following "direction" by the use of the words *immobilization*, *mobilization*, or *restriction*—there will be even more clear information about what that direction really means. Is it to

gain PIP extension (mobilize), to rest (immobilize) the PIP in extension, or to block a portion of PIP extension (restriction)?

Intent: Immobilization, Mobilization, and Restriction

Intent, the next level of the MOCS, refers to the overall function or primary purpose of the orthosis, which is generally **immobilization**, **mobilization**, or **restriction**. Adding the orthosis' purpose to the description provides the fabricator with a clearer understanding of what is being requested. For example, a prescription for an RF PIP extension mobilization orthosis tells the fabricator that an extension force needs to be exerted on the PIP joint of the RF. The purpose of an RF PIP extension immobilization orthosis, on the other hand, is to immobilize the PIP joint in extension. Finally, an RF PIP extension restriction orthosis restricts full extension of the PIP joint but allows active flexion (as often requested for management of a finger with a swan-neck deformity).

In Section II, the orthoses are organized according to their most common purpose, although additional functions are also defined. For example, the RF PIP immobilization orthosis is discussed in Chapter 7. However, because it is essentially the same pattern used for an RF PIP extension mobilization orthosis (serial static design), this use is referenced under the heading "Additional Functions." The cross-reference list provided in this book will also help in quick pattern location.

Design Descriptors

The design descriptor improves understanding of the type of orthosis that is requested. In this text, the descriptors are used as an aid whenever necessary. Design descriptors include non-MOCS nomenclature that is still widely used by hand surgery and hand therapy specialists throughout the world; some examples are *gutter*, *spica*, *static*, *dynamic*, *static progressive*, and *serial static*. These terms are discussed separately later in this chapter.

In the MOCS, design descriptors, which are selectively included, appear in parentheses after the name of the orthosis. In this book, however, the descriptors are most often found at the beginning of the name to help readers with critical thinking and decision-making processes. The descriptive terms include the following:

- Digit-based: Originating from the digit, allowing MCP joint motion, and possibly extending to the distal phalanx
- Hand-based: Originating from the hand, allowing wrist motion, and possibly extending to the distal phalanx
- Thumb-based: Originating from the thenar eminence or thumb and incorporating one or more joints of the thumb
- Forearm-based: Originating from the forearm, allowing full elbow motion, and possibly extending to the distal phalanx
- Arm-based: Originating from the upper arm and possibly including the wrist, elbow, and/or shoulder joints
- Circumferential: Encompassing the entire perimeter of a body part

- Gutter: Including only the radial or ulnar portion of a body part
- Radial: Incorporating the radial aspect of a body part
- Ulnar: Incorporating the ulnar aspect of a body part
- Dorsal: Traversing the dorsal aspect of the hand or forearm
- Volar: Traversing the volar aspect of the hand or forearm
- Anterior: Traversing the anterior aspect of a body part
- Posterior: Traversing the posterior aspect of a body part

Non–Modified Orthosis Classification System Nomenclature

The widely used terms *static*, *serial static*, *dynamic*, and *static progressive* are not included in the MOCS. These terms designate choices of designs that a therapist can incorporate to achieve immobilization, mobilization, or restriction of the intended structure(s). These choices are noted under "Common Names" in Section II and are listed in the book's index.

Static Orthoses

Static orthoses have a firm base and immobilize the joint(s) they cross. They can be used to facilitate dynamic functions, for example, by blocking one joint to encourage movement of another. In some cases, a static orthosis is considered to be nonarticular—having no direct influence on joint mobility—while providing stabilization, protection, and support to a body segment, such as the humerus or metacarpal. Static orthoses may be the most common orthosis that therapists are called on to make. They can be used as an alternative to mobilization devices when ease of application and compliance are potential issues (Riggs, Lyden, & Chung, 2011).

Serial Static Orthoses

Serial static orthoses or casts are applied with the tissue at its near maximum length; they are worn for long periods to accommodate elongation of soft tissue in the desired direction of correction. They are remolded or new devices are made by the therapist to maintain the joint(s), soft tissue, and/or muscle–tendon units they cross in a lengthened position. Serial static orthoses are constructed to be circumferential and nonremovable. This option provides for greater patient compliance and assures the therapist and physician that the tissue is being continually stressed without the risk of the tissue rebounding, which could happen if the orthoses were removed (Brand & Thompson, 1993; Colditz, 2011a; Schultz-Johnson, 2003a).

Dynamic Orthoses

Dynamic orthoses generate a mobilizing or supportive force on a targeted tissue that results in passive gains or passive-assisted range of motion (ROM) (Fess & Phillips, 1987; Glascow, Tooth, Fleming, & Peters, 2011). Dynamic orthoses have a static base that provides the foundation for some type of outrigger attachment. Controlled mobilizing forces are applied via a dynamic (elastic) assist, which may be rubber bands, springs, neoprene, or wrapped elastic cord. The dynamic force applied through the orthosis continues as long as the elastic component can contract, even when the shortened tissue reaches the end of its elastic limit (Schultz-Johnson, 1992, 2003b). As soon as appropriate, dynamic forces should be applied to the targeted tissue because this provides better opportunity for contracture resolution and/or tissue elongation. The less mature the scar tissue, the better the tissue will respond to the intermittent force application of a dynamic orthosis (Colditz, 2011b; Glascow et al., 2011). Mature, dense scar tends to respond more favorably to a prolonged static progressive force (Colditz, 2011b). A dynamic orthosis can also be used as an active-resistive exercise modality against its line of pull.

Static Progressive Orthoses

Static progressive orthoses achieve mobilization by applying unidirectional, low-load force to the tissue's maximum end ROM until the tissue accommodates. Construction is similar to dynamic orthoses, except these use nonelastic components to deliver the mobilizing force, including, but not limited to, nylon cord, strapping materials, screws, hinges, turnbuckles, and nonelastic tape (Sueoka & DeTemple, 2011). Once the joint position and tension are set, the orthosis does not continue to stress the tissue beyond its elastic limit (Schultz-Johnson, 1992, 2003a, 2003b). The force can be modified only through progressive adjustments. Some patients may tolerate static progressive application better than dynamic application, perhaps because the joint position is constant while the tissue readily accommodates to the tension and is less subject to the influences of gravity and motion (Colditz, 2011b; Schultz-Johnson, 1992, 1996, 2002, 2003b).

Function of Orthoses and Objectives for Intervention

This section reviews the objectives for orthotic intervention and provides appropriate clinical examples for immobilization, mobilization, and restriction. Remember that not all orthoses can be simply classified, and the primary objective may not always be clear-cut. There may be multiple objectives for orthotic intervention. For example, a wrist/hand immobilization orthosis (WHFO) for a patient with rheumatoid arthritis may be designed to immobilize inflamed arthritic joints while placing the MCP joints in near extension and a gentle radially deviated position to minimize ulnar drift and periarticular deformity.

The discussion that follows covers general and common examples to emphasize how critical thinking is necessary when fabricating orthoses. Experienced therapists recognize that managing complex injuries requires much overlap and problem solving in order to determine the best approach.

Immobilization Orthoses

Although the **immobilization orthosis** is the most common and simplest form of orthotic intervention, it can be used for the most complex of injuries. Static orthoses are considered immobilization orthoses because they do not allow motion of the joints to which they are applied. Immobilization orthoses can be considered either articular or nonarticular, immobilizing the joints they cross (articular), or stabilizing the structure to which they are applied (nonarticular), as in the case of a humerus orthosis (Fig. 1–6).

The common objectives for immobilization are as follows:

- Provide symptom relief after injury or overuse
- Protect and properly position edematous structure(s)
- Aid in maximizing functional use of the hand
- Maintain tissue length to prevent soft tissue contracture
- Protect healing structures and surgical procedures
- Maintain and protect reduction of a fracture
- Protect and improve joint alignment
- Block or transfer power of movement to enhance exercise
- Reduce tone and contracture of a spastic muscle

These objectives and examples of orthotic intervention are discussed in the following sections.

• Provide Symptom Relief

An immobilization orthosis can provide significant pain relief when applied as soon as possible after injury. The injured structures should be placed in a resting, nonstressed position, minimizing movement that can influence pain. This orthosis is initially worn day and night and may be removed for only short periods of exercise and hygiene. After the initial symptoms have subsided, orthosis use is decreased; eventually, the orthosis may be used only for preventing the risk of reinjury. For example, a person who has sustained a wrist sprain may present with exquisite pain when wrist motion is attempted. The use of a wrist immobilization orthosis (WHO custom or prefabricated) is appropriate for approximately 1 month or until pain subsides. After the period of immobilization, the orthosis may be used for only sleeping and/or at-risk activities (Fig. 1–9).

EXAMPLE: WRIST/HAND IMMOBILIZATION ORTHOSIS (WHO) (Fig. 1–9)

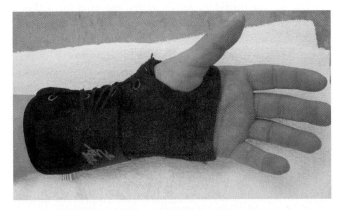

FIGURE 1–9 Wrist/hand immobilization orthosis: (WHO). A simple prefabricated wrist orthosis can be used to stabilize a painful wrist when a custom design is not warranted or feasible.

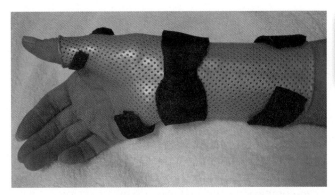

FIGURE 1–10 Wrist/thumb immobilization orthosis: (WHFO). Immobilization of the thumb and wrist can provide relief for a patient with acute deQuervain's tenosynovitis.

A radial wrist/thumb immobilization orthosis (WHFO) can assist in decreasing inflammation and pain within the first dorsal compartment (deQuervain's tenosynovitis) by preventing simultaneous wrist ulnar deviation and thumb flexion. The wrist is positioned in neutral to 20° extension with 0 to 5° of ulnar deviation. This position keeps the extensor pollicis brevis (EPB) and the abductor pollicis longus (APL) tendons in alignment with the radius as they exit the pulley about the radial styloid (Eaton, 1992). The thumb carpometacarpal (CMC) joint is positioned in slight abduction, and the MP joint is included in a slightly flexed, comfortable position (Fig. 1–10). The orthosis is generally worn full time for 3 to 4 weeks, and then use is gradually reduced to nights only once the day symptoms have resolved. The orthosis is discontinued when the patient is asymptomatic to provocative (painful) positioning.

EXAMPLE: WRIST/THUMB IMMOBILIZATION ORTHOSIS (WHFO) (Fig. 1–10)

• Protect and Position Edematous Structures

Edema is often the first observable reaction to injury yet not always the first addressed. Its immediate reduction is critical to facilitate proper healing with minimal complications (such as tight joint capsules and ligaments, which could lead to joint and soft tissue contracture). An edematous hand may be a painful hand that has associated injuries that must be considered before orthosis application. For example, consider fabricating an orthosis that places the digital joints in a safe position (MCP flexion, IP extension) and can be donned and doffed easily to allow access for wound and pin care. Attention to joint positioning in the orthosis, elevation, massage, compression wraps, and gentle active ROM of adjacent structures (if appropriate) all contribute to reducing edema and preventing deformity (e.g., MCP extension and PIP flexion contractures).

Compression bandages or gloves (e.g., Coban™ and Isotoner® gloves) can be worn under the orthosis for edema reduction and can complement the device's effectiveness. However, caution is necessary when donning and doffing these compression devices to avoid injury or reinjury of the healing bones, tendons, and/or ligaments. Furthermore, the therapist must carefully consider the type and placement of the straps. A narrow strap placed across an edematous area may cause pooling of edema proximal and distal to the strap and may irritate superficial sensory nerves. Circumferentially wrapping or encompassing the orthosis, distal to proximal, with an elasticized wrap or compressive garment (e.g., Ace™ wrap, elasticized stockinette, or Coban™) may help distribute pressure evenly along the extremity and aid in minimizing edema.

In addition, patient education regarding the importance of the use of an orthosis, in conjunction with other edema management methods, facilitates early reduction of edema. Crush injuries are often complex and may involve one or more structures, including bone, ligament, tendon, and nerve. Patients often do well during the initial stages of healing with a simple wrist/hand/thumb immobilization orthosis to keep the involved structures positioned, supported, and protected. Therapists working with these patients should strive to achieve optimal joint positioning. One of the most important goals is to maintain the antideformity position of the hand (also referred to as the intrinsic plus or safe position): MCP flexion, IP extension, and thumb palmar abduction. If this is not accomplished early after injury, MCP joint collateral ligament shortening and PIP joint volar plate contracture may occur, which can result in MCP extension and PIP flexion contractures. Optimal joint positions may be difficult to achieve initially owing to stiffness, pain, and significant edema. Be persistent, fabricate the orthosis within a comfortable ROM, monitor, and serially adjust the orthosis as pain allows (Fig. 1–11).

EXAMPLE: WRIST/HAND/THUMB IMMOBILIZATION ORTHOSIS (WHFO) (Fig. 1–11)

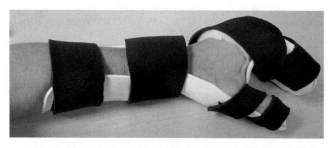

FIGURE 1–11 Wrist/hand/thumb immobilization orthosis: (WHFO). A simple wrist/hand/thumb immobilization orthosis (traditionally named a resting hand splint) can provide the support, proper positioning (MCP flexion, IP extension, thumb palmar abduction), and healing environment that crush injuries require.

• Aid in Maximizing Functional Use

An orthosis can enhance function by correctly positioning and supporting structures that are injured or unstable. During the day, these supportive, lightweight, functional orthoses can often help patients use their hands to engage in vocational, academic, or recreational activities. Without support, function is diminished and deforming forces may dominate. Figures 1–12A–D shows a patient with advanced scleroderma and how a small, light orthosis can allow the simple act of turning a key. These orthoses can be fabricated to position and support with minimal bulk (Fig. 1–12C,D). The bulkier the orthosis, the more likely it will interfere with functional use.

EXAMPLE: INDEX FINGER RADIAL DEVIATION ORTHOSIS (HFO) (Fig. 1–12)

A thumb CMC joint that becomes subluxed and painful when a pinch is attempted may benefit from the use of a well-molded first CMC immobilization orthosis (Colditz, 1995a; Sillem, Backman, Miller, & Li, 2011). Function and comfort are gained by careful attention to molding and pressure distribution about the base of the first metacarpal bone and the CMC joint. These types of orthoses (rigid or soft) offer a degree of stabilization to a thumb CMC joint and places the first metacarpal bone in a better anatomical position of abduction. Small devices such as the one shown in Figure 1–13B can significantly relieve pain during active use of the thumb and enable the patient to grasp and pinch more effectively (Fig. 1–13A,B).

EXAMPLE: THUMB CMC IMMOBILIZATION ORTHOSIS (HFO) (Fig. 1–13)

• Maintain Tissue Length

Orthoses can preserve tissue length when applied carefully and accurately and within the appropriate time frame. Contractures of soft tissue can occur from many sources. One such cause is nerve injury, resulting in muscle–tendon imbalances in the hand. Left untreated, these imbalances often result in tendon–ligament shortening, which in turn may create some degree of joint contracture.

During the initial stages of injury, the goal for orthotic intervention should be to place the joints in a position that inhibits tissue shortening and enables functional use. During the end stages of scar maturation (3 to 6 months or longer), the goal may be to keep the tissue at its achieved maximum length to prevent regression of tissue tightness (Genova, Lester, & Walsh, 2010; McFarlane, 1997). At this stage, the orthosis is not influencing the tissue length but is maintaining the desired and previously achieved ROM. Gains attained in therapy sessions and at home can be maintained with a balanced program of proper immobilization and exercise.

Adduction contractures of the thumb can occur after injury to or repair of the median nerve. To prevent this, an orthosis should be applied as soon as possible after nerve repair. The orthosis can be forearm-based, with the wrist slightly flexed, intimately molded into the first web space, and extending distally to the thumb IP joint crease. Care should

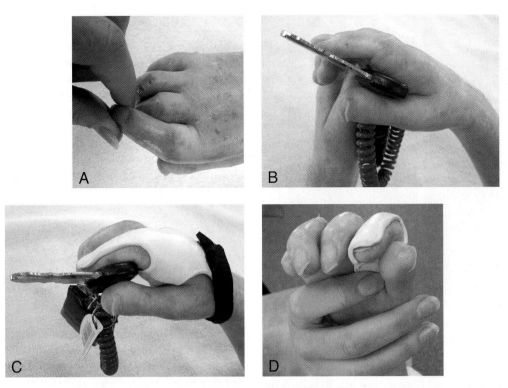

FIGURE 1–12 **Digit immobilization orthosis: (HFO). A,** Severe MCP/PIP instability and ulnar deformity of the index finger makes it nearly impossible for this patient with scleroderma to **(B)** turn a key. **C,** A small orthosis holding the index finger in neutral deviation allows for a stable post for the thumb to hold the key against. **D,** Note how the material wraps along the ulnar border, keeping the volar–radial border free for tactile input.

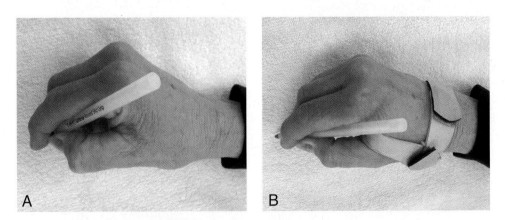

FIGURE 1–13 **Thumb immobilization orthosis: (HFO). A,** A thumb CMC immobilization orthosis is being used for stabilization of this joint while writing is attempted. This small device is only one of many design options available that can help prevent subluxation of the first CMC joint during functional use. **B,** Note the thumb posture before application of the orthosis.

be taken to avoid undue stress on the ulnar collateral ligament of the thumb MP joint during fabrication. This orthosis position maintains the thumb in maximum abduction, preventing a possible adduction contracture while placing the nerve repair in a shortened position to allow for healing (Fig. 1–14A). As the nerve heals and greater extension of the wrist is allowed, a small hand-based device can be made to fit over a wrist immobilization orthosis. This can be worn at night to maintain tissue length of the first web space. This may be an option for patients who want to attempt functional use of the hand during the day (Fig. 1–14B). Whatever option is chosen, the goal is to prevent an adduction contracture of the first web space.

EXAMPLE: WRIST/THUMB CMC PALMAR ABDUCTION IMMOBILIZATION ORTHOSIS (WHFO) (Fig. 1–14)

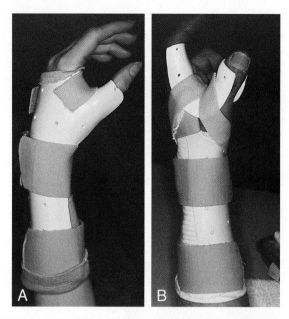

FIGURE 1–14   Wrist/thumb CMC palmar abduction immobilization orthosis: (WHFO). A, A wrist/thumb CMC palmar abduction immobilization orthosis used to prevent adduction contractures of the first web space after median nerve injury or repair. It can be fabricated to incorporate the wrist and first web space as shown here. **B,** As the nerve heals and wrist extension is allowed, a removable spacer can be made directly over a simple wrist orthosis and applied at night or when the hand is not being used.

• Protect Healing Structures and Surgical Procedures

A therapist may be called on to fabricate an immobilization orthosis to rest and protect an extremity that has undergone an operative procedure. This may involve a simple orthosis or an intricate one that must immobilize several structures in specific positions because of a complex injury or surgical repair. For postoperative orthotic fabrication, close communication with the surgeon is critical to guide proper selection of orthosis. Consideration needs to be given to fabricating the orthosis around or over drains, wounds, external pins, or skin grafts. These issues, as well as the pain level and psychological trauma of injury and surgery, make fabrication of the orthosis in the postoperative extremity quite a challenge.

Support, comfort, and protection of a patient's status after a Dupuytren's contracture release can be achieved by using a hand immobilization orthosis. This orthosis is applied after the bulky dressing is removed, new hand and digit dressings are reapplied, and the orthosis is then fabricated over these dressings. The patient is able to take the device off and perform the exercise regime dictated by the therapist/surgeon (Fig. 1–15A–C).

EXAMPLE: HAND/DIGIT IMMOBILIZATION ORTHOSIS (HFO) (Fig. 1–15)

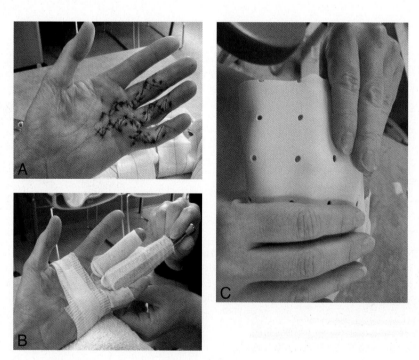

FIGURE 1–15   Hand/digit immobilization orthosis: (HFO). A hand and digit immobilization orthosis is applied after a Dupuytren's contracture release. The orthosis supports the MCP and IP joints of the involved digits in a comfortable extension postoperatively. **A,** Dressings are removed. **B,** New dressings are applied. **C,** The material is applied over the dressings and molded to the patient's tolerable digit extension end range.

• Maintain and Protect Reduction of a Fracture

An orthosis can provide fracture stabilization and maintain reduction when applied by an experienced therapist and supervised by a physician. There are times when casting is not appropriate for a patient and an orthosis can be used as an alternative. The use of thermoplastic material can often provide an intimate fit around detailed areas, such as the metacarpal heads and phalanges, which may be harder to achieve with traditional casting materials. Some patients are more comfortable with the lighter thermoplastic material and better functional use of the hand that comes with orthotic intervention versus casting.

Stable fractures, such as some fifth metacarpal fractures, may be treated effectively with an RF–SF MCP immobilization orthosis (Fig. 1–16). This type of orthosis, when molded intimately and carefully, provides continued alignment and protection for the healing fracture, maintains the RF–SF MCP collateral ligaments in a lengthened position, and allows for active ROM of the proximal and distal joints. The position of the fourth and fifth MCP joints is generally 60° of flexion, with the wrist, PIP, and DIP joints often left free. Because the fourth and fifth metacarpals are mobile compared to the second and third metacarpals, the hand portion of the orthosis should encompass the second and third metacarpal bases to improve stability and provide adequate purchase of the orthosis on the hand (Colditz, 2011a).

EXAMPLE: RF–SF MP FLEXION IMMOBILIZATION ORTHOSIS (HFO) (Fig. 1–16)

• Protect and Improve Joint Alignment

An orthosis can be fabricated to align subluxed and/or deviated joints to an improved anatomical position. In certain conditions, such as rheumatoid arthritis, joint laxity and/or tendon ruptures may disrupt proper joint mechanics, resulting in significant functional loss. Immobilization orthoses may work well to provide support and protection; they also redirect and attempt to position ligaments properly during healing (Beasley, 2011; Dell & Dell, 1996; Philips, 1995).

Patients with arthritis can wear a comfortable and supportive wrist and hand immobilization orthosis at night; the orthosis aids in maintaining proper joint alignment, protects against deforming forces, and prevents or minimizes soft tissue contractures. Not only can the orthosis be molded to support the larger joints involved but strategically directed soft straps can also aid in repositioning the small joints of the digits within the design. Without attention to corrective positioning, joint deformity and limitation of function may occur sooner rather than later. The person with arthritis often welcomes the rest and support that the immobilization orthosis provides (Fig. 1–17A,B).

EXAMPLE: WRIST/HAND/DIGIT IMMOBILIZATION ORTHOSIS (WHFO) (Fig. 1–17)

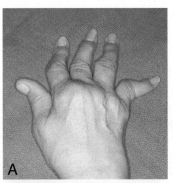

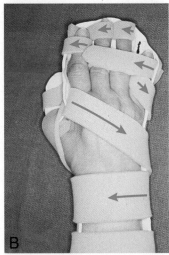

FIGURE 1–17 Wrist/hand/digit immobilization orthosis: (WHFO). A, The hand of patient with psoriatic arthritis. **B,** An immobilization orthosis with carefully positioned straps provides support to and maintains near optimal positioning of the involved joints during rest periods.

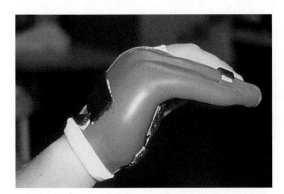

FIGURE 1–16 RF–SF MCP flexion/IP extension immobilization orthosis: (HFO). An orthosis used for treatment of a fifth metacarpal head fracture and PIP joint sprain. The pressure applied through the volar–dorsal nature of this device during the molding process minimizes the tendency for the bone fragments to shift.

• *Block or Transfer the Power of Movement*

Applying a cast or orthosis to an individual joint can be used to block or transfer the power of movement to another joint in the same plane of motion. By blocking movement at a particular joint, the power of that movement is then transferred either proximally or distally. This can be especially useful when the goal is to glide a tendon through scar tissue or facilitate movement of a stiff joint. These devices are often used in the field of hand rehabilitation as a home exercise tool.

A circumferential orthosis or cast to block PIP joint motion, leaving the DIP free, transfers the force of flexion to the DIP joint. The PIP orthosis acts as a mechanical block, eliminating flexor digitorum superficialis function and encouraging the flexor digitorum profundus tendon to work independently to move the distal phalanx (Fig. 1–18). This same concept can be applied to the DIP joint. If the DIP joint is held in extension, the forces of flexion are then transferred to the PIP joint. If the other digits are held in extension, the orthosis will help block flexor digitorum profundus motion and isolate flexor digitorum superficialis glide.

EXAMPLE: PIP IMMOBILIZATION ORTHOSIS (FO)
(Fig. 1–18)

• *Reduce Tone and Contracture of a Spastic Muscle*

There is controversy in the literature regarding which design and therapeutic approaches are most effective for inhibiting tone in a spastic muscle. However, most therapists agree that early orthotic intervention is beneficial for decreasing

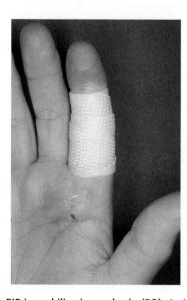

FIGURE 1–18 PIP immobilization orthosis: (FO). A simple cylindrical orthosis (here fabricated with QuickCast2) can be used to isolate and promote flexor digitorum profundus glide.

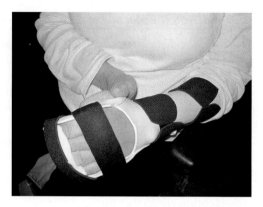

FIGURE 1–19 Wrist/hand immobilization orthosis: (WHFO). A wrist/hand immobilization orthosis (volar–dorsal approach) is often a common choice for managing high tone in the wrist and hand and to prevent skin breakdown.

muscle tone, preventing or reducing contractures, and preventing maceration of skin in the palm (Botte, Kivirahk, & Kinoshita, 2011; Mathiowetz, Bolding, & Trombley, 1983; McPherson, 1981; Neuhaus, Ascher, & Coullon, 1981; Rose & Shah, 1987).

The choice of design is influenced by the severity of the muscle tone, any existing contracture(s), and the ability to position the patient for the actual fabrication. Two people may be needed to fabricate these orthoses. Tone-reducing techniques performed before orthosis application often helps. See Chapter 21 Adult Neurologic Dysfunction for details regarding options for orthoses and patient positioning for ease of fabrication. There are many prefabricated orthoses available that provide support and alignment to the upper extremity and can be applied with greater ease for the patient. These may be better choices for patients that live alone or are dependent on others to don and doff the orthosis. These can be found and further described in Chapter 11 Prefabricated Orthoses.

Fabrication of orthoses to address contractures (or prevent the development of) due to an increase in tone can be challenging. The use of additional materials such as hard cones, finger spreaders, or neoprene straps (attached or incorporated into the orthosis) can sometimes aid in better positioning of the digits, thumb, and wrist while fabricating the device (Fig. 1–19).

EXAMPLE: WRIST/HAND/THUMB IMMOBILIZATION
ORTHOSIS (WHFO) (Fig. 1–19)

Mobilization Orthoses

The rationale of fabricating **mobilization orthoses** is based on a physiologic theory that controlled tension applied over a long period of time alters cell proliferation. Brand and others have well described and documented the benefits of using different forms of mobilization techniques as a treatment modality (Bell-Krotoski, 1995; Bell-Krotoski & Breger-Stanton, 2011; Bell-Krotoski & Figarola, 1995; Brand & Thompson, 1993; Colditz, 1995b; Fess,1995, 2011; Fess & McCollum, 1998; Flowers & LaStayo, 1994, 2012; Glascow et al., 2011; Gyovai & Wright Howell, 1992; Krotoski, 2011; Prosser, 1996; Rose & Shah, 1987; Tribuzi, 1995). The effectiveness of mobilization of tissue using an orthosis is not based on the concept of stretching tissue but relies on actual cell growth. The target tissue lengthens when the living cells of the contracted tissues are stimulated to grow. The stimulation occurs when consistent external tension is applied through the orthosis over time (Brand & Thompson, 1993; Krotoski, 2011). The living cells recognize the tension placed on them, permitting the older cells of collagen to be actively absorbed and replaced with new collagen cells oriented in the direction of the applied tension.

This concept of tissue growth has been demonstrated in several African groups for whom it is deemed fashionable to stretch out certain body parts, such as earlobes, lips, and necks. For example, a small dowel is placed in the earlobes of a young child; the diameter of the dowel is serially increased as the tissue expands and accommodates to each new size (Fig. 1–20).

Mobilization orthoses can be challenging to plan and to fabricate. The therapist has many options (dynamic, serial static, static progressive) when contemplating which type of mobilization orthosis is most appropriate to produce the desired result. The integration of specific information gathered in the initial assessment—for example, age, motivation, psychological status, associated trauma or disease, avocational or vocational demands, quality of the joint's end ROM (soft, hard, elastic), length of time since injury or surgery, active versus passive ROM, and function—contributes to the decision-making process. For example, a patient with a dense, long-standing PIP joint flexion contracture may be better served with a serial static or static progressive orthosis than

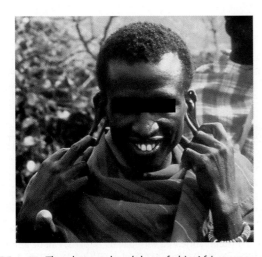

FIGURE 1–20 The elongated earlobes of this African man are the result of stretching owing to the lifelong use of graded ear dowels.

with a dynamic orthosis. Serial static or static progressive orthoses maintain the PIP joint in extension for a set period of time. A dynamic orthosis may not offer enough time within the orthosis (because it is removable) or enough force to overcome a dense contracture (Bell-Krotoski & Breger-Stanton, 2011; Colditz, 2011b; Flowers, 2002; Schultz-Johnson, 2002).

Dynamic and static progressive orthoses differ only in the way mobilizing forces are applied and delivered to the target tissue. Tension through both types of orthoses is initially set by the therapist and can be adjusted by the well-informed patient. The patient may be instructed to decrease the tension for night comfort and to increase the tension between treatment sessions. With dynamic orthoses, the effectiveness of the dynamic forces (especially rubber bands) may diminish over time because of the tendency of the elastic properties of the bands to fatigue under tension. Gravity may also adversely affect the elasticity of the dynamic force by progressively stretching out the bands.

The use of dynamic orthoses through the night is generally not encouraged. The nature of this orthosis is to deliver continuous tension to the target structure, even though the tissue may have reached its maximum tolerable length. Most patients cannot endure this persistent tension at night and end up removing the device (Schultz-Johnson, 1996, 2002, 2003b). Furthermore, sleeping with a dynamic orthosis may be awkward and cumbersome, and there is a possibility that the line of pull could get caught up in bedding or clothing. When applied properly, static progressive and serial static orthoses may be worn throughout the night; these devices hold the target structure at or close to maximum tolerable length but not beyond this position (Bell-Krotoski & Breger-Stanton, 2011; Schultz-Johnson, 1996).

Patients are able to remove both dynamic and static progressive orthoses for hygiene, completion of active exercise, and functional use. Serial static casts are generally fabricated to be nonremovable. They can be changed when the tissue has accommodated to the tension placed on them. Generally, this occurs between 3 and 6 days. Some serial static orthoses are made to be worn for a long period of time (e.g., throughout the night) but allow for periods of exercise and rest. For patients who require an uninterrupted stretch in one direction (as in a PIP flexion contracture secondary to a central tendon injury), an orthosis that is removable may **not** be the best choice. Once the orthosis has been removed, the tissue is able to rebound back to its original resting position, and the gains that were achieved may be at least partially lost. A nonremovable circumferential serial static cast should be considered in these situations.

Attempts should be made to measure and document all forces applied to the hand. Too much tension can cause discomfort, edema, and tissue reaction; too little tension may not be effective. Various force gauges can be used to document tension applied through a "dynamic" orthosis (see Chapter 4 Mechanical Principles). The tension should be measured and adjusted on a consistent basis because the forces may lessen as the hand heals and tissues relax. Observation and clinical judgment are important means of assessing tension parameters; however, patient education is paramount. A patient wearing an MP extension mobilization orthosis following an MP joint arthroplasty will require significantly less tension than a patient whom the clinician is attempting to elongate contracted tissues (Fess, 2005; Jacobs & Austin, 2003). This information needs to be clearly communicated with the patient and/or family members. If not, great harm can occur.

Orthosis wearers should be aware of the signs of too much tension (e.g., blanching skin, pain, numbness/tingling, and color changes) and what they should perceive (e.g., slight discomfort or a mild stretching sensation) (Fig. 1–21). If redness persists (does not fade) 30 minutes after removal of the orthosis, tension/position will need to be adjusted. Too much tension that has been generated over a short duration of time may create microtearing of soft tissue structures. This in turn will increase inflammatory and proliferative activity of cells resulting in increased scar tissue (Bell-Krotoski & Breger-Stanton, 2011; Brand & Thompson, 1993; Fess, 2005, 2011; Schultz-Johnson, 2002, 2003a, 2003b).

Initially, a general rule of thumb may be to attempt to wear the orthosis for 1 hour. If there is no discomfort or sign of tissue distress, gradually increase the wearing time by 1 hour per day. If none of the warning signs have been noted, yet the patient perceives a slight stretching sensation, continue the regimen until the goal time is achieved. Chapter 15 Stiffness, provides more detailed information.

The common objectives for mobilization orthoses are as follows:

- Remodel long-standing, dense, mature scar tissue
- Elongate soft tissue contractures, adhesions, and musculotendinous tightness
- Increase passive joint ROM
- Realign and/or maintain joint and ligament profile
- Substitute for weak or absent motion
- Maintain reduction of an intra-articular fracture with preservation of joint mobility
- Provide resistance for exercise

These objectives and examples of orthotic intervention are discussed in the following sections.

• Remodel Long-standing, Dense, Mature Scar Tissue

A soft tissue contracture can often be addressed with some form of mobilization using an orthosis. The choice of orthosis types depends on many factors, including information obtained from the physician such as bony union or neurovascular status, maturity of the scar, end feel of the tissue, and the patient's anticipated compliance and motivation level. Mature scar tends to respond well to serial casting or orthosis fabrication (Bell-Krotoski & Breger-Stanton, 2011; Schultz-Johnson, 1992, 2002, 2003a). Softer, less mature scar may respond better to dynamic forces, which are applied with proper mechanical principles (Fess, 2011; Fess & Phillips, 1987; Flowers & LaStayo, 1994, 2012). Soft tissue contracture that is associated with Dupuytren's disease and contractures secondary to fibrotic tissue do not respond to mobilization with an orthotic device.

A cylindrical extension mobilization orthosis (cast) applied to a long-standing, dense PIP flexion contracture may be effective in elongating the contracture and maintaining the desired lengthened position (Colditz, 2011b). Therapeutic techniques (e.g., heat, ultrasound, joint mobilization, passive stretching, and massage) used before casting or fabrication of an orthosis may aid in preparing the tissue's responsiveness to stretch. As the tissue lengthens or the ROM increases, the serial static orthoses or casts are changed to support the joint in the new position. Each new device helps remodel the tissue to a further lengthened position (Fig. 1–22). The cast or orthosis is changed every 3 to 6 days, depending on individual protocols, until the contracture is resolved (Flowers, 2002; Flowers & LaStayo, 1994, 2012; Glascow et al, 2011, 2012; Means, Saunders, & Graham, 2011).

EXAMPLE: PIP EXTENSION MOBILIZATION ORTHOSIS (FO)
(Fig. 1–22)

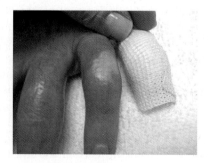

FIGURE 1–21 Note the blanching of the skin from too much localized force on the dorsum of the PIP joint of this serial static PIP extension mobilization cast. Once pressure areas have been resolved, wearing time can be gradually reintroduced.

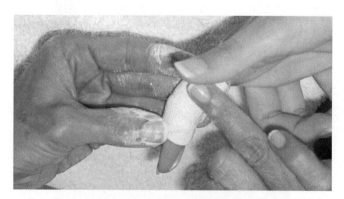

FIGURE 1–22 **Digit extension mobilization orthosis: (FO).** Intimately molded cast (here fabricated with plaster of paris) can be applied and changed frequently to allow for tissue remodeling. Serial casting can be effective in resolving PIP joint contractures.

• Elongate Soft Tissue Contractures, Adhesions, and Musculotendinous Tightness

Several factors are thought to contribute to the outcome of contracture resolution and soft tissue elongation when using an orthotic device. Some of these include the amount and quality of pretreatment stiffness and intervention, diagnosis, time since injury, age, gender, insurance status, and family support (Glascow et al., 2011, 2012; Glascow, Wilton, & Tooth, 2003). Fabrication of an orthosis for mobilization can be effective in elongating contracted soft tissue and stretching adhesions and tight muscle–tendon units during the proliferative stage of scar formation. Judiciously and incrementally applied tension during this phase of wound healing can greatly enhance tissue accommodation (see Chapter 3 Tissue Healing, for details). Preparing the tissue, usually by heating and stretching before the orthotic application, maximizes the device's benefit.

Forearm, wrist, and digit motion can be significantly limited by soft tissue adherence after flexor tendon injury and repair. A wrist/hand extension mobilization orthosis is one treatment option for addressing flexor tendon adhesions and musculotendinous extrinsic tightness in the volar forearm (Fig. 1–23). The static progressive nature of the orthosis holds tension at the wrist and digit's maximum extension ROM, thereby longitudinally stressing the volar forearm's contracted soft tissue structures. Orthosis adjustments occur only when the tissue response allows. This type of orthosis can be taken off for hygiene purposes or to work on active and/or passive ROM.

EXAMPLE: WRIST/HAND EXTENSION MOBILIZATION ORTHOSIS (WHO) (Fig. 1–23)

• Increase Passive Joint Range of Motion

Orthosis fabrication is one of the most effective ways of increasing passive mobility of stiff joints. It has been shown that the amount of increase in passive ROM of a stiff joint is proportional to the amount of time the joint is held at its end ROM (Colditz, 2011b; Flowers, 2002; Flowers & LaStayo, 1994, 2012; Schultz-Johnson, 2002). Serial static and static progressive mobilization devices may accomplish this goal effectively (Schultz-Johnson, 1996). Both types of orthoses are applied after the joint has been prepared (warmed and stretched in therapy) at the tissue's near maximum end range and held there until the tissue response allows repositioning to accommodate a change in length (Glascow, Tooth, & Fleming, 2008). This should be a comfortable, tolerable position for the patient.

An MCP flexion mobilization orthosis can be effective in increasing the passive ROM of the MCP joints. This orthosis addresses MCP collateral ligament tightness that can occur after bony or soft tissue injury to the hand or cast immobilization that hinders full MCP motion. Before applying flexion forces to the MCP joint(s), check with the physician regarding possible issues such as bony union, neurovascular status, and/or tendon repair strength. This orthosis applies flexion forces to the tight MCP joints via two different static progressive approaches. The therapist should be certain that the distal volar border of the orthosis clears the distal palmar crease, allowing for unrestricted MCP flexion (Fig. 1–24).

EXAMPLE: FOREARM-BASED MCP FLEXION MOBILIZATION ORTHOSIS (WHFO) (Fig. 1–24)

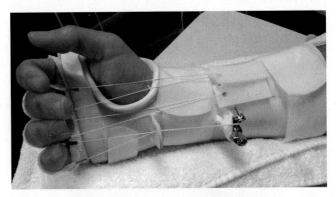

FIGURE 1–24 Forearm-based MCP flexion mobilization orthosis: (WHFO). An MCP flexion mobilization orthosis using two different methods for a static progressive approach. A MERiT™ static progressive component is used for the small digit, and simple loop to hook with static line is used for the ring and middle digits. This orthosis is aimed at improving MP joint flexion secondary to collateral ligament shortening. The MERiT™ was chosen for the small digit because of the severity of the extension contracture.

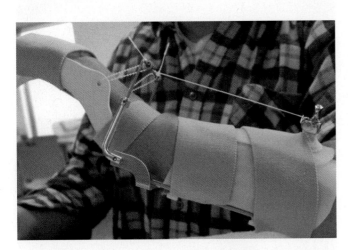

FIGURE 1–23 Wrist/hand extension mobilization orthosis: (WHO). A static progressive wrist/hand extension mobilization orthosis using a Phoenix wrist hinge and simple soft strapping influences adherent volar forearm soft tissue.

• *Realign and/or Maintain Joint and Ligament Profile*

When ligaments surrounding a joint become tight, stretched, or damaged from disease or injury, the joint may sublux or deviate. This process causes an alteration of joint mechanics. Patients may experience pain, may note an inability to use the hand, and often develop harmful substitution patterns. Surgical intervention, such as an MCP arthroplasty or extensor tendon rebalancing, can be a treatment option for these patients. After surgery, a therapist may fabricate a mobilization orthosis. Correctly applied, a postsurgical orthosis can maintain joint–tendon alignment, thereby decreasing previous substitution patterns and deforming forces while increasing the functional capabilities of the hand during the course of healing.

An MCP extension mobilization orthosis is often used in the postoperative care of a patient who has undergone MCP joint arthroplasty. The orthosis gives support to the wrist, provides a stable base for outriggers to assist the weakened digital extensors, and prevents undue stress on the reconstructed joints (Swanson, 1995). The orthosis should be fabricated only after the operative procedure, integrity of the joints/surrounding soft tissue, and ligament reconstruction have been discussed with the surgeon. The purpose of this device is to provide well-controlled guided motion to the MCP joints and to allow for training of the new capsule with proper balance between stability and motion (Fig. 1–25).

The force applied to the MCP joints should be just enough to position them in passive extension with some degree of radial deviation yet allow for gentle active digital flexion. The force used here is much less than the amount used to elongate a soft tissue contracture. Reconstruction of the radial collateral ligament to the index finger (IF) MCP joint is commonly seen in association with MCP arthroplasty. A radially placed outrigger (also known as a supinator attachment) can be added to the orthosis to correct any IF pronation deformity (Bell-Krotoski & Breger-Stanton, 2011; DeVore, Muhleman, & Sasarita, 1986; Philips, 1995).

EXAMPLE: FOREARM-BASED MCP EXTENSION MOBILIZATION ORTHOSIS (WHFO) (Fig. 1–25)

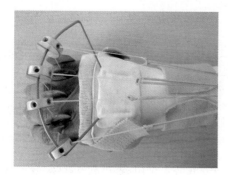

FIGURE 1–25 **Forearm-based MCP extension mobilization orthosis: (WHFO).** This MCP extension mobilization orthosis is used after an MP joint arthroplasty. Slings can be adjusted on the outrigger to guide alignment of the MCP joints into slight radial deviation while maintaining proximal phalanx alignment.

• *Substitute for Weak or Absent Motion*

A mobilizing force through an orthosis may aid functional use of the hand by substituting for absent musculature or assisting in the motion of weak muscles. The dynamic force replaces or assists the motion performed by specific musculature. However, a primary goal when using these orthoses is to preserve good passive motion (Fess, 2011; Fess & McCollum, 1998; Fess & Phillips, 1987). Orthoses that take advantage of the natural tenodesis action of the hand are commonly fabricated to assist functional use after nerve injury. Such substitution orthoses can greatly enhance function, prevent joint contracture, and minimize the overstretching of involved muscle–tendon units (see Chapter 19 Peripheral Nerve Injuries, for details).

An orthosis that addresses the loss of radial nerve function was first fabricated at the Hand Rehabilitation Center (Chapel Hill, NC) and later described by Colditz (1987). The orthosis has a thermoplastic component that rests on the dorsum of the forearm but does not cross the wrist joint. By using a static line directed from the forearm base to the proximal phalanges, the MCP joints are suspended in extension. This orthosis re-creates the tenodesis action of the hand by allowing passive wrist extension through active finger flexion as well as passive finger extension via active wrist flexion. It enables the digits to extend, span, and grasp and release light objects—critical motions for functional use (Fig. 1–26A,B).

EXAMPLE: RECIPROCAL WRIST EXTENSION, MCP FLEXION/WRIST FLEXION, MCP EXTENSION MOBILIZATION ORTHOSIS (WHFO) (Fig. 1–26)

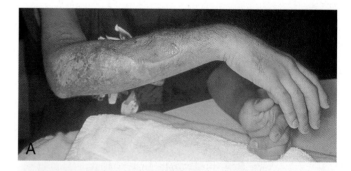

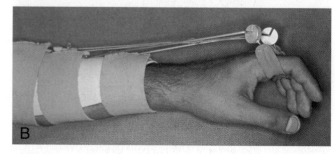

FIGURE 1–26 **A,B, Reciprocal wrist extension/MCP flexion, wrist flexion/MCP extension mobilization orthosis: (WHFO). A,** A patient with radial nerve injury. **B,** An orthosis that uses the Phoenix outrigger kit allows partial functional use of the hand via tenodesis action.

• Maintain Reduction of an Intra-articular Fracture

The application of a gentle traction force to a healing intra-articular fracture site during monitored, controlled ROM maintains fracture alignment, facilitates healing, and contributes to the preservation of joint mobility (Dennys, Hurst, & Cox, 1992; Schenck, 1986; Wong, 1995). Such orthoses are often fabricated in the operating room or shortly thereafter and are most often created by an experienced therapist who has close, ongoing communication with the surgeon.

Intra-articular PIP fractures can be selectively managed with external traction using an orthosis. Schenck (1986) originally developed and described one such traction orthosis. The surgeon places a wire horizontally through the middle phalanx leaving the ends of the wire protruding. The wire is bent to hold rubber bands or springs that are then attached to a hoop that extends from the orthosis base. The rubber band or spring attachment is commonly made with a bent aluminum device or thermoplastic material that can easily glide along the hoop. The traction from the PIP joint to the hoop can be cautiously moved through a specific degree of motion hourly or as prescribed by the physician. The completed orthosis should be checked by the surgeon to ensure proper fracture alignment and force application (Fig. 1–27). This method may be applied to other joints, such as the MCP joint, and many variations of this orthosis have been described since Dr. Schenck's original article (Dennys et al., 1992; Schenck, 1986; Wong, 1995).

EXAMPLE: CIRCULAR TRACTION (SCHENCK DESIGN) PIP INTRA-ARTICULAR MOBILIZATION ORTHOSIS (WHFO) (Fig. 1–27)

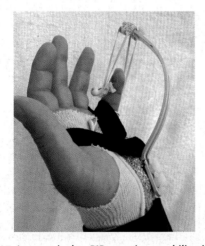

FIGURE 1–27 Intra-articular PIP traction mobilization orthosis: (WHFO). This modified version of the original Schenck-designed intra-articular orthosis maintains gentle traction and fracture alignment while allowing guarded, controlled passive motion of the PIP joint.

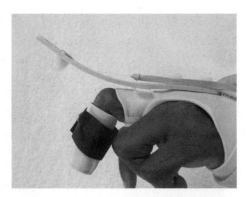

FIGURE 1–28 PIP extension mobilization orthosis: (HFO). A PIP extension mobilization orthosis being used for controlled resistance to an adherent flexor digitorum superficialis tendon. The DIP is held in extension by a small circumferential cast/orthosis to eliminate any action of the flexor digitorum profundus tendon. Increasing flexor digitorum superficialis tendon glide and gentle strengthening are the goals of this orthosis.

• Provide Resistance for Exercise

Dynamic orthoses can be used as an exercise tool to apply resistance in the opposite direction of the patient's active force. This can be a useful way to facilitate tendon excursion through scar, gain tensile strength of specifically targeted muscles, and provide resistance to adherent tendons.

Providing resistance to an adherent tendon, such as a flexor digitorum superficialis or flexor pollicis longus, can facilitate tendon gliding through scar and contribute to increasing tensile strength once a strengthening program has begun. To facilitate flexor digitorum superficialis glide, the orthosis is fabricated to position the MCP joint in extension, and the DIP is held in extension via a cast or with thermoplastic material. A sling is then applied to the middle portion of this DIP cast (Fig. 1–28). Resistance to the line of pull is felt when PIP flexion is attempted.

EXAMPLE: PIP EXTENSION MOBILIZATION ORTHOSIS (HFO) (Fig. 1–28)

Restriction Orthoses

Restriction orthoses limit a specific aspect of joint mobility. These orthoses can be a challenge to fabricate, especially when made for patients who have multiple injuries with a combination of needs. Static orthoses, dynamic orthoses, and forms of taping are considered types of restrictive orthoses because they can be made to restrict some portion of joint motion while allowing the rest of the joint to move freely. A therapist may be asked to fabricate a device that completely immobilizes a joint and creatively allows motion or partial motion of other joints. This scenario requires integration of problem-solving skills, clinical judgment, critical thinking, and understanding of how wound healing stages apply to specific tissues. Careful attention to the construction and fit of

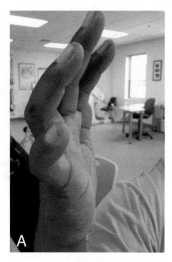 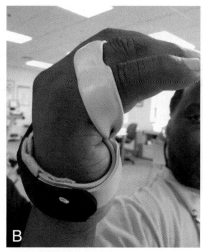 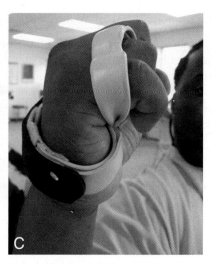

FIGURE 1–29 RF–SF MCP extension restriction orthosis: (HFO). After low ulnar nerve injury, preventing hyperextension at the MCP joints facilitates extension at the IP joints. The fourth and fifth MCP joints are generally positioned between 45 and 70° of flexion to optimize function within the orthosis while awaiting nerve regeneration. **A,** Subtle claw deformity noted **(B)** full IP extension and **(C)** near composite digit flexion.

these orthoses is crucial because of the expected motion and use of the extremity within the orthosis.

The common objectives for restriction orthoses are as follows:

- Limit motion after nerve injury or repair.
- Limit motion after tendon injury or repair.
- Limit motion after bone–ligament injury or repair.
- Provide and improve joint stability and alignment.
- Assist in functional use of the hand.

These objectives and examples of orthotic intervention are discussed in the following sections.

• Limit Motion after Nerve Injury or Repair

Restrictive orthoses can effectively block potentially deforming and abnormal forces to the hand secondary to nerve injury. They allow the healing nerve or reinnervated nerve to glide within a protected ROM, minimizing tension at the repair site, decreasing the risk of adherence to soft tissue structures, increasing blood flow, and improving the nutritional environment. Chapter 19 provides specific design details.

A restriction orthosis can prevent the common claw deformity of the ring and small digits that occurs after low ulnar nerve injuries (Fig. 1–29A–C). Such an orthosis restricts extension motion at the MCP joints by applying well-distributed pressure at the dorsum of the proximal phalanxes and allowing the transfer of force from the extrinsic extensors to the dorsal hood mechanism of the digits. By placing the MCP joints in some degree of flexion, extension of the IP (PIP and DIP) joints is made possible in the absence of the ulnar innervated intrinsic muscles by means of the radial nerve–innervated extrinsic extensors. This position provides the extensor tendons with a mechanical advantage

that greatly enhances composite grasp and release, which is quite awkward and difficult without the orthosis.

EXAMPLE: RF–SF MCP EXTENSION RESTRICTION ORTHOSIS (HFO) (Fig. 1–29)

• Limit Motion after Tendon Injury or Repair

After soft tissue injury or surgical repair, limited motion is often necessary to promote tissue healing, prevent joint contractures, maintain tissue length, and facilitate gliding of structures to minimize adhesion formation. There are numerous protocols that address orthotic intervention for these types of injuries, and only one technique is discussed here. Refer to Chapter 20 Tendon Injuries, for a discussion of various tendon protocols.

Extensor tendon injuries in zones V to VII can be managed with a restrictive orthosis (Fig. 1–30). The wrist is held in static extension (35 to 45°) while the MCP joints are passively extended using rubber band traction. Active MCP flexion against the rubber bands can be performed to a set volar block. Initially, the block is restricted to approximately 30° of MCP joint motion. Gradually, as healing progresses, the block is adjusted to allow greater MCP flexion. The adjustments are generally done each week as long as the tendon healing allows (Evans, 2011; Evans & Burkhalter, 1986; Thomas, Moutet, & Guinard, 1996). This type of orthosis promotes early protected motion and tendon excursion for optimal healing with less risk of adhesion formation and tendon rupture.

EXAMPLE: WRIST EXTENSION IMMOBILIZATION, DIGIT EXTENSION MOBILIZATION/FLEXION RESTRICTION ORTHOSIS (WHFO) (Fig. 1–30)

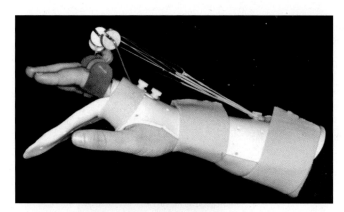

FIGURE 1–30 Wrist extension immobilization, MCP extension mobilization/flexion restriction: (WHFO). This restrictive orthosis (using a Phoenix outrigger kit) immobilizes the wrist in slight extension while providing dynamic MCP flexion to a predetermined range. The patient actively flexes the digits to the volar block, allowing passive excursion of the extensor tendons. Dynamic forces, via the rubber bands, return the digits to full extension.

• Limit Motion after Bone–Ligament Injury or Repair

After fracture reduction or surgical fixation, an orthosis that allows a restricted ROM can be used to promote bone growth, healing of associated ligaments, joint mobility, and soft tissue/tendon gliding. The initial amount of joint restriction depends on the surgical procedure, the severity of the fracture dislocation, the extent of ligament involvement, and the physician protocol. The therapist

and/or physician monitor the amount and degree of allowed extension or flexion exercise and gradually may increase the limits of motion as healing progresses. The permitted, restricted arc of motion promotes healing of the injury or repair and aids in minimizing tendon adherence (Blazer & Steinberg, 2000; Gallagher & Blackmore, 2011; Kadelbach, 2006; Schenck, 1986).

Limiting full extension after a posterior elbow dislocation is the key to preventing reinjury. A static or dynamic orthosis can minimize lateral movement of the elbow, decrease motions of pronation and supination, and restrict elbow extension. The degree of elbow extension restriction is determined by the severity of the fracture dislocation and the position required, preventing subluxation. The position may be altered as the involved structures heal and the physician permits. Care is taken to minimize the risk of flexion contracture by carefully extending the motion allowed as healing progresses. By applying an elbow extension restriction orthosis, the distal forearm straps may be removed to allow unrestricted functional elbow flexion while limiting elbow extension to the confines of the device (Fig. 1–31A,B). A hinged extension restriction orthosis includes an elbow hinge applied to forearm and humerus circumferential "cuff." The hinge is locked to prevent a specific degree of extension while allowing unrestricted elbow flexion (Fig. 1–31C). The degree of extension block is determined by the physician protocol.

EXAMPLE: ELBOW EXTENSION RESTRICTION ORTHOSIS (EWHO) (Fig. 1–31)

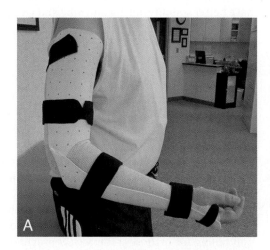
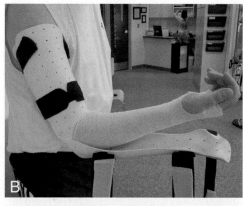
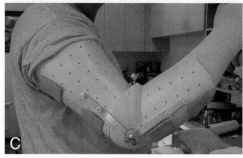

FIGURE 1–31 Elbow extension restriction orthosis. A, Immobilization (EWHO): When this elbow extension restriction orthosis' distal straps are removed, the patient is able to **(B)** slide the wrist out and flex the elbow within the orthosis' parameters. **C,** Mobilization (EO): This elbow extension restriction orthosis (with a Phoenix elbow hinge component) limits the amount of elbow extension yet allows unimpeded flexion.

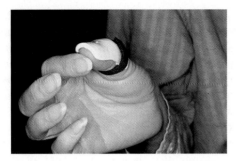

FIGURE 1–32 Thumb IP immobilization orthosis: (FO). This thumb IP extension restriction orthosis provides stability and protection to an unstable IP joint. The block prevents deviation and hyperextension at the joint but allows limited flexion for light activities that require pinching.

• *Provide and Improve Joint Stability and Alignment*

A restrictive orthosis, such as an IF–SF MCP ulnar deviation orthosis, can help support and realign subluxed and/or deviated joints to an improved anatomical position while preserving some functional use of the extremity. Such restrictive devices can block or restrict harmful movement patterns that place undue stress on joints, ligaments, and tendons. Functional orthoses often allow patients to use their hands in a natural way while limiting pain and edema and without contributing to further joint or soft tissue breakdown.

A small dorsal thumb IP joint orthosis can limit the IP hyperextension and lateral IP deviation deformities sometimes seen in the patient with rheumatoid arthritis (Fig. 1–32). This orthosis creates an extension block with lateral borders (a hood) to allow IP flexion. This positioning greatly improves stability during pinch. An elastic wrap is recommended for securing the proximal portion of the orthosis about the proximal phalanx of the thumb; the distal hood can be left free (Terrono, Nalebuff, & Philips, 1995). Applied in this way, the orthosis allows functional IP flexion with minimal deforming forces. Therapy should also include gentle ROM exercises to avoid soft tissue contractures, intrinsic muscle tightness, and collateral ligament shortening.

EXAMPLE: THUMB IP EXTENSION/LATERAL DEVIATION RESTRICTION ORTHOSIS (FO) (Fig. 1–32)

• *Assist in Functional Use of the Hand*

Orthoses are an excellent way to assist and ready the hand for functional use (Deshaies, 2008; Sillem et al., 2011). Chronic, improper positioning as a result of a poorly fit orthosis can lead to contractures, functional lengthening or shortening of tendons, pain, and prolonged edema. Orthosis fabrication can be used advantageously to position joints and tendons while preventing the possible consequences. The key to independence is maintaining function for as long as possible.

A small lightweight orthosis can be used to manage a supple swan-neck deformity (PIP hyperextension, DIP flexion). Such a device balances digital extension by applying

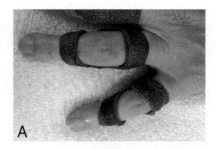

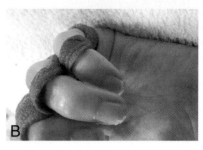

FIGURE 1–33 PIP extension restriction orthosis: (FO). A small PIP extension restriction orthosis worn during functional use to manage long standing swan-neck deformities. **A,** Digit extension. **B,** Digit flexion.

three-point pressure about the PIP joint (Fig. 1–33A). Dorsal pressure applied proximal and distal to the PIP joint limits the joint's extension; volar pressure directly supports the joint. Hyperextension is not permitted; however, flexion of the digit is preserved (Fig. 1–33B). Intervention should also include a program of intrinsic stretching and ROM exercises for the wrist and uninvolved joints. Patients can manage quite well with these small devices, which allow them to have better stability during pinching and grasping activities.

EXAMPLE: PIP EXTENSION RESTRICTION ORTHOSIS (FO) (Fig. 1–33)

Conclusion

This chapter describes the blended nomenclature important to all therapists working with upper extremity patients. It also provides practical clinical examples of various orthoses, outlines common objectives for intervention, and offers insight in the use of L-Codes in billing for orthoses. The MOCS provides clarity and a mechanism to define orthoses through a sequence of analytic steps that combines historical nomenclature, the CMS coding language, and parts of the ASHT splint classification system. The editors and authors of this publication strongly believe that unified terminology is paramount when referring to orthotic devices in every aspect of our professions.

Fabricating orthoses for the injured extremity is only one part of a comprehensive rehabilitation program. For successful orthotic intervention, the clinician must help the patient (and/or caregiver) understand the importance of compliance and make certain they are aware of the orthosis function; why are they wearing it? The orthosis must be comfortable to wear, convenient to apply, and should have an acceptable aesthetic appearance for the wearer. The orthosis needs to be accepted into the patient's lifestyle; otherwise, it may have a detrimental effect (Callinan, 2008; Deshaies, 2008; McKee & Rivard, 2004; McKee & Rivard, 2011; Sandford, Barlow, Lewis, 2008).

Chapter Review Questions

1. Explain the terms:
   A. Orthotic
   B. Orthosis
   C. Orthoses
   D. Splint

2. What is an L-Code?

3. What is the difference between a mobilization orthosis and a restrictive orthosis?

4. What are the three basic mobilization orthoses and how do they differ from each other?

5. What must a clinician take into consideration when choosing the most appropriate orthosis for a patient?

Anatomical Principles

Noelle M. Austin, MS, PT, CHT

Chapter Objectives

After study of this chapter, the reader should be able to:

- Appreciate the normal architecture of the hand and upper extremity.
- Name the three arches that comprise the arch system in the hand and describe the importance of including these arches within a molded orthosis.
- Recognize the precautions related to orthosis application and how this relates to patient education.
- Give examples of the various bony prominences and superficial nerves that are at risk for irritation from orthosis application.

Key Terms

Acromioclavicular joint
Articular capsule
Articular cartilage
Axillary artery
Axillary nerve
Brachial artery
Brachial plexus
Carpometacarpal (CMC) joints
Collateral ligaments
Deep palmar arterial arch
Deep venous arch

Distal palmar crease
Distal radioulnar joint
Distal transverse arch
Glenohumeral joint
Humeroradial joint
Humeroulnar joint
Longitudinal arch
Median nerve
Metacarpophalangeal joints (MCP)
Palmar creases
Proximal palmar crease

Proximal radioulnar joint
Proximal transverse arch
Radial artery
Radial nerve
Radiocarpal joint
Superficial arterial arch
Superficial venous arch
Thumb interphalangeal joint (IP)
Ulnar artery
Ulnar nerve

Introduction

The anatomy of the upper extremity is composed of a complex arrangement of bones, joints, nerves, muscles, and vascular structures, which work together to permit a wide range of functional capabilities. To be effective as clinicians, therapists must have a comprehensive understanding of how these structures function conjointly under normal and abnormal conditions, such as injury and disease. This chapter focuses on the anatomical structures of the upper extremity and notes how they are specifically related to issues of orthotic fabrication.

Please see anatomy tables on thePoint companion website.

The Bones and Joints of the Upper Extremity

The skeletal structure of the upper extremity is defined proximally by the shoulder girdle and distally by the finger joints (Fig. 2–1A,B). This complex configuration of bones allows each joint to move in specific ways, permitting mobility and function of the hand in space. Dysfunction of even one joint in the upper extremity can affect the ability of the other joints to function normally (Calliet, 1994).

Except for the scapulothoracic joint, the joints of the upper extremity are considered synovial joints, which have a joint cavity, **articular cartilage** lining the bony ends, and an **articular capsule** containing synovial fluid (Fig. 2–2) (Moore, 2011; Moore, Agur, & Dalley, 2011). Synovial joints are categorized by their bony configuration and the amount of motion they allow. Each type of synovial joint is represented in the upper extremity (Fig. 2–3A–F) (Moore, 2011; Moore et al., 2011). Ligaments are composed of thick connective tissue that emanates from the joint capsule; they provide stability to the joint. The ligaments of each joint are shown in the figures throughout this chapter.

Wherever the patient's problem lies—from the shoulder to the distal interphalangeal joint—the therapist's goal is to appreciate normal joint mechanics; to preserve, as much as possible, the normal anatomical alignment; and to provide the opportunity for maximal functional use. Therapists must understand how the upper extremity structures interact under normal and abnormal conditions and must ultimately be aware of how therapy intervention can influence the final outcome.

The Shoulder

In the proximal upper extremity, the **shoulder complex** includes the sternoclavicular, **acromioclavicular**, scapulothoracic, and **glenohumeral joints**. The first three of these joints are discussed here because they link the upper extremity to the trunk and their status can affect the ultimate function of the limb. The sternoclavicular joint is a saddle joint consisting of the medial end of the clavicle and the lateral aspect of the manubrium; it allows motion in several directions (Fig. 2–4) (Moore, 2011; Moore et al., 2011). The acromioclavicular joint is a **plane joint** formed by the lateral end of the clavicle and medial portion of the acromion; it permits rotation and anterior to posterior movement of the acromion on the clavicle (Fig. 2–5) (Moore, 2011; Moore et al., 2011). The articulation between the scapula and thorax is considered a pseudo joint (false joint); it allows the scapula to glide along the thoracic wall as the arm moves in space (Fig. 2–6) (Kapandji, 1982). The ball-and-socket arrangement of the glenohumeral joint is formed by an articulation between the glenoid fossa of the scapula and the head of the humerus. This loose configuration provides a highly mobile arrangement; however, mobility is achieved by sacrificing stability. The joint allows the arm to move freely in extension and flexion, abduction and adduction, and internal and external rotation (Fig. 2–7A–D) (Kapandji, 1982; Moore, 2011; Moore et al., 2011).

The Elbow

The **elbow joint** is composed of the **humeroulnar** and **humeroradial joints** (Moore, 2011; Moore et al., 2011). The humeroulnar joint consists of the trochlea of the distal humerus as it joins the trochlear notch of the proximal ulna. The humeroradial joint is made up of the capitulum of the distal humerus and the head of the radius. The elbow joint is generally considered a hinge joint, which allows extension and flexion (Fig. 2–8A–D). There is a normal valgus carrying angle of 5° in males and 10 to 15° in females (Hoppenfeld, 1976). When fabricating elbow orthoses with the forearm positioned in supination, the therapist must incorporate the valgus angle into the design to ensure an appropriate fit.

The Forearm

The **proximal radioulnar joint** consists of the articulation of the radial head with the radial notch of the ulna. The **distal radioulnar joint** (DRUJ) is made up of the ulnar notch of radius and the head of the ulna. These articulations are both considered pivot joints; they permit the radius to rotate about the ulna during supination and pronation (Fig. 2–9A–C) (Moore, 2011; Moore et al., 2011). Stability is provided proximally by the annular and quadrate ligaments and distally by the anterior and posterior radioulnar ligaments along with the triangular fibrocartilage complex (TFCC) (Levangie & Norkin, 2011; Tubiana, Thomine, & Mackin, 1996). The interosseous membrane helps bind the radius and ulna together by virtue of its fiber orientation from the radius to the ulna (Levangie & Norkin, 2011). Therapists applying forearm-based orthoses must appreciate the variation in muscle bulk during forearm rotation and compensate for this by rotating the forearm at the end of the molding process to ensure adequate fit.

The Wrist

The wrist complex incorporates the radiocarpal and midcarpal joints. The **radiocarpal joint** is a condyloid joint created by the connection between the distal radius with the scaphoid and lunate. The midcarpal joint is a plane joint formed by the intimate union of the proximal (scaphoid, lunate, triquetrum, and pisiform) and distal (trapezium, trapezoid, capitate, and hamate) carpal rows (Moore, 2011; Moore et al., 2011). In combination, the radiocarpal and midcarpal joints allow extension and flexion,

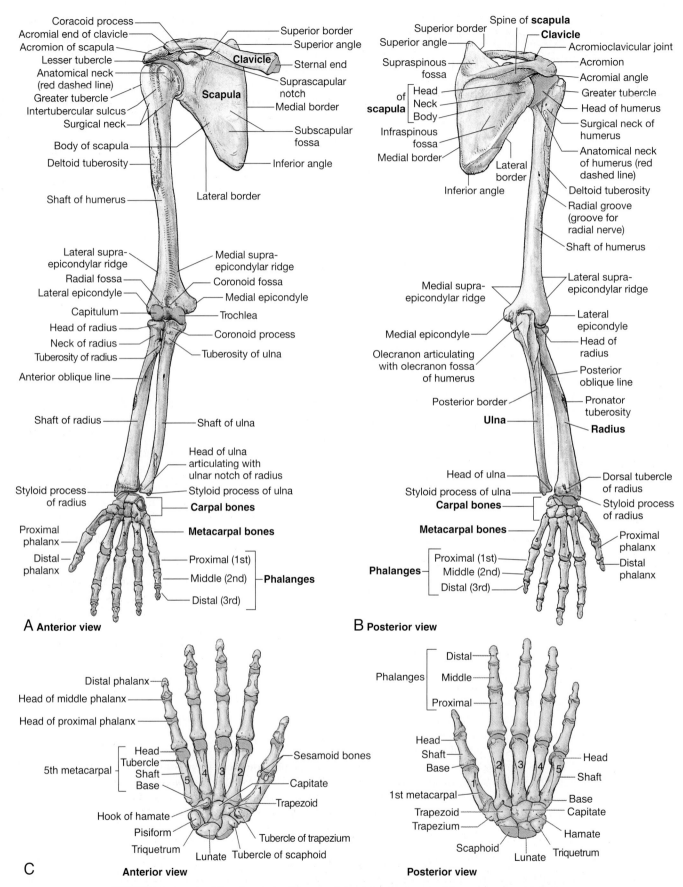

FIGURE 2–1 Anterior **(A)** and posterior **(B)** views of the skeletal structure of the upper extremity. **C,** Anterior and posterior views of the skeletal structure of the hand. Reprinted with permission from Moore, K. L., Agur, A. M., & Dalley, A. F., II. (2011). *Essential clinical anatomy* (4th ed.). Baltimore, MD: Lippincott Williams & Wilkins.

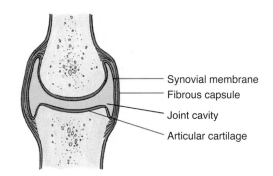

FIGURE 2–2 A joint cavity, which contains synovial fluid, separates the two bones of a synovial joint. A fibrous articular capsule encloses the synovial membrane and the bones' ends, which are covered with cartilage. Synovial joints are the most common and important type of functional joint, providing free movement between the bones they join. Reprinted with permission from Moore, K. L., Agur, A. M., & Dalley, A. F., II. (2011). *Essential clinical anatomy* (4th ed.). Baltimore, MD: Lippincott Williams & Wilkins.

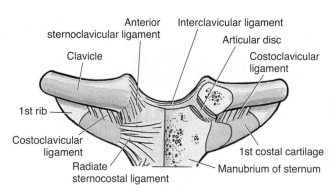

FIGURE 2–4 **The sternoclavicular joint.** Reprinted with permission from Moore, K. L., Agur, A. M., & Dalley, A. F., II. (2011). *Essential clinical anatomy* (4th ed.). Baltimore, MD: Lippincott Williams & Wilkins.

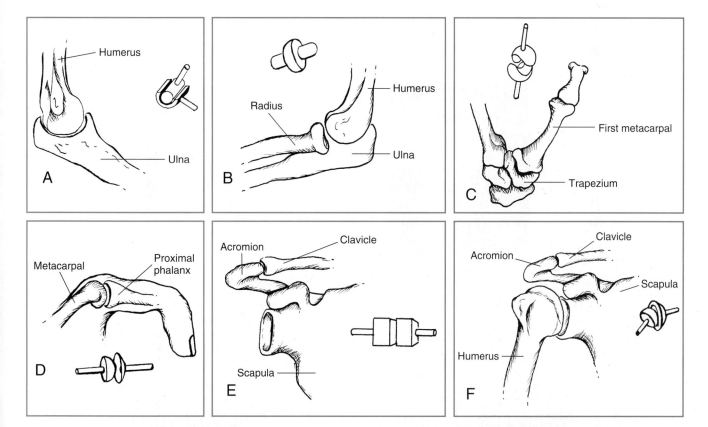

FIGURE 2–3 **Types of upper extremity synovial joints. A,** Uniaxial hinge joints, such as the humeroulnar joint, permit only flexion and extension. **B,** Uniaxial pivot joints, such as humeroradial joint, allow rotation. A round process on one bone fits into a ligamentous socket in the other bone. **C,** One bone of a biaxial saddle joint, such as the trapeziometacarpal joint, is concave and the other is convex at the point of articulation. **D,** Biaxial condyloid joints, such as the metacarpophalangeal joint, permit flexion and extension, abduction and adduction, and circumduction. **E,** Plane joints, such as the acromioclavicular joint, permit gliding or sliding movements. **F,** Multiaxial ball-and-socket joints, such as the glenohumeral joint, permit flexion and extension, abduction and adduction, medial and lateral rotation, and circumduction. The rounded head of one bone fits into a concavity in the other bone. Adapted with permission from Moore, K. L., Agur, A. M., & Dalley, A. F., II. (2011). *Essential clinical anatomy* (4th ed.). Baltimore, MD: Lippincott Williams & Wilkins.

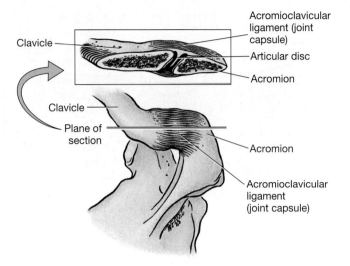

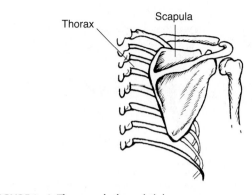

FIGURE 2–6 The scapulothoracic joint.

FIGURE 2–5 Acromioclavicular joint. Reprinted with permission from Moore, K. L., Agur, A. M., & Dalley, A. F., II (2011). *Essential clinical anatomy* (4th ed.). Baltimore, MD: Lippincott Williams & Wilkins.

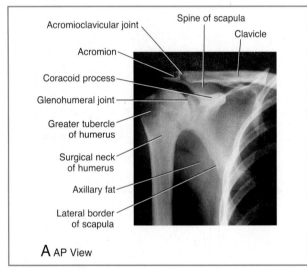

A AP View

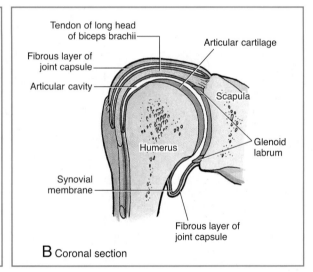

B Coronal section

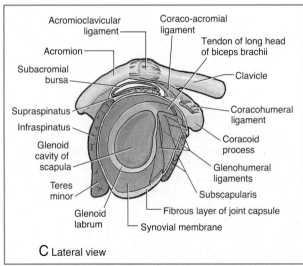

C Lateral view

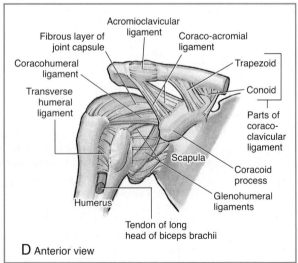

D Anterior view

FIGURE 2–7 Glenohumeral joint. Anteroposterior **(A)**, coronal section **(B)**, lateral **(C)**, and anterior **(D)**. Reprinted with permission from Moore, K. L., Agur, A. M., & Dalley, A. F., II (2011). *Essential clinical anatomy* (4th ed.). Baltimore, MD: Lippincott Williams & Wilkins.

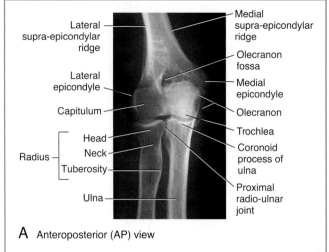

A Anteroposterior (AP) view

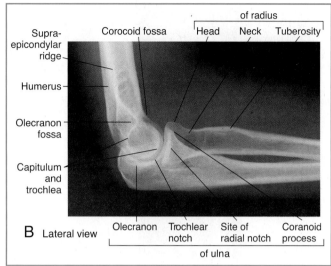

B Lateral view

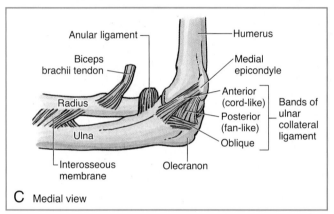

C Medial view

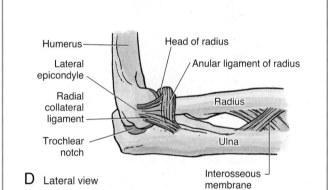

D Lateral view

FIGURE 2–8 Elbow joint. Anteroposterior **(A)**, lateral **(B)**, medial **(C)**, and lateral **(D)**. Reprinted with permission from Moore, K. L., Agur, A. M., & Dalley, A. F., II. (2011). *Essential clinical anatomy* (4th ed.). Baltimore, MD: Lippincott Williams & Wilkins.

radial and ulnar deviation, and a small amount of circumduction (Fig. 2–10A–C and Table 2–1).

The Hand

The **carpometacarpal (CMC) joints** of the digits are considered plane joints; they provide minimal motion at the index and middle fingers and progressively more mobility in the ring to small fingers (Moore, 2011; Moore et al., 2011). This arrangement allows humans to grasp objects tightly (Fig. 2–10A–C). The CMC joint of the thumb, formed by the articulation of the trapezium with the base of the first metacarpal, is considered a saddle joint. It permits radial abduction and adduction, palmar abduction and adduction, and opposition (Fig. 2–10A–C) (Moore, 2011; Moore et al., 2011).

The digital **metacarpophalangeal (MCP) joints** are condyloid joints formed by the union of the metacarpal heads with the base of the proximal phalanges. They allow flexion and extension, abduction and adduction, and circumduction (Fig. 2–11A–C and Table 2–2) (Moore, 2011; Moore et al., 2011). The thumb MP joint is unique in its ability to allow a few degrees of abduction and rotation, which improves precision pinch function (Fess & Philips, 1987).

Distally, the digital proximal interphalangeal (PIP), distal interphalangeal (DIP), and **thumb interphalangeal (IP) joints** are considered simple hinge joints, allowing only extension and flexion (Fig. 2–11A–C) (Moore, 2011; Moore et al., 2011). Therapists must appreciate the tension placed on the ligamentous structures when applying orthoses to the digits. The MCP joint **collateral ligaments** are taut in flexion and slack in extension, but the opposite is true for the palmar plate (taut in extension; slack in extension). Therefore, the MCP joints should be positioned in flexion to place these ligaments at maximal length and to prevent shortening and extension contractures (Fig. 2–11B,C) (Fess & Philips, 1987; Pratt, 2011a). Similarly, when addressing the IP joints, the therapist

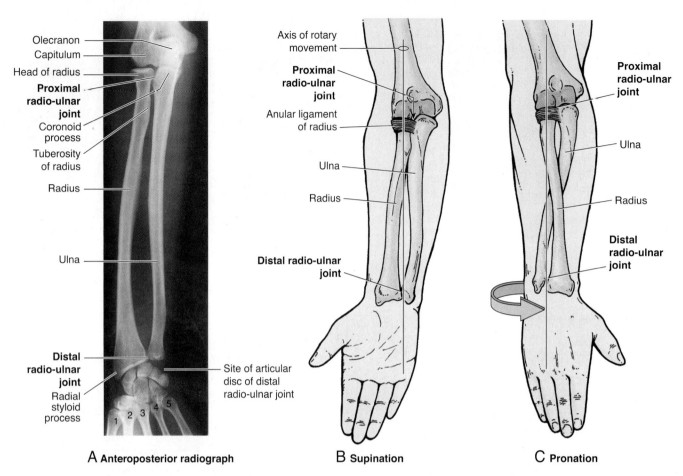

FIGURE 2-9 Proximal and distal radioulnar joints. Anteroposterior radiograph **(A)**, supination **(B)** and pronation **(C)**. Reprinted with permission from Moore, K. L., Agur, A. M., & Dalley, A. F., II. (2011). *Essential clinical anatomy* (4th ed.). Baltimore, MD: Lippincott Williams & Wilkins.

must remember that the volar plate is taut in extension and slack in flexion. Ideally, these joints are positioned in full extension to prevent shortening and flexion contractures (Fig. 2–12).

Arches of the Hand

The bony architecture, along with the muscles of the hand, contributes to the formation and maintenance of the arches in the hand (Fig. 2–13A,B) (Bowers & Tribuzi, 1992; Fess & Philips, 1987; Pratt, 2011a; Tubiana et al., 1996). The **proximal transverse arch** is a rigid arrangement at the level of the distal carpal bones. In comparison, the **distal transverse** and **longitudinal arches** are mobile and add depth to the hand. The distal transverse arch is located at the level of the metacarpal heads and provides the ability of the hand to grasp objects of different sizes. The mobility afforded by the ring and small finger CMC joints allows for this mobile arch. The longitudinal arch courses from the carpal level through the four digital rays. This highly mobile arch adapts to meet the needs of specific grasping activities. For example, when fabricating orthoses for metacarpal fractures, the

therapist must appreciate the differences in mobility of the CMC joints. For example, small finger metacarpal fractures require inclusion of the middle and ring finger metacarpals to gain adequate purchase, stability, and immobilization of the fracture.

When the hand is injured, the arch system can be compromised, altering hand function. For example, ulnar nerve injury and the subsequent loss of intrinsic function (active MCP flexion/IP extension) disrupts the normal arch system, causing virtual collapse (Fig. 2–14A–C). Therapists must appreciate the mobility and stability that the arches provide and should incorporate them into each orthosis to maximize the functional potential of the hand. In addition, a well-contoured orthosis that incorporates the arches minimizes migration of the orthosis on the body and better stabilizes a mobilization orthosis on the extremity when force is applied (Fig. 2–15A,B).

Creases of the Hand

Palmar creases are distributed throughout the hand in a relatively consistent pattern (Bowers & Tribuzi, 1992; Fess & Philips, 1987; Pratt, 2011b). These creases form in direct

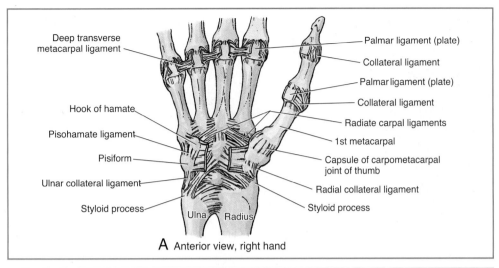

A Anterior view, right hand

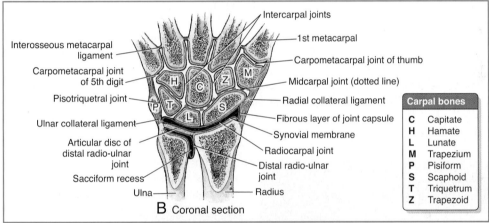

B Coronal section

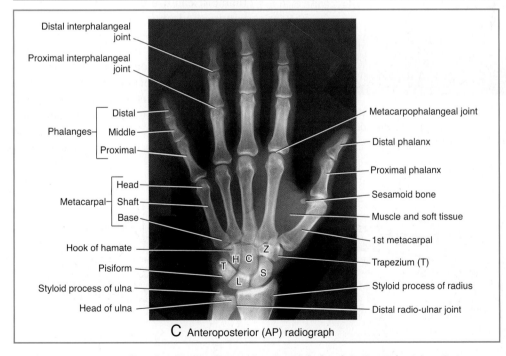

C Anteroposterior (AP) radiograph

FIGURE 2–10 Joints of hand and wrist. A, Anterior view, right hand. **B,** Coronal section. **C,** Anteroposterior (AP) radiograph. Reprinted with permission from Moore, K. L., Agur, A. M., & Dalley, A. F., II. (2011). *Essential clinical anatomy* (4th ed.). Baltimore, MD: Lippincott Williams & Wilkins.

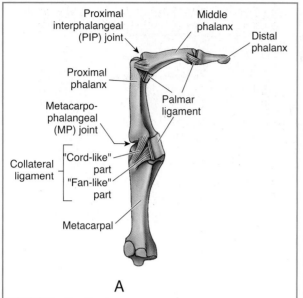
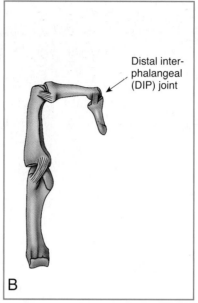
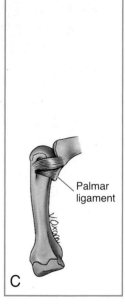

FIGURE 2–11 Metacarpophalangeal (MCP) and interphalangeal (IP) joints. A, Collateral ligaments and palmar ligaments (plates). MCP joint collateral ligaments are lax in extension **(B)** and taut in flexion **(C)**. Reprinted with permission from Moore, K. L., Agur, A. M., & Dalley, A. F., II. (2011). *Essential clinical anatomy* (4th ed.). Baltimore, MD: Lippincott Williams & Wilkins.

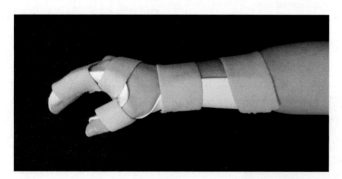

FIGURE 2–12 In the antideformity position, the MCP joints are flexed and the IP joints are extended with the thumb CMC joint midway between palmar and radial abduction.

relation to the underlying structures and the functional demands placed on those structures. To appropriately apply orthoses to the hand, the therapist must gain an appreciation for which specific joints underlie each crease (Fig. 2–16). The therapist can use the creases as boundaries when making patterns and fabricating orthoses. To permit motion distally, the orthosis must clear the creases proximally (Fig. 2–17A–C). For example, wrist orthoses must clear the **proximal palmar crease** (PPC) and **distal palmar crease** (DPC) to allow a full digital range of motion. (To maintain wrist position, the orthosis should extend distally as far as possible in the palm.) Differences in metacarpal length contribute to the obliquity of the PPC and DPC, requiring an oblique angle at the distal edge of a volar wrist orthosis (Fig. 2–18A,B). An additional

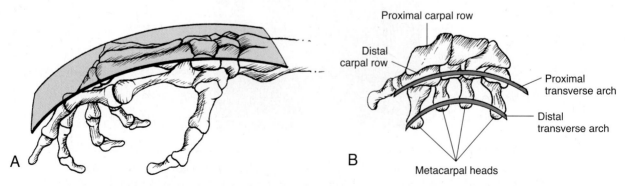

FIGURE 2–13 A, The longitudinal arch of the hand spans the length of the rays and carpus. **B,** The proximal and distal transverse arches of the hand.

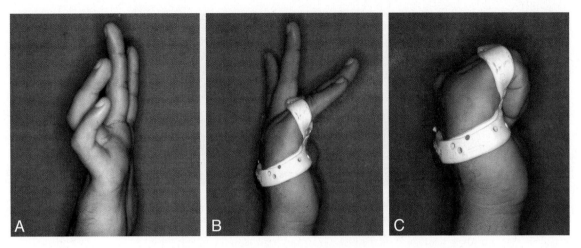

FIGURE 2–14 **A,** After ulnar nerve injury, there is a loss of the arch system. MCP extension restriction orthosis during active digit extension **(B)** and active digit flexion **(C).**

consideration involves the importance of recognizing each patient's individual anatomical characteristics. For example, in one patient, clearing for the DPC on the radial side of the palm may be enough to allow full motion of the MCP joints; but in another patient, the orthosis must clear the PPC to allow full motion.

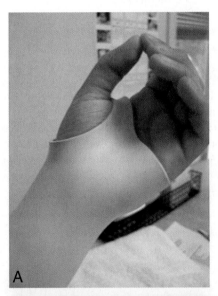

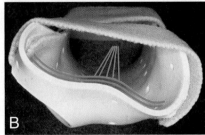

FIGURE 2–15 **A,** Gently opposed position helps to capture arches during the molding process. **B,** A wrist immobilization orthosis that includes the transverse and longitudinal arches to ensure a stable fit.

Orthotic Implications

Bony prominences exist throughout the upper extremity skeleton, and they must be taken into consideration when molding an orthosis (Fess & Philips, 1987; Pratt, 2011b). These areas tend to be vulnerable because of minimal soft tissue covering. Avoiding pressure over these areas by the orthotic material and strapping is of extreme importance, along with educating the patient about what to watch for in terms of warning signs. Signs of too much pressure include pain, redness, and possible skin necrosis (breakdown) from ischemia. The

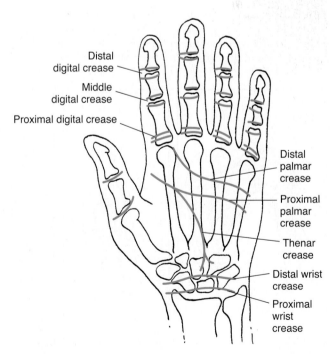

FIGURE 2–16 The relationship between the palmar creases and their underlying joints.

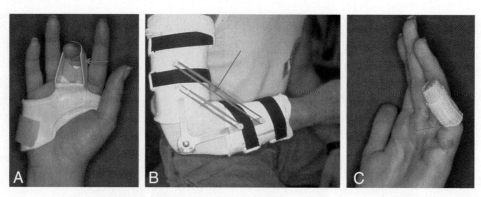

FIGURE 2–17 **A,** A PIP flexion mobilization orthosis that clears the middle digital crease to allow unimpeded PIP flexion. **B,** An elbow extension restriction/flexion mobilization orthosis with clearance at the anterior aspect. **C,** A DIP immobilization orthosis that extends too far proximally to allow full flexion of the PIP joint.

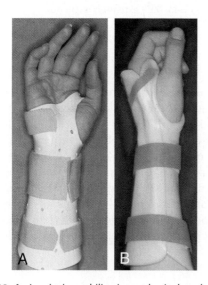

FIGURE 2–18 **A,** A wrist immobilization orthosis that clears the DPC and PPC to allow the digits full range of motion. **B,** A wrist immobilization orthosis with inadequate clearance of the PPC, impeding the range of motion at the index MCP joint.

primary prominences to consider include the following (Fig. 2–19A–D):

- Clavicle
- Spine of scapula
- Acromion
- Olecranon
- Medial and lateral epicondyles
- Radial and ulnar styloid processes
- Base of first metacarpal
- Dorsal thumb MP and IP joints
- Dorsal MCP, PIP, and DIP joints
- Pisiform

Clinical Example

A well-molded orthosis that disperses the area of pressure application can prevent the aforementioned complications by providing a custom fit with accommodations, such as padding or flaring of the orthosis' edges in the at-risk areas (Fig. 2–20A–G). For example, when molding the ulnar bor-

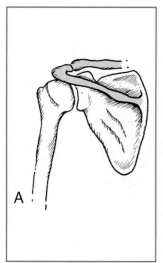
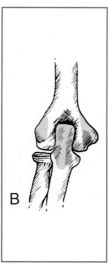
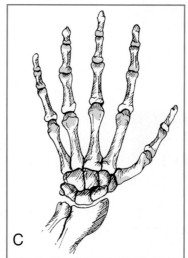
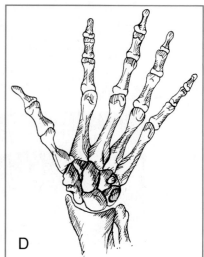

FIGURE 2–19 Bony prominences of the shoulder **(A)**, elbow **(B)**, dorsal wrist and hand **(C)**, and volar wrist and hand **(D)**.

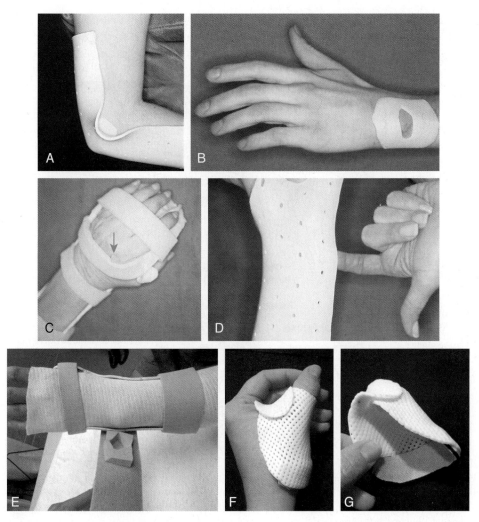

FIGURE 2–20 **Accommodations for bony prominences. A,** Prepadding at lateral epicondyle for a posterior elbow immobilization orthosis. **B,** Prepadding with a donut at the distal ulna. **C,** Padding of the strap that traverses the index MCP joint. **D,** Flaring at the distal ulna on a wrist immobilization orthosis. **E,** Padding on wrist strap with donut for sensitive distal ulna. **F and G,** Neoprene adhered to base of CMC joint immobilization orthosis.

der of a volar wrist support, the therapist should flare the edge adjacent to the ulnar styloid process to help prevent the bone from abutting the hard orthotic material during forearm rotation motions.

Nerves and Muscles of the Upper Extremity

The nerve supply to the upper extremity arises from the **brachial plexus** (Fig. 2–21 and Table 2–3) (Moore, 2011; Moore et al., 2011). The plexus originates from the cervical level of the spinal cord via the brachial plexus, receiving contributions from the ventral rami of spinal nerves C5–T1.

Variations may exist with some contribution from C4 and T2. These five nerve roots combine to form the **superior**, **middle**, and inferior trunks. Posterior to the clavicle, the three trunks in turn divide into the three anterior divisions and three posterior divisions. The divisions then give rise to the **posterior**, **lateral**, and medial cords of the plexus. The cords are named according to their relationship to the axillary artery. The cords provide the origin for the terminal nerve branches: **musculocutaneous**, **axillary**, **radial**, **median**, and **ulnar nerves**. Figure 2–21 and Table 2–3 outline the specific origins of the small branches throughout the plexus.

Each terminal nerve branch traverses through the upper extremity, passing through and innervating specific muscles along its path toward the hand (Fig. 2–22A–E and Table 2–4) (Rayan, 1992; Spinner, 1995; Wolfe, Pederson,

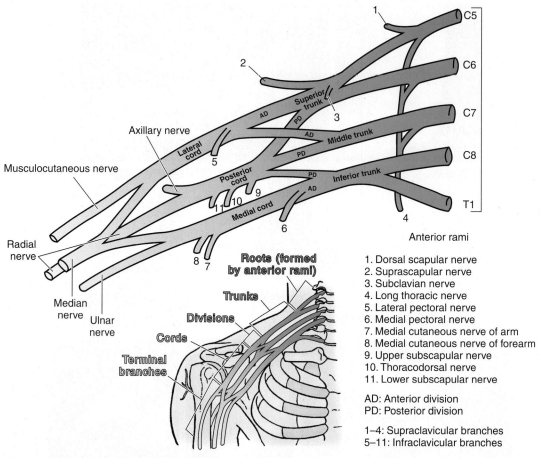

FIGURE 2–21 Branches of the brachial plexus. Note that the musculocutaneous, median, and ulnar nerves are arranged like the limbs of a capital M. Reprinted with permission from Moore, K. L., Agur, A, M., & Dalley, A. F., II. (2011). *Essential clinical anatomy* (4th ed.). Baltimore, MD: Lippincott Williams & Wilkins.

Hotchkiss, & Kozin, 2010). (Chapter 19 includes a detailed discussion of nerve anatomy, including pathways, innervations, and compression sites.) In general, the radial nerve innervates the dorsal extensor muscles of the elbow, forearm, wrist, and hand. The median and ulnar nerves provide innervation to the volar flexor muscles and the intrinsic muscles of the hand. Sensation of the upper extremity is provided by various cutaneous nerves as shown in Figure 2–22. Throughout each nerve's individual pathway, areas exist in which the nerves are vulnerable to compression by other anatomical structures, such as muscles and ligaments. These nerves are also vulnerable to external forces, such as those associated with wearing an orthosis.

Therapists must have a working knowledge of peripheral neuroanatomy, along with full comprehension of the muscular and cutaneous innervations in the upper extremity. Table 2–5 lists the muscular attachments, innervations, and actions and serves as a handy reference when making decisions about orthotic fabrication and rehabilitation of a patient. The muscles of the anterior compartment of the forearm are divided into three layers (Fig. 2–23A–C). The extrinsic digital flexors pass through the carpal tunnel region as they enter the hand (Fig. 2–23D). The muscles of the posterior compartment are arranged in two layers. (Fig. 2–24A,B). These extrinsic muscles traverse the dorsal wrist in separate compartments within the extensor retinaculum (Fig. 24–C,D). Chapter 18 on "Tendon Injuries" provides a detailed discussion of the muscular anatomy of the forearm and hand.

Orthotic Implications

Therapists must avoid excessive compression of the superficial nerves while molding the orthosis and again when applying straps or mobilization components (Fess & Philips, 1987). Similar to educating patients regarding bony prominences, the therapist must explain to the patient the symp-

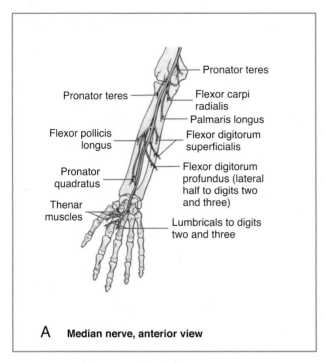

A **Median nerve, anterior view**

Pronator teres
Pronator teres
Flexor carpi radialis
Palmaris longus
Flexor pollicis longus
Flexor digitorum superficialis
Pronator quadratus
Flexor digitorum profundus (lateral half to digits two and three)
Thenar muscles
Lumbricals to digits two and three

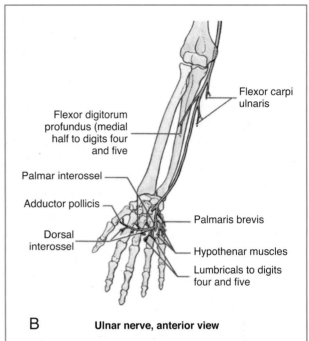

B **Ulnar nerve, anterior view**

Flexor carpi ulnaris
Flexor digitorum profundus (medial half to digits four and five
Palmar interossei
Adductor pollicis
Dorsal interossei
Palmaris brevis
Hypothenar muscles
Lumbricals to digits four and five

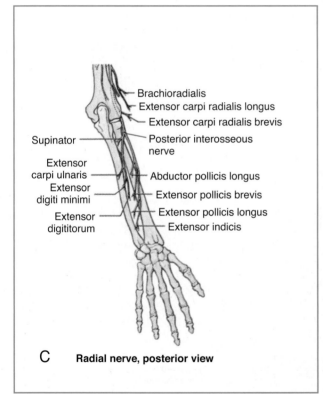

C **Radial nerve, posterior view**

Brachioradialis
Extensor carpi radialis longus
Extensor carpi radialis brevis
Supinator
Posterior interosseous nerve
Extensor carpi ulnaris
Extensor digiti minimi
Abductor pollicis longus
Extensor pollicis brevis
Extensor digititorum
Extensor pollicis longus
Extensor indicis

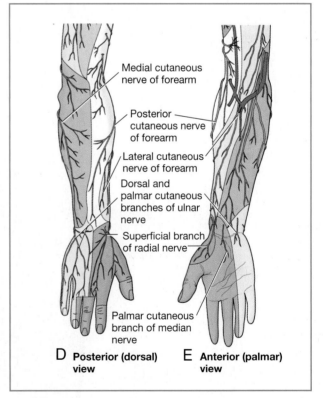

D **Posterior (dorsal) view**   E **Anterior (palmar) view**

Medial cutaneous nerve of forearm
Posterior cutaneous nerve of forearm
Lateral cutaneous nerve of forearm
Dorsal and palmar cutaneous branches of ulnar nerve
Superficial branch of radial nerve
Palmar cutaneous branch of median nerve

FIGURE 2–22 **Nerves of the forearm and hand. A,** Median nerve (anterior view). **B,** Ulnar nerve (anterior view). **C,** Radial nerve (posterior view). Distribution of cutaneous nerves in the upper extremity posterior **(D)** and anterior **(E)**. Reprinted with permission from Moore, K. L., Agur, A. M., & Dalley, A. F., II. (2011). *Essential clinical anatomy* (4th ed.). Baltimore, MD: Lippincott Williams & Wilkins.

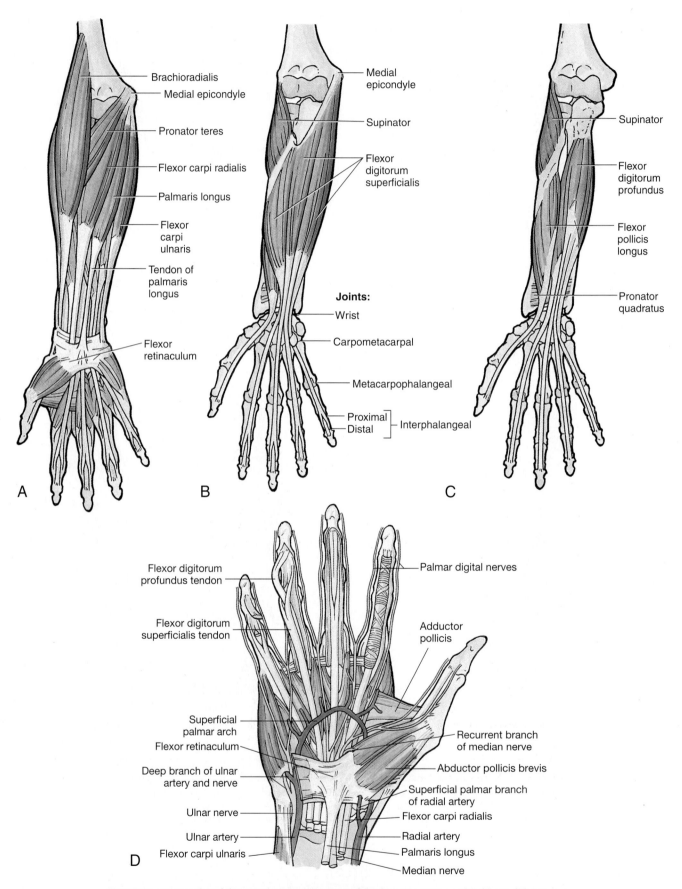

FIGURE 2–23 **Muscles of the anterior compartment of the forearm. A,** Superficial layer, **(B)** intermediate layer, **(C)** deep layer, and **(D)** volar view of hand showing path of flexors from carpal tunnel to the fingertips. Reprinted with permission from Moore, K. L., Agur, A. M., & Dalley, A. F., II. (2011). *Essential clinical anatomy* (4th ed.). Baltimore, MD: Lippincott Williams & Wilkins.

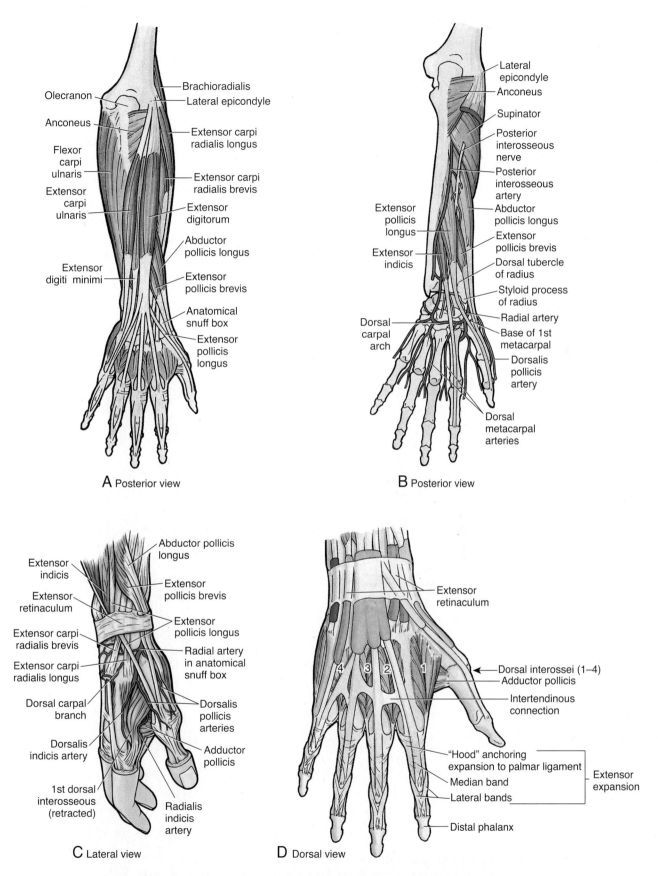

FIGURE 2–24 Muscles of the posterior compartment of the forearm. A, Superficial dissection, **(B)** deep dissection, **(C)** anatomical snuffbox region at radial wrist and **(D)** dorsal view of hand with extensor retinaculum at the wrist and extensor expansion at the digit level. Reprinted with permission from Moore, K. L., Agur, A. M., & Dalley, A. F., II. (2011). *Essential clinical anatomy* (4th ed.). Baltimore, MD: Lippincott Williams & Wilkins.

toms of nerve compression and what to do if they occur. Symptoms of nerve irritation include numbness, paresthesias (tingling), burning, motor control changes, and/or pain. Timely orthotic modification or strap adjustment is necessary if the patient reports any of these signs. Patient education regarding this matter is the key to preventing long-term nerve damage and ensuring maximal compliance with orthosis wearing. Patients are more inclined to wear a comfortable orthosis than one that is causing undue symptoms. Specific nerves that are vulnerable to compression because of their superficial location include the following (Fig. 2–25A,B):

- Suprascapular nerve
- Axillary nerve
- Radial nerve at radial groove
- Ulnar nerve at cubital tunnel
- Superficial branch of ulnar nerve
- Superficial branch of radial nerve
- Median nerve at wrist
- Digital nerves

Clinical Example

When fabricating an orthosis, the therapist must be aware of the underlying anatomy and anticipate any potential nerve irritation to prevent the aforementioned complications. Accommodations include applying padding, flaring the orthosis edges, and using straps and slings of adequate width to disperse pressure about the at-risk areas (Fig. 2–26A–D). For example, when applying a dorsal wrist and hand immobilization orthosis to a patient who has sustained a flexor tendon injury, the therapist must recognize that the superficial branch of

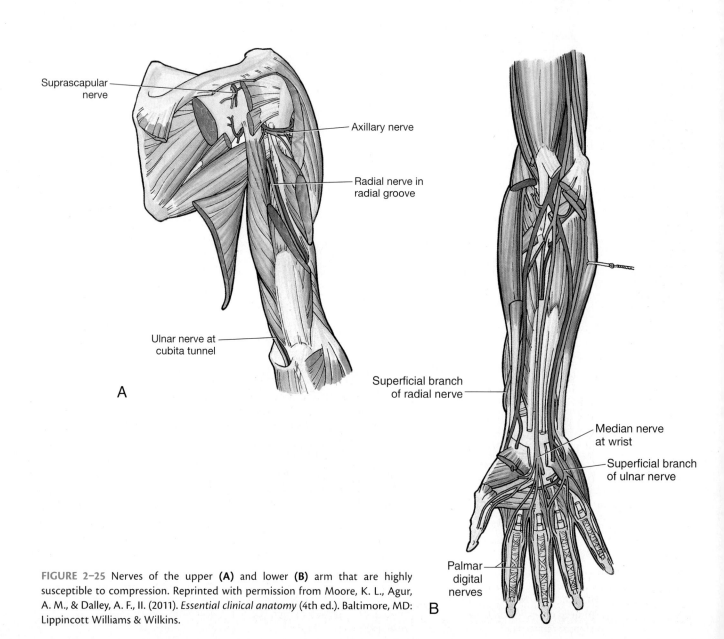

FIGURE 2–25 Nerves of the upper **(A)** and lower **(B)** arm that are highly susceptible to compression. Reprinted with permission from Moore, K. L., Agur, A. M., & Dalley, A. F., II. (2011). *Essential clinical anatomy* (4th ed.). Baltimore, MD: Lippincott Williams & Wilkins.

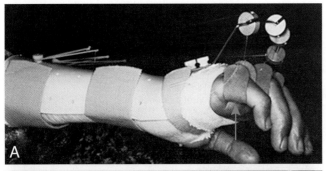

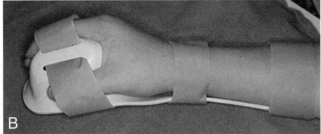

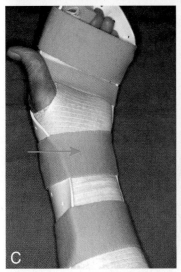
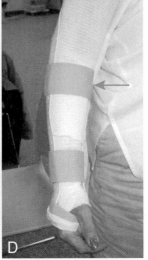

FIGURE 2–26 A, This orthosis puts the digital nerves at risk for compression volarly as the weight of the fingers pulls the slings. **B,** The wrist strap on this antispasticity orthosis is not wide nor made of soft flexible material enough; thus, the radial sensory nerve is at risk for irritation. **C,** The wrist strap on this wrist/hand immobilization orthosis, if placed too tightly, combined with the necessary wrist flexed positioning, can place undue pressure on the median nerve at the carpal tunnel level. **D,** The proximal strap on this forearm rotation restriction orthosis can result in ulnar nerve irritation with distal paresthesias on the ulnar side of the hand.

the radial nerve is highly susceptible to irritation at the radial wrist. The nerve may be irritated by both the wrist flexion position along with the dorsally applied material. Furthermore, the orthosis must be worn on a full-time basis. The therapist must be sure there is no excess pressure along the dorsal and radial forearm over the path of this nerve. Any signs of skin redness or patient

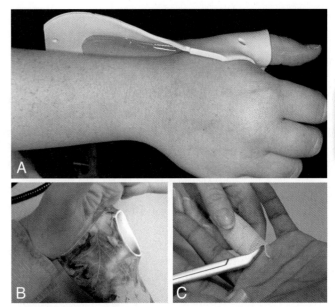

FIGURE 2–27 A, Lining underneath this radial-based thumb orthosis with gel to protect a hypersensitive radial sensory nerve. **B,** The palm of the orthosis fabricator is being used to 'flare and smooth' the distal rim of this orthosis. **C,** Trimming edge of PIP joint cast to prevent sharp edge from irritating digital nerves.

complaints of numbness or paresthesias in the dorsoradial hand indicate the need for timely intervention by the therapist. Modifications or adjustments to the orthosis include flaring away from the nerve, padding the area with soft foam or gel, and being sure to trim away any offending material (Fig. 2–27A–C).

Vascular Supply of the Upper Extremity

The blood supply to the upper extremity arises proximally from larger vessels that bifurcate to form smaller vessels that provide circulation distally throughout the extremity (Fig. 2–28A–C and Table 2–6) (Moore, 2011; Moore et al., 2011). In the shoulder area, the **axillary artery** originates from the subclavian artery at the border of the first rib. The axillary artery in turn continues as the brachial artery, passing the inferior border of the teres major. The **brachial artery** provides the main blood supply to the arm. In the inferior portion of the cubital fossa, at the level of the neck of the radius, the brachial artery divides to form the **radial artery** and the larger **ulnar artery**. These arteries descend through the forearm into the hand to unite and form the **superficial** and **deep palmar arterial arches**. The ulnar artery primarily forms the superficial arch, whereas the radial artery primarily forms the deep arch. The superficial and deep palmar

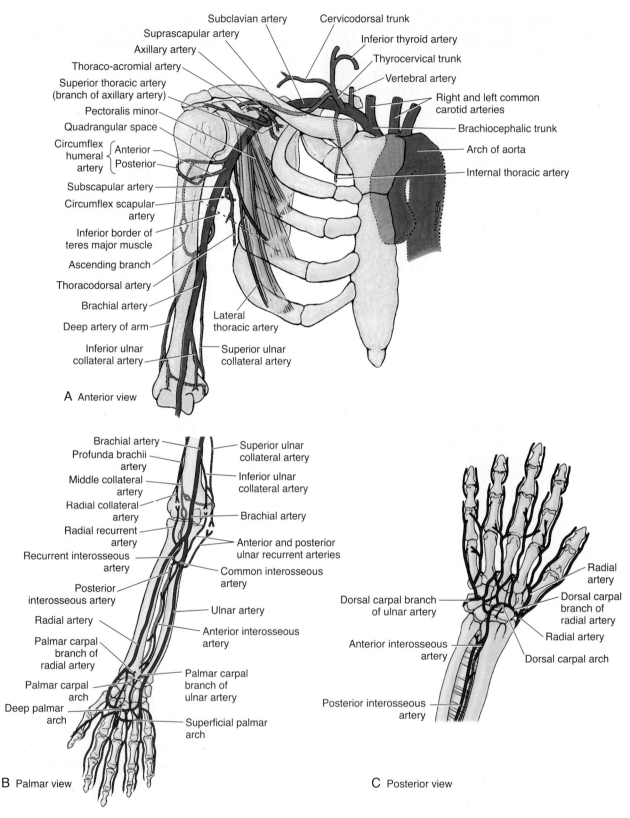

FIGURE 2–28 Arteries of the shoulder and upper arm **(A)**, forearm **(B)**, and hand **(C)**. Reprinted with permission from Moore, K. L., Agur, A. M., & Dalley, A. F., II. (2011). *Essential clinical anatomy* (4th ed.). Baltimore, MD: Lippincott Williams & Wilkins.

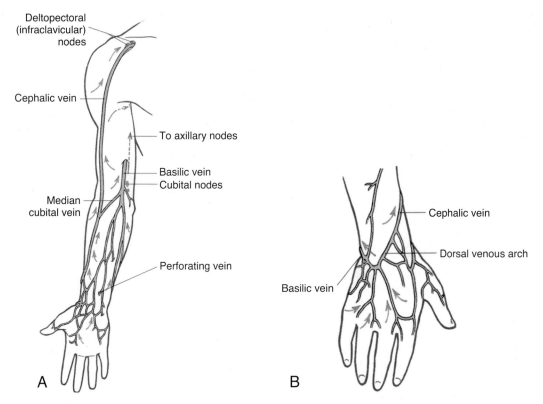

FIGURE 2–29 **Superficial venous and lymphatic drainage of upper limb. A,** Anterior view showing the cephalic and basilic veins and their tributaries. *Red arrows,* superficial lymphatic drainage to lymph nodes. **B,** Dorsal view showing dorsal venous arch. Reprinted with permission from Moore, K. L., Agur, A. M., & Dalley, A. F., II. (2011). *Essential clinical anatomy* (4th ed.). Baltimore, MD: Lippincott Williams & Wilkins.

arches provide circulation to the hand and give rise to the digital arteries.

Superficial and **deep venous arches** lie close in relation to the superficial and deep arterial arches. The dorsal digital veins drain into the dorsal metacarpal veins, forming the dorsal venous network. This network continues as the **cephalic** and basilic vein**s** proximally (Fig. 2–29A,B). The therapist must be familiar with the circulation of the upper extremity when forming orthoses, especially for patients with injury to, surgical repair of, or compromise of these structures.

Orthotic Implications

When orthoses, straps, casts, or edema wraps are applied too tightly, circulation to a tissue may be compromised (Fess & Philips, 1987). Therapists must educate their patients on the signs of impaired blood flow: color changes (deep red, blue, or blanched), temperature changes (cool/cold or extreme warmth), or an excessive throbbing sensation. Prompt alterations must be made to correct the problem. There may also be vascular problems related solely to the position of the body part in the orthosis. For example, in a patient who has undergone surgical arterial repair, the therapist must carefully position the joints above and below the repair to prevent undue tension at the surgical site.

Clinical Example

Careful application of circumferential orthoses, wraps, and straps is imperative to prevent disruption of blood flow to and from the body part (Fig. 2–30 A–C). An edema response follows trauma from injury, surgery, or both. One of the therapist's primary goals is to decrease edema to prevent the problematic sequelae of stiffness and adhesion formation. Therapists commonly use these elasticized compression products for management of edema. These items must be applied judiciously, and the patient should be informed regarding any adverse signs. The problem may be resolved by simply adjusting the amount of tension on the wrap or by changing the wear schedule to intermittent use.

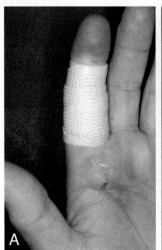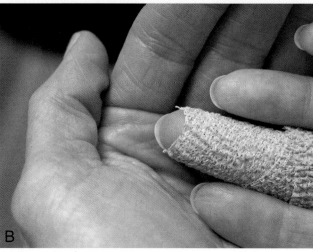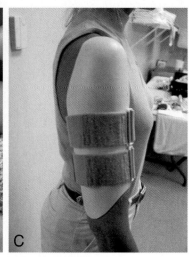

FIGURE 2–30 **A,** Note change in color of fingertip with this circumferential cast indicating excess pressure on the digital blood supply. **B,** When any circumferential wrap is applied to a body part, the patients should remain in the clinic to monitor for any vascular changes so timely adjustments can be made prior to sending them home. **C,** Patients wearing circumferential orthotic designs, such as this humerus orthosis, should be educated regarding signs and symptoms of neurovascular compromise. Oftentimes, these designs can be modified into a bivalve or clamshell-type design with a strapping system as shown here to allow for easy adjustments.

Conclusion

The anatomy of the upper extremity is an intricate arrangement of bones, muscles, vessels, and other soft tissue structures that interact to allow for functional use of the upper limb. To appropriately apply orthoses, the therapist must understand how these structures function together and how they interact with orthoses.

Chapter Review Questions

1. What are the three arches in the hand?

2. How can the creases of the hand be used during the orthotic fabrication process?

3. Describe two techniques to accommodating for bony prominences.

4. What are the signs of nerve irritation?

5. What precautions must a therapist educate a patient to be aware of when dispensing these devices?

3 Tissue Healing

Richard A. Bernstein, MD*

Chapter Objectives

After study of this chapter, the reader should be able to:

- Define the three stages of tissue healing.
- Understand which types of orthoses are appropriate to apply at each stage of wound healing.
- Explain how lifestyle factors can influence a patient's ability to heal.
- Give a minimum of one diagnosis and the most appropriate orthosis intervention for each of the following; immobilization, restriction and mobilization of healing tissue.
- Recognize the impact preexisting medical conditions have on the healing process.
- Discuss the importance of patient education regarding precautions for orthosis wear.

Key Terms

Antideformity position
Collagen synthesis
Edema
Elastic behavior
Fibroblasts
Fibroplasia and proliferative stage
Granulation tissue

Infections
Inflammatory stage
Macrophages
Maturation and remodeling stage
Osteoblasts
Osteoclasts
Plastic behavior

Primary closure
Secondary intention
Stages of tissue healing
Tensile strength
Tissue oxygenation
Tissue remodeling
Viscoelastic properties

Introduction

The biology of soft tissue healing is paramount to the treatment of hand and upper extremity disorders. Whether trauma or elective surgery, understanding the biologic processes involved is important to predict patient outcomes. Both the surgeon and therapist need to understand and to a large degree predict how the tissue will respond to the injury. This guides the patients' rehabilitation, use of orthoses, modalities, and progression of functional tasks. The **stages of tissue healing** influence the use and extent of orthotic intervention and therapy; the status and stage of a healing wound directs the specifics of orthotic selection, fabrication, and patient use.

---

*This chapter is based on the first edition chapter written by Steven Wenner, MD, and Ellen Smithline, RN.

Stages of Wound Healing

The stages of tissue healing are inflammation, fibroplasia (proliferative), and scar maturation (chronic stage or remodeling) (Fig. 3–1). The response to injury is proportional to the nature and severity of the trauma, associated injuries, and tissue contamination. For instance, a sharp laceration with a "clean" knife through nerve and tendon will respond acutely and chronically different than a 50-lb dirty weight crushing a finger and transecting the nerve and tendon. Sharp injuries do better than crush and clean better than contaminated. Inflammation sometimes has a negative connotation, but inflammation is a necessary biologic response to injury. Scavenger cells such as **macrophages** and **osteoclasts** are brought into the area to biologically debride the injured tissue, and the inflammatory response also brings in healing cells such as **fibroblasts** and **osteoblasts**.

Tissue oxygenation is essential for wound healing. Oxygen is carried in the blood, dissolved in the plasma, and bound to hemoglobin. Biologic function and tissue processes are dependent on adequate tissue oxygenation, which requires adequate blood flow (Stotts & Wipke-Tevis, 1997). Orthoses and edema management products need to help stabilize the tissue environment, allow adequate blood flow, and be careful not to impede arterial inflow and venous outflow, which affects tissue oxygenation.

Inflammatory Stage

The first stage, which lasts for less than 1 week, that of inflammation, is characterized by an influx of white blood cells, especially macrophages, and an increase in local vascularity (Fig. 3–1). These scavenger cells help cleanse the area of bacteria, necrotic debris, and foreign material. Edema occurs from the body's inflammatory response to injury, increased vascularity, and often some degree of venous congestion (Smith & Dean, 1998; Strickland, 1987, 2000). At this stage, rest is more important than exercise; immobilization orthoses are useful for protecting, supporting, and resting the injured part (Fig. 3–2A–C). Because of the tendency for venous congestion, elevation can help improve the tissue congestion, and orthoses help decrease the stress or tension on a surgically repaired structure, such as bone, tendon, or nerve. The orthosis should maintain the injured part in the position that is most advantageous position for subsequent restoration of function. Classically for a hand injury, this involves the **antideformity position**: slight wrist extension along with metacarpophalangeal (MCP) joint flexion and proximal interphalangeal (PIP) joint extension (Fig. 3–3A,B). This posture puts the collateral ligaments of the MCP joints and volar plates at the PIP joints at maximal stress to help counteract scarring and contracture that can subsequently impede motion (risk of MCP extension and PIP flexion contracture). By placing these soft tissue structures at maximal tension,

once therapy begins, one does not need to counteract tissue tightness. Simultaneously, adjacent structures should be positioned to prevent unwanted deformity and to facilitate prompt return to function (Smith & Dean, 1998).

Fibroplasia and Proliferative Stage

The second stage of fibroplasia begins 4 or 5 days after the injury occurs and lasts for 2 to 6 weeks (Fig. 3–1). Fibroblasts enter the wound and begin synthesizing collagen, which ultimately becomes scar tissue. Whereas bone is the only tissue to regenerate itself, collagen proliferation, although on the positive side augments healing, on the negative side interferes with the normal anatomical tissue. **Granulation tissue**, the foundation of the wound, depends on adequate angiogenesis and tissue oxygenation. Early in the fibroplastic stage, immobilization allows neovascularization and protects the newly deposited immature collagen fibers, thereby facilitating an increase in tensile strength of the wound. Between weeks 3 and 6, cellularity diminishes; and the extracellular matrix, largely collagen, increases both in volume and in tensile strength (Smith & Dean, 1998; Strickland, 1987, 2000). During this stage, appropriately applied stress can facilitate tissue growth (Fig. 3–2D,E). Mobilization orthoses, which take advantage of tissue's elasticity and responsiveness to external stress, are useful. A balance must be achieved between applying enough stress to encourage positive scar remodeling and avoiding excessive stress, which could cause further tissue damage (Fig. 3–4A,B).

Maturation and Remodeling Stage

During the stage of scar maturation (Fig. 3–1), the collagen fibers become better organized and remodel along the lines of stress, thus enhancing the **tensile strength** of the healing wound. The load per cross-sectional area that can be sustained by the wound is referred to as tensile strength, which occurs at a rate equal to the pace of **collagen synthesis** (Fess & McCollum, 1998; Strickland, 1987, 2000). Therefore, understanding a tissue's tensile strength influences the decision process of orthotic intervention and therapy (Fig. 3–2F,G). Bone, tendon, and nerve healing occurs at varying rates and influence the therapy protocol.

In a well-nourished immunocompetent patient, a surgically sutured wound is at its weakest 2 weeks postsurgery. Tensile strength is 30% in 3 weeks, 60% in 6 weeks, and 90% in 6 months (Fig. 3–5). Therefore, the use of orthoses and therapy regimen needs to keep these tissue factors in mind during the rehabilitative process (Kane, 1997). For a fresh flexor tendon repair, early tendon gliding diminishes scarring within the flexor tendon sheath; however, until suture material and repair techniques can counteract the active forces generated by the flexor muscles, active exercises are typically restricted until the 6-week point. Although tensile strength of the flexor tendon is still

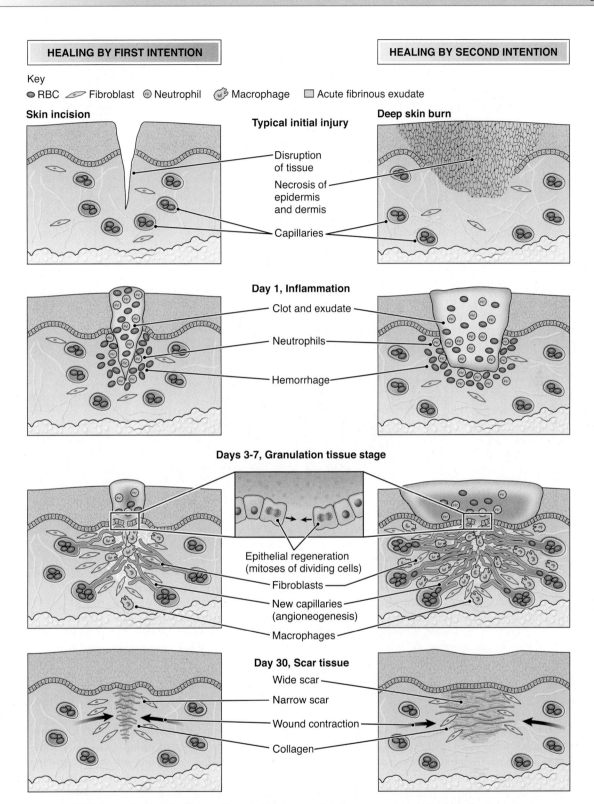

HEALING BY FIRST INTENTION

HEALING BY SECOND INTENTION

Key
RBC   Fibroblast   Neutrophil   Macrophage   Acute fibrinous exudate

Skin incision

Typical initial injury

Deep skin burn

Disruption
of tissue
Necrosis of
epidermis
and dermis
Capillaries

Day 1, Inflammation

Clot and exudate
Neutrophils
Hemorrhage

Days 3-7, Granulation tissue stage

Epithelial regeneration
(mitoses of dividing cells)
Fibroblasts
New capillaries
(angioneogenesis)
Macrophages

Day 30, Scar tissue

Wide scar
Narrow scar
Wound contraction
Collagen

FIGURE 3–1 Healing by first and second intention. Small, narrow wounds heal by first intention **(left),** usually in less than a week, and leave a small scar. Large wounds heal by second intention **(right),** have more inflammatory tissue, take several weeks to heal, and leave a larger scar. Borrowed with permission from McConnell, T. H. (2007). *The nature of disease: Pathology for the health professions.* Philadelphia, PA: Lippincott Williams & Wilkins.

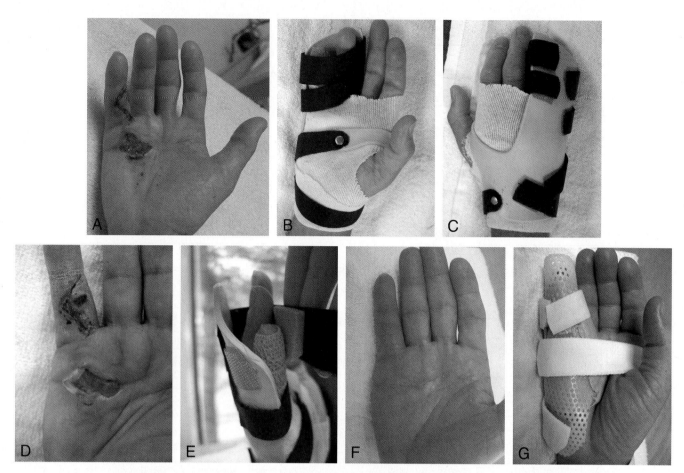

FIGURE 3–2 A, Inflammatory stage of healing characterized by fibrin depositing and forming the initial gel of the wound matrix. First day postoperative Dupuytren's release, notice skin closed in digit with sutures while the palm was left open to heal by secondary intention. **B and C,** Hand-based ring and small finger immobilization orthosis used postoperatively to position digits in maximal extension. Note use of elasticized wrap to control edema. **D,** Proliferative stage of healing during which collagen is laid down, giving the wound strength. Shown is 10 days postoperative—sutures have been removed and open palm area is beginning to close. **E,** Orthosis modified by adding foam to provide gentle extension stretch to the PIP joint, counteracting tendency for flexion contracture. **F,** Scar maturation stage shown when collagen, responsible to structure and integrity of the wound, is formed in a generally random manner. Note complete wound closure at 6 weeks postoperative. **G,** Volar orthosis with Elastomer™ included for scar management; used at night for 6 additional months.

diminished in the first 6 weeks postoperatively, with current surgical techniques, a supervised active protocol is typically begun during this period. (Refer to Chapter 18 on *Tendon Injuries* for additional information.)

Although scars soften during the maturation and remodeling stage, they also contract and shorten. In certain circumstances, such as a partial fingertip amputation, wound contracture is a favorable process. Amputations without exposed bone measuring less than 1 cm^2 heal favorably by **secondary intention**. However, for instance, in a laceration perpendicular to a flexor crease, this contracture can lead to a permanent, painful scar. With shortening, the scar's elasticity decreases; thus, stretching and corrective orthoses are

valuable for preventing unwanted contractures (Fig. 3–6A,B). The length of the maturation phase depends on several factors, including age, comorbidities (such as diabetes or rheumatoid arthritis), genetic background, location of the wound, and length and intensity of the inflammatory phase. Scar maturation is a continual process, and remodeling can occur for up to a year (Smith & Dean 1998; Strickland, 1987, 2000).

The stages of wound healing are a fluid process, not necessarily segmental as staging suggests (Fig. 3–7). Just as the healing stages overlap, so do the time frames for using specific orthoses (Fig. 3–8). For example, immobilization orthoses may be indicated throughout the healing process

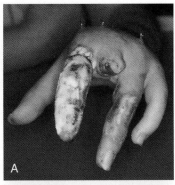

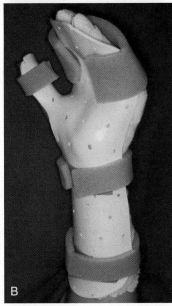

FIGURE 3-3 **A,** A press injury led to the amputation of the middle finger and replantation of the index and ring fingers. **B,** A simple immobilization orthosis promotes healing by providing a safe position for the joints: wrist extension, MCP joint flexion, IP joint extension, and thumb palmar abduction.

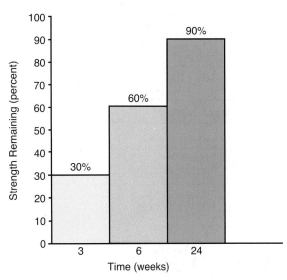

FIGURE 3-5 Tensile strength at 3 weeks, 6 weeks, and 6 months.

but typically more in the inflammatory phase. In subsequent phases, immobilization orthoses may have a role, especially during sleep; but mobilization orthoses are often used during the later stages (Colditz, 2011; Fess, Gettle, Phillips, & Janson, 2005).

Effect of Orthoses on Tissue Healing

During the inflammatory and early fibroplastic stages, certain tissues such as bone and nerve are best managed with immobilization orthoses; protection is more important than exercise (Fig. 3-9A,B). Fractures need protection until callous begins to stabilize the bone; nerves repaired

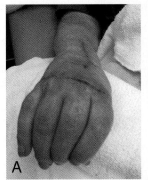

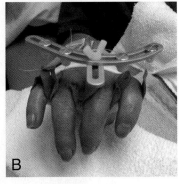

FIGURE 3-4 **A and B,** RA patient 10 days after MCP arthroplasty using mobilization orthosis during the encapsulation process to promote optimal collagen alignment (Digitec Outrigger System, Patterson Medical, Warrenville, IL).

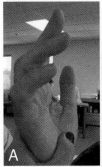

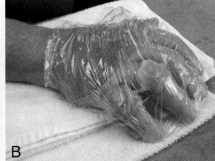

FIGURE 3-6 **A and B,** Patient with long-standing PIP joint flexion contractures caused by ulnar neuropathy using prefabricated PIP extension mobilization orthoses in conjunction with paraffin/heat application. This preconditioning of joints is helpful prior to manual therapy intervention.

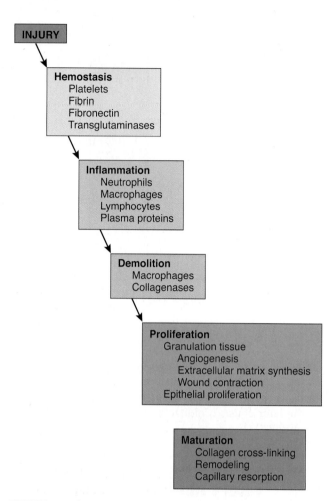

FIGURE 3–7 **The repair cascade.** Repair can be viewed as a chain of events, each stage completing the previous one and initiating the subsequent one. Borrowed with permission from Rubin, E., & Farber, J. L. (1999). *Pathology* (3rd ed.). Philadelphia, PA: Lippincott Williams & Wilkins.

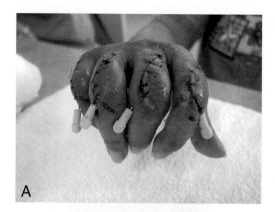

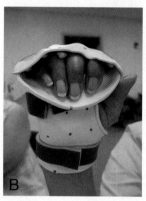

FIGURE 3–9 **A and B,** Patient with RA 2 days following PIP joint reconstruction to reverse swan-neck deformities; immobilization orthosis used to rest and protect reconstruction. Note position of MCP flexion to prevent collateral ligament shortening.

microsurgically need protection based on the intraoperative findings of the degree of tension at the repair site. When edema subsides, mobilization orthoses may be appropriate. Stress should be applied to the healing tissue to the degree that it favorably influences scar remodeling but not so much that it further damages tissues (Fig. 3–10). However, timing

FIGURE 3–8 Orthotic management for the patient should be based on the current stage of healing. The most common orthotic intervention is shown here; however, special conditions may require deviation from these guidelines.

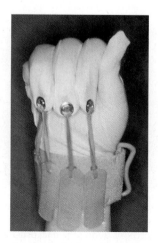

FIGURE 3–10 Use of a simple flexion glove to impart gentle dynamic stretch to stiff digits.

requires balance with biology; the degree of tissue trauma, persistent contamination or infection, or an immunocompromised host can prolong the inflammatory phase and retard healing.

Healthy healing tissue will benefit from early therapy and will respond favorably to continuously applied gentle stress. Edema and pain should diminish, and function should increase if the mobilizing orthosis is appropriately applied and working. However, the overly aggressive use of mobilization orthoses (dynamic, static progressive, or serial static) during the fibroplastic stage or their premature use may reinjure healing tissues and retard recovery. For example, unstable fractures and torn collateral ligaments are injuries for which active range of motion (ROM) and accompanying mobilizing orthoses should be delayed until the likelihood of disruption of healing owing to a repeat injury is diminished (Fess & McCollum, 1998; Strickland, 1987, 2000).

For most tissues, the stress that can be safely applied and the degree and duration of the force increase at approximately 6 weeks after injury, when generally speaking tensile strength is 60% normal. At this point, the scar maturation or remodeling stage commences, and it is the sensible time to introduce serial static or static progressive orthoses if necessary (Fig. 3–11).

Tissue Remodeling

Soft tissue is alive and possesses **viscoelastic properties** that allow it to lengthen and shorten within a certain anatomical range. When soft tissue has shortened, perhaps as a consequence of scar contracture, orthotic and casting techniques are useful adjuncts for stretching the tight tissue.

Tissue remodeling may be favorably encouraged by gentle stretching over a period of time, allowing an alteration in cellular structure and alignment in response to the

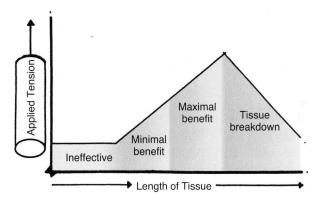

FIGURE 3–12 Length–tension curve depicting elastic and plastic behaviors of tissue.

applied forces. Old cells are phagocytosed and new cells are created, orienting themselves in the direction of the tension. Through remodeling, the length of the previously contracted tissue increases—termed ***elastic behavior***. On the other hand, tissue fibers that are stretched beyond their elastic limits will exhibit ***plastic behavior*** and tear or rupture. When the tissue and cells are injured in this manner, enzymatic proteins are released from the cells and more scarring can occur (Brand & Thompson, 1993) (Fig. 3–12).

Clinical Considerations

During the rehabilitation of injured tissue, the goal is gaining length of contracted tissue without causing further tissue damage, which results in inflammation, hemorrhage, and further scarring. This may occur with an overzealous stretching program or excessive force applied with an orthosis. Such tissues become reactive, stiff, and painful, possibly leading to problems such as a complex regional pain syndrome (CRPS), previously known as reflex sympathetic dystrophy (RSD). Brand and Thompson (1993) noted that if tissue is held stretched to its tolerable limit for a longer time, it has a greater chance of undergoing permanent remodeling and lengthening. When using mobilization orthoses, using a tolerable tension (lower stress) for a longer period of time is more beneficial than increasing the tension (high stress) for short periods of time (Brand & Thompson, 1993; Fess et al., 2005).

Conditions and Factors That Influence Tissue Healing

Tissue healing and remodeling are influenced by several factors, including the magnitude of soft tissue trauma, the extent of bony involvement, tissue contamination and infection, and vascular injury on both the venous and arterial sides. A stable skeletal platform is critical for healing; if one fails to achieve bony stability, soft tissue healing can be compromised. Revascularization allows the influx of

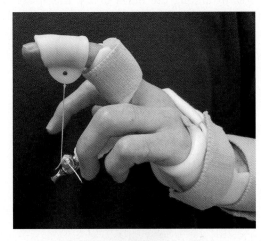

FIGURE 3–11 Middle finger PIP flexion mobilization orthosis used 8 weeks after a proximal phalanx fracture. A MERiT™ component provides the static progressive force. Note the extended outrigger on which the MERiT™ device rests. This allows for an accurate 90 degree angle of force application (Patterson Medical).

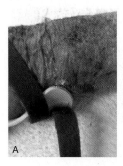
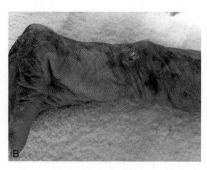

FIGURE 3–13 **A and B,** Skin breakdown at distal ulna from edge of orthosis rubbing against skin in this elderly patient.

macrophages to remove debris, and increased tissue oxygenation aids cellular proliferation. Rigid internal fixation is the gold standard to treat unstable fractures; this not only provides the best biomechanical construct to allow bony healing but also helps diminish the stresses on the soft tissue envelope. Plates or screws are most often utilized; Kirschner wires can also provide stability but not the same rigid mechanical construct. In the most extreme conditions, temporary or definitive treatment can be obtained through external fixation.

Some injuries include nerve damage that may lead to a loss of protective sensation. Once the orthosis is applied, the patient, family, medical staff, and therapist need to understand the importance of monitoring the extremity for possible skin irritation or breakdown caused by the orthosis (Fig. 3–13A,B). Often, patients cannot fully appreciate the orthosis' contact with the skin, and pressure areas can develop. Any redness, erythema, or potential for skin breakdown needs to be immediately addressed to avoid frank ulceration. For patients at risk, the orthosis should be of lighter weight, incorporate protective padding, or are made with soft-lined materials to aid in protecting the at-risk tissue. Edges need to be smoothed and sharp or jagged borders avoided. Wide, soft, and strategically placed straps may aid in minimizing shear and compression stresses along the orthosis–skin interface and is of particular importance when applying an orthosis to an individual with vascular insufficiency.

Age

Age strongly influences the healing process. The younger the patient, the more likely the tissue(s) involved will heal quickly and without complications. In general, younger patients wear orthoses and casts for shorter periods of time, and ROM is initiated earlier than for older patients. Stotts and Wipke-Tevis (1997) noted, "fetal wound healing is virtually scarless." Comorbidities also increase with age. Diabetes, vascular insufficiency, steroid use, and associated peripheral neuropathies increase with age and are associated with a poorer prognosis.

Lifestyle Factors

Nutrition

Dietary factors have a profound effect on wound healing. On the most simplistic level, a diet with an appropriate balance of fat, proteins, and carbohydrates are essential. Caloric requirements are dramatically elevated after trauma; however, with massive trauma, often, a patient's ability to eat may be compromised. Parenteral nutrition can help if the gastrointestinal tract is poorly functioning. Measuring serum albumin levels can help guide a patient's nutritional status while high caloric supplements are often necessary. A deficient diet may contribute to weight loss, an increased risk of infection, and poor wound healing (Pinchocofsky-Devin, 1997). In thin patients or those with minimal subcutaneous fat, consider using soft prefabricated orthoses or orthotic materials made of neoprene; straps should be placed away from bony prominences, especially in cachectic or malnourished individuals.

Tobacco Use

Nicotine is a vasoconstrictor and restricts blood flow to the skin, thereby creating low oxygen levels and markedly diminishes the body's ability to heal. Nicotine, carbon monoxide, and hydrogen cyanide are inhaled with each puff and clearly cause delayed wound healing (Jenson, 1991; Silverstein, 1992; Smith & Feske, 1996). At the microvascular level, nicotine results in increased blood viscosity and platelet aggregation. At the bone marrow level, nicotine decreases the formation of red blood cells, fibroblasts, and macrophages (the cellular elements required to repair wounds). Carbon monoxide, the inhaled by-product of smoking, has 300 times the affinity for hemoglobin than does oxygen. When it binds with hemoglobin, oxygen transport is decreased and thus there is less oxygen within the tissues. This leads directly to slower wound healing; for many reasons notwithstanding the index injury, therapists should review with each patient the effects of continued nicotine use on healing rates (Fig. 3–14).

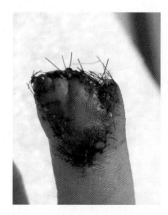

FIGURE 3–14 Necrotic flap noted in patient who is a heavy smoker.

Alcohol Use

Excessive alcohol intake can also impair the immune system, lead to malnourishment, and cause liver damage (Rund, 1997). Malnutrition is common in alcoholics: albumin and protein levels are diminished, and the bodies' reserves to heal are severely impaired. Delirium tremens, commonly known as "DTs," can occur with abrupt alcohol withdrawal. Orthoses need to be protective and carefully placed, especially if restraints are required in an inpatient setting. As with tobacco use, patient education is paramount.

Medical Conditions

Connective tissue disorders and systemic diseases not only have a generalized effect on the body but also may be associated with impaired tissue oxygenation, which can delay local tissue healing (LeRoy, 1996). With any of the medical conditions mentioned in this chapter, orthotic intervention should be only one aspect of the medical and therapeutic intervention. When an orthosis is fabricated for a patient who has a medical condition that affects tissue healing, vascular compromise, or impaired sensation, both the therapist and the patient should inspect the skin frequently. The therapist should adjust the orthosis and modify the straps as soon as any signs of redness or irritation occur. Affected patients may not perceive the discomfort of the orthosis on the body part owing to nerve and/or vascular involvement.

Buerger's Disease

Buerger's disease, thromboangiitis obliterans, is characterized by progressive inflammation and thrombosis of small and medium arteries and veins of the hands and feet associated with tobacco smoking. Affected individuals frequently have nonhealing ulcerations; arterial and venous occlusion may occur. Cessation of smoking is paramount, although many patients with Buerger's are highly addicted. Initially, nonhealing ulcers occur; subsequently, gangrene is unfortunately common. If vascular problems persist, these individuals may have to undergo amputation later in the course of the disease.

Raynaud's

Raynaud's is a condition caused by spasticity or occlusion of the digital arteries, with blanching and numbness in the digits (Fig. 3–15) (LeRoy, 1996). Three different conditions exist, Raynaud's syndrome, Raynaud's disease, and Raynaud's phenomenon. Raynaud's syndrome is *secondary* to immune-mediated inflammatory arthritis or an autoimmune connective tissue disease. Raynaud's disease is the name given when the findings are not associated with either condition. Finally, the term Raynaud's phenomenon is used when the cause is unknown. Initially, patients report cold sensitivity, sometimes from simple exposure such as reaching for food in a freezer. In advanced stages, the skin may become firm, thickened, and leathery. Flexion contractures can develop because the skin becomes tightly bound to the underlying subcutaneous tissue. Cold temperatures and autoimmune

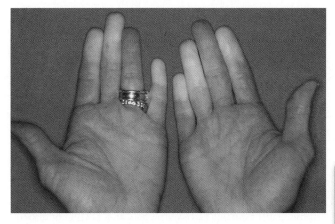

FIGURE 3–15 Note the blanching of the digits because of Raynaud's syndrome, a vasospastic disorder triggered by cold temperatures.

diseases are among the many factors that precipitate the onset of symptoms. Orthotic materials that are soft, flexible, and contribute to retaining warmth (e.g., neoprene) may be a sensible option for these patients.

Systemic Lupus Erythematosus

Systemic lupus erythematosus (SLE) is an autoimmune disease that can affect any major organ and occurs more predominantly in women, with a variable course of symptomatology (LeRoy, 1996). As with other autoimmune diseases, the body's own immune system attacks the body's normal cells and tissue, resulting in inflammation and tissue damage. The course of the disease is unpredictable, but musculoskeletal manifestations are common, specifically affecting joints and skin. The disease can wax and wane with periodic "flares" of illness balanced with periods of remission. Not only is the disease itself pertinent to this discussion but also treatment. Corticosteroids, immunosuppressants, and medications commonly used in the treatment of cancer are often used in lupus patients. These medications significantly retard the function of the immune system and interfere with healing.

Diabetes

Patients with diabetes may be one of the most difficult groups of patients to treat and apply orthoses. Patients are typically subclassified as insulin-dependent diabetes mellitus (IDDM) and non–insulin-dependent diabetes mellitus (NIDDM). The former have a much more severe form of the disease and, consequently, greater difficulty with wound healing (Davidson, 1999). Peripheral neuropathy is also more common, leading to a loss of protective sensation. Retarded wound healing occurs based on tissue ischemia and neuropathy. Glucose control is critical; individuals with poor blood sugar control, commonly known as "brittle diabetics," are at greater risk of complications. Diabetic neuropathy demands attention to the details of orthotic fabrication. Patients may lack protective sensation; orthotic pressure may, therefore, cause unnoticed skin injury (Fig. 3–16). It is important

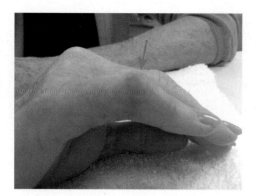

FIGURE 3–16 Reddened area over PIP joint caused by pressure from orthosis. Patient did not perceive this sore area because of diabetic neuropathy and did not inspect the skin as instructed. If the orthosis was not modified, this could have resulted skin breakdown.

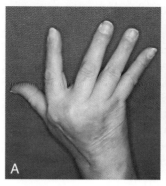 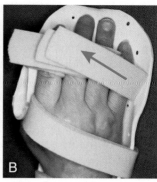

FIGURE 3–17 A, RA with ulnar deviation deformity at MCP joints. **B,** A night wrist and digit immobilization orthosis maintains the MCP joints in a neutral position and supports the wrist and thumb.

that the patient and therapist perform frequent, regular inspection of the area for early signs of pressure and redness.

Rheumatoid Arthritis

Rheumatoid arthritis (RA) is a systemic immunologic disorder primarily affecting synovial tissue, although most major organ systems can be directly or indirectly affected. Synovial tissue commonly surrounds joints and tendons and, in the normal situation, aids in tissue nutrition, oxygenation, and lubrication. In RA, the autoimmune response causes synovial proliferation producing excess fluid and the fibrous tissue hyperplasia can form "pannus." Destructive enzymes produced by the hypertrophic synovium can be destructive to the articular cartilage, ligaments, and joint. Because of the high incidence of small joint involvement, orthotic fabrication of the hands and wrists are common. Orthoses have an important role not only during a period of exacerbation to protect inflamed painful joints but also have, in the long term, to prevent further joint deformity (Fig. 3–17A,B).

Pharmacologic treatment often involves medications that retard healing; corticosteroids, for instance, inhibit the normal development of tensile strength in a healing wound and should be taken into account when formulating a treatment plan. Corticosteroids also inhibit the natural inflammatory response and patients are at higher risk of infection. When possible, thin, lightweight, soft, and flexible materials should be used to fabricate orthoses. Many patients have fragile skin and require additional protection at the orthosis–skin interface. Refer to Chapter 17 on *Arthritis* for further information.

Sickle Cell Disease

Sickle cell disease is a group of inherited blood diseases that can cause severe pain, damage to vital organs, and occasionally death in childhood or early adulthood (Sickle Cell Disease Research Foundation, 1999). The geometrically deformed red blood cells cannot pass easily through the blood vessels, creating a sludging effect and preventing oxygen from reaching the tissues. This results in severe pain and damage to the organs; wound healing is also inhibited. Orthoses fabricated for these patients should be made with caution; straps and other materials should not compress tissue, which could further impede vascular flow.

Peripheral Vascular Disease

Patients with peripheral vascular disease (PVD) are at risk for impaired wound healing because of tissue hypoxia (Fig. 3–18A,B). Improvement in arterial circulation and/or venous drainage improves wound healing; therefore, any signs of orthotic compression should be addressed promptly. Orthosis straps should be applied firmly enough to secure the orthosis on the body part but not so tight that circulation is affected.

Medical Treatment and Complications

Radiation Therapy

Radiation therapy has a dramatic benefit in curing or controlling certain cancers but also can have damaging effect on previously healthy tissue. Vascular deterioration occurs, creating a hypoxic environment for the tissue; and the

FIGURE 3–18 A, Tissue breakdown and slow wound healing after open reduction internal and external fixation for metacarpal fracture in this patient with PVD. **B,** Wrist and ring/small finger immobilization orthosis with light gauze dressing covering open area.

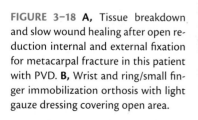 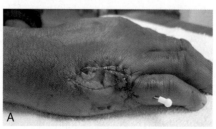

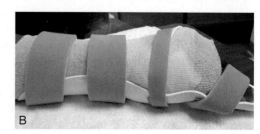

adverse consequence of radiation therapy may not become apparent until several years after treatment. Management of these wounds is difficult because of circulatory compromise. Orthoses and straps should be applied cautiously to these areas for the reasons described previously.

Steroids

Corticosteroid use can impair all phases of wound healing. Because these drugs slow the healing process, they increase the risk of infection; but the signs and symptoms may be masked by the suppressed inflammatory response (Stotts & Wipke-Tevis, 1997). Patients on chronic steroids often suffer from thinning of the skin, giving it a tissue paper–type appearance and are prone to skin tears and breakdown. Therapists need to evaluate potential areas of friction or pressure when applying orthoses to patients who are using steroid medications. Steroids, like tobacco and alcohol, slow the healing process and increase the risk of skin breakdown. Daily skin inspection and timely orthotic modification can accommodate the risks associated with steroid use.

Edema

Tissue **edema** is the physiologic response to injury often resulting from tissue congestion, diminished venous drainage, and decreased capillary blood flow (Fig. 3–19A,B). The increase of interstitial fluid may decrease oxygen diffusion to the tissues. Edema can result from the overly aggressive manipulation of healing tissue by manual techniques or orthotic fabrication methods; and, if occurring, the therapy protocol should be modified. Caution should be taken when applying a mobilization orthosis to a severely edematous part (Fess et al., 2005). Rest, by use of an immobilization orthosis along with edema management techniques/products, may be a better plan until the edema has subsided enough to allow for more aggressive techniques.

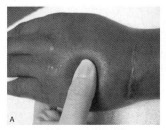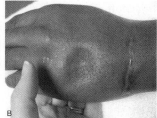

FIGURE 3–19 A and B, Pitting edema characterized by remaining indentation as shown.

Techniques to reduce edema before orthotic application include elevation, massage, compression garments (Isotoner® gloves), circumferential bandages (Ace™ or Coban™ wrapping), or therapeutic elasticized taping methods (Fig. 3–20A–C). These can be worn under orthoses, and straps can be modified to prevent window edema (swelling between straps) (Villeco, 2012). Circumferential dressings should be rewrapped periodically during the day to avoid specific areas of increased pressure and to allow progressive control of edematous tissue. However, too much compression may decrease arterial blood flow, thereby creating vascular compromise to the limb. Circulation should be monitored after and during the application of compression garments and circumferential bandages, and patients should be informed about the signs and symptoms of diminished arterial blood flow (e.g., dusky or blue nail beds; numbness, tingling, or coolness of skin). As edema diminishes, the orthosis will need to be remolded to ensure an adequate fit.

Edema itself can cause significant restriction in the ROM of the joint. Reactive, stiff, painful, edematous tissue does not permit motion; the therapeutic program must be modified to restore tissue homeostasis (Brand & Thompson, 1993). More rest and less movement of the injured part are usually appropriate, and any stress applied to the healing tissue by the orthosis should be monitored closely.

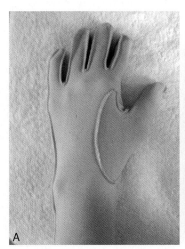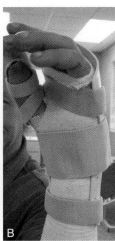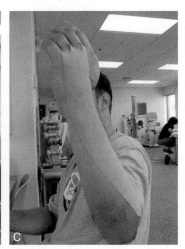

FIGURE 3–20 Edema management techniques including **(A)** compressive glove, **(B)** compression via circumferential wrapping with Coban™ for the thumb and elasticized stockinette, and **(C)** use of Kinesio® Tex Tape for edema control.

Infection

Infections involve the invasion of tissue by microorganisms: viruses, bacteria, fungi, or atypical organisms (Thompson & Taddonio, 1997). Infection increases oxygen demand and decreases oxygen delivery to tissues secondary to edema and collagen breakdown. These changes prolong and accelerate the inflammatory phase of wound healing. Common signs of infection include erythema, purulence, and wound drainage but also may include wound discoloration, friable granulation tissue, pain or tenderness out of proportion, and delayed wound healing. Infected tissue interferes with the normal cascade of wound healing, and immobilization through orthotic application helps diminish motion that consequently aids in the body's natural ability to treat the infection. Orthoses should be carefully applied to allow access and free drainage of open areas as well as ease of application and removal to facilitate wound care. Consider using perforated thermoplastic materials to increase air exchange under orthoses that have dressings.

Vacuum-Assisted Wound Closure

A great advance in the treatment of open wounds is commonly referred to as "wound vac treatment" (Von Der Heyde & Evans, 2011; Webb, 2002). Once surgically debrided, a specially designed sponge is contoured to cover the open area; sealed with an impervious cover; and finally, negative pressure is applied through a closed system. With suction applied, exudates, serous fluid, and edema are removed from the wound, facilitating wound granulation and reepithelialization. Wounds previously requiring rotational flaps, free flaps, and skin grafting can often be treated without further surgery as healing occurs through secondary intention. Appropriately placed orthoses help protect the injured area, facilitating drainage and allowing the growth of healthy granulation tissue. Orthoses should protect the extremity and avoid kinking of the suction apparatus.

Orthotic Application for Specific Tissues

For the therapist and surgeon to treat the condition and to correct it, they must understand the integrity of the anatomical structures: the articular surfaces, bones, ligaments, capsules, tendons, nerves, vessels, skin, and subcutaneous tissues. The type of orthotic application (static, serial static, static progressive, or dynamic), the technical considerations for designing the orthosis, and the pattern used depend on the specifics of the tissue pathology (Strickland, 1987, 2000).

Skin

Wounds heal by either primary or secondary intention. With **primary closure**, wound healing occurs when wound edges are anatomically aligned and held by suture, "steri-strips,"

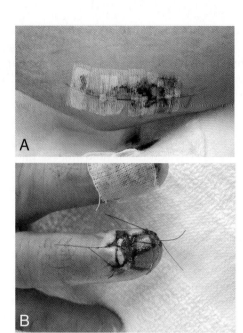
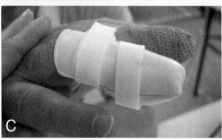
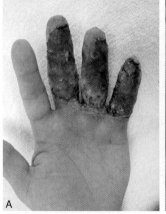

FIGURE 3–21 A, Skin closure using running suture and steri-strips post ulnar nerve release at the elbow. **B and C,** Sutured nail bed repair and protective orthosis.

or skin glue (Fig. 3–21A–C). With adequate approximation, collagen synthesis binds the edges together, accelerating the healing curve.

Healing by secondary intention refers to the process of a wound closing from the inside out (Fig. 3–22A,B). The wound

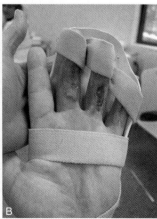

FIGURE 3–22 A and B, Burn injury healing by secondary intention, with orthosis keeping gentle extension positioning during collagen formation.

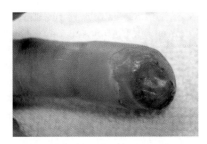

FIGURE 3–23 Partial fingertip amputation healing by secondary intention may result in less sensory deficits versus surgical repair.

base fills with granulation tissue and then covered with epithelial cells. As this occurs, the wound edges are gradually drawn centripetally until closure has been achieved. This method may be chosen if the wound is contaminated or infected and when there may be inadequate skin coverage. Wound healing by secondary intention is often advantageous as in partial, superficial fingertip amputations (Fig. 3–23). Wounds less than 1 cm^2 can often be treated with this technique; it avoids the general risks associated with surgery as well as donor site morbidity from harvesting skin grafts. In the author's experience, it allows better reinnervation and return of sensation and, often, a better cosmetic appearance. Secondary wound healing was used by McCash (1964) in his so-called open palm technique of Dupuytren's fasciectomy and has seen resurgence in utilization (Fig. 3–2). A transverse palmar incision is made to debride the pathologic palmar fascia and is then left open at the conclusion of surgery. This diminishes the risk of hematoma formation, seroma, and obviates the need for skin grafting or undo tension on the surgical wound.

Skin grafts and flaps demand specific dressing and orthotic application measures to ensure their survival (Levin, 2011) (Fig. 3–24A–E). A partial- or full-thickness skin graft obtains its nutrition initially by diffusion from the surrounding tissues. Vascularized granulation tissue enters the graft from its bed, and capillaries enter the sutured wound edges and allow its incorporation as living skin. The incorporation of grafts depends on the health of the granulation bed, the host's nutritional and metabolic status, comorbidities, and age and takes approximately 2 weeks during which time the graft must be held close to the underlying bed. Surgically placed stents, dressings, and orthoses should minimize motion at the graft site to facilitate incorporation. Generally speaking, the orthosis should only rigidly immobilize the grafted area; adjacent joints should be unencumbered and free to move to prevent adjacent joint stiffness and arthrofibrosis. For example, a skin graft

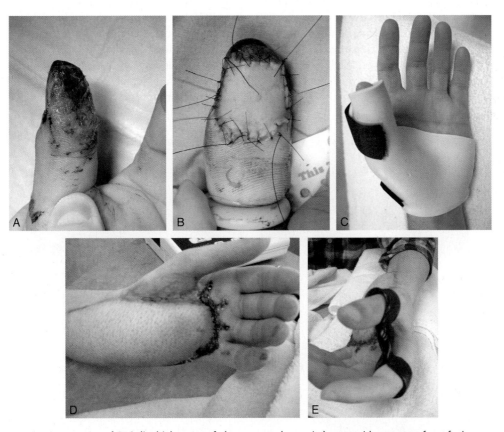

FIGURE 3–24 **A and B,** Split-thickness graft (upper arm donor site) to provide coverage for soft tissue loss at thumb. **C,** Protective thumb immobilization orthosis to protect graft from external forces. **D,** Flap coverage in distal forearm/palm following extensive burn injury. **E,** Thumb CMC immobilization orthosis to prevent first web space contracture: this unique design prevents need for any contact on healing flap.

used for a Dupuytren's fasciectomy should be immobilized to facilitate revascularization of the graft, but the adjacent joints released as part of the surgery should be free and mobilized to obtain the desired surgical and therapeutic result.

Skin and soft tissue flaps require specific attention to their pedicles, the source of arterial inflow and venous outflow. The pedicle must not be compromised, compressed, or kinked by the position of the operated site in the orthosis or by the straps.

Tendon

Tendon healing occurs because of intrinsic and extrinsic contributions (Gelberman, Khabie, & Cahill, 1991; Lundborg, 1976; Lundborg, Holm, & Myrhage, 1980; Lundborg & Rank, 1980). Intrinsic healing, which depends on cells bridging the injury site directly, relies on vincular blood flow; blood flow from the proximal synovial fold in the palm and the bone insertion distally; and diffusion of synovial fluid (and the nutrients it contains) (Fig. 3–25A–C). At one point in time, it was believed that flexor tendon healing occurred via extrinsic fibroblast ingrowth and thus required rigid immobilization. The consequence was dense adhesions between the tendon and fibroosseous canal. Lundborg (1976) has shown that flexor tendon healing occurs intrinsically via the intratendinous vascular arcade. Although tenosynovial fluid undoubtedly provides an anatomically conducive milieu, fibroblastic ingrowth from the tendon sheath is counterproductive to the desired end result: a strong tendon junction free of external adhesions. Adhesions cause scar at the site of tendon injury; if the adhesions are too thick or inelastic, they restrict tendon gliding and often require further surgeries such as a tenolysis (Wang, 1998).

The stages of tendon healing are the same as for other wounds—inflammatory, fibroplastic, and remodeling—and the timing is also similar to that described previously. However, the critical need to restore tendon gliding, to regain active digital motion, and the nature of the healing present challenges to the surgeon and therapist. The surgeon must create a repair that has maximum strength, permits early motion, and minimizes bulk at the repair site to ease gliding. The therapist must then initiate an early ROM program to establish gliding of the tendon in its fibroosseous canal. The orthosis must facilitate exercise but limit stress on the repair (Wang, 1998) (Fig. 3–26A–D). Tendons that are mobilized soon after repair heal with fewer and less restrictive adhesions, achieve greater tensile strength sooner, and establish better gliding than immobilized tendons. Multiple clinical studies reflect this favorable biology of healing and are beyond the context of this chapter.

The precise rehabilitation program depends on the surgeon's and therapist's experience, the nature of the injury, technical factors of the tendon repair (integrity of repair, suture strength), and presence of associated injuries. Current trends favor a modified Duran (early passive mobilization), Kleinert-type program with rubber band-type traction (early passive mobilization), or, most currently, an early active mobilization protocol including place hold exercises (Duran, Houser, Coleman, & Stover, 1978; Evans, 2012; Lister, Kleinert, Kutz, & Atasoy, 1977; Pettengill, 2005; Trumble, 2010). In all situations, the custom-fabricated orthosis should protect the repair, with slight wrist and MP joint flexion. The Kleinert protocol can be more labor intensive to make and requires a very precise orthosis that adequately protects the repair with biomechanically appropriately placed bands and pulleys. Common to all

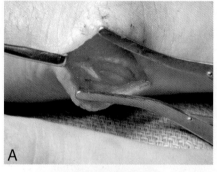

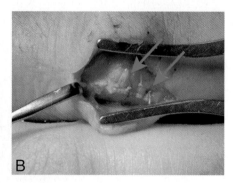

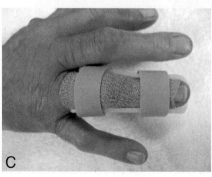

FIGURE 3–25 **A and B,** Repair of extensor mechanism at lateral PIP joint. **C,** Digit immobilization orthosis initial weeks of rehabilitation.

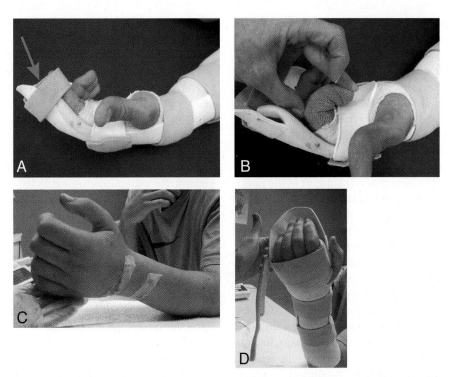

FIGURE 3–26 A and B, Index finger flexor tendon repair with wrist/hand immobilization orthosis in place. Note use of Coban™ for edema and thermoplastic palmar strap (verses a loop strap) to better maintain position of hand in orthosis. Additional piece of thermoplastic added dorsal and distal to MCP joint to allow digit strap to impart gentle extension stretch at PIP joint, which was developing a flexion contracture. **C and D,** Extensor tendon repair at wrist level and wrist/hand immobilization orthosis with removable hand segment to allow IP joint motion for exercise.

protocols though, is the focus on reestablishing early tendon gliding. Significant advances in tendon surgery have occurred in the last decade. Traditionally, a two-strand core suture was used; current trends and research uses four-, six-, and eight-strand repairs. The greater number of strands across the repair site helps increase the initial strength of the repair to allow the therapists to institute active tendon protocols at an earlier stage. The dilemma is how many core strands is optimal. When one is striving for strength, a greater number of sutures of greater suture caliber is favored. However, the negative consequence is first, the more strands crossing the repair site diminishes the cross-sectional area of actual tendon available for healing. Second, theoretically, more foreign body can cause more peritendinous scar tissue, greater adhesions, and poorer gliding. Finally, advances have been made in the epitendinous sutures regarding suture technique—for example, locking. The epitendinous sutures have two significant purposes: first, it helps "tidy" the repaired tendon to minimize bulk and aid gliding; and second, despite the small caliber of suture used, it does provide significant increased strength to the repair. The pulley system is an important component when addressing a flexor tendon injury. Doyle and Blythe (1977) demonstrated the critical importance of the A2 and A4 pulleys; but, when possible, all pulleys should be preserved and surgically induced trauma minimized. When possible, the pulleys should be left in situ; however, current

surgical techniques emphasize pulley maintenance, venting, repair, or reconstruction when necessary. Refer to Chapter 18 on "Tendon Injuries" for further information.

Periarticular Soft Tissue

Joint stiffness results either from direct injury to the articular surfaces, capsule, and ligament apparatus; or secondarily from edema, scar formation, and contracture affecting the soft tissues around the joint and its associated muscle–tendon units. Anatomical restoration of joint congruity and soft tissue support and the elimination of edema help prevent such joint stiffness. Several questions must be addressed to achieve successful treatment of a stiff joint. First, what was the extent of traumatic damage to the joint and how well was it restored? Simple articular fractures, especially in younger individuals, often involves a minimally or noncomminuted injury through the joint. In contrast, the elderly may have significant comminution with multiple small fragments often too small to reconstruct requiring removal. How was the fracture addressed? How well was the articular surface restored? Was a small amount of displacement accepted and treated nonoperatively? If it required operative treatment, was it done open or closed? With closed reduction techniques, additional soft tissue damage is lessened. However, anatomical restoration is paramount; open treatment usually requires a surgical incision (and subsequent scar) around the tendon, ligaments, and joint capsule. Finally, was rigid internal fixation applied? Screw or plate fixation generally holds the reduction better; but not only the implants but also the soft tissue dissection can lead to more scar formation. When open reduction internal fixation (ORIF) techniques are used, the goal is to obtain rigid stability to allow a more aggressive postoperative rehabilitation protocol. However, in some situations, fragment size or fracture pattern is not conducive and K-wires or sutures may be used but do not have the same mechanical stability. How much damage occurred to the soft tissue support of the joint, specifically ligaments, capsule, and for the PIP joint, the volar plate? If the trauma disrupted any or all of these structures, were they allowed to heal with closed treatment or, if operated, were they surgically released to treat the fracture and/or were they repairable at closure? What was the extent of the trauma and the extent of surgical treatment to the supporting musculotendinous units? The early response of the soft tissue will often predict the tissue's and patients' response to treatment. The patients' affect is also an important determining factor in how aggressive the team can be with therapy. Recurrent inflammation may demand a less aggressive approach, whereas a more rapid improvement in the clinical situation may necessitate a change in the precise configuration of the orthosis. As edema changes, as motion improves, and as radiographs delineate progressive healing, orthoses might require frequent modifications to accommodate changes in status. In certain instances, a contracted ligament will lengthen just so much; further increases in joint motion may be the result of a hinge-open effect rather than to concentric articular gliding (Brand & Thompson, 1993; Strickland, 1987, 2000).

Commonly encountered contractures include elbow flexion, wrist flexion, MCP joint extension, PIP joint flexion, and thumb adduction. Such contractures may be the result of direct joint trauma (e.g., intra-articular fractures), periarticular crushing, sprains, articular surface contusions (e.g., jammed finger), and other injuries. However, contractures may also occur secondarily from edema, improper positioning, and subsequent soft tissue contracture that follow injury elsewhere in the upper extremity. These and other contractures may respond to a therapy program that includes edema control, exercise, and application of a mobilization orthosis (usually dynamic, static progressive, or serial static) (McKee, Hannah, & Prignac, 2012) (Fig. 3–27A–C). Occasionally, in the multiple traumatized patient, the extremities are neglected while the major organ system damage is addressed. Education is important with other health-care providers that early application of orthoses in a trauma patient can minimize contractures and aid in minimizing the need for future rehabilitation intervention. When a contracture is severe and unresponsive to therapy and orthotic application, surgical release is sometimes required, after which a resumption of therapy, with orthoses, is indicated (Slade & Chou, 1998). Refer to Chapter 15 on "Managing Stiffness of the Hand" for further information.

Bone and Cartilage

Fracture healing follows the same sequence as the healing of other tissues (Fig. 3–28). Inflammation, edema, and hemorrhage occur at the time of injury. The fibroplastic stage is characterized cellularly by migration of both scavenger osteoclasts and healing osteoprogenitor cells from their endosteal and periosteal origins adjacent to the fracture site. The initial inflammatory response is critical to the healing cascade; anti-inflammatories have been shown in spine fusion models to interfere with bony healing and fusion rates and consequently should be avoided. The collagen matrix deposited by osteoblasts eventually calcifies. The

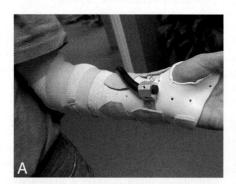

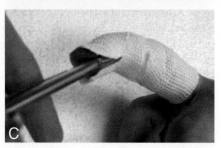

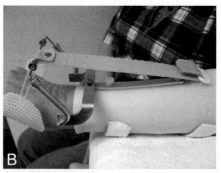

FIGURE 3–27 Types of mobilization orthoses: **(A)** dynamic forearm supination (Rolyan® Dynamic Pronation/Supination Kit), **(B)** static progressive wrist extension (Phoenix Wrist Hinge), and **(C)** serial static PIP extension (QuickCast 2) (All products available through Patterson Medical).

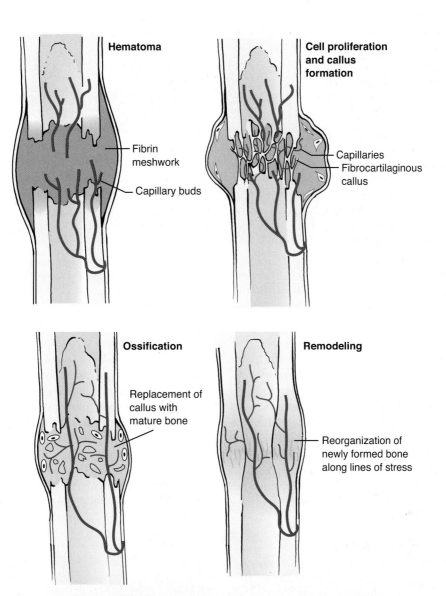

FIGURE 3–28 The stages of bone healing. The hematoma stage provides the fibrin meshwork and capillary buds needed for subsequent cellular invasion. Cellular proliferation and callus formation represent the stages during which osteoblasts enter the area and form the fibrocartilaginous callus that joins the bone fragments. The ossification stage involves the mineralization of the fibrocartilaginous callus, and the remodeling stage involves the reorganization of mineralized bone along the lines of mechanical stress. Borrowed with permission from Porth, C. M. (2005). *Pathophysiology concepts of altered health states* (7th ed.). Philadelphia, PA: Lippincott Williams & Wilkins.

developing callus remodels during the scar maturation stage and responds to the controlled application of stress. As bone healing progresses, the requirements of external immobilization change. In nonsurgically treated fractures, casts, and subsequently, orthoses protect the bone to allow osseous consolidation (Fig. 3–29A–D). As healing progresses, it is important to allow stress and/or joint mobility, so orthoses should be lessened during callous maturation and remodeling (Slade & Chou, 1998). Orthoses are usually less bulky and can be contoured more precisely than casts. Their use with fractures permits earlier and more complete mobilization of nearby joints. This can lessen fracture site, distal limb,

and digit edema with its concomitant fibrosis, ligament and capsular contracture, and tendon adherence. Refer to Chapter 16 on "Fractures" for further information.

Nerve

Nerve injury results in degeneration of the axon and the myelin sheath distal to the wound and for a short distance proximally (Wallerian degeneration) (Fig. 3–30A–E). During the inflammatory stage of nerve healing, macrophages clear the cellular debris. Subsequently, axonal buds migrate proximally through the endoneural tube, and Schwann cells

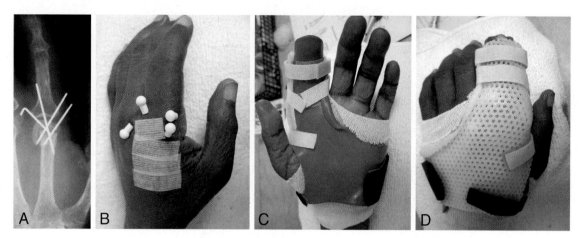

FIGURE 3–29 A and B, Metacarpal fracture with closed reduction and external pinning. **C and D,** Hand-based index finger immobilization orthosis with dorsal clamshell segment for protection of protruding pins. Perforated dorsal material chosen to allow air exchange.

envelop the axon in a new myelin sheath as the stage of fibroplasia progresses.

During the fibroplastic stage, protection of the nerve repair against tensile forces is crucial. The surgeon must observe intraoperatively the effect of movement of nearby joints on tension at the site of the repair because this will guide the early postoperative rehabilitation program of the nearby joints. If only a nerve repair was performed, the area was immobilized 3 to 4 weeks; however, Chao et al. (2001) demonstrated that without undue tension on the repair site, nerves can be mobilized earlier in conjunction with tendon repair protocols. Advances in nerve grafting techniques have provided alternatives to a nerve repair under tension. Biocompatible collagen tubes are available in various lengths and diameters and are useful in cases of segmental nerve loss. The conduits provide a biologically conducive milieu for axonal regeneration. Occasionally, autogenous nerve grafts taken from the sural, posterior, interosseous, or antebrachial cutaneous nerve or nerve allografts are also available. A study by Evans, Bain, Mackinnon, Makino, and Hunter (1991) suggested that actually leaving a 5-mm gap between nerve ends can aid in the correct realignment of motor and sensory nerve fibers in mixed nerve repairs. Refer to Chapter 19 on "Peripheral Nerve Injuries" for further information.

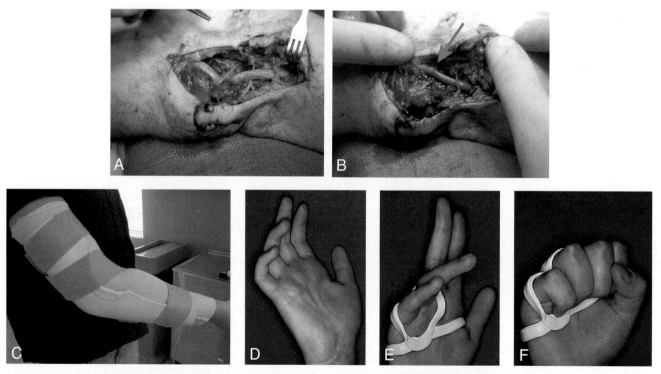

FIGURE 3–30 A and B, Ulnar nerve laceration and repair at level of the elbow. **C,** Postoperative positioning in an elbow immobilization orthosis. **D and E,** Distal orthosis used once claw deformity became evident, allowing full functional flexion and extension via the long extensors (radial nerve innervated).

Conclusion

Knowledge of the sequence of events of tissue healing is critical for understanding how and when to intervene—both surgically and conservatively. The selection of a particular treatment program by the surgeon and therapist, including the timely use of specific orthoses, is determined by the nature of the injury and its repair, the techniques used in treatment, the stage of tissue healing, factors that may influence the healing process, and the response of the tissues to previous therapeutic measures.

Chapter Review Questions

1. What are the three stages of tissue healing?

2. Describe the importance of the antideformity position.

3. Should a patient be placed immediately into a digit mobilization orthosis 2 days after wrist fracture repair if he or she presents with swollen and stiff fingers? Why or why not?

4. What factors may negatively influence a patient's ability to heal?

5. What precautions should be stressed when dispensing an orthosis for a patient with diabetes and rheumatoid arthritis?

4 Mechanical Principles

Gary P. Austin, PT, PhD
MaryLynn Jacobs, MS, OTR/L, CHT

Chapter Objectives

After study of this chapter, the reader should be able to:
- Understand the basic terminology of mechanics related to the application of an orthosis on the upper extremity.
- Appreciate the various types of force and stress that relate to orthotic fabrication.
- Describe the three lever systems and the term "mechanical advantage" as it relates to the design and fit of an orthosis.
- Be able to determine which type of force delivery is best for a given outcome.
- Evaluate the proper fit and function of an immobilization and a mobilization orthosis.

Key Terms

Angle of application	High-profile designs	Rotational force
Axis of rotation	Hysteresis	Second-class lever
Bending	Levers	Shear stress
Compression	Linear force	Stress
Creep	Low-profile designs	Tensile stress
Effort arm	Magnitude	Third-class lever
Elastic force	Mechanical advantage	Torque
First-class lever	Moment of force	Torsion
Friction force	Pressure	Translational Force
Fulcrum	Resistance arm	

Introduction

Orthotic intervention is the intentional application of external loads to specific anatomical structures to manipulate the internal reaction forces and thus enhance or restore function of the extremity. Mechanics is the science that addresses the effects of forces on structures. Ideally, the effective therapist integrates basic mechanical concepts into all facets of design and fabrication of an orthosis.

A potential barrier to understanding and incorporating these concepts is the confusing mechanical terminology. Therefore, the purposes of this chapter are twofold: to define the fundamental mechanical terms and concepts pertinent to the design and fabrication of an orthosis and to discuss the clinical relevance and application of these basic principles using specific examples.

Force

As clinicians and students interested in the therapeutic application of force, it is essential that the concept of force be clearly defined. Force is an action or influence that either arrests, produces, or changes the direction of motion (LeVeau, 1992). A force can be sufficiently described using the following parameters:

- Nature: the type or kind of force (e.g., push or pull)
- **Magnitude**: the amount or quantity of influence present
- Line or angle of application: the path or direction along which the force acts
- Point of application: the location on the structure at which the line of force acts

An unbalanced force with a point of application other than the center of the object results in the rotation of an object around a fixed axis. Such a force is referred to as a **moment of force**, or **torque**. An example of torque is pulling down on a lever to open a door (Fig. 4–1A). A force with a point of application directly through the center of the object results in the translation of an object along a straight or curvilinear path. This is referred to as **linear force**. An example of linear force is the act of pushing a box along a floor (Fig. 4–1B). Although it may appear that **rotational force** should be the principal focus when discussing orthotic intervention, in fact, most motions incorporate both rotational and **translational** components.

As will become evident, an orthosis is fundamentally the sum of translational and rotational forces acting on anatomical structures for a specific therapeutic purpose. Thus, the different applications of force and force systems must be appreciated. Although it might seem that two forces equal in magnitude would have the same therapeutic effect, this is rarely the case. Furthermore, therapists must understand that the system with the greater force does not always yield the greatest benefit.

There are different forms or types of force. The most pertinent forces for the design and fabrication of orthoses are torque (moment of force), elastic force, and friction force.

Torque

The vast majority of articulations in the human body consist of segments or levers assembled around an **axis of rotation**, that is, the proximal and distal segments rotate around a joint axis. By virtue of this structure, the point of application of force is at a distance from the joint axis, producing joint motion that is rotational in nature. Rotational motion is produced, changed, or prevented by force applied in the form of torque. Torque, or the moment of force, is the potential for a force to produce the rotation of a lever around an axis.

The magnitude of torque is a function of two components: the magnitude of applied force and the perpendicular distance from the axis of rotation to the point of application of the force, otherwise known as the moment arm. More specifically,

$$\tau = F \times d$$

where τ is torque, F is force, and d is the perpendicular distance from the axis of rotation to the point of application (Fig. 4–2A). It is important to note that the torque about an axis, or joint, can be modified by manipulating either the distance from the axis of rotation at which the force is applied (Fig. 4–2B) or the quantity of the applied force (Fig. 4–2C). Increases in the force and/or distance produce increases in torque; in other words, torque is directly proportional to both force and distance.

Lever Systems and Mechanical Advantage

For orthoses, torque is commonly applied to a joint via leverage. **Levers** are rigid structures through which a force can be applied to produce rotational motion about a fixed axis. A lever system is composed of a **fulcrum**, or fixed axis, and two arms: the **effort arm** (EA) and the **resistance arm** (RA). The effort arm, also referred to as the force arm, is the segment of the lever between the fulcrum and the effort force (EF) that is attempting to stabilize or mobilize a structure. With respect to orthotic fabrication, the fulcrum typically coincides with the anatomical axis of the target joint, the effort arm is the segment of the orthosis that applies the effort force, and the resistance arm is the segment of the limb that resists the effort force. The effort force and resistance force (RF), in acting about a fixed axis, create opposing torques about the fulcrum (Fig. 4–3).

The components of the lever system can be arranged to create different types, or classes, of levers, each with a characteristic mechanical advantage or efficiency. The **mechanical advantage** (MA) of a lever system is defined by the relation

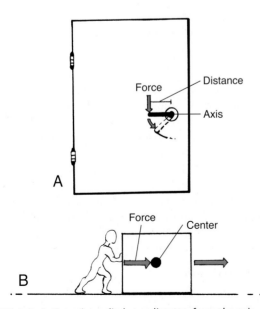

FIGURE 4–1 **A,** Force is applied at a distance from the axis, causing a rotation of the lever. **B,** Linear force is applied directly through the center of the box, causing a translation across the surface.

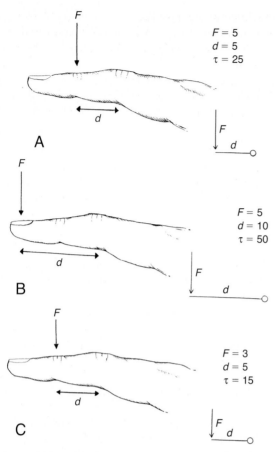

FIGURE 4–2 The torque (τ), or moment of force, can be affected by changes in either the distance (d) from the axis of rotation at which the force (F) is applied or the magnitude of the force applied. **A,** F = 5, d = 5, τ = 25. **B,** F = 5, d = 10, τ = 50. **C,** F = 3, d = 5, τ = 15.

between the length of the effort arm and the length of the resistance arm:

$$MA = EA/RA$$

Thus, there are three possible relations and three classes of lever systems (Fig. 4–4A–C). Examples of a **first-class lever** system are a seesaw, a pair of scissors, pliers, and a crowbar. Because the fulcrum is between the effort and the resistance

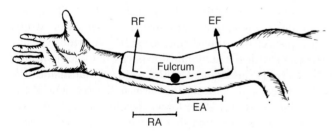

FIGURE 4–3 In this anterior elbow immobilization orthosis, the effort arm (*EA*) is the proximal segment of the orthosis, which applies the effort force (*EF*); the resistance arm (*RA*) is the distal segment of the limb, which applies the resistance force (*RF*). These forces, acting about the elbow joint axis, create opposing torques.

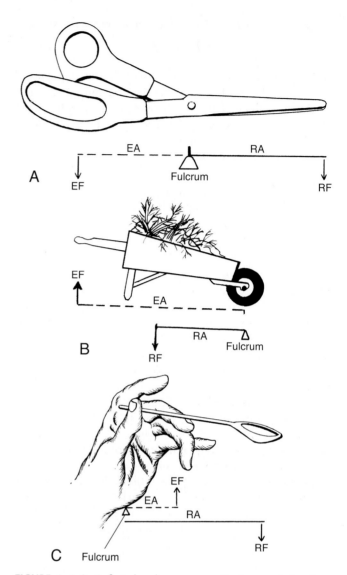

FIGURE 4–4 **A,** A first-class lever system. **B,** A second-class lever system. **C,** A third-class lever system.

arms, the mechanical advantage can be greater than, less than, or equal to 1. Common **second-class lever** systems include the wheelbarrow and the nutcracker. In each of these, the mechanical advantage is greater than 1 because the resistance is between the effort force and the fulcrum. Examples of **third-class lever** systems are a spoon, a fork, tweezers, a shovel, and a fishing rod. In this case, the effort force is applied between the fulcrum and the resistance force; because the effort arm is shorter than the resistance arm, the mechanical advantage is less than 1. Note that the majority of orthoses are first-class lever systems.

Clinical Considerations

The goal when designing an orthosis (i.e., a lever system) is to deliver the intended therapeutic stress to the target structure in the most efficient manner. The length of the resistance arm greatly influences the mechanical advantage

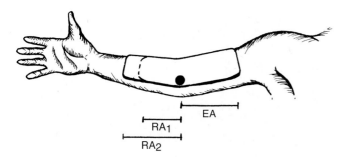

FIGURE 4–5 When the resistance arm (RA_2) is lengthened, less force is required to generate sufficient torque to prevent elbow joint movement. When the resistance arm (RA_1) is shortened, greater force is required to immobilize the elbow joint.

of the applied force. The effort arm of the orthosis can also affect the mechanical advantage by the manner in which it is molded to the body part. Both the effort and the resistance arms should conform to the structures they contact and should incorporate adequate surface area for proper pressure distribution. The net effect of the forces acting on a joint or structure should result in an optimal therapeutic effect and minimal negative effects. If the opposing force (effort arm) is not properly distributed relative to the distal force (resistance arm), the orthosis may become uncomfortable and thus ineffective. Therapists can create mechanical advantages through meticulous orthosis fabrication techniques and the judicious application of basic mechanical principles.

- The longer the resistance arm, the less force required to generate sufficient torque (Fig. 4–5). And, conversely, the shorter the resistance arm, the more force required to produce sufficient torque.
- The effort arm is most comfortable when adequate length and depth are incorporated into the orthosis (Fig. 4–6A,B). A short, narrow, and shallow effort arm is likely to create excessive pressure and discomfort; a well-molded effort arm more effectively dissipates pressure.
- The greater the force generated through the resistance arm, the broader and longer the shape of the effort arm.

As a clinical example, consider fabricating an orthosis to mobilize a stiff proximal interphalangeal (PIP) joint in the direction of flexion. The effort arm (on the volar proximal phalanx) is fabricated in the direction of extension. If the surface contact area of the effort arm is not of adequate length, circumference, and/or contour, this may result in localized shear and compression stress and potential migration of the orthosis (shear and compression stress are discussed later in this chapter). When the proximal segment migrates or shifts, the resistance arm is not able to provide a perpendicular angle of pull to the PIP joint axis of rotation, causing the resistance arm to alter the sling's fit on the middle phalanx (Fig. 4–7A–C).

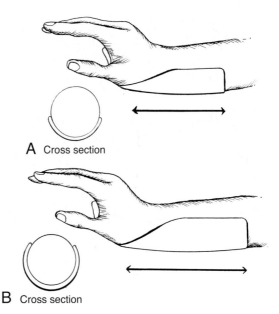

A Cross section

B Cross section

FIGURE 4–6 **A,** An orthosis with a short, narrow, and shallow effort arm is likely to cause discomfort from inadequate pressure distribution. **B,** An orthosis with a longer, broader, and deeper effort arm adequately distributes pressure and thus increases comfort. The depth of the orthosis should encompass two-thirds of the circumference of the body part, not only adding strength but also allowing for adequate placement of straps without the risk of compressing soft tissue.

Angle of Application

The **angle of application** of the moment of force or torque is critical to the proper design and fabrication of orthoses. Ideally, the force should be applied so that the angle of application is oriented 90° to the lever. This maximizes the therapeutic effect of the external force because the total force influencing the target segment acts in the intended direction. When the force is applied in a purely perpendicular orientation to the target segment, there are no forces in other directions (Fig. 4–8A–C). However, at an angle other than 90°, a portion of the force acting on the segment is applied in a direction other than the desired trajectory (either compression or tension), thereby effectively diminishing the perpendicular component and decreasing the therapeutic torque (Fig. 4–8D,E). Thus, when the angle of application is either greater or less than 90°, the beneficial effect of the application of torque cannot be optimized and potentially damaging compression and/or shear stress is applied.

Design Considerations

GENERAL

- To achieve a near 90° angle of application, use line guides and pulleys to aid in the orientation (Fig. 4–9A–E).
- To prevent undue torque or stress on the surrounding soft tissues, view the orthosis from all angles to ensure that the pull of the line is directed centrally over the digit or limb and oriented properly in all planes (Fig. 4–9B).

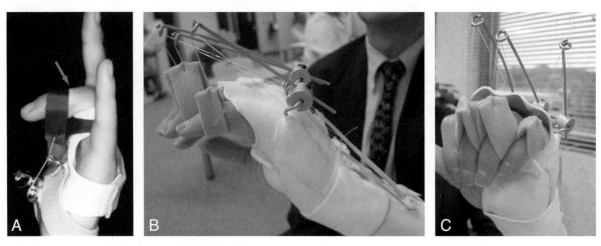

FIGURE 4–7 A, Shear stress is created on the proximal dorsal edge of this sling, secondary to a change in the angle of pull. In addition, improper fit and shifting of the effort arm in the proximal segment of the orthosis contribute to the loss of the 90° angle of application (MERiT™ component; Patterson Medical, Warrenville, IL). **B,** There is a potential for shear stress at the distal orthosis/dorsum of small finger (SF) interface. **C,** However, when viewed during digital flexion, the distal portion of the orthosis is molded to accommodate for the convex/concave nature of the dorsum of the digits. This design distributes the shear stress adequately (Rolyan® Adjustable Outrigger Kit; Patterson Medical).

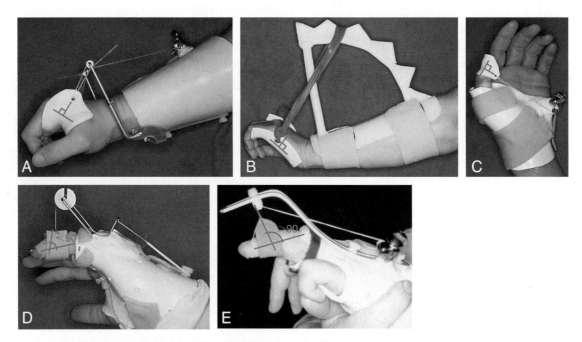

FIGURE 4–8 Demonstrating the optimal 90° angle of application with Phoenix Wrist Hinge (Patterson Medical) **(A)**. A homemade wrist extension mobilization orthosis, nicknamed the "Dinosaur orthosis" is shown here with a near 90° angle of application. For a true 90° angle, the TheraBand® would need to move one segment proximally (Patterson Medical) **(B)**. A thumb IP flexion mobilization orthosis (Splint-Tuner™; North Coast Medical, Morgan Hill, CA) **(C)**. **D,** The angle of force application is less than 90° in this hand-based PIP extension mobilization orthosis, causing shear stress at the distal volar edge of the sling (Phoenix Single Finger Outrigger; Patterson Medical). **E,** The angle of force application is greater than 90° in this orthosis, leading to shear stress at the proximal volar edge of the sling (Base 2™ Outrigger Kit; North Coast Medical).

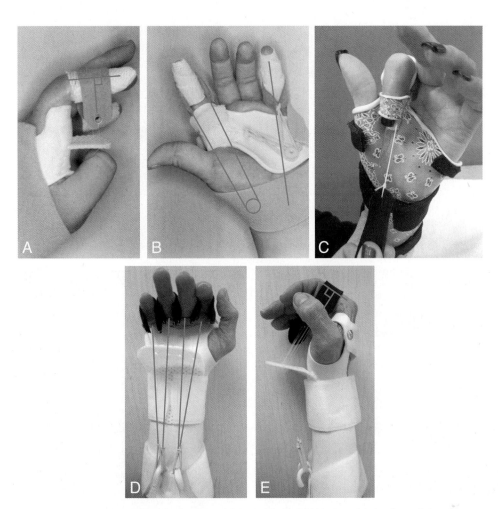

FIGURE 4–9 A, Lateral view of the 90° angle of application of a hand-based index finger (IF) PIP flexion mobilization orthosis. The thermoplastic line guide (perforated material) allows for simple orthosis adjustments as the range of motion improves. Note the small cast that aids in distributing pressure across the middle phalanx. **B,** Volar view highlighting the line of force application directed toward the scaphoid. Note the two monofilament lines originating from the IF sling and traversing through the perforated material. The small finger loop is addressing a stiff MCP joint. Because of the relative shortness of the small finger, a cast applied to the IP joints creates a longer, more effective lever arm to concentrate the flexion force to the MCP joint. **C,** With this isolated IF composite IP flexion mobilization orthosis, the convergence of the line of application is toward the base of the thumb/scaphoid. **D,** During the simultaneous mobilization of all digits into flexion, the lines of application tend to spread out more secondary to the anatomical fourth and fifth metacarpal length and mobility and bulk of loop material between each digit. These circumstances contribute to the convergence of the lines in a more proximal orientation on the forearm rather than tightly gathered toward the thumb base (radial middle third of the forearm) (Fess, 2004). **E,** Note the radial view with a 90° angle of force application.

- With a few exceptions, the general rule of thumb when using a mobilization orthosis to improve flexion of the digits, the anatomical configuration of the hand requires that the line of application converge toward the scaphoid (Fig. 4–9B). If this orientation is not incorporated into the orthosis design, excessive stress will be placed on the metacarpophalangeal (MCP) joints, causing discomfort and potential harm.
- Fess (1989, 2004) describes the importance of differentiating single finger versus multiple finger flexion alignment while considering the construction of a mobilization orthosis. It is recommended that the reader further study this work (Fess, 1989, 2004, 2011).
- Isolated, *individual* finger flexion converges toward the thumb base/scaphoid bone (Fig. 4–9C).
- During *simultaneous* finger flexion, the merging of the digits point to the radial middle third of the forearm. The dorsal rotation of the fourth and fifth metacarpals changes the alignment of the longitudinal axis of the ulnar digits away from the direction of the scaphoid and to an ulnarly directed position (Fig. 4–9D,E).

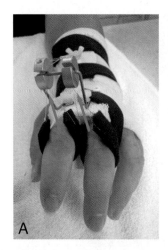
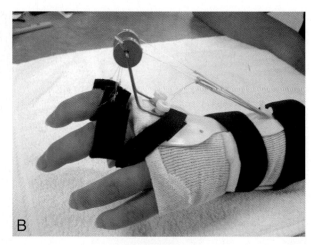
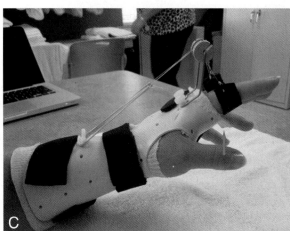
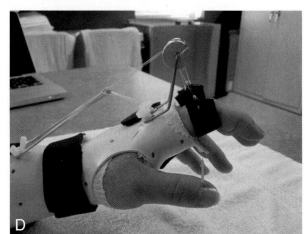

FIGURE 4–10 A–D This MCP IF/middle finger (MF) extension mobilization orthosis has a radially directed pull to protect the reconstruction of the radial collateral ligaments of the MCP joints and the silicone implant arthroplasties in this young patient with rheumatoid arthritis. **C and D,** Radial view of MCP digit extension and digit flexion to the thermoplastic block that is incorporated into the orthosis (Phoenix Single Finger Outrigger; Patterson Medical).

- Occasionally, a force applied in either a radial or ulnar direction is indicated, for example, after MCP joint arthroplasties or sagittal band repairs (Fig. 4–10A–D). (Except for special circumstances such as these, the line of application should be centrally located over the longitudinal axis of the bone being mobilized.)

HIGH-PROFILE DESIGN

- **High-profile designs**—mobilization orthoses that have high vertical outriggers—are commonly thought to require fewer adjustments to maintain the optimal 90° angle of application than a low-profile orthosis. However, this conjecture has been called into question, and the actual deviations from 90° line of pull are roughly 1° for each degree of motion gained (Austin, Slamet, Cameron, & Austin, 2004). Adjustments must be made when large improvements are seen in joint motion; otherwise, the line of pull will no longer be at 90°. Deviation of the line of pull from 90° results in

both a reduction in the therapeutic corrective force and an increase in the dangerous shear component of the applied force (Austin et al., 2004).
- Patient compliance is often a challenge because the orthosis is large. The dimensions of the high-profile design can make it cumbersome to engage in activities of daily living, such as putting the arm through a shirt sleeve.
- When using high-profile designs, the therapist should be careful to attach the outrigger sturdily on the orthosis base because this attachment site has the potential of low stability.

LOW-PROFILE DESIGN

- With **low-profile designs**—mobilization orthoses that have low, close to the surface outriggers—the force required to mobilize a joint may be uncomfortable and difficult to tolerate for extended periods of time.
- Low-profile designs may be cosmetically appealing. However, when greater resistance is necessary, such

as when mobilizing a dense 60° PIP flexion contracture, it may be more appropriate to incorporate a higher outrigger into the orthosis design. In such a situation, the force is applied at a greater distance from the joint axis to produce a greater amount of torque on the contracture.

- A low-profile design is an excellent choice for an orthosis that is used to substitute for weak or absent musculature, as seen when managing a radial nerve injury. Typically, less torque is needed to hold the distal segments (wrist and MCP joints in this case) in the proper position to substitute for the loss of muscle action than is needed to try to mobilize a stiff joint. For this purpose, only minimal adjustments are necessary, and the low-profile design tends to enhance function.

- Although dynamic orthoses require periodic adjustments to maintain an optimal 90° angle of pull, many make the unsubstantiated claim that high-profile dynamic orthoses require less frequent adjustment of the outrigger than do low-profile dynamic orthoses. However, it appears that it may be best to assume that the actual deviation from 90° line of pull is quite small for both low- and high-profile devices and these likely require adjustments at the same frequency to maintain the optimal 90° line of pull on the target segment (Austin et al., 2004, Fig. 2).

- Low-profile orthosis designs can be less cumbersome for performance of activities of daily living and often fit under loose clothing.

- Low-profile outriggers may undergo alternations in alignment more rapidly when applied for the purpose of correcting a contracture because of the short angle of application (Fess, 2011)

Elastic Force

Elastic force is the influence on the motion of an object or segment that is the result of the amount of applied stretch. Elastic force is directly proportional to both the stiffness of a structure and the amount of displacement present. Specifically,

$$F = -k\Delta l$$

where F is elastic force, k is stiffness, and Δl is the change in length or displacement. Elastic force can be increased by increasing the stiffness of the structure and/or increasing the amount of displacement or stretch. Stiffness is the relationship between the amount of force produced and the applied stretch:

$$-k = \frac{F}{\Delta l}$$

In other words, a stiffer structure produces a large amount of resistance to a small stretch, whereas a less stiff structure offers little resistance in response to the same stretch.

Clinically, when a therapist fabricates an orthosis to influence tissue response, he or she must consider the elastic nature of both the target tissues and the materials used to make the orthosis. The therapist should be familiar with the properties of the materials, including such factors as resistance to stretch, rigidity, and conformability (see Chapter 5 on "Equipment and Materials" for more information).

Torque-Angle Measurement

The notion of elastic force and stiffness applies not only to the materials used to produce external loads (e.g., rubber bands, elastic cord, and spring coils) but also to the internal reaction forces of the limb. An example is the torque-angle measurement proposed by Brand and Hollister (1993), in which torque is measured at several joint angles. These measurements provide the clinician with information regarding the magnitude of resistance to motion at particular joint angles throughout an arc of movement. A stiff hand, for example, offers more resistance at different angles than does a "normal" hand.

Clinical Considerations

When using elastic force to mobilize stiff structures, the therapist must take into account the clinical objectives. Is the goal to mobilize a mature, dense joint contracture or to stabilize the MCP joints in extension after MCP joint arthroplasty? Both situations may employ an elastic force; however, the amount of force and the materials used to achieve these goals may differ considerably.

To date, there is no documented ideal amount of elastic force for optimal mobilization of a specific structure. However, the amount of force applied depends on such factors as individual tolerance, diagnosis, stage of tissue healing, chronicity of the problem, severity of the contracture, density of the contracture, patient's age, lifestyle factors (smoking, alcohol use), and other health-related issues. A range of 100 to 300 g has been suggested for mobilization of the small joints of the hand, whereas higher parameters (350+ grams) seem to be more effective for larger structures (Bell-Krotoski & Figarola, 1995; Brand & Hollister, 1993; Flowers & LaStayo, 1994, 2012; Giurintano, 1995; Glasgow, Tooth, Fleming, & Hockey, 2012; Glasgow, Tooth, Fleming, & Peters, 2011). The estimate of 300 g is based on what is tolerated per unit of surface area of the skin, not on the tolerance of the contracted tissue to tension. Therefore, in most cases, skin tolerance becomes the limiting factor in determining appropriate orthosis tension, not the specific targeted tissue. "While the optimum force has yet to be calculated, the amount of force applied to the tissues must be determined relative to the tissues that are contracted. A force of 800 grams may be on the high end of the spectrum for the PIP joint but is a relatively small amount when considering remodeling at the elbow or shoulder" (Bell-Krotoski & Figarola, 1995, p. 135).

The therapist can almost always rely on the tissue's response to the tension to help determine the effectiveness of the mobilizing forces. Signs of too much stress include edema, skin blanching, vascular changes, and complaints of pain. With tools such as tension gauges (e.g., Haldex gauge), the therapist can obtain a general estimate of the amount of

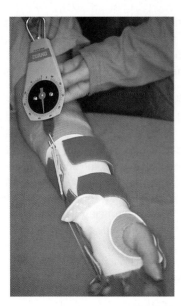

FIGURE 4–11 A tension gauge applied to a mobilization orthosis determines the approximate forces on the intended tissue.

tension a dynamic orthosis is applying to the involved area (Fig. 4–11). A few of the common devices a therapist can use to generate an elastic force for mobilizing soft tissue are discussed in the next sections.

RUBBER BANDS

The length and thickness of a rubber band determine its effectiveness when used for fabrication of a mobilizing orthosis. Thinner (narrow) rubber bands tend to elongate more easily than do thicker ones (i.e., narrow bands are less stiff). A rubber band, made of latex and rubber, does not return to its exact original shape after being *stretched, relaxed, and then restretched*. This phenomenon is called **hysteresis**.

If a rubber band has been held in a *constant* stretched position for a long period of time, eventually, there will be a *permanent* change in length. The structure of the rubber band has been permanently altered, this is called **creep**. The clinician should appreciate that rubber bands do not behave exactly like a spring and will undergo some degree of hysteresis and creep as the orthosis is worn. Therefore, attention to the rubber band's effectiveness should be monitored and reassessed accordingly.

The therapist must consider the purpose of the orthosis when selecting the properties of the rubber band (i.e., thickness, length, width). For example, a narrow rubber band may not be stiff enough to aid in mobilizing a dense PIP flexion contracture but may generate adequate force to maintain a PIP joint in extension after an extensor tendon repair.

WRAPPED ELASTIC CORD

Wrapped elastic cord is made of a light layer of cotton wrapped around an elastic cord. It provides a greater degree of resistance or stiffness when stretched. With this type of material, less stretch is required to generate movement of a stiff joint than with a rubber band; therefore, caution should be used.

SPRING COILS

Spring coils can produce an elastic force as well. They are available in various sizes (diameters and lengths) that offer different degrees of resistance. The composition, stiffness, and length of the coil aid the therapist in the appropriate selection for the tissue involved. Spring coils produce a consistent controlled force with little material breakdown, an advantage over rubber bands. However, they are more costly and less readily available than rubber bands.

Friction Force

Friction force is a type of **translational force**, sometimes referred to as either static friction or kinetic friction. Friction opposes movement between two surfaces and acts parallel to the surfaces. The force of friction (F_x) is proportional to the coefficient of friction (μ) and the contact force (F_c):

$$F_x = \mu F_c$$

The coefficient of friction is specific to each material. At rest, the opposing force of friction is categorized as static and depends on the coefficient of static friction (μ_s) and F_c. When motion occurs, friction is classified as kinetic, or moving, friction and depends on the coefficient of kinetic friction (μ_k) and F_c.

In situations of either motion or equilibrium, friction is directly proportional to (1) the coefficient of friction specific to the material(s) and (2) the amount of contact force. The therapist, therefore, can minimize friction by using materials with lower coefficients of friction, such as smooth, nonperforated thermoplastics (instead of gel or foam-lined thermoplastic materials). In addition, friction can be reduced by decreasing the contact force generated by rubber bands and straps. Often, friction must be minimized to prevent skin irritation or breakdown, such as chaffing or blistering. Sources of potential harmful friction include orthosis borders, poor-fitting straps, attachments that rub against the skin (e.g., the underside of rivets or rubber band posts), and edges that extend beyond joint creases.

Clinical Considerations

Friction may be desired to prevent the migration of an orthosis along the skin. In such cases, friction can be increased by applying straps to increase the contact force or by simply lining the orthosis with thin foam strips or a tape (e.g., Microfoam™ Tape, Patterson Medical) to increase the coefficient of friction.

At times, a small amount of orthosis migration is inevitable; for example, a wrist immobilization orthosis causes some degree of friction along the orthosis–skin interface as the patient moves the digits and elbow. An attempt must be made to decrease this friction force; it can be lessened by covering the involved area with materials such as cotton stockinette, TubiGrip™, or TubiPad® (Patterson Medical).

Friction, also referred to as drag, may be present in the pulley systems used for dynamic mobilization orthoses. As the monofilament line passes through the line guide or pulleys, the point of contact can be a source of friction,

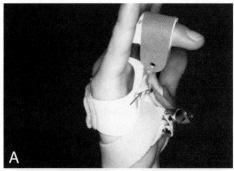

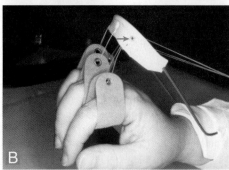

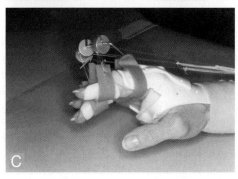

FIGURE 4–12 Examples of monofilament line guides that approach at different angles. Note the point of contact and potential sites of friction: commercial line guide **(A)**, thermoplastic material with punched hole **(B)**, and Phoenix Outrigger Kit (Patterson Medical) **(C)**.

thereby increasing unwanted resistance through the orthosis. This can be the result of the coefficient of friction of the monofilament, the orthosis line, or the line guide itself (Fig. 4–12). The amount of friction present is increased when the angle at which the monofilament line enters one of these devices is increased.

Most manufactures of orthosis fabrication components have attempted to address these issues. For example, the Phoenix outrigger has a tubular plastic insert in which the monofilament line passes, and the Rolyan® adjustable outrigger is completely rounded and smooth to reduce dragging of the line as it traverses the outrigger (see Chapter 5 on "Equipment and Materials" for additional information). Therapists should be aware of this problem when fabricating homemade line guides. Friction can be minimized by smoothing and rounding the edges and by carefully monitoring the angles of force application.

Stress

When designing and fabricating orthoses, the therapist must understand the **stress** produced by external forces. By definition, stress is the response of, or resistance offered by, a surface to the deformation caused by an externally applied force or moment (Nordin & Frankel, 2001; Soderberg, 1986). Stress (σ), often simply referred to as pressure, is described according to the amount of force (F) per unit area (A), specifically:

$$\sigma = \frac{F}{A}$$

Stress, therefore, is directly proportional to F and inversely proportional to A. In other words, stress is increased when either the magnitude of the force applied to the surface area is increased or the amount of area over which the force is applied is decreased (Fig. 4–13). Stress can occur in different forms, the most important of which are compression, shear, tensile, bending, and torsion.

Compression

Compression, often mistakenly referred to simply as **pressure**, is the special case of stress in which opposing loads push toward one another along the same line of application (Fig. 4–14). A compressive stress (σ) is distinguished by the perpendicular angle of application of the load. Usually, compression results in a squeezing type of force, causing a broadening and flattening of the object (Nordin & Frankel, 2001). Compressive stress is maximized by the perpendicular nature of the force application. Notably, pure compression lacks a force component parallel to the surface (defined as shear). Compression is proportional to

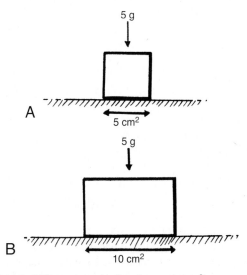

FIGURE 4–13 Different magnitudes of stress (g/cm²) can result from the application of a 5-g force to different-sized areas. **A,** Small area (5 cm²): stress = 1 g/cm². **B,** Large area (10 cm²): stress = 0.5 g/cm².

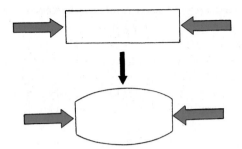

FIGURE 4–14 To maximize compressive stress, force should be applied in a perpendicular fashion.

the perpendicular force (F_{perp}) and inversely proportional to the surface area:

$$\sigma_c = \frac{F_{perp}}{A}$$

For a constant magnitude of force, compression can be minimized by increasing the surface area over which the force can be distributed. For a constant surface area, compression can be reduced by decreasing the perpendicular force.

Clinical Considerations

The therapist must be sure to fabricate the base of an orthosis with sufficient length, depth, and contour. In addition to offering greater mechanical advantage, a longer orthosis base provides greater surface area over which to distribute the contact force. A wider and deeper orthosis base is not only stronger but also minimizes shear stress and maximizes pressure distribution.

Optimizing the conformity of materials to the shapes, contours, and curvatures of the body part being immobilized can minimize compressive stress. If care is not taken to meticulously pad vulnerable areas such as the ulnar or radial styloid and pin sites, increased compressive stress can result in discomfort, possible pin migration, and probable noncompliance.

Straps—although necessary to secure the orthosis firmly on the extremity—can be sources of compressive stress. A narrow strap width, especially in conjunction with shallow orthoses (less than two-thirds of the circumference), can produce high compressive stresses on the soft tissue it lies on. This can lead to an uncomfortable, ill-fitting orthosis (Fig. 4–15). Increasing the width and conformability of the straps aids in distribution of the compressive forces over a greater surface area and helps minimize orthosis migration.

Orthosis borders should be fabricated so that they lie flush with the skin surface that the strap traverses. The strap should not bridge the two borders of the orthosis; it should, in fact, actually come in light contact with the skin. For example, the lateral borders of a volar forearm orthosis base should be just at the level of the dorsal forearm. The strap(s) can then be applied to rest lightly on the dorsal forearm. As previously mentioned, if the lateral borders of the orthosis do not rise high enough to reach the dorsal skin surface, the straps cannot lie flush; they instead wrap around the dorsal skin and underlying soft tissue structures, causing

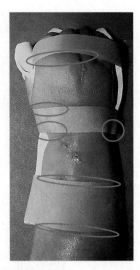

FIGURE 4–15 Improper selection and placement of straps can create high and uncomfortable compressive and shear forces. The borders of this orthosis are inadequate (too low) in order to support the bulk of the hand and forearm. The narrow straps are also a source of high compressive stress.

potential neurovascular compression, pinching of the skin against the orthosis border, and discomfort for the wearer.

Too high orthosis borders can cause a "bridging" of the straps where there is no contact with the skin surface beneath the strap. This type of closure will not adequately secure the orthosis onto the extremity. There will be too much room left between the orthosis strap and the skin, allowing unwanted movement of the immobilized part (Fig. 4–16A–F).

The therapist should remember that slings and loops can also be sources of compression stress. Several techniques help the orthosis fabricator avoid compression to the lateral, dorsal, or volar aspects of the digit (or body part in the sling or loop). One orthosis line can be attached to each side of a sling (two pieces of line) and then joined after they pass through the pulley. This prevents the circumferential compression created when one line is threaded through both ends of the loop, an important consideration when addressing a digit with edema or neurovascular issues (Fig. 4–17A). Alternatively, a well-contoured cuff fabricated from thermoplastic, plaster, or QuickCast may be placed under the sling as a support. The thermoplastic cuff with a soft sling disperses the compressive forces applied through the sling by lifting the borders away from the skin and increasing the area of force application (Fig. 4–17B). Circumferential cuffs can also be fabricated to maximize pressure distribution (Fig. 4–17C,D).

Shear

Shear stress results from force being applied parallel to the surface and produces a tendency for an object either to deform or to slide along the surface. This can occur in two instances: when two parallel opposing forces are applied in the same plane (coplanar) but not along the same line

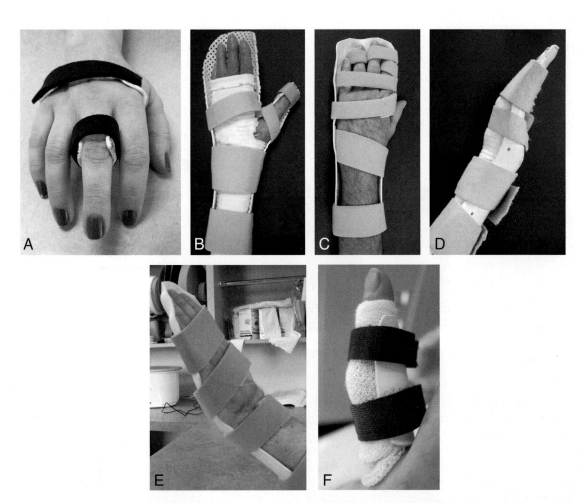

FIGURE 4–16 A, Note the floating straps on this hand-based MF MCP immobilization orthosis. **B,** When the orthosis borders are too generous, the straps tend to "float" between the lateral borders and hardly braze the skin, leaving room for unintended motion. Although the strap widths in this figure are appropriate, the borders on this orthosis are too high in order to properly secure the wrist and forearm into the device. Note the use of adhesive foam between the strap and skin in order to "absorb" the extra room. **C,** When adjustment of the orthosis borders is not an option, originating the strap from a lower spot on the inside of the orthosis may offer better purchase and effectiveness of the strap as it traverses the tissue it is intended to hold in place. This technique is often used for the patient with rheumatoid arthritis (as shown here) because it can assist in managing the zigzag forearm and hand deformity often seen in these patients. **D,** This orthosis demonstrates appropriate border height and strap placements. **E,** Note how the straps have the potential to "push" the skin against the low border. The narrow width and "too" proximal placement of the wrist strap can contribute to discomfort during wear. **F,** This small PIP extension immobilization orthosis has been fabricated with low lateral borders that inadequately support the proximal and middle phalanges. The dorsal straps need to push the digit into the orthosis, leading to possible compression stress and edema pooling between straps.

(noncollinear) and when two oblique opposing forces share the same point of application but are neither parallel nor perpendicular (Fig. 4–18). In the first case, shear stress is high owing to the parallel force and compressive stress is negligible in the absence of perpendicular force. In the second case, in which the angle of application does not equal 90°, there exists both a parallel component (shear) and a perpendicular component (compression). Although difficult to measure, the amount of shear in the latter case can be inferred from the angle of application. Shear is inversely proportional to the angle of application: As the angle approaches 0° (as in the former case), the shear dominates; and as it becomes more perpendicular, it decreases.

Shear is often accompanied by other stresses, for example, compression, tension, and torsion (as seen in orthoses that attempt to mobilize forearm rotation). In addition, static or kinetic friction may be present as a counterforce to the shear stress. If static friction is high, it may impart high shear stresses to the subcutaneous tissue interfaces. For example, ineffective strapping on a posterior elbow immobilization orthosis

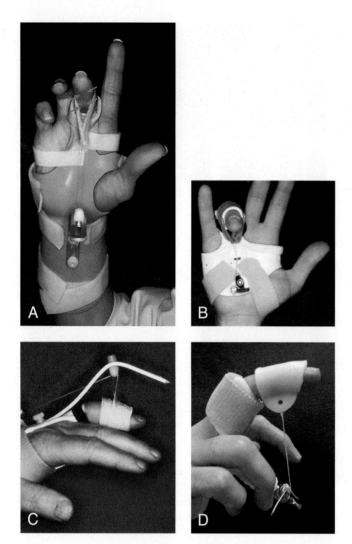

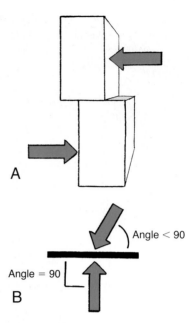

FIGURE 4–18 Shear stress results from force being applied parallel to the surface and can occur when two parallel opposing forces are applied in the same plane (coplanar) but not along the same line (noncollinear) **(A)** and when two oblique opposing forces share the same point of application but are neither parallel nor perpendicular **(B)**.

FIGURE 4–17 **A,** A forearm-based PIP flexion mobilization orthosis with one monofilament line converging at the volar aspect of the digit creating compressive stress along the dorsum and lateral aspect of the digit. **B,** A hand-based PIP flexion mobilization orthosis with a custom-molded thermoplastic cuff (under the sling) on the middle phalanx. This technique can be used to decrease compression of the lateral borders of the digits by lifting the sling borders off the middle phalanx. Circumferential slings constructed with QuickCast 2 (Patterson Medical) **(C)** or with thermoplastic material **(D)** can maximize surface area. (Base 2™ Outrigger Kit and Splint-Tuner™; North Coast Medical).

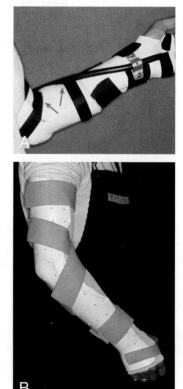

may quickly lead to noncompliance because of discomfort. If 1″ traditional loop straps (instead of conforming soft or elasticized straps) are applied in an oblique fashion to secure the anterior elbow into the orthosis, the loop strap edges are likely to rub along the skin. Rather than applying a direct compressive stress (i.e., perpendicular), the straps impart an oblique compressive stress and produce shear stress in the tissues over which they traverse (especially in the presence of high static friction) (Fig. 4–19). In such cases, the therapist should consider using soft, conforming 2″ straps (e.g., made from neoprene, or soft foam such as Rolyan® SoftStrap®,

FIGURE 4–19 **A,** The 1″ straps, placed just proximal and distal to the elbow crease, place high shear and compression stress to the tissue beneath (Rolyan® Dynamic Supination Pronation Kit; Patterson Medical). **B,** Conforming, soft 2″ straps better distribute the force and improve patient comfort.

Patterson Medical) or a circumferential wrap that is applied along the entire length of the orthosis for even compression.

Clinical Considerations

The therapist should use care to smooth out, roll, and/or flare uneven or sharp orthosis edges. This is especially important near joint creases where movement will occur (e.g., the volar distal portion of a wrist immobilization orthosis where the MCP joints are free to move).

When using circumferential bandages or wraps to assist in the molding of an orthosis (e.g., when a second set of hands is needed), the therapist should avoid applying them too tightly. During the wrapping process, orthosis borders may inevitably be pushed in toward the body part. This makes it difficult to smooth the borders away from the skin and may cause shear stress along the entire length of the orthosis–skin interface (Fig. 4–20).

When fabricating a mobilization orthosis, the therapist must consider both compression and shear stresses. Mobilizing forces, which are attached to the proximal orthosis base, usually traverse the length of the orthosis and terminate distally to the intended joint(s). If the proximal base of the orthosis is not adequately secured to the limb, motion at the distal joints will result in an undesirable migration or dragging and shearing of the proximal base over the skin. The amount of shear stress depends on the coefficient of friction of the materials used and the direction and amount of force necessary to make the change at the intended joint(s) (Fig. 4–21A–C).

The therapeutic effect of a mobilization orthosis is to increase the range of motion, thereby causing the angle of application to shift from 90° (Fig. 4–8E). Alterations in the angle of application through a sling can create an uneven pull, resulting in shear stress proximally on the orthosis base and distally on the sling. The patient may cease to use the orthosis because of discomfort. When tissue is changing rapidly owing to the use of a mobilization orthosis, the

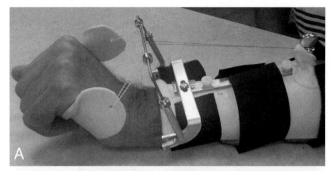
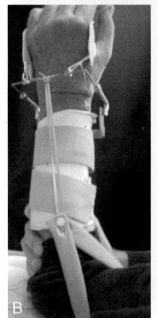
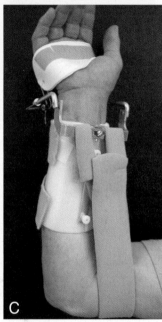

FIGURE 4–21 **A,** Wrist extension mobilization orthosis using a Phoenix Wrist Hinge (Patterson Medical). This static progressive approach uses the adjustable MERiT™ component (Patterson Medical). Shear stress is increased proximally as the mobilizing force drags the orthosis base distally. Although there is some natural mobility of the skin (proximally and distally), this mobility is increased with the force generated through the orthosis **and** if the orthosis is not adequately contoured and secured. Therefore, the base has no choice but to migrate/translate distally. **B and C,** These are similar mobilization orthoses using an elastic (dynamic) force. Consider either of these proximal strap techniques; the straps are applied from the proximal base of the orthosis to above the elbow joint. These strategies can minimize the distal migration of the orthosis.

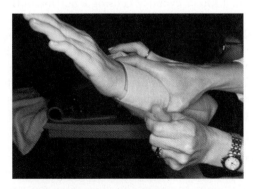

FIGURE 4–20 Use caution when applying a circumferential wrap to secure an orthosis while molding. The wrap can cause shear at the borders if not applied carefully; this can be avoided by leaving a small border of thermoplastic material outside the wrap so that this edge will not be pushed into the skin by the bandage. Wrap the orthosis lightly and uniformly.

patient should visit the clinic frequently so the therapist can adequately monitor the orthosis line and adjust it as necessary to ensure a 90° angle of force application. Commercially available outriggers make adjustment simple.

Orthosis bases must be fabricated to the correct length and circumference. The proximal orthosis border of a short forearm-based orthosis is likely to pivot on the volar aspect of the forearm (because of attempted distal movement by the patient), causing shear stress at the proximal orthosis border and irritation of the superficial sensory nerves and skin (Fig. 4–22).

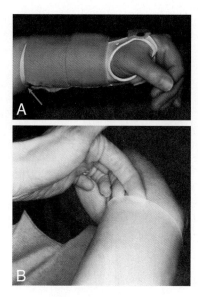

FIGURE 4–22 A, The proximal border of this short forearm-based orthosis is pivoting on the volar aspect of the forearm and digging into the skin. **B,** The proximal borders should be flared away from the skin as they are cooling during the fabrication process.

Tensile

Tensile stress is opposite in nature to compressive stress and is the result of opposing loads pulling away from a surface along the same line of application (Fig. 4–23). Tensile stress, also referred to as tension and distraction, results in stretching as evidenced by the lengthening and narrowing of an object to which it is applied. As is true with compression, tensile stress is the greatest when the force is applied perpendicular to the surface. Thus, to optimize the effect of tensile stress, the pulling force should be applied at a 90° orientation to the target surface.

Clinical Considerations

When the goal of orthotic fabrication is to gain thumb abduction, the therapist may find it challenging to optimize tensile stress. Force applied to the proximal phalanx does not deliver tensile stress to the tight first dorsal interossei or to the adductor pollicis (thumb web); rather, it produces excessive

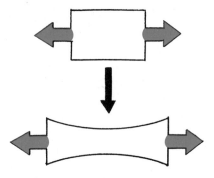

FIGURE 4–23 Tensile stress results from opposing forces pulling away from a surface along the same line of application. It is also referred to as tension, distraction, and stretching.

stress at the ulnar collateral ligament of the thumb MP joint. The therapist should take care when fabricating an orthosis that delivers tensile stress directly to the distal aspect of the first metacarpal. The sling should conform around the head of the first metacarpal (which may cause discomfort in the web space if not molded well), and the angle of application should be directed 90° from the long axis of the first metacarpal (Fig. 4–24).

Tensile stress can be used to maintain reduction of an intra-articular fracture while preserving joint mobility. The application of a gentle traction force to a healing intra-articular fracture site can help maintain bone alignment, facilitate healing, and preserve joint range of motion. An example is the circular traction PIP intra-articular mobilization orthosis designed by Schenck (1986). The surgeon places a wire horizontally through the bone proximal to the fracture site, leaving the ends of the wire protruding. The wire is bent to place rubber bands or springs, which are then attached to a hoop extending from the orthosis base. Tensile stress is then delivered from the wire to the hoop via the rubber band or spring. The hoop allows for segmental changes in range of motion while maintaining consistent stress throughout the range. These orthoses are often fabricated during the immediate postoperative period (Fig. 4–25A–D).

Bending and Torsion

Compression, shear, and tensile stresses can be present in two particular combinations. **Bending** is the application of loads to a structure in such a manner that the object simultaneously undergoes tension, compression, and shear as it bends about a transverse axis (Fig. 4–26). Compression develops on the concave aspect of the structure, and tension forms across the convex aspect. In addition, shear stress develops as a result of the opposing parallel forces producing the bending (LeVeau, 1992). The bending stress is directly proportional to both the magnitude of the force and the distance from the transverse axis at which it is applied.

Torsion is stress produced when a rotational force is applied to a rod or cylinder, causing a portion of the structure to turn around the longitudinal axis (Fig. 4–27) (Nordin & Frankel, 2001). Torsion, also referred to as twisting, is directly proportional to the distance from the longitudinal to the point of application of the force. To generate greater torsion, apply the force farther from the axis about which the intended twisting will occur. Torsion results in the simultaneous generation of compression, tension, and shear forces.

Clinical Considerations

BENDING

A clinical example of the effects of bending stress is when a therapist attempts to elongate an elbow extension contracture by using an elbow flexion mobilization orthosis. The therapist must appreciate the tensile stress present along the posterior aspect of the elbow while compression stress is applied to the soft tissue structures along the anterior aspect of the elbow (Fig. 4–28A–C). Shear stress simultaneously may occur at the

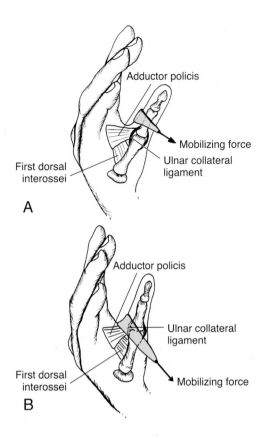

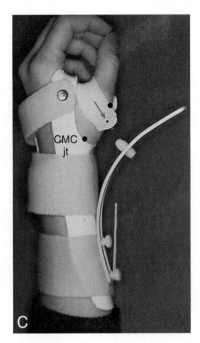

FIGURE 4–24 **A,** An incorrectly applied thumb sling stressed the ulnar collateral ligament at the thumb MP joint. **B,** A correctly applied thumb sling mobilizes the first dorsal interossei and the adductor pollicis muscles. **C,** A QuickCast 2 (Patterson Medical) sling was molded to orient stress to the distal portion of the first metacarpal instead of the ulnar collateral ligament (Digitec Outrigger System; Patterson Medical).

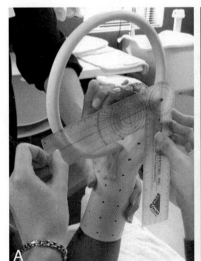
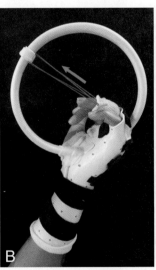
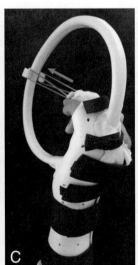
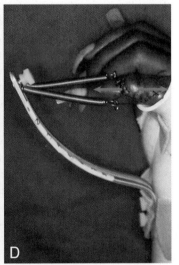

FIGURE 4–25 **A,** The clinician is shown here measuring the distance from the distal pin site on the middle phalanx to the traction point on the "hoop." **B,** Completed design using elastic "rubber band" traction. **C,** A dorsal to volar view to appreciate the role of the attachment device on the hoop. This small device plays a significant role in the ability to gently and segmentally change angles while keeping the tension uniform throughout the range. **D,** Variation of a PIP intra-articular orthosis. Note the perpendicular line of application via the spring coils attached to a surgically placed horizontal wire through the middle phalanx. Gentle tension is applied to the PIP joint, maintaining ligament length and bone alignment while providing supervised periods of limited joint range of motion (Components of the Digitec Outrigger System used, Patterson Medical).

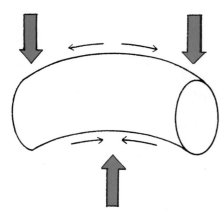

FIGURE 4–26 Bending is the application of force in such a manner that the object simultaneously undergoes tension, compression, and shear as it bends about a transverse axis.

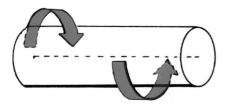

FIGURE 4–27 Torsion stress, or twisting, is produced when a rotational force is applied to a rod or cylinder, causing a portion of the structure to turn around the longitudinal axis.

skin–orthosis interface of both the humeral and forearm cuffs owing to orthosis migration. The force applied through the device attempts to mobilize the distal segment (forearm cuff) in the direction of elbow flexion. In doing so, the proximal segment tends to migrate distally, whereas the distal segment migrates proximally. This shifting of the orthosis can cause shear stress along the orthosis–skin interface.

TORSION

The concept of torsion stress is demonstrated by a supination–pronation mobilization orthosis used to gain forearm rotation (Shah, Lopez, Escalante, & Green, 2002). To appreciate this concept, the therapist must first understand that forearm rotation is created by the simultaneous effort of both the proximal and the distal radioulnar joints. The nature of this design imparts a torsion stress along the entire length of the forearm, which is considered the axis of rotation. Therefore, the principles of adequate orthosis length, pressure distribution, and precise orthosis molding along the entire forearm are critical for the construction of these orthoses (Fig. 4–29). The potential pressure points include the proximal and distal ends of the orthosis where the force originates and terminates (elbow and wrist joints). With this orthosis, compression and shear stresses and distal migration (the result of a linear force) are inevitably present at the orthosis–skin interface during force application. The effectiveness of this type of orthosis depends on proper fit, which requires careful monitoring by the therapist along with education of the patient.

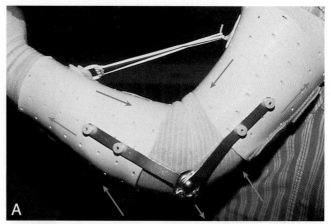

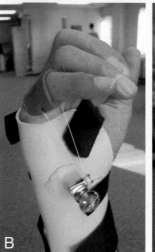
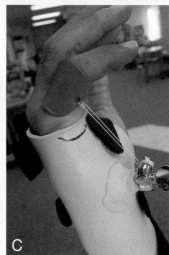

FIGURE 4–28 **A,** An elbow flexion mobilization orthosis uses bending stress to increase elbow flexion (Phoenix Elbow Hinge; Patterson Medical). **B,** An SF MCP flexion mobilization orthosis in which the bending stress is noted at the volar MCP. **C,** Adjustments to be made (see black line) in this orthosis to clear the MCP crease and allow unimpeded bending with significantly less stress (MERiT™ component; Patterson Medical).

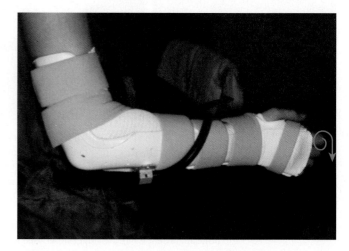

FIGURE 4–29 A forearm supination–pronation mobilization orthosis uses torsion stress to increase the supination of the forearm (Rolyan® Dynamic Supination Pronation Kit; Patterson Medical).

Conclusion

The application of an orthosis enhances or restores function of the extremity via the intentional application of external loads to manipulate the internal reaction forces of specific anatomical structures. This chapter defined and clarified the fundamental mechanical terms and concepts pertaining to the design and fabrication of orthoses. In addition, the clinical relevance of these terms and concepts were discussed in light of specific clinical application. The effective therapist successfully integrates basic mechanical concepts into all facets of orthosis design and fabrication.

Chapter Review Questions

1. What is the optimal angle of force application and how can a therapist ensure this is maintained in an orthosis?

2. Give an example of compressive stress and how it relates to orthotic application.

3. Why should orthoses be fabricated as long and wide as possible?

4. What is the difference between a high- and a low-profile design?

5. Name two potential areas of friction force in a typical wrist immobilization orthosis.

Equipment and Materials

Noelle M. Austin, MS, PT, CHT

Chapter Objectives

After study of this chapter, the reader should be able to:

- Name the various tools to have in the clinic for orthotic fabrication.
- Recognize the importance of different thermoplastic characteristics and how these influence optimal material selection.
- Appreciate the various types of strapping and lining/padding materials and understand how to choose appropriately.
- Understand the basic components of mobilization orthoses.

Key Terms

Bonding
Combination plastic and rubber-like materials
Conformability
Drape
Elastic materials
Finger loops
Finger slings
Fingertip attachment
Hand drills
Heat guns
Heating pans

Heating time
Hinges
Hook
Line connector
Line guide
Line stops
Lines
Lining material
Loop
Low-temperature thermoplastic orthotic materials
Memory

Mobilization force
Nonperforated Materials
Outrigger systems
Perforated Materials
Plastic materials
Proximal attachment device
Resistance to stretch
Rigidity
Rubber materials
Rubber-like materials
Working time

Introduction

This chapter presents the fundamentals of orthotic fabrication, including reviews of the equipment and materials needed to create orthoses effectively and efficiently. With today's rising health-care costs, it has become increasingly important to be economical. Thus, therapists have been forced to change the way they buy and use rehabilitation products. They must educate themselves about what is available and use their local sales representatives as resources regarding new products. Such measures can help therapists make more fiscally prudent decisions. If therapists take the time to research a particular item, they will usually be able to find a lower cost or less-expensive substitute. The constant innovation in orthotic fabrication techniques and methods has spurred the need for consumers to be discriminating when purchasing products. Experimenting with new materials and providing feedback to vendors can promote positive changes in the available rehabilitation products.

Before fabricating an orthosis, the therapist must be sure to have the necessary equipment, tools, materials, and accessories readily accessible. These products can be purchased from rehabilitation vendors (see Appendix A for contact information). To provide patients with the best orthotic options, therapists must be aware of what is currently available. Therapists should be familiar with the major rehabilitation catalogs and their Web sites. These Web sites often include links to videos or other resources demonstrating how best to use the product. Also spend some time browsing local hardware and hobby stores for creative ideas and products to incorporate into orthoses and/ or rehabilitation. When attending continuing education courses, therapists should visit vendors' booths and make an effort to obtain hands-on experience with new or unfamiliar products; these measures increase the therapists' comfort with using various products. Note that each vendor has its own version of common rehabilitation items and mobilization component kits. Vendors may offer the same products as their competitor, or something very similar, but they may call the item by a different name. Other invaluable resources are hand therapy journals featuring practical information on orthosis fabrication and unique ideas/hints from fellow therapists often presented in case study format.

Essential Equipment

This section discusses the equipment needed to fabricate upper extremity orthoses efficiently and effectively. In Section II, the Clinical and Pattern Pearls provide detailed information and helpful hints on how to use specific products and offer alternative and cost-containing strategies.

Heating Sources

Thermoplastic materials need to be heated to a softened state before they can be molded to the body part. Heating pans and heat guns provide the most common means to warm the material for orthotic fabrication.

Orthotic Heating Pans

Ideally, dedicated **heating pans** are used to heat materials; however, if they are not available, electric frying pans will suffice. Drain water and dry pan thoroughly at the end of each clinic day to prevent any water contamination issues. This will also help preserve the bottom surface of the pan, preventing the breakdown of nonstick coating or the adherence of hard water deposits. Although hot pack heaters are readily available in most clinics, their use to soften thermoplastics includes the following disadvantages: inability to control water temperature, difficult to remove materials without overstretching (especially if attempted in a vertical manner), and possibility of contamination from dirty water.

Commercial heating pans are available in several sizes, ranging from a pan that is large enough to accommodate large pieces of orthotic material to a small household electric frying pan (Fig. 5–1). Small pans may be easier to manage in the clinic because they are easy to clean, quick to heat, and do not require too much counter space. Each type of orthotic material must be heated to a specific temperature per the manufacturer's specifications to take advantage of that

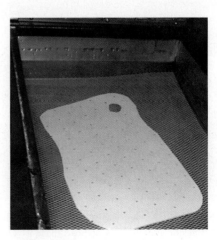

FIGURE 5–1 A large heating pan.

material's specific properties. The water temperature should be adjusted accordingly. Some of the newer pan designs have thermal regulators; a thermometer can also be used to check the temperature before heating the material. Be aware that owing to the location of the heating coils, materials may be heated unevenly when using a heating pan. This can be avoided by moving the material around the pan during the heating process.

There are several ways to prevent orthotic material from sticking to the bottom and sides of the pan, including keeping the material moving by use of a spatula and the addition of a drop of liquid hand soap, dish washing liquid, or lotion to the water. Another trick is to employ the use of pan netting. Not only does this stop material from sticking to the pan but it also protects the hands from being burned, prevents the overstretching of softened materials, and eases the task of removing the heated material from the water. Remember that netting may leave an imprint on material that is very contouring. An alternative is to layer the bottom of the pan with paper towels. Spatulas help when removing heated material from the pan and prevent imprints in the material. Consider adding a liquid disinfectant when changing the water to prevent contamination.

Heat Guns

Heat guns are a source of dry heat that can be used to spot warm specific areas of thermoplastic material. Care must be taken when using this device to adjust an orthosis; inadvertent overheating of adjacent regions can cause irregular surfaces and the loss of contour or fit of the orthosis (especially problematic when using materials with memory). Special nozzles are available to direct the heat to a small area; the Precision Point Heat Gun provides a concentrated source of heat (North Coast Medical, Morgan Hill, CA) (Fig. 5–2). Minor changes in contour and edge finishing can be accomplished with a heat gun as well.

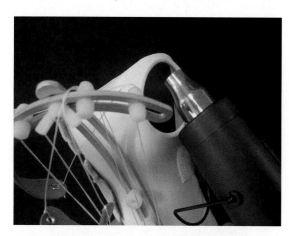

FIGURE 5–2 A Precision Point Heat Gun being used to adjust web space in MCP flexion mobilization orthosis (Base 2™ Outrigger Kit, North Coast Medical).

The heat gun can be used to prepare the surface of the thermoplastic material for bonding, as when applying components such as outriggers. These guns are particularly useful when heating components before applying them to the orthosis, allowing them to be embedded into the thermoplastic. In addition, if experiencing difficulty with adherence of adhesive hook material onto the thermoplastic, heating the adhesive just to the point of getting tacky prior to application can ensure that it will be strongly attached.

Orthotic Tools

The use of high-quality tools is extremely important when fabricating orthoses. Using tools that are not appropriate for the specific task can be frustrating and ineffective, making the fabrication process more difficult than otherwise. In the long run, an initial investment in quality products saves time and money. Well-maintained tools help avoid the need for replacement and guard the therapist against developing a repetitive stress injury.

In addition to cutting devices, other mandatory tools include pliers, hole punches, hand drills, wire cutters, and benders. Many other tools can assist in making the fabrication process easier. The therapist should browse through rehabilitation catalogs to learn about other tools and how they are used in the fabrication process.

Cutting Devices

Thermoplastic materials are available in large sheets, which need to be cut into specific shapes or patterns for a particular design. Many types of cutting devices are found in manufacturers' catalogs. When cutting unheated materials, use a utility knife or heavy-duty shears or snips. Some distributors offer time-saving precut thermoplastic materials (to be discussed in detail later in this chapter), eliminating the need to cut up large sheets; these precut forms are ready to be warmed in the water and molded onto the body part.

Using dull, improperly chosen scissors to cut out orthotic patterns from warmed material can be frustrating. Invest in a quality pair of scissors such as Gingher Super Shears (Patterson Medical, Warrenville, IL) that are comfortable to use (Fig. 5–3A). Designating a "thermoplastic-material only" pair of scissors can help prevent adhesive from sticking to the blades, which causes the warm material to stick to the scissors' blades later. Assign the use of other, less-expensive scissors for cutting adhesive-backed materials, such as hook, lining, and padding. Special Non-Stick Scissors are coated to minimize adhesives from sticking to the blades (Patterson Medical) (Fig. 5–3B). Adhesive can be removed from the scissors with solvent, Goo Gone®, rubbing alcohol, or nail polish remover. Sharpen the blades frequently to maintain sharp, smooth edges; ask a local fabric or craft store about sharpening services. Furthermore, sharp blades will help protect the therapist from developing overuse syndromes, which can result from making the repetitive, forceful strokes needed to operate dull scissors.

When cutting with scissors, practice using *smooth, long strokes* rather than short snips, which cause multiple irregular sharp edges and can lead to an uncomfortable,

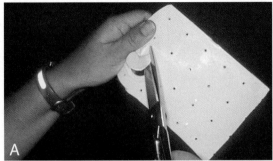

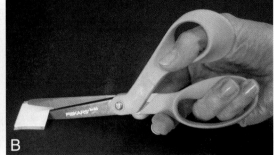

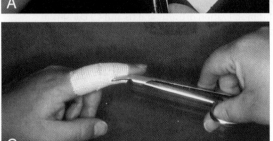

FIGURE 5–3 **A,** To obtain a smooth cut edge, the scissors should be sharp and the material should be warm— Gingher Scissors (Patterson Medical). **B,** Special Non-Stick Scissors shown here trimming adhesive-backed foam product (Patterson Medical). **C,** A Serial Cast Cutter Scissors is used to remove a serial static finger cast (North Coast Medical).

unsightly orthosis. All borders and corners should be smooth and slightly rounded to maximize patient comfort, provide an aesthetically pleasing result, and add strength and rigidity to the orthosis.

Other scissors may be useful in the clinic. Bandage scissors, which remove surgical or wound dressings, have a protective blunt tip to prevent injury to the patient. Mini Serial Cast Cutter Scissors (North Coast Medical), designed to remove digit casts, are essential when using serial casting techniques for digit flexion contractures (Fig. 5–3C). They provide a safe way to remove a finger cast effectively and without risk of cutting the skin. Joyce Chen Scissors allow for precise trimming techniques (North Coast Medical).

Pliers

Pliers are important for various fabrication tasks, including bending wire for outriggers, embedding small components such as eyelets into warm thermoplastic material, setting speedy rivets in place, and holding components or adhesive hook to warm over a heat gun. Various types of pliers are available in a range of styles and sizes, although the most common are blunt- and needle-nose pliers. Having both types on hand in the clinic is essential to manipulate various components.

Hole Punches

A high-quality hole punch with a range of hole sizes is necessary for creating holes in soft materials for strapping or custom finger loops/slings and also for punching holes in hard thermoplastic materials for straps application, outriggers, rivets, and hinge components (Fig. 5–4). When the tubes on the tool grow dull, it becomes difficult to punch a hole; therefore, it is wise to buy a heavy-duty tool with replaceable tubes.

Hand Drills

Electric **hand drills**, such as the Dremel® (available with a cord or rechargeable battery pack), can be used to make

holes in an orthosis in locations that the traditional hole punch cannot reach, such as applying an elbow hinge to a humeral and/or forearm cuff (Fig. 5–5A). This prevents the potentially dangerous task of heating a sharp device, such as an awl, over a heat gun to make the hole. The drill can be used to add custom perforations to specific regions of an orthosis, which help prevent skin maceration or rash caused by excess perspiration. Slits can also be drilled into thermoplastic materials to allow for custom strapping of individual digits (Fig. 5–5B,C).

Wire Cutters and Benders

Wire cutters and benders provide a way to customize an outrigger for specific anatomical requirements (Fig. 5–6). When component kits are not available or appropriate for a patient, the therapist must fabricate the orthosis from

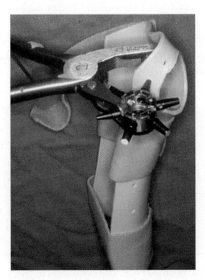

FIGURE 5–4 A hole punch is needed to prepare material for a rivet.

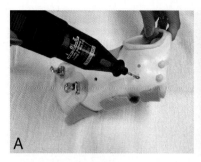
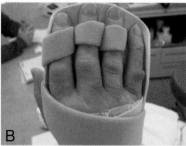
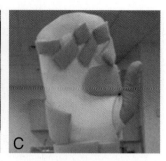

FIGURE 5–5 Dremel® used to **(A)** create a hole in this mobilization orthosis and **(B and C)** cut slits in material to allow for customization of strapping system.

scratch, using outrigger wire and ingenuity to create the desired effect. By bending the wire, the therapist can create a customized orthosis to accommodate a difficult anatomical configuration or situation, for example, fabricating over postsurgical dressings, wounds, casts, or external pins or fixators.

Low-Temperature Thermoplastic Orthotic Materials

Numerous types of **low-temperature thermoplastic orthotic materials** are available through rehabilitation vendors (AliMed, 2012; Chesapeake Medical Products, 2012; DanMic Global, 2012; DeRoyal Industries, 2012; North Coast Medical, 2012; Orfit Industries America, 2011; Patterson Medical, 2013; see Table 5–1 for contact information). Many therapists are justifiably confused about how to choose the right material for a specific orthosis. Unfortunately, there is no easy answer. Therapists must use their clinical knowledge and experience when making these decisions. Often, sorting through the options is just a matter of learning more about the products and not being afraid to try different options. During the planning stage, consider which types of materials have the best handling and physical features for that particular orthotic application. The key handling characteristics include resistance to stretch and memory. The important

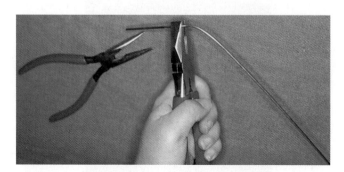

FIGURE 5–6 Blunt-nosed pliers help bend wires to create homemade outriggers.

TABLE 5–1
Distributors of Thermoplastic Materials

AliMed
297 High Street, Dedham, MA 02026
Phone: 800-225-2610
Fax: 800-437-2966
www.alimed.com

Chesapeake Medical Products
9629 Philadelphia Road, Suite 110, Baltimore, MD 21237
Phone: 888-560-2674
Fax: 410-574-9349
www.chesapeakemedical.com

DanMic Global
2188 Vizcaya Circle, Campbell, CA 95008
Phone: 408-626-0153
Fax: 408-628-4731
www.danmicglobal.com

DeRoyal Industries
200 DeBusk Lane, Powell, TN 37849
Phone: 800-251-9864
Fax: 800-543-2182
www.deroyal.com

North Coast Medical
18305 Sutter Blvd, Morgan Hill, CA 95037
Phone: 800-821-9319
Fax: 877-213-9300
www.ncmedical.com

Orfit Industries America
350 Jericho Turnpike, Suite 101, Jericho, NY 11753
Phone: 888-673-4887
Fax: 877-935-8505
www.orfit.com

Patterson Medical
28100 Torch Parkway, Suite 700, Warrenville, IL 60555
Phone: 800-323-5547
Fax: 800-547-4333
www.pattersonmedical.com

physical qualities consist of bondability, thickness, and perforations/colors. Assessing these factors in advance will improve the ability of the orthosis to meet that particular patient's needs.

A single type of material is not suitable for all orthoses or for all patients; there are many factors that must be taken into account when it comes to selecting the appropriate material. Therapists must recognize each material's unique characteristics (e.g., conformability and resistance to stretch) and understand the desired function of the orthosis in terms of the required rigidity and ventilation. In addition, they need to appreciate the particular nuances of each patient in terms of diagnosis, compliance, and age as well as recognize the limitation of their own fabrication skills and experience.

The novice therapist should develop a comfort level with a few types of materials before venturing on to others. The more experienced therapist who is comfortable using only a few types of materials, however, should broaden his or her selection choices by experimenting with other available materials. Expanding material options ultimately benefits the patients. Remember, however, that material selection may also be limited by other factors, including availability, budgetary constraints, and physician preferences.

To help the therapist begin to understand the multitude of orthotic material options, the following sections introduce the terms used to describe the materials' characteristics (i.e., drapability and resistance to stretch). Later sections discuss the general categories of orthotic materials (i.e., plastic and rubber-like). Specific brand name materials are not examined in depth because the availability of materials often changes; refer to manufacturers' catalogs and Web sites for current availability. If the therapist understands the particular characteristics and general categories of orthotic materials, he or she should be able to select the correct one from almost any vendor.

Some distributors describe a material's conformability, whereas others label this same factor as drapability or moldability. This can be confusing for a therapist who is trying to decide which material to use. The two largest companies that offer thermoplastic materials, North Coast Medical and Patterson Medical, both describe their thermoplastic product line in relation to the resistance to stretch, allowing for some comparison between their products. It can be more challenging to relate the smaller company's products because there is variability with the descriptive terms used. The following sections simplify the nomenclature as much as possible and present broad concepts and key points to aid the selection of a particular orthotic material.

Handling Characteristics

Conformability and Resistance to Stretch

To meet the requirements of a specific patient, the therapist must choose a material with the optimal conformability and resistance to stretch for that particular orthosis.

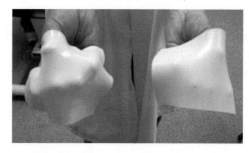

FIGURE 5–7 Demonstration of resistance to stretch: material on left with least resistance to stretch, and material on right with maximal resistance to stretch—notice difference in conformability.

Conformability or **drape** is the degree to which a heated material is able to mold well and produce an intimate fit that encompasses the contours and irregularities of the body part (North Coast Medical, 2012; Patterson Medical, 2013). **Resistance to stretch** is the degree to which a heated material is able to counteract being stretched or pulled, giving the therapist valuable information on how much handling the material can tolerate (North Coast Medical, 2012; Patterson Medical, 2013). Resistance to stretch is generally inversely related to the degree of conformability (Breger Lee & Buford, 1992). Ranging from minimum to maximum, thermoplastics can be sorted on a continuum of resistance to stretch (Fig. 5–7). To demonstrate this property, thoroughly heat a small piece of material in water and try to pull it apart. Resistance to stretch determines the degree of conformability. The more resistance to stretch, the less conformable the material will be when applied; less resistance to stretch results in more conformability and contouring during application. Refer to Table 5–2 for more information on how thermoplastic materials from various companies are organized on a continuum of resistance to stretch.

HIGH CONFORMABILITY/LOW RESISTANCE TO STRETCH

- Requires only light handling during the molding process to achieve a precisely formed orthosis
- Best used when gravity can assist in the orthotic fabrication process (Fig. 5–8)
- Often the material of choice for the skilled therapist because little handling is needed during the molding process
- Recommended when the patient is best approached with minimal handling (i.e., the patient who is postsurgical, extremely painful, or arthritic)
- Recommended for smaller orthoses (i.e., finger and hand) because the therapist can achieve a precise fit, maximizing patient comfort and preventing orthosis migration

LOW CONFORMABILITY/HIGH RESISTANCE TO STRETCH

- Requires firm handling during the molding process to obtain a well-conformed orthosis
- Can be used when the orthosis cannot be formed with the assistance of gravity

CHAPTER 5

TABLE 5–2

Thermoplastic Materials

Company Name			Resistance to Stretch		
	Minimum		**Moderate**		**Maximal**
AliMed	Multiform™		Multiform™ Clear Elastic		
Chesapeake	Excel™		Infinity™		FiberForm® Stiff
			FiberForm® Soft		Marque-Easy™
			Rebound™		
			Colours™		
DanMic Global	Danmic Aqua™				Danmic Ortho™
DeRoyal	LMB Drape™		LMB Blend™		
North Coast Medical	Clinic®	Encore™	Vanilla	Omega™ Max	Omega™ Plus
		Preferred®	Spectrum	Solaris	
			Prism™		
Orfit	Orfit® Drape		Orfit® NS Soft		Orfit® NS Stiff
			Orfit® Natural NS		Bluelight™
			Orfit® Colors™ NS		Orfit® Ortho
			Orfit® Classic Soft		Orfit® Classic Stiff
			Orfilight™		Orfibrace™
			Soft-Fit® NS		
			Orfit® Ease		
Patterson Medical	Polyform®		Polyflex II®		Ezeform®
			Kay-Splint II®		
			Orthoplast® II		
	Aquaplast® ProDrape-T™		Aquaplast®-T		Aquaplast®-T Resilient
			Aquaplast® Original		Aquaplast® Original Resilient
			Aquaplast® Watercolors™		Synergy®
			TailorSplint™		San-Splint®
			Kay-Splint III®		Orthoplast®

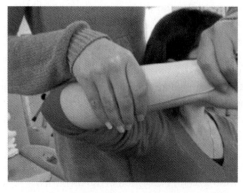

FIGURE 5–8 A forearm-based ulnar wrist orthosis is molded with the assistance of gravity.

- Comfortable for the novice therapist, who may feel more in control with a hands-on approach
- Circumferential wraps may be used to aid in the molding process when fabricating without an assistant, molding against gravity, or applying material to a large area. Wrapping too tightly may cause the orthotic borders to dig and results in skin irritation (Fig 5–9)
- Recommended for larger orthoses (i.e., forearm, elbow, and shoulder) for which an intimate fit is not crucial and a greater degree of control may be needed

Memory

Memory is the degree to which a material is able to return to its original shape once molded and then reheated (DeRoyal

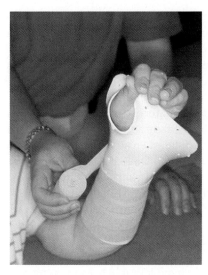

FIGURE 5–9 A forearm-based wrist orthosis is molded with a proximal wrap to allow hands-on positioning distally.

Industries, 2012; North Coast Medical, 2012; Patterson Medical, 2013). This quality ranges from 100% to 0% (no) memory (Fig. 5–10A,B).

HIGH-MEMORY MATERIAL

- Recommended when fabricating an orthosis that will require frequent remolding (i.e., a serial static orthosis); once the material is reheated, it tends to return to the shape of the original pattern.
- Cost-efficient to remold an existing orthosis instead of making a new one to accommodate for any change in tissue status.

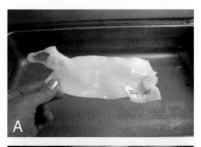

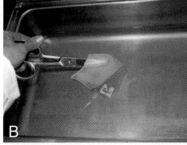

FIGURE 5–10 Demonstration of material memory: material was heated and stretched out (**A**), then reheated and shrunk back to original shape (**B**).

- Recommended for novice therapists; they can place the material back in the water and start over if a mistake is made during the molding process.
- Do not remove the molded orthosis from the body part until it is completely set or it will return to its original shape. This may alter the final fit of the orthosis, which is especially consequential when the material is wrapped circumferentially, as in a thumb immobilization orthosis. If the material is removed too soon, shrinking can occur and the patient may not be able to don the orthosis after setting is complete.
- Be careful when using a heat gun for spot heating; ridges can form, which may adversely affect the comfort and fit of the orthosis.

Rigidity

Rigidity is the ultimate stiffness or strength of a material or the degree to which a molded orthosis is able to resist deformation when external forces are applied (DeRoyal Industries, 2012; North Coast Medical, 2012). This quality ranges from highly rigid to highly flexible (Fig. 5–11).

- High-rigidity materials are recommended when the potential forces placed on the orthosis will be significant (i.e., a hand orthosis for a construction worker who applies excessive force to the hands).
- Thicker materials ($^1/_8''$) are more rigid than thinner materials ($^1/_{16}''$).
- Overstretching during the fabrication process creates weakened areas in the orthosis, which may decrease rigidity.
- Specific diagnoses (i.e., metacarpal fractures) require more rigid materials to support the healing structures.
- A circumferential design provides a more rigid support than a volar or dorsal approach even if the material is thin.

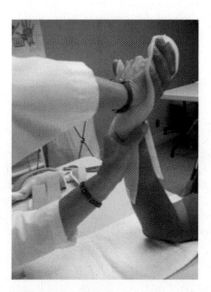

FIGURE 5–11 When fabricating an orthosis that needs to withstand potentially high forces, such as this serial static wrist and digit mobilization orthosis, choose a material that is rigid (thick and solid).

Bonding

Bonding is the ability of a material to adhere to itself once heated (DeRoyal Industries, 2012; North Coast Medical, 2012; Patterson Medical, 2013). Bondability refers to the presence of coating, which acts as a barrier to prevent unwanted adherence. Some materials are available with or without this coating—be sure to read the specific description before placing an order. If there is "mystery material" in your clinic, consider experimenting with small pieces to determine whether a coating is present and label accordingly. When in doubt, assume there is no coating and be cautious with overlapping using techniques described in the following text to prevent inadvertent sticking. Some manufacturers offer specific hints for best handling their materials, such as Orfit products. To decrease surface tackiness and improve handling ability, they recommend rubbing talcum powder on the surface of the thermoplastic prior to heating and adding liquid soap to the heating pan water.

- Coated thermoplastic does not bond to itself unless overheated, overstretched, scratched, or treated with solvent.
- Coated material does not bond to itself when heated. For example, this helps when fabricating thumb orthoses, allowing the therapist to create a trap door to ease removal (Fig. 5–12A).
- Coated material also allows for temporary bonding when two heated pieces are overlapped, which can assist with the fabrication process. Once the material has cooled completely, this area can easily pop apart as long as the material was not overstretched (Fig. 5–12B).
- Coated material has a reduced tendency to adhere to the patient's skin, hair, and wound dressings. It is generally easier to clean as well.
- Coated material is easier to clean than noncoated material because it is less porous; this is especially helpful for patients who require long-term orthosis use.

- Do not overstretch coated material; this weakens the coating and may cause the material to adhere to itself.
- The coating may be removed with a solvent or by aggressively scratching the surface with an emery board/sandpaper or awl/scissors if adherence to another piece of material is required.
- Uncoated material adheres to itself when both areas are heated fully and pressed together, which is especially helpful when attaching outriggers or when using an extra piece of material to reinforce a particular area of the orthosis. Using a heat gun to make the thermoplastic slightly tacky can help ensure a strong bond.
- Use a stockinette liner over the dressing when molding with uncoated material to prevent sticking to dressings and superficial skin.
- When coated material is unavailable, use a wet paper towel or hand lotion between two pieces of uncoated material to prevent adherence (Fig. 5–12C).

Heating and Working Times

Each material has an optimal heating temperature (ranging from 140° to 170°F), **heating time** (ranging from 0.5 to 2 minutes), and **working time** (from 1 to 7 minutes). Specific information can be found in manufacturers' catalogs and literature that accompanies sheet material (AliMed, 2012; Chesapeake Medical Products, 2012; DeRoyal Industries, 2012; North Coast Medical; Orfit Industries America, 2011; Patterson Medical, 2013). The working time refers to the time in which the heated material can be molded onto the body part before the orthosis sets.

- All materials should be partially heated (for approximately 30 seconds) before the specific pattern is cut out. Material is heated partially when lifting the edge with scissors or spatula reveals moderate stiffness with slight bending. This partial heating can save the therapist's thumb from the forceful cutting of hard material.

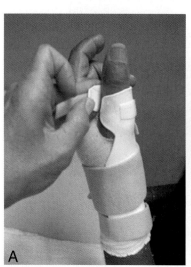
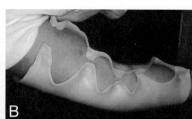
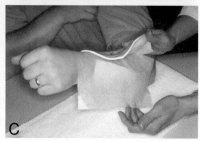

FIGURE 5–12 A, Coated material allows overlapped pieces to pop open, which can accommodate, for example, an enlarged thumb IP joint. **B,** A posterior elbow immobilization orthosis applied with the pinch-and-pop technique. The edges will be trimmed to form smooth borders anteriorly. **C,** A wet paper towel placed between uncoated materials prevents adherence.

- Some materials provide a self-sealing edge for a smooth finish after being cut while warm, preventing the need for edge finishing later.
- When making large orthoses, the novice therapist may want to hold one edge of the material while the other edge is partially heated for cutting; this allows the therapist to maintain control of the material at all times.
- Thin or highly perforated materials have a shorter working time; thick, solid materials have a longer working time.
- Elastic and rubber-like materials tend to have longer working times than plastic materials.
- Do not remove the material from the body part too soon or the shape and fit may be lost, causing buckling or ridges to form in the orthosis.
- Materials with longer working times are recommended for complex orthoses requiring multiple joints in specific positions, such as commonly encountered with neurologically involved patients.
- Materials with shorter working times are recommended for patients who are unable to hold a specific position for a long period (i.e., pediatric patients).
- Sometimes, it is necessary to hasten the setting time (i.e., for a patient who is in pain). Note that this cannot be done using material with memory because the final fit may be altered.
- Accelerate the cooling by wrapping the material with an elastic wrap that has been soaked in ice water or with a TheraBand® that has been stored in the freezer (Patterson Medical). Note that wrapping may cause irritation if it causes the edges to dig into the skin.
- Accelerate the cooling by using cold spray or by removing a partially set orthosis and placing it under cold running water. Note that the cold spray technique may irritate the skin or eyes, so do this away from the patient.
- Avoid overheating the material (leaving in water too long, placing in water too hot), which can alter its properties and lead to overstretching, thinning, and material fatigue, which in turn can decrease the rigidity of the completed orthosis.
- Always dry off any excess water on the material prior to applying to the body part.
- Before applying the material to the patient's body part, check the material's temperature against the therapist's skin.
- Be extra careful to avoid overheating or burning the skin of patients who have any sensory involvement including loss of sensation or skin hypersensitivity (commonly seen after cast removal). Use a stockinette over the body part to minimize heat.

Physical Characteristics

Thickness

Materials are available in several thicknesses, most commonly $^1/_{16}''$, $^3/_{32}''$, $^1/_{12}''$, $^1/_8''$, and $^3/_{16}''$ thick (Fig. 5–13)

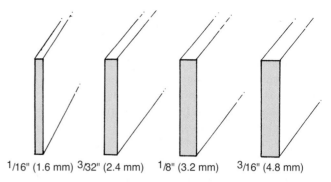

$^1/16''$ (1.6 mm) $^3/32''$ (2.4 mm) $^1/8''$ (3.2 mm) $^3/16''$ (4.8 mm)

FIGURE 5–13 Materials of different thicknesses.

(AliMed, 2012; DeRoyal Industries, 2012; North Coast Medical, 2012; Patterson Medical, 2013). Commonly, therapists get in the habit of using $^1/_8''$ material for all orthoses, but this is not always necessary. The therapist may choose a specific thickness based on the orthosis' function. In general, $^1/_8''$ is suitable for arm, forearm, elbow, and wrist orthoses; $^3/_{32}''$ and $^1/_{16}''$ are appropriate for hand-based and pediatric designs. To create the lightest and least bulky device, the therapist should choose the thinnest material possible that provides the required support and rigidity. Thicker materials tend to provide more rigid support. Thinner materials offer a less bulky, lighter weight alternative. When thin materials are used for circumferential orthoses, they can create adequate rigidity if the therapist takes advantage of contouring. For example, circumferential forearm fracture orthoses may be best created with $^3/_{32}''$ or $^1/_{16}''$ material instead of $^1/_8''$ material, which creates a bulky orthosis that can impede function. Thinner materials can be cut more easily, which can decrease the strain on the therapist's hands.

Perforations

Almost all thickness and types of material are available in **perforated** and **nonperforated** forms. The density of perforations can range from 1% to 42% (Fig. 5–14) (North Coast Medical, 2012; Patterson Medical, 2013). Perforated materials allow air exchange, which helps decrease the incidence of skin problems such as rash, excessive sweating, and/or maceration (Breger Lee & Buford, 1991, 1992). Orthoses fabricated from perforated materials are lighter in weight and also more flexible, which can make donning/doffing easier with circumferential designs.

The therapist must decide whether providing a lightweight orthosis with increased ventilation is worth the sacrifice in rigidity. This downside must be weighed carefully

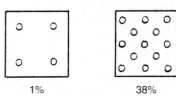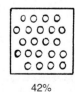

1%   38%   42%

FIGURE 5–14 Density of perforations.

to ensure that the orthosis provides an adequate amount of rigidity or support. For example, an orthosis to support a fracture requires a more rigid support than one applied for tendinitis. In most cases, a $^3/_{32}''$ lightly perforated material in a circumferential design can adequately support a distal radius fracture while allowing air exchange.

Because perforations help decrease the orthosis' weight, they may improve wear compliance. Extra perforated materials may need to be edged with extra-thin material to provide a smooth, reinforced border. Do not overstretch heated perforated materials because the holes elongate and the material may thin out unevenly.

Colors

Orthotic materials are available in an assortment of colors. Bright colors may help maximize compliance in a young patient or aid in a quick retrieval among bed linens in a nursing home. On the other hand, some patients may feel the colors draw unwanted attention to themselves and their condition. In these cases, skin tones are the more appropriate choice. Darker colors, such as black, help hide dirt and are best worn by patients who work in an industrial environment. Patterson Medical offers the Rolyan® Imprints® line, which includes patterns on one side of the thermoplastic to further allow customization of the orthosis (Fig. 5–15).

Coating

To decrease odors and microorganisms in orthoses used long term or with patients who sweat a lot, thermoplastics are available with antimicrobial built in (AM™ Built In, Patterson Medical). This added component can increase the

longevity of the orthosis and improve wear compliance. Note that the materials with this protective coating are slightly more resistant to stretch than regular version.

Categories

The most commonly used thermoplastic materials can be categorized in and described by the following terms: plastic, rubber or rubber-like, combination plastic and rubber-like, and elastic (Patterson Medical, 2013) (Fig. 5–16). These groupings help the therapist keep track of each type of material and its workable characteristics. Refer to Table 5–1 for current thermoplastic material selections. Thermoplastic materials are traditionally sold in 18″ by 24″ sheets; however, some manufacturers now sell materials in smaller sheets, allowing for easier storage and less cutting in the clinic. Label the thermoplastic sheets upon delivery and as the sheet is being cut down so there is no question in the future what type of material it is. Otherwise, as the material gets used, it may be confusing what types of material are left over.

Plastic

Plastic materials are generally highly conformable and have minimal resistance to stretch (e.g., Polyform and Multiform) (AliMed, 2012; Berger Lee & Buford, 1992; DeRoyal Industries, 2012; North Coast Medical, 2012; Patterson Medical, 2013). These materials are best used with gravity's assistance and by an experienced therapist because the material can be challenging to control. The ability to make minor adjustments in an orthotic pattern by stretching the material can help ensure a better fit. Small orthoses requiring a well-molded precise fit are best made with these materials. Plastic materials contour nicely when molding over pins or bony prominences (Fig. 5–16).

The therapist may leave fingerprints in the material if he or she uses a too aggressive hands-on approach during the

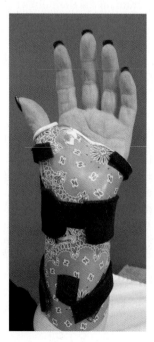

FIGURE 5–15 Wrist and thumb immobilization orthosis fabricated using patterned material: Rolyan® Imprints® Blue Bandana Polyform® (Patterson Medical).

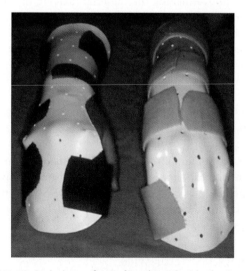

FIGURE 5–16 An intimate fit can be achieved with plastic materials (**right**); note the detail of the contours obtained across the dorsum of the MCP joints. Rubber-like materials tend to mold to the shape of the hand with less detail (**left**).

molding process. Gentle handling with smooth, light strokes is the best way to work with these materials. Overheating can make plastic materials too soft, leading to overstretching and making them difficult to control. To minimize overstretching, handle these materials horizontally on pan netting rather than vertically. These are not suggested for novice therapists because of the material's high degree of conformability.

Rubber or Rubber-Like

Rubber or **rubber-like materials** offer a good degree of control at the expense of conformability owing to their high resistance to stretch (i.e., Rolyan® Ezeform®, Patterson Medical; Omega™ Plus, North Coast Medical). These materials do not drape and contour as well as plastic materials; thus, the final fit is sometimes less detailed (Fig. 5–16). Larger orthoses that do not require an intimate fit, such as a wrist/hand immobilization orthosis worn over wound dressings, are best made with these materials. Rubber materials offer a significant degree of control with minimal stretching or fingerprinting. Novice therapists may find these materials easy to work with because they are forgiving and tolerate repeated handling and manipulation; firm handling is required to achieve a contoured fit. Cut rubber-like materials when still slightly warm to obtain extremely smooth edges.

Combination Plastic and Rubber-Like

Perhaps the most versatile fabrication products are those with moderate resistance to stretch or those in the middle of the continuum; **combination plastic and rubber-like materials** tend to offer the best of both worlds in terms of conformity and stretch (i.e., Rolyan® TailorSplint™, Patterson Medical; Preferred®, North Coast Medical). These "blended" materials can be used for virtually all types of orthoses and are an excellent choice for a multi-use material in the clinic. These materials produce an orthosis with a well-molded fit while allowing the therapist some degree of control during the molding process. Many therapists find these materials to be useful for a wide variety of orthoses, including forearm- and hand-based designs (large and small). The specific characteristics depend on the proportions of rubber and plastic in the thermoplastic base.

Elastic

All **elastic materials** have some amount of memory with varying degrees of resistance to stretch (i.e., Aquaplast®, Patterson Medical; Prism™, North Coast Medical; and Orfit® products, Patterson Medical & North Coast Medical) (Fig. 5–12A). As noted earlier, this characteristic is best used in situations in which there is a need for frequent remolding to accommodate for changes in tissue. Some of these materials are available uncoated, which allows them to adhere to the body part; this may help in achieving a precise, intimate fit by acting as a second pair of hands. The degree of conformability and stretch depends on the specific material's chemical composition.

When pinched together lightly, coated elastic materials can provide a temporary bond that can be popped apart once the orthosis is set. This technique can be helpful when fabricating without the assistance of gravity (Fig. 5–12B). It is easy to determine when most elastic materials are heated fully because they turn transparent (except for some colored elastic materials, which turn opaque). This transparency provides visualization of sites where potential irritation can occur and allows for accommodations of these hot spots during the molding process. Therapists generally deem these materials as quite versatile and use them successfully for a multitude of orthoses.

Elastic materials do have some disadvantages. If the molded orthosis is removed when the material is still slightly warm, the material will continue to set, causing further tightening or shrinking and altering the final fit. Obtaining a well-contoured orthosis with $^1/_8''$ material may be troublesome because of the material's tendency to shrink during its setup time. Elastic materials have a longer setup time than plastic materials and can be frustrating when time efficiency is an issue. In addition, the novice therapist may find it difficult to achieve a smooth edge with these materials. Accurate pattern creation, along with cutting the pattern out while the material is warm, can help therapist to achieve smoother edges.

Precut and Preformed Orthoses

Precut forms can help save time and money as well as decrease material waste. These precut forms come in various material types, thicknesses, perforation patterns, colors, and sizes to satisfy most orthotic fabrication needs (Fig. 5–17A). They are heat pan ready, avoiding the time needed to create and cut out patterns. In some instances, the precuts may not meet the needs of the therapists; they may not be their preferred pattern. Patterson Medical offers a Custom Pre-Cut Program; this is a cost- and time-saving option for therapists working in a busy hand clinic. The therapists can create their own precut form, customizing the shape, material type, thickness, and perforations. These forms are then given an item number and can be ordered in batches just as the catalog precuts are.

Rolyan® AquaForm™ Zippered Splints (Patterson Medical), thermoplastic precuts with a zipper sewn in for closure, provide the therapist with a valuable option for addressing a multitude of diagnoses (Fig. 5–17B,C). They are commonly used for fractures and as the base for a mobilization orthosis. Refer to Section II for more specific information including fabrication tips.

The other options include preformed orthoses (prefabricated into a specific shape and size); these are offered in a wide range of orthosis types, sizes, and materials (Fig. 5–17D). Once heated, most of these can be modified to provide a custom fit. This is a great option for the therapists challenged with fabricating general orthoses in a setting where they do not have either the skills or time to fabricate the orthosis from scratch (i.e., acute care or rehabilitation setting).

Other

Thermoplastics in pellet form are available; these can be used for adaptations of tools and utensils improving function with activities of daily living (Fig. 5–18A). Simply soften

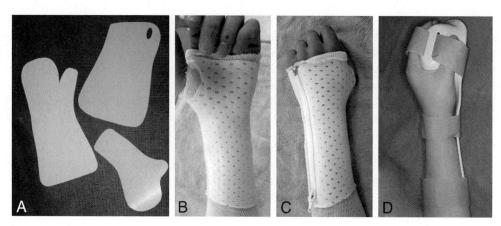

FIGURE 5–17 A, Precut orthosis forms. **B and C,** Rolyan® AquaForm™ Zippered Wrist Splint (Patterson Medical). **D,** Preformed Rolyan® Neutral Position Hand Splint (Patterson Medical).

them in a cup of hot water and then mold around the item to form a handle. Other sheet material choices currently available include lined materials (i.e., ProPlast, Patterson Medical; Trio™ Composite Thermoplastic, North Coast Medical) (Fig. 5–18B), mesh-type thermoplastic materials (i.e., X-Lite®, Patterson Medical) (Fig. 5–18C), and neoprene for soft restrictive orthoses (see Chapter 14 on "Neoprene Orthoses")

(Fig. 5–18D). Casting techniques provide an option for some forms of orthotic intervention. Casts require the use of plaster of paris, fiberglass, Delta-Cast® Casting Tape (BSN medical Inc.), QuickCast 2 (Patterson Medical), and Orficast™ (North Coast Medical) materials (see Chapter 12 on "Casting as an Alternative to Thermoplastics") (Fig. 5–18E) (Colditz, 2002). Various taping products are gaining popularity for

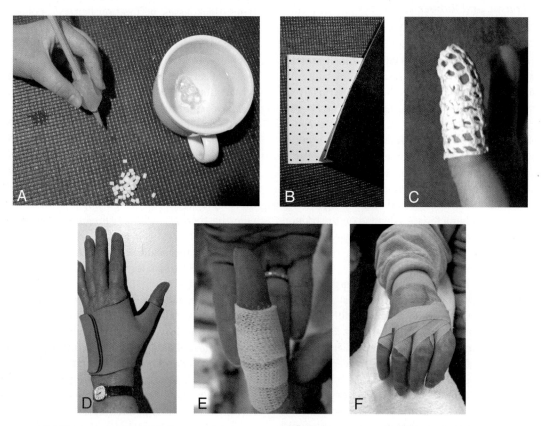

FIGURE 5–18 A, Thermo-Pellets™ used to form pencil grip (North Coast Medical). **B,** ProPlast in sheet form (Patterson Medical). **C,** X-Lite® used for this DIP orthosis (Patterson Medical). **D,** Custom neoprene carpometacarpal (CMC) restriction orthosis. **E,** QuickCast 2 to address PIP flexion contracture (Patterson Medical). **F,** Kinesio® Tex Tape used to minimize tendency for MCP joints to ulnarly deviate following MCP arthroplasty.

immobilizing or restricting a joint or body part, including the McConnell Taping method, elastic therapeutic taping (Kinesio® Tex Tape) (see Chapter 13 on "Taping Techniques") (Fig. 5–18F). As noted earlier, therapists must be diligent in keeping up with new materials and techniques.

Additional Equipment

Strapping Materials

Strapping is used to secure an orthosis to a body part. The proper application of straps is crucial to ensure the orthosis serves the intended purpose. Commonly, therapists focus on molding the thermoplastic material to the patient and obtaining a contoured fit. They tend to minimize the importance of strapping as it relates to proper orthosis fit. Careless use of straps can ultimately lead to an ineffective device. Like thermoplastic materials, numerous types of strapping systems are available. As therapists, we must challenge ourselves to look beyond the traditional **hook** and **loop** for specific situations. First, therapists must appreciate the mechanics of orthotic fabrication. The wider the strap, the better the force will be distributed. However, straps should not be so wide that they inhibit full motion. Narrow straps can potentially cause redness and irritation of the underlying soft tissue. When applying straps over bony regions, consider using foam to further distribute the pressure. Be mindful to maximize the mechanical advantage of the orthosis. Use the length of the orthosis when fastening the straps. You can mold the orthosis optimally, yet if the strapping is not secured at the proximal and distal edges, the best possible mechanics may never be realized.

The most common method to secure an orthosis to a body part is with hook-and-loop straps. Velcro® is the most familiar brand name; however, other versions are available. Usually, the adhesive-backed hook strip is attached to the orthosis and the loop strip is wrapped around the body part. Hook-and-loop straps are available in several widths ($^1/_2''$ to $2''$) and colors. Precut strapping is convenient, reducing waste and speeding up the fabrication process. Adhesive-backed hook strips are available in precut lengths, which can eliminate sticky scissors. Many patients, especially children, enjoy choosing their own strap colors, and involving the patient can help maximize compliance. Spot heating the adhesive-backed hook before applying it to the orthosis increases adherence and provides a firm attachment.

When a hook strip is used to secure a circumferential loop strap, the therapist must decide whether to use one or two pieces of hook strip (Fig. 5–19). A disadvantage of using two smaller pieces is the increased risk of detachment with repeated donning and doffing of the orthosis. Two pieces, however, may better accommodate a bulky forearm, as when applying straps proximally. An advantage of one longer strip of hook material is the increased surface area of attachment,

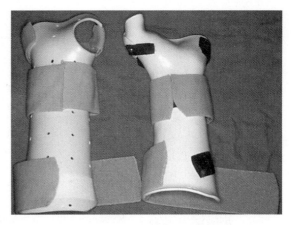

FIGURE 5–19 Methods of applying adhesive-backed hook strips to a wrist orthosis. Using two separate strips proximally as seen on the right prevents any hook from remaining uncovered and catching on clothing.

lowering the chance that the strap will come off the orthosis. However, this method requires more hook-and-loop material, which can be costly. Remember to allow enough loop strip to cover the hook strip fully; otherwise, the hook strip tends to stick to clothing and bedding. Round the edges of the loop strip to prevent snagging and inadvertent detachment on clothing; in addition, rounded edges are more aesthetically pleasing.

In addition to the conventional hook-and-loop material, therapists can use an elasticized loop to secure the orthosis firmly to the patient. Soft foam and neoprene straps are available; they may be more comfortable against the skin than traditional hook-and-loop tape. These materials conform nicely to the contours of the extremity and allow for some fluctuations owing to edema. These straps are not as durable as hook-and-loop material and thus may increase the cost of an orthosis. In specific situations, using these more expensive straps may be the best choice. Specialized strapping may be beneficial in terms of comfort and function. For example, when fabricating an orthosis for a patient with arthritis, soft strapping such as Rolyan® SoftStrap® Strapping Material (Patterson Medical) may be the optimal choice (Fig. 5–20A). Be aware that these materials have less "repetitions" than traditional loops; just flip the strap over to double the use. For patients using the orthosis during functional use, it may be beneficial to choose an elasticized loop such as RStretch™ (Patterson Medical) or a neoprene strap (Fig. 5–20B). These stretchable straps accommodate muscle contraction/relaxation better than stiffer loop material. When applying small finger orthoses, consider RThin™ (Patterson Medical) loop material because its low profile minimizes bulk between the digits (Fig. 5–20C).

Many other strapping systems exist, including hook-and-loop strips combined on one strap. This material works well for patients with limited use of an extremity. For the pediatric population, systems are available that provide the extra strength needed to secure orthoses adequately to

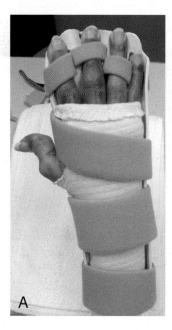

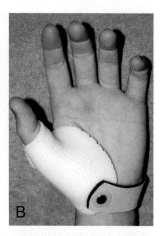

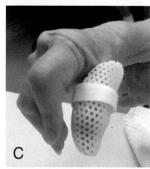

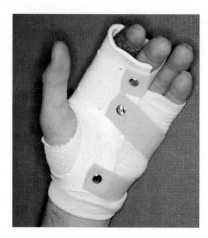

FIGURE 5–21 This hand orthosis includes rivets to secure the straps volarly.

FIGURE 5–20 **A,** Rolyan® SoftStrap® used to secure digits in this wrist and hand immobilization orthosis used after extensor tenosynovectomy. **B,** Neoprene strap used to accommodate muscle movement in this MP immobilization orthosis during functional use. **C,** Thin loop strapping used for a thumb orthosis.

active children (i.e., Dual-Lock® Fastening System, Patterson Medical). D-rings and buckles are options for securing straps that need to control the tension; these are especially beneficial for circumferential orthoses used as fracture bracing.

A rivet can be used to secure one end of the strap permanently to a small area of the orthosis where an adhesive-backed hook strip would be inefficient. A hole punch and blunt-nosed pliers are all that is needed to set these rivets. Riveting one end may also help keep patients (pediatric, geriatric) from losing their straps (Fig. 5–21). Be sure to cover the underside of the rivet with a small piece of lining material or tape to protect the skin; rusting can occur as a result of excessive moisture.

Therapists must be creative when designing strapping systems for an orthosis, taking into account each patient's unique needs. For example, a patient with severe arthritis may benefit from specialized loops on the straps to ease donning and doffing of the orthosis and the strategic placement of the straps to aid in improving joint alignment. Patient education regarding the proper application of straps is imperative. Taking a photo with a cell phone of the orthosis in place can help with proper application later. Have patients don and doff the orthosis in the clinic to be sure they are confident in proper placement of the straps. The adhesive hook

should act as a "road map" for proper placement of loop material. Numbering of the straps may be helpful. Patients should be aware of potential problems associated with improper application such as neurovascular compromise and bony/soft tissue irritation. The strapping should be snug enough to hold the orthosis in place but not so tight it causes tissue irritation. If there is an issue of significant edema, and the potential for "window edema" between the straps is present, perhaps using a circumferential wrap may be beneficial while the edema subsides. Proper orthotic strapping is commonly overshadowed by the focus on thermoplastic selection and the molding process itself. Strapping selection is a crucial step in the orthotic fabrication process and can assist in maximizing the effectiveness and final outcome. There are multiple options available, and we need to use critical thinking to challenge ourselves to come up with the optimal strapping solution.

Helpful hints in the form of Clinical and Pattern Pearls are provided throughout Section II to highlight where and why straps should be placed in specific areas. Keep the following general principles in mind when considering where to place straps on an orthosis.

- Wider straps offer better force distribution than narrow ones (Bell-Krotoski & Breger-Stanton, 2011; Brand & Hollister, 1999; Fess, Gettle, Philips, & Janson, 2005). Increasing the area of pressure contact helps prevent soft tissue irritation. However, straps should not be so wide that they impair the range of motion at unaffected joints.
- Use self-adhesive foam in conjunction with the strap to prevent uneven pressure distribution and tenderness at bony regions (Fig. 5–22A). Uneven pressure can result from placing a strap across a bony area, such as the ulnar styloid process.
- To make the straps sit flush against the skin, they must be placed at an angle to accommodate the shape of the body part. For example, when applying straps to a forearm, the therapist must take into account the

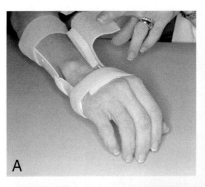
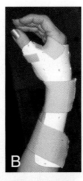
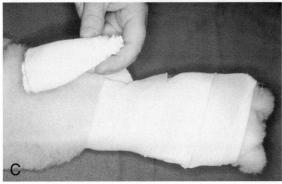

FIGURE 5–22 **A,** Foam placed across the wrist strap can prevent irritation of bony prominences. **B,** Notice angle of proximal strap to accommodate the bulk of the forearm musculature. **C,** A bias-cut wrap secures resting support for a patient with severe edema. The lining of Dacron batting helps maintain a dry environment within the orthosis.

provides a more even pressure distribution across the entire area. When the edema subsides, the wrap can be replaced with traditional hook-and-loop strips.

- Soft straps can be fringed to improve pressure distribution, increase comfort, and aid in edema control. Patients should always be told to watch for signs of swelling (especially distal to and between straps), vascular compromise, sensory changes, and improper fit. They should be instructed to loosen the straps appropriately.
- As a cost-saving measure, consider purchasing 1″ adhesive hook, which should meet all of your fabrication needs. Patients appreciate that this narrow width allows full hook coverage, preventing the hook from sticking to clothes and bedding.
- To save time, keep on hand a supply of precut hook tabs in the most common lengths.
- To minimize ordering multiple widths, consider keeping 2″ loop strapping in stock and cut it down as needed.
- Keep all scraps of loop material for future use. This will allow for full use of all loop material.
- Ordering multiple colors can allow for ultimate orthosis customization and could aid in orthotic wear compliance.

Lining and Padding Materials

Occasionally, therapists find it beneficial to line the inside of an orthosis partially or completely with a **lining material** to improve comfort, especially for older patients with thin, sensitive skin that may get irritated by direct contact with the thermoplastic (Fig. 5–23A,B). Be judicious with adhering permanent linings within an orthosis because they cannot be washed. Linings often become malodorous and discolored from the perspiration that inevitably occurs when airflow is prevented. Skin integrity can be compromised when subjected to a prolonged moist environment; rashes, macerations, or actual skin breakdown may be seen. Adhesive-backed liners are difficult to remove and frequent changes can be frustrating and expensive. Padding and lining materials are available in various thickness and textures; keeping a few in the clinic's inventory should be sufficient.

Orthotic liners may be permanent (adhesive on one side) or removable (completely separate from the orthosis itself). With most orthoses, use a removable liner, which can be washed to avoid potential hygiene issues that could become problematic with the more permanent types. There are some specific clinical situations when permanently applying a liner within the orthosis may improve the comfort and, likely, the compliance with a wearing schedule. In these cases, choosing a product that can be easily removed and replaced (low tack) would be advantageous. Possible hygiene issues such as excessive moisture (caused by sweating, wound exudates, etc.) or sloughing

tapered shape of the body part. This is especially applicable when securing an orthosis on a patient with large forearms (Fig. 5–22B).

- Straps should be tight enough to hold the orthosis securely in place but not so tight that circulation is impaired. Pinching the skin against the borders can irritate superficial sensory nerves and should be avoided. Educating the patient regarding signs of neurovascular compromise is imperative.
- Remember to maximize the mechanical advantage of an orthosis by securing straps in specific areas (Brand & Hollister, 1999; Fess et al., 2005). For example, the proximal strap on a wrist support should be placed as close to the proximal edge as possible and the middle strap should be attached just proximal to the axis of the immobilized wrist joint to prevent the patient from flexing out of the orthosis.
- To make the orthosis less likely to be removed by a questionably compliant patient, use a circumferential bandage to secure the device.
- If the straps have caused window edema (swelling between the straps), try applying a bias-cut wrap (commercially available nonelasticized material cut on the bias) from distal to proximal as well as elevation to decrease swelling (Fig. 5–22C). This technique

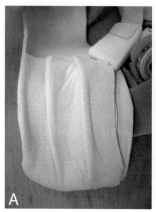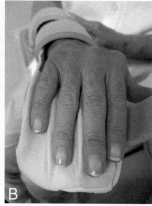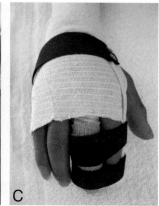

FIGURE 5–23 **A and B,** Adhesive foam lining is used to form individual troughs so that the fingers can rest within them. **C,** Notice use of removable elasticized sleeve for hand/forearm and digit wrap to address edema.

of skin can be avoided by changing the liner frequently. Choosing a liner that is "closed cell" (impenetrable by liquid and easy to clean but does not permit air exchange) versus "open cell" (allows the absorption of liquid) can provide an environment that is easily cleansed. Open-cell products are somewhat breathable, absorbing any excess moisture, which could create a potentially unhealthy environment for the affected hand. There are materials that have a permanently attached liner within the thermoplastic such as foam in Rolyan® AirThru™ (Patterson Medical). Excessive moisture is commonly an issue when patients need to wear an orthosis full time in warm, humid climates. Helpful options include using a perforated material to allow increased ventilation or using a thin layer of polyester quilting batting (available in craft stores) between the skin and thermoplastic. Removable polyester (Dacron) batting effectively wicks the moisture away from the skin (Fig. 5–22C). Do not use cotton batting, which allows the wetness to remain against the skin. The batting should be changed at least daily to prevent skin problems.

In terms of removable products, cotton stockinette is the most common and economical product available. These can be removed, washed, and reused, providing a suitable interface between the skin and orthosis. If the patient has a problem with excessive moisture within the orthosis, polypropylene stockinette is an option; it has a wicking action to keep the area dry. For patients with edema, consider providing an elastic sleeve such as TubiGrip™ or SurgiGrip®; for those requiring padding, consider TubiPad® (Fig. 5–23C) (Patterson Medical). For digit orthoses, cotton stockinette (SurgiTube®) or elasticized wraps (Coban™ or CoFlex®) can be used as a liner; just remember to apply the product to the area prior to molding to allow for extra room within the orthotic design (Patterson Medical). For patients who require long-term use of an orthosis or request a thicker liner, the durable Terry-Net™ liner may be the best option (Patterson Medical). Liners that include the

thumb are available for application beneath thumb orthoses. If a sewing machine is accessible in the clinic, thumb components can be sewn into stockinette liners. Instruct patients to change the liner daily, wash by hand, and air dry.

Use orthotic padding material sparingly, if at all. Remember, a well-molded, properly fitting orthosis does not generally need padding. There is no substitute for a well-molded orthosis; therefore, it is not appropriate to pad to improve the fit after the molding process. Adding padding after fabrication alters the orthosis fit and can create shear and compression stresses to adjacent areas (Brand & Holister, 1999; Fess et al., 2005). The increased bulk over the padded area may cause an increase in pressure. On the other hand, padding in orthoses can be beneficial if used correctly. Padding can be valuable over areas where excessive pressure may create potential "hot spots" such as bony prominences or superficial nerves. When applying padding to the thermoplastic, anticipate the potential trouble areas and prepad that region (Fig. 5–24A). Mold the thermoplastic directly over this padding and finish by inverting the padding back into the formed orthosis. If a patient returns to the clinic with complaints of a pressure point, avoid applying padding after the molding process; this can cause a shifting of the orthosis, producing a different pressure point in another region. Instead, prepad the irritated area and heat/remold the entire orthosis. When choosing padding for an orthosis, therapists must consider the thickness as well as the texture. Generally, choose a padding that is as thin as possible but still meets the needs of the patient to protect the area. As an alternative to foam-based products, therapists may find gel padding effective in protecting a sensitive area, especially if there is a scar present (Fig. 5–24B). Padding can be applied not only on the thermoplastic segment of the orthosis but to the strapping system as well. This can be especially helpful when straps traverse over one of those potential "hot spots."

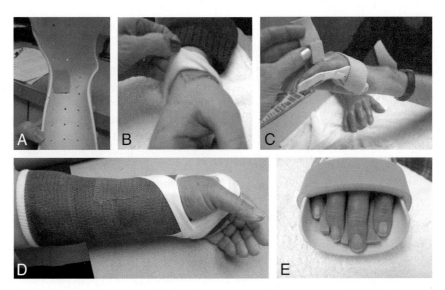

FIGURE 5–24 **A,** The padding was placed prior to molding this dorsal wrist and hand orthosis to minimize pressure at the distal ulna. **B,** Gel used to protect hypersensitive radial sensory nerve. **C,** Foam adhered to strapping will encourage optimal PIP joint position in extension. **D,** Microfoam™ Tape used to line this wrist cast. **E,** Foam cut into triangles adhered to orthosis for separating digits for a patient with arthritis to wear at night.

Padding incorporated into straps at specific areas can be used to provide gentle feedback to optimally position joints (Fig. 5–24C). This is particularly helpful when immobilizing in the antideformity position: metacarpophalangeal (MCP) joint flexion/proximal interphalangeal (PIP) joint extension. Padding over the PIP joints can aid in maintaining this position. Padding may help prevent or gently stretch joint contractures by imparting a gentle stretch to the tissue: just be sure that the diagnosis allows for this type of stress on the tissue. Alternative products that are helpful in the clinic include Microfoam™ Tape and hook-receptive neoprene (Patterson Medical). Microfoam™ Tape is a low-tack foam tape that can be applied to pad specific areas of an orthosis, very useful around the first web space (Fig. 5–24D). This tape has a nonskid quality that can be helpful in preventing orthosis migration: apply longitudinal strips within the orthosis. Neoprene can be used as an alternative to traditional padding materials. This soft and contouring material is comfortable against the skin: attach within an orthosis via hook or permanently bond to noncoated thermoplastics during the molding process. Foam pieces can also function as finger separators in resting orthoses (Fig. 5–24E).

Scar management techniques can be incorporated directly into the orthotic design by employing the use of gel, Putty Elastomer™, or Otoform™ products (Patterson Medical). Gel is available in sheets or pads (Fig. 5–24B). Form the heated material over the scar and mold to allow for accommodation of the product within the confines of the orthosis (Fig. 5–25A,B). These products need to be reformed as the scar changes, at which time the orthosis must be remolded to adjust for this alteration in dimension. Using a thermoplastic material that is conducive to frequent reheating, such as one from the elastic group, is the best choice. Some materials on the market have a layer of gel laminated to the thermoplastic material, providing another means of scar management (Silon-STS®, Patterson Medical).

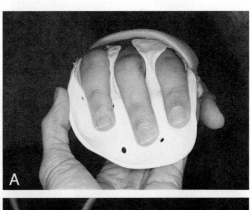

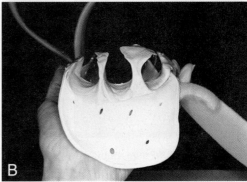

FIGURE 5–25 **A and B,** This volar orthosis has an incorporated scar mold for a patient with a contracted palmar scar.

Components

This section presents the orthotic components needed to fabricate a mobilization orthosis (dynamic and static progressive). The specific systems as well as fabrication instructions are discussed in Section II. Because there are frequent innovations in orthotic fabrication techniques and products, it is important to read current catalogs and journals to stay abreast of what is on the market.

Outrigger Systems

The outrigger portion of an orthosis is an extension from the orthotic base that acts as an anchor to apply a mobilizing force (Fig. 5–26A). **Outrigger systems** must be adjustable devices that allow the therapist to maintain the optimal 90° angle of pull. Each rehabilitation catalog offers numerous outrigger systems to meet specific therapy needs (AliMed, 2012; North Coast Medical, 2012; Orfit Industries America, 2011; Patterson Medical, 2013) (refer to Appendix A for a complete listing of vendors).

To determine which is the most appropriate option for a given patient, the therapist must carefully consider many factors: the therapist's preference, the patient's unique needs, and product availability. For example, when presented with a patient who needs a digit extension mobilization orthosis, the therapist must determine which design to use: hand or forearm based; single or multiple digits; high or low profile; custom or prefabricated; and static progressive, serial static, or dynamic (Austin, Slamet, Cameron, & Austin, 2004) (Fig. 5–26B). In general, the accessories for a specific system—line guides, pulleys, and proximal attachment devices—can be purchased separately to allow custom-fabricated orthoses.

When a commercial outrigger kit is not appropriate or available, the outrigger can be easily made from wire, rolled thermoplastic, or thermoplastic tubing (see Section II for details) (Fig. 5–26C,D). Copper or aluminum wire can be cut with pliers or snips and bent using a vice, pliers, or a bending bar. A small piece of perforated thermoplastic material can be molded to the frame to allow the line to glide through. Thermoplastic tubes can be easily shaped into outriggers after they have been softened in warm water. To attach a custom outrigger to the orthotic base, use a big enough piece of thermoplastic material to adequately cover the proximal

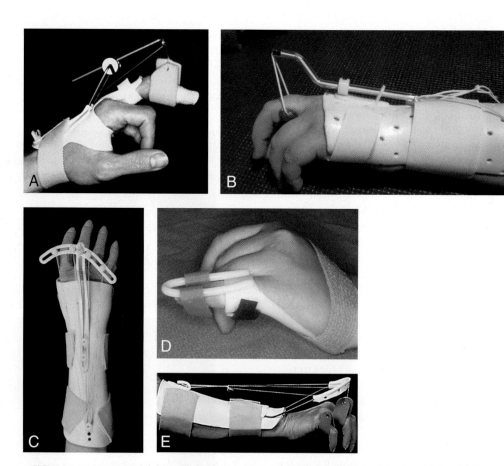

FIGURE 5–26 Outriggers: **(A)** Hand-based PIP extension mobilization orthosis with a dorsal Rolyan® Adjustable Outrigger Kit. Notice the DIP extension immobilization cast to isolate the forces of extension to the PIP joint (Patterson Medical). MCP extension mobilization orthoses using **(B)** Orfitube™ system (North Coast Medical) and **(C)** Digitec Outrigger System (Patterson Medical). Homemade outriggers using **(D)** Rolyan® Aquatubes® (Patterson Medical) and **(E)** bent wire with scrap thermoplastic to create pulley system.

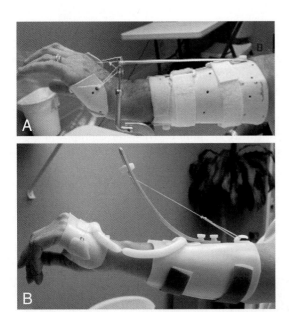

FIGURE 5–27 Wrist extension mobilization orthoses: **(A)** Phoenix Wrist Hinge (Patterson Medical) and **(B)** custom hinge using Rolyan® Aquatubes® (Patterson Medical). Also shown is Digitec Outrigger System (Patterson Medical).

portion of the outrigger. The higher the outrigger, the less stable the attachment site; be sure to provide adequate proximal length for attaching to the orthotic base. To form a strong bond, use solvent to remove any coating on the material. If no wire or tubing is available, heat a strip of thermoplastic material and create a rolled tube, which can then be formed into an outrigger.

Hinges

Rehabilitation catalogs offer **hinges** for addressing the wrist and elbow joints. Hinges allow motion in one plane of movement. They are extremely versatile, satisfying various orthotic fabrication needs (Fig. 5–27A). They can be used for immobilization by creating a static situation when locked to prevent motion, restriction by blocking a portion of the available range of motion, and mobilization by using a dynamic component or static line to stretch the joint or soft tissue structures. Hinges are helpful for mobilization orthoses to prevent migration; for example, in a dynamic elbow flexion orthosis, the hinge prevents the proximal and distal cuffs from being drawn together by the rubber band traction. If kits are not available, handmade versions can be fashioned from a crimped piece of thermoplastic tubing or by loosely attaching two pieces of thermoplastic material together with a large rivet or rubber band post (Thomes & Thomes, 1999) (Fig. 5–27B).

Accessories

FINGERTIP ATTACHMENTS

Mobilization orthoses of the digits frequently requires a way to apply force directly from the fingertips via a **fingertip**

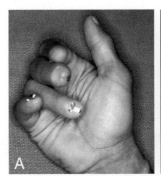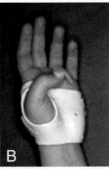

FIGURE 5–28 Fingertip attachments for the application of mobilization forces include **(A)** dress hooks glued to the nails and **(B)** hook material glued to the nails.

attachment. The options available include fingernail hooks, adhesive-backed hooks, and wrap-on hooks (Trueman, 1998) (Fig. 5–28A,B). Fingernail hooks and adhesive-backed hooks require the use of glue on the nail to provide a secure attachment. To prepare the surface of the nail for a secure bond, scratch with an emery board and then clean with alcohol. The devices are detached by using nail polish remover. Removable wrap-on hooks provide a means of attaching a mobilization force without disrupting the nail; they are lined with a slip-resistant material. Kinesio® Tex Tape can also be trimmed to create a means to attach line to a fingernail. When using these products, be mindful not to compress the digit's neurovascular structures.

FINGER SLINGS AND LOOPS

Finger slings and **loops** can be purchased in various materials, including suede, leather, and soft material, the choice of which depends on preference. For cost containment, use strap material scraps to make custom slings and loops. The small finger can be challenging to fit with a prefabricated sling, commonly needing trimming for both length and width. A sling is an open trough in which each end of the fabric has its own line; those lines may or may not converge. A loop is a closed trough in which the two ends of the fabric converge to a single line (Fig. 5–29A–C). Loops are easier and quicker to apply because only one line needs to be secured, whereas a sling requires two lines. Caution should be taken not to compromise vascularity in the digit when applying finger slings and loops. Slings decrease the compressive forces on the digit. Educate the patient on the signs and symptoms of impaired circulation. See Chapter 4 for details about designing line attachments to minimize compressive and shear forces on the digit (Bell-Krotoski & Breger-Stanton, 2011; Brand & Hollister, 1999; Fess et al., 2005). A digital cuff fabricated from thermoplastic material can also help prevent unnecessary forces under the sling. The same mechanical principles are applicable when designing a mobilization orthosis for the wrist or elbow; the distal cuff is analogous to the finger sling or loop.

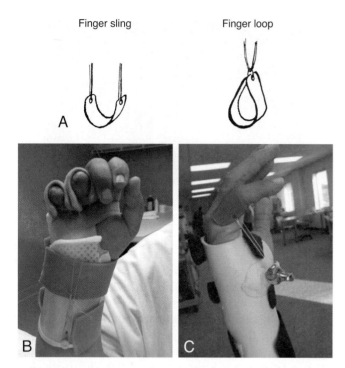

FIGURE 5-29 A, Finger sling and finger loop. Homemade using scraps of **(B)** soft strapping material for MCP flexion mobilization (dynamic) and **(C)** thermoplastic material for static progressive MCP flexion mobilization orthosis (MERiT™, Patterson Medical).

LINES

Static **lines**, which connect the distal attachment to the more proximal connection, can be fashioned using nonelastic monofilament or nylon cord (Fig. 5–30A). These materials create a line that is resistant to drag, which is especially important when they are gliding through line guides or pulleys. The length should be sufficient to allow unobstructed gliding through the pulleys. Because these lines are nonelastic, they can be effectively used for fabricating static progressive orthoses (Schultz-Johnson,

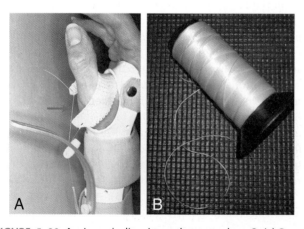

FIGURE 5-30 A, A static line is used to attach a QuickCast 2 (Patterson Medical) sling to the elastic force for a first web space mobilization orthosis with a Base 2™ Outrigger Kit (North Coast Medical). **B,** Spool of Nymo Cord (Patterson Medical).

2002). Traditionally, fishing line was used by therapists; however, this can be challenging to manage and keep knots tied because of its smooth texture. Nymo Cord (Patterson Medical) offers a better option that is easier to handle when knotting and guiding through pulley systems (Fig. 5–30B).

LINE GUIDES

A **line guide** or pulley gives the therapist a means to change the direction of a force. Maximizing the angle of application, ideally at 90°, improves the effectiveness of the orthosis (Bell-Krotoski & Breger-Stanton, 2011; Brand & Hollister, 1999; Fess et al., 2005) (refer to Chapter 4 on "Mechanical Principles" for details). There are many types of commercially available guides (Fig. 5–31A,B). The

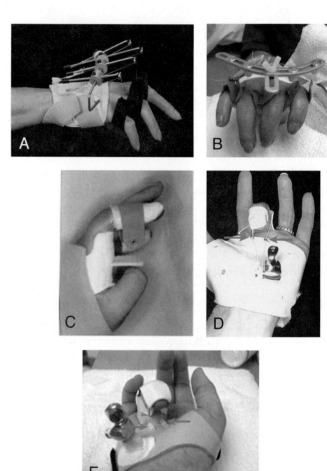

FIGURE 5-31 Pulley systems: **(A)** Rolyan® Adjustable Outrigger Kit with pulleys over proximal phalanges; hand based for MCP extension mobilization following loss of digit extension after posterior interosseous nerve injury (Patterson Medical). **B,** Digitec Outrigger System is highly adjustable, allowing for easy modification of pulley position (Patterson Medical). **C,** Homemade pulley using scrap of perforated thermoplastic material. **D,** Safety pins were bent, heated, and embedded into the thermoplastic material to act as line guides for the static progressive force. **E,** Rolyan® Aquatubes® were cut and embedded within this version of a similar orthosis (Splint-Tuner™ shown in **D and E**; North Coast Medical).

therapist can fashion one by using a scrap piece of thermoplastic material and punching a hole in it to allow the line to pass through. Perforated materials are user friendly; the therapist can easily change the angle of pull by choosing from the many existing holes (Fig. 5–31C). Metal eyelets and safety pins offer yet more options; they are inexpensive and can be easily bent, heated, and embedded in the thermoplastic material (Fig. 5–31D). Thermoplastic tubes can also be used to create line guide (Fig. 5–31E).

LINE CONNECTORS AND STOPS

Line connectors provide an alternative to knots for attaching the line to slings or mobilization forces. They allow the therapist to adjust tension in a dynamic orthosis easily by changing the placement of the connector rather than becoming frustrated with tying and retying knots that frequently loosen. Connectors are simply crimped with pliers.

Line stops provide a means to control the available range of motion allowed in a restrictive-type orthosis (Fig. 5–32). Stops are applied to the line proximal to the line guides or pulleys at a specific point determined by the desired motion restricted. They can be removed and reapplied to change the available range. Tape can also be used on the line to restrict the range of motion.

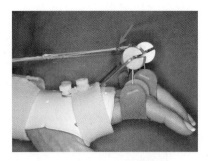

FIGURE 5–32 When rehabilitating an extensor tendon repair, line stops can be used with a dynamic digit extension orthosis to restrict MCP flexion (Phoenix Outrigger Kit, Patterson Medical).

MOBILIZATION FORCES

The therapist can apply a **mobilization force** to a body part in several ways. For dynamic orthoses, choose from stretchy forces, such as graded rubber bands, wrapped elastic cord (Fig. 5–33A), elastic thread, elasticized loop, pajama elastic, neoprene, elasticized wrap, graded springs/coils, and TheraBand® or TheraTubing® products (Mildenberger, Amadio, & An, 1986) (Fig. 5–33B–G). Replace elastic products frequently to ensure an accurate

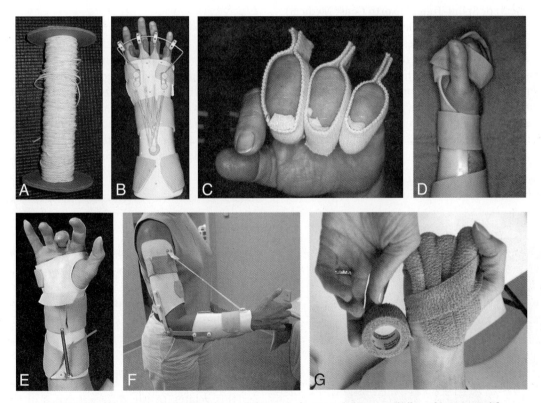

FIGURE 5–33 Dynamic mobilization forces: **(A)** Spool of wrapped elastic cord allows for easy modification of force applied. **B,** Rubber bands provide the MCP extension force on this Phoenix Outrigger Kit (Patterson Medical). **C,** Pajama elastics are easily stapled into a loop to create this PIP/DIP strap. Note use of foam to soften stress on nails. **D,** Strap of neoprene material provides final flexion stretch in this digit mobilization orthosis. **E,** Spring coil delivering MCP flexion force. **F,** Thera-Tube® for force application with this elbow flexion mobilization orthosis (Phoenix elbow hinge, Patterson Medical). **G,** Elasticized wrap used for a quick way to apply general flexion stretch to digits.

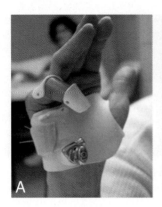
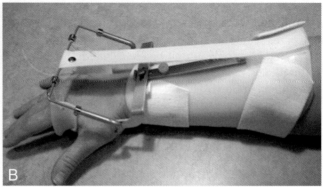

FIGURE 5–34 Static progressive forces: **(A)** MERiT™ (Patterson Medical) and **(B)** homemade using traditional hook-and-loop material allowing for adjustments of static tension (Phoenix Wrist Hinge, Patterson Medical).

generation of force on the tissue. These force-generating components may be connected distally by means of a static line. Consider using a force or tension gauge to measure the applied force to prevent the sling from being too aggressive with the tissue.

Static progressive orthoses use a nonelastic means of applying a mobilization force. Turnbuckles can be fashioned to provide this static force. Components such as the MERiT™ (Patterson Medical) or Splint-Tuner™ (North Coast Medical) provide an adjustable means of static force application that can be used in a multitude of orthoses (Fig. 5–34A). A thumb screw on the device provides a way to progressively change the static tension. A homemade option includes the use of hook-and-loop material that can be progressively changed to impart a greater stretch. Loop strips allow easy adjustment; the strip is simply attached to a different place on the hook material to alter the tension (Fig. 5–34B).

PROXIMAL ATTACHMENT DEVICES

A distally applied dynamic or static force requires a **proximal attachment device** for connecting to the orthosis (Fig. 5–35A,B). Dynamic forces can be attached with rubber band posts or hooks made from scrap thermoplastic material. Static progressive forces can be secured through the use of adjustable devices as noted earlier.

Conclusion

It is imperative for the therapist to keep abreast of current available equipment and materials to provide patients with the most effective orthotic intervention. Therapists with the knowledge and skills required for orthotic fabrication are able to respond to the individual needs of each patient by blending creatively this knowledge base to fabricate the most appropriate orthosis.

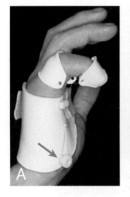
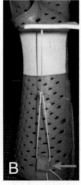

FIGURE 5–35 **A,** A rubber band post acts as convenient proximal attachment device for this low-profile final-flexion orthosis. Note line guides made from Rolyan® Aquatubes® (Patterson Medical). **B,** Homemade hook from scrap thermoplastic material used on this MCP flexion mobilization orthosis.

Chapter Review Questions

1. Why is having a good pair of scissors so important with orthotic fabrication?

2. What other tools are helpful to have in the clinic for orthotic fabrication?

3. Describe the term *resistance to stretch* and how this relates to the different types of thermoplastic materials.

4. When is using padding or lining material appropriate in an orthosis?

5. What are the best ways to stay abreast of the new component systems available?

6 Fabrication Process

Noelle M. Austin, MS, PT, CHT
with additional contributions by:
   Gary P. Austin, PT, PhD
   Gail Garfield Dadio, MHSc, OTR/L, CHT, CLT
   Pat McKee, M.Sc., OT Reg. (Ont.), OT(C)

Chapter Objectives

After study of this chapter, the reader should be able to:

- Appreciate the importance of therapist–physician communication.
- Name and describe the different segments of a comprehensive upper extremity examination.
- Recognize the importance of evidence-based practice.
- Develop an understanding of the PROCESS of orthotic fabrication.
- Integrate the results of the examination into a comprehensive treatment plan including the role for orthosis intervention.
- Appreciate the various frames of reference and how they influence orthosis application.

Key Terms

Bio-occupational approach
Disabilities of the Arm, Shoulder, and Hand (DASH)
Evidence-based practice
Frames of reference
Goniometers

Grip dynamometers
Numerical Rating Scale (NRS)
Person, Environment, Occupation (PEO) Model
Pinch gauges
PROCESS

Rehabilitative approach
Upper Limb Functional Index (ULFI)
Visual Analog Scale (VAS)
Volumeter

Introduction

This chapter presents the process of orthotic fabrication, from receiving the physician's orders to issuing the orthosis to the patient. Discussion includes information needed from the physician, items to include on the upper extremity examination, interpretation of the findings, and the establishment of an appropriate intervention plan. Finally, this chapter introduces the unique style of Section II of this book, which details a specific approach to orthotic fabrication. This format uses the acronym **PROCESS**, which provides the reader with a systematic method for creating orthoses and makes the description of each orthosis simple to follow and easy to understand. All the chapters in Section II follow this format; therefore, it is critical for the reader to be familiar with the PROCESS concept.

Referral

A patient is generally referred to the therapist by a physician for fabrication of an orthosis and/or therapy. The referral should include as much of the following information as possible:

- Patient name
- Diagnosis and/or surgical procedure
- Date of injury and/or date of surgery
- Precautions
- Orthosis specifications
  - Purpose (i.e., immobilization)
  - Type (i.e., immobilization orthosis to rest a body part)
  - Desired joint position(s) (i.e., antideformity position: wrist at 30° extension, metacarpophalangeal [MCP] joints at 40° flexion, proximal interphalangeal [PIP] joints and distal interphalangeal [DIP] joints at 0°)
  - Goal (i.e., allow tendons to heal)
  - Wearing schedule (i.e., at all times, except bathing and exercise)

Obtaining a copy of the operative report is extremely helpful, especially for complicated cases in which multiple procedures were performed that require protection in specific positions. Understanding what structures were injured and how they were repaired dictates the postoperative rehabilitation and orthotic management approach. Viewing radiographs and other special studies (i.e., magnetic resonance imaging [MRI], computed tomography [CT] scans, and nerve conduction velocity studies) is also beneficial to gain a greater insight about the patient's condition.

Although the therapist may not always have the opportunity to see test results or operative reports before examining the patient, it remains imperative that the therapist has a full understanding of the diagnosis and prescribed intervention before rendering treatment. If there are questions or concerns, do not hesitate to call the physician's office to receive clarification of orders. When in doubt, be conservative with positioning; orthoses can always be modified once the physician is contacted.

Ideally, therapists should strive to establish a strong relationship with their referring physicians. Appreciate that each doctor has his or her own philosophy on treatment approach. Communicating effectively with the referral source promotes a professional relationship full of mutual respect and trust. Physicians are more apt to return phone calls and respond to requests when they have thoughtful interactions with the therapist. Always organize questions and concerns before speaking with the physician; his or her time is valuable and often limited. Asking intelligent, relevant questions helps instill confidence in the therapist's skills and provides for optimum patient treatment.

Sometimes general referrals are sent, giving the therapists some latitude to decide on the orthosis to be made.

Therapists are then challenged to use their clinical skills to provide patients with the most appropriate device. As the patient's conditions evolve, their orthotic needs most likely change. It then becomes essential for patients to follow up with their doctor to receive an updated referral or signed therapy progress note with new orders that reflect the change in status.

Examination

The examination provides the basis for all critical thinking and therapy intervention. All patients must be evaluated so the most appropriate orthosis can be chosen. Appendix B includes a sample upper extremity examination. Orthotic fabrication should not be approached as a rote intervention; each patient should be viewed as a unique case, and the therapist should appreciate that no two patients are alike in terms of rehabilitation and orthotic needs despite similar diagnoses. Even when patients are referred for a one-time visit, therapists must perform at least an abbreviated yet comprehensive version of an examination. Therapists are challenged to gather and integrate all the pertinent information that will allow them to make decisions that are in the best interest of the patient.

During the examination process, the therapist not only establishes a rapport with the patient but also gains some insight into the issues of compliance and motivation. Note the resting posture of the injured part and how freely the patient uses or moves the extremity. Addressing signs of neglect early on to prevent long-term disuse is essential. At the other extreme, the overzealous patient should be cautioned when the diagnosis requires complete rest or limited use. Keep in mind that some patients, owing to diagnostic precautions, may not tolerate a complete examination; thus, portions of the examination (range of motion and strength) may not be appropriate to assess (status post multiple flexor tendon repairs). As healing progresses, these segments of the examination should be addressed.

This section briefly reviews the subjective and objective information that the therapist should obtain from the patient as part of the examination process, highlighting some key points related to orthotic application. For more details, see one of the many available upper extremity rehabilitation texts. The sources listed as suggested reading for this chapter offer more in-depth information.

Subjective Information

Age

The therapist must take into consideration the age of the patient because the approach to orthotic fabrication differs for an infant, child, young adult, middle-aged adult, and older patient. For example, when applying orthoses to infants, it is important to be sure that there are no small parts that can potentially loosen and present a choking hazard. Thin thermoplastic material, 3/32″ or 1/16″, generally provides sufficient strength for their small hands. Consider taking advantage of the available hard-to-remove strapping systems when designing a device for a pediatric patient. Compliance of the older child may be enhanced if he or she is given an orthosis that is colored or decorated to the child's taste (Fig. 6–1A). Chapter 22 gives more specific information on addressing the pediatric patient.

A strong, durable material that is easy to clean is generally the appropriate choice for a young athlete. When addressing geriatric patients who have fragile, sensitive skin, consider using lightweight, perforated materials. Strapping systems for the older population should be constructed to allow for easy, independent donning and doffing. Soft straps that are gentle on the skin and superficial bony prominences may aid in wear compliance (Fig. 6–1B).

Hand Dominance

Hand dominance becomes especially important when considering the functional needs of a patient. Patients may require instruction and specific training on how to modify activities of daily living (ADLs) to compensate for orthosis constraints. Adaptations to the orthosis can be incorporated during fabrication—for example, to provide built-up handles on tools or utensils to be used in combination with the orthosis—to maintain function of the dominant hand (Fig. 6–2).

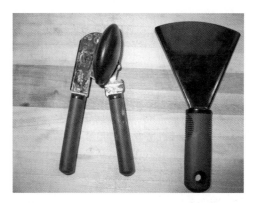

FIGURE 6–2 Large-handled kitchen gadgets can make cooking less stressful for hand joints.

Past Medical History

Consideration should be given to past medical history, including unrelated medical conditions and how they can influence the present upper extremity diagnosis. Note previous surgeries and any known allergies. Inquire about any previous injuries or surgeries in the affected area. A listing of current conditions and medications should be obtained for the medical record. For example, a patient with diabetes may suffer from decreased circulation, which can lead to prolonged healing times and sensory changes (Fig. 6–3). This condition mandates frequent and vigilant inspection of the skin under the thermoplastic material and straps to check for skin changes. Chapter 3 provides further information on how specific diseases can affect the healing process. Last, understand that medical problems can mimic or contribute to upper extremity conditions; be sure to conduct a thorough screening starting with reviewing medical history (Goodman, 2010).

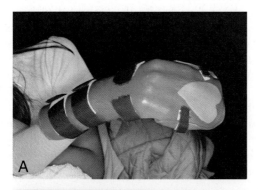

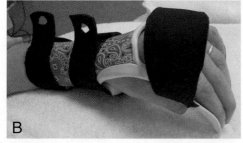

FIGURE 6–1 **A,** Pediatric dorsal wrist and hand immobilization orthosis used after a flexor tendon repair. Note the thermoplastic heart applied to the distal portion. **B,** Notice how the soft straps used on this wrist and hand immobilization orthosis have loops dorsally to allow for independent donning and doffing of the device in this elderly patient.

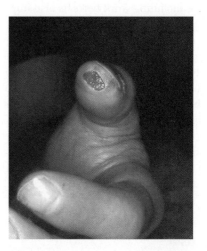

FIGURE 6–3 This diabetic patient unknowingly burned his thumb in the oven and did not realize it because of lack of sensation.

History of Present Condition

Questioning the patient regarding the history of the present condition should include factors such as the onset of symptoms, mechanism of injury, previous therapeutic intervention, surgical history, and postoperative management. This information can guide the therapist in making decisions about how to treat the patient most effectively. During the interview process, the therapist should begin to think about the rehabilitation options. However, the therapist must realize that an orthosis is only one part of the treatment regime and is best complemented by other modalities, such as exercise and patient education. For example, a patient with conservatively managed carpal tunnel syndrome may benefit from an orthosis to position the wrist in neutral while sleeping. But if that patient does not make complementary lifestyle changes, such as creating an ergonomic workstation, the symptoms of the syndrome will likely remain problematic. A thorough screening for proximal issues is essential because symptoms originating in the neck and shoulder region can overlap and interact with more distal diagnoses (Yung & Asavasopon, 2010).

Social and Vocational History

The home environment can affect a patient's ability to comply with a rehabilitation regime. Obtaining information regarding the level of assistance a patient has at home (from family members or other caregivers) becomes pertinent when there is a question about the patient's ability to don and doff the orthosis independently and to follow through with a home program or activity limitations. For example, a patient who is supposed to wear an orthosis full time while acting as the sole caretaker of three children may have difficulty functioning within the constraints of the device. Therapists need to consider the patient as a whole person, not just a diagnosis. Find out if the patient is a smoker because this can impact healing of bone and soft tissue. Document alcohol use as well; this relates to overall general health.

Interviewing the patient regarding his or her work environment, including work tasks, is also important, especially if the patient must wear the orthosis during work hours. Functional demands help dictate the material and design of the orthosis. Regarding orthotic selection, for example, thicker materials (⅛″) may be the most appropriate choice for individuals who work at labor-intensive jobs. Adaptations may be needed to allow maximal function (Fig. 6–2). The same is true when considering a patient's avocational interests. For example, if the patient participates in athletic competition, the orthosis must abide by sports-specific regulations to be acceptable during play. Exterior padding may be required to prevent injury to others.

Objective Information

Functional Level

Discussing the patient's current functional level is important to ascertain how the injury or surgery has affected his

or her life. In addition to the detailed history, standardized testing of dexterity and coordination can help the therapist assess functional performance (Apfel, 1990; Jebson, Taylor, Trieschmann, Trotter, & Howard, 1969; McPhee, 1987; Smith, 1973; Tiffin & Asher, 1948; Totten & Flinn-Wagner, 1992). Completion of a simple questionnaire that asks the patient to grade his or her functional ability to complete specific tasks (e.g., no assistance through minimal, moderate, or maximal assistance or unable to complete) is another way to gather information. These data help the therapist establish functional goals and provide a means to mark progress. The **Disabilities of the Arm, Shoulder, and Hand (DASH)** and the **Upper Limb Functional Index (ULFI)** are two commonly used questionnaires to assess functional status (Cox, Spaulding, & Kramer, 2006; Gabel, Michener, Burkett, & Neller, 2006; Gabel, Yelland, Melloh, & Burkett, 2009; Lehman, Sindhu, Shechtman, Romero, & Velozo, 2010).

Dexterity refers to the skill or ability to use one's hands for completion of tasks related to ADLs. There are numerous tests available to quantify the level of dexterity, including the Jebsen Taylor Hand Function Test; Purdue Pegboard Test; Nine Hole Peg Test; and Minnesota Rate of Manipulation Tests, Crawford Small Parts Dexterity Test, and O'Connor Peg Board Test to name a few (Desrosiers, Hébert, Bravo, & Dutil, 1995; Fess, 2011; Mathiowetz, Weber, Kashman, & Volland, 1985). These tests of dexterity and coordination can be chosen depending on the individual patient and his or her ability level.

Involve the patient in setting up functional goals. Integrating personal goals into the treatment plan is a great way to maximize compliance. For example, a patient may be discouraged with his or her inability to play the piano after a trigger finger release. Acknowledging this frustration and establishing goals that include the return to playing the piano may make the patient more apt to follow the prescribed treatment regime.

Patients must have a clear understanding of their limitations while wearing an orthosis (Fig. 6–4). For example, a patient who underwent an extensor tendon repair requires full-time immobilization and is thus unable to use that

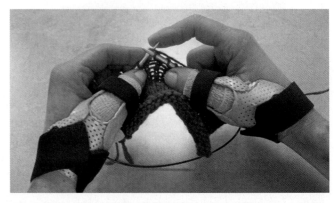

FIGURE 6–4 Bilateral functional hand use with MP joint immobilization orthoses for osteoarthritis.

hand during the early stages of healing. This patient may require assistance with tasks such as bathing, dressing, and food preparation. The therapist must fully discuss with the patient the precautions and risks associated with the diagnosis, surgical procedure, and therapy program (including use of orthosis) to maximize compliance and reduce chance of rupture or attenuation of the surgical repair.

Therapists can offer patients helpful hints on how to improve independence and function for ADLs. Simple modifications such as using kitchen utensils with built-up handles can ease the stress and pain of arthritic joints. These modifications can be used simultaneously with an orthosis or a device can be fabricated for use with a specific functional task. For example, cylindrical foam, elastomer, or thermoplastic material can be used to modify writing utensils.

Pain

The therapist should ask the patient to describe pain in terms of quality, degree, and location (Chapman, Schimek, Colpitts, Gerlach, & Dong, 1985; Echternach, 1993; Melzack, 1975; Schultz-Johnson, 1988a). Changes in degree can be determined by using a scale: **Visual Analog Scale (VAS)** or **Numerical Rating Scale (NRS)**, usually 0 (*no pain*) to 10 (*pain as bad as it can be*) (Sindu, Shechtman, & Tuckey, 2011). Mapping out the pain on an illustration of the upper extremity may help define the location. Avoid placing patients with moderate to severe pain in mobilization orthoses. Aggressive mobilization may aggravate pain and increase edema. If mobilization orthoses are ordered for such a patient, contact the physician to discuss any concerns. Oftentimes, waiting a few days can make a big difference in terms of reduction of inflammation and increased tolerance to mobilization. Pain may also influence the choice of materials used; highly

drapable materials may be easier to apply because they conform without much hands-on manipulation. Orthoses can be fabricated to accommodate the electrode pads often used to modify pain (transcutaneous electrical nerve stimulation [TENS] or high volt).

Visual Inspection and Palpation

Inspect the affected area and take note of any masses, swelling, deformities, atrophy, scars or wounds (Rayan & Ackelman, 2011) (Fig. 6–5A,B). Following visual inspection, begin to gently palpate the region; commence this portion of the examination in an area away from the focal point (Fig. 6–5C,D). In some clinical situations, physically palpating the area may not be indicated. If applicable, view both extremities simultaneously to compare the two sides. This is an opportune time to gain rapport with the patient, being gentle and confident with this hands-on interaction. In addition, note the posture of the hand and the patient's willingness to move.

Edema

Quantify edema whenever possible by measuring volume or circumference. Use a **volumeter** to measure the volume of the limb or a measuring tape to quantify circumference (Fig. 6–6A) (Brand & Wood, 1977; Villeco, 2011; Schultz-Johnson, 1988b). The therapist must fully describe the quality (e.g., pitting, brawny) and location. In the early stages of healing of an acutely injured or postoperative extremity, edema is frequently an issue that requires therapy intervention (Fig. 6–6B). Edema may be reduced by an orthosis that correctly positions the extremity; compression garments (gloves, elasticized wraps, and sleeves); and education regarding elevation, ice, and exercise (if appropriate) (Fig. 6–6C) (Villeco, 2012).

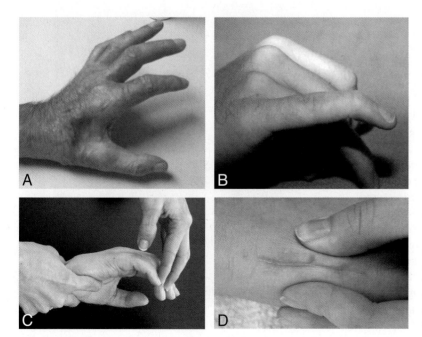

FIGURE 6–5 A, Patient presents with atrophy of first dorsal interossei following prolonged ulnar nerve compression at the elbow. **B,** Lack of terminal tendon function indicated by flexed posture at the DIP joint. **C,** Gentle passive ROM used to determine soft tissue extensibility. **D,** Palpation of scar reveals adherence to the underlying tissue.

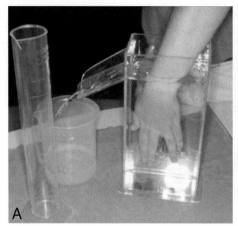
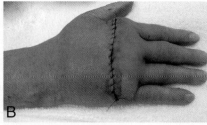
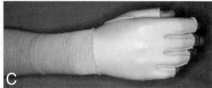

FIGURE 6–6 **A,** A volumeter quantifies edema. Measure the contralateral limb for comparison. **B,** Dorsal hand edema following MCP joint arthroplasties. **C,** Edema management may include the use of a compression glove and an elasticized tubular bandage.

Edema may increase after the use of orthoses, especially with mobilization tissue. Consistent, repeated evaluation provides the therapist with information about how the tissue is tolerating the therapy and orthotic intervention. If the extremity becomes edematous and reactive, the approach should be modified. For example, if edema is aggravated by a mobilization orthosis, consider resting and immobilizing the area for a few days. Once the edema has decreased, cautiously reintroduce the mobilization orthosis, monitoring for any edema response.

Fluctuations in edema should influence the strapping choice. Window-type edema, which occurs between two straps, may be avoided by wrapping the limb circumferentially or by applying a compressive sleeve under the orthosis. Circumferential wraps (e.g., Coban™ or Ace™ wraps), applied distal to proximal, impart an even pressure to an edematous limb. Circumferential orthoses should be used cautiously with patients who have an edematous extremity; if applied too tightly, problematic pooling of edema distal to the orthosis can occur. In select cases, these orthoses may help reduce edema; Chapter 12 provides more information.

Sensibility

Assessing **sensibility** is essential when conducting an upper extremity examination (Bell-Krotoski, 2011; Bell-Krotoski, Weinstein, & Weinstein, 1993; Callahan, 1995; Dellon, 1981; Moberg, 1958; Novak, Mackinnon, Williams, & Kelly, 1992; Tan, 1992). Monofilament examination and two-point discrimination testing are the most common methods for evaluating sensation (Fig. 6–7A,B). A monofilament examination, considered a threshold test, is administered by applying graded forces of filaments to the testing area (Bell-Krotoski & Tomancik, 1987). Two-point discrimination, considered an innervation density test, involves the ability to distinguish between two stimuli applied to the skin at specific locations (Dellon, 1978; Dellon, Mackinnon, & Crosby, 1987; Mackinnon & Dellon, 1985). Quick screening for light touch may be adequate if the patient has no complaints or signs of nerve involvement.

The therapist must consider impaired sensation in order to provide the patient with a properly fitting orthosis and to prevent tissue irritation. Every effort should be made to increase the surface area of application to disperse the pressures on sensory-impaired regions. When applying an orthosis to a limb with impaired sensation, the therapist must review the precautions with the patient. Any complaints of numbness or paresthesias should be dealt with immediately. Because they lack complete sensory feedback, such patients must learn to perform frequent visual examinations of the affected extremity, looking for any signs of excess pressure.

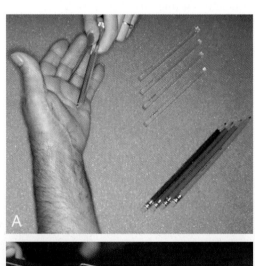
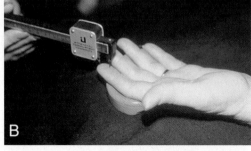

FIGURE 6–7 **A,** A monofilament set. **B,** A two-point discriminator.

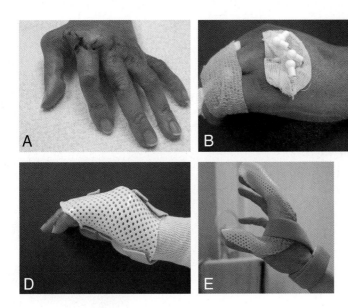
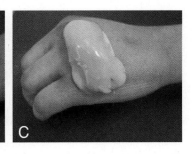

FIGURE 6–8 **A,** Open MCP joint after removal of implant because of infection. **B–D,** Application of Elastomer Putty over pins to create protective bubble in orthosis. Notice use of Xeroform over pins beneath putty to protect pin sites. **E,** CMC abduction orthosis with Elastomer mold used to maximally disperse pressure at the first web space.

Soft Tissue and Wound Status

Therapists should assess the soft tissue and wound status. Document any wounds or surgical incisions and quantify with measurements and descriptions (Evans, 1991; Von Der Heyde & Evans, 2011; McCulloch & Kloth, 1990) (Fig. 6–8A). Digital photos offer a valuable way to document changes in a wound status. Maceration, rashes, and skin breakdown can result when the skin is subjected to prolonged orthosis wear or excessive moisture. Perforated materials are a good choice for application over wounds because they allow air exchange between the thermoplastic and skin.

Therapists frequently need to be creative when applying orthoses over wound dressings and/or surgical hardware, such as pins or external fixators. To mold material directly over exposed pins, prepad the area and then apply the warm thermoplastic material. Consider using solid, highly drapable material for this type of orthosis (Fig. 6–8B–D). For sensitive scars, gel-lined materials are available. Scars can also be prepadded with gel or a scar management product such as elastomer or Otoform™ (Fig. 6–8E).

Vascularity

Color and temperature differences between the involved and uninvolved side should also be noted to address the vascular status of the limb. Altered sympathetic response may present with color and temperature changes of the skin. Assessment becomes of extreme importance when vascular structures have been injured or surgically repaired (Ashbell, Kutz, & Kleinert 1967; Levinsohn, Gordon, & Sessler, 1991) (Fig. 6–9A). Orthoses, straps, or slings that are applied too tightly may impede circulation, manifested by a change in color and/or temperature (Fig. 6–9B). Wide straps and slings may dissipate pressure on the affected part by increasing the area of force application (Brand & Hollister, 1999; Fess, Gettle, Philips, & Janson, 2005). Chapter 4 provides a more detailed discussion of these concepts.

Circumferential designs are not the best choice for patients who have undergone vascular repair or who have possible vascular compromise. Such orthoses may not provide enough room for fluctuations in edema. When edema increases, the pressure within the device may also increase, leading to impaired circulation.

Range of Motion

Goniometers are used to measure active and passive range of motion (ROM) (Fig. 6–10) (Boone et al., 1978; Cambridge-Keeling, 1995; Hamilton & Lachenbruch, 1969). Active ROM provides information about a patient's willingness or ability to move. Gaining insight regarding the soft tissue and joint status of the musculotendinous unit is important (e.g., tendon adherence, tendon continuity, and nerve innervation). Joint stiffness and musculotendinous tightness can be assessed with passive ROM measurements.

Ongoing evaluation of ROM becomes imperative when introducing an orthosis to mobilize tissue. ROM is a way of measuring gains and provides feedback for the orthotic intervention effort. If no improvements are evident, the regime must be changed accordingly. For example, if no gains are

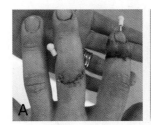
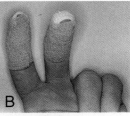

FIGURE 6–9 **A,** DIP joint open dislocation with pinning and surgical repair of vascular structures along with terminal tendon. Note dusky appearance distal to injury. **B,** When a circumferential wrap is applied to a body part, the patient must monitor for any throbbing or color/temperature changes.

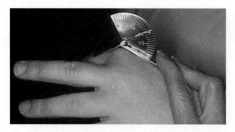

FIGURE 6–10 A small finger goniometer is a convenient way to measure the small joints of the hand.

made from use of a dynamic PIP extension orthosis, the therapist should consider changing to a serial static treatment approach or perhaps using both day and night orthoses. ROM measurements can also indicate that joints are getting tighter, as is sometimes seen at the MCP joints when a wrist cast extends too far distally, impeding full MCP motion.

Strength

Grip dynamometers, **pinch gauges**, and manual muscle testing (MMT) provide ways to assess muscle function and nerve innervation (Fig. 6–11A,B) (Bechtol, 1954; Hislop & Montgomery, 2007; Kendall, McCreary, & Provance, 2005; Mathiowetz, Volland, Kashman, & Weber, 1985; Mathiowetz, Weber, Volland, & Kashman, 1984; Schmidt & Toews, 1970). Three types of pinch may be tested: lateral or key pinch, three point (three-jaw chuck), and thumb tip to index-finger tip (tip pinch) (Fig. 6–12A–F) (Casanova & Grunert, 1989). Quantifying changes in strength is helpful when justifying the need for continued therapy. Repetitive grip testing has been used by therapists to attempt to quantify sincerity of effort (Shechtman, Guiterrez, & Kokendofer, 2005; Sindhu, Shechtman, & Veazie, 2012).

Strength testing may be contraindicated in many cases, depending on the diagnosis and healing timeframe. For example, elbow flexion strength testing should be deferred in the early stages of healing after a biceps tendon repair owing to the high risk of rupture immediately after surgery. Strength

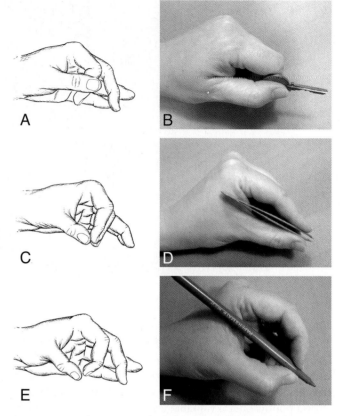

FIGURE 6–12 Three types of pinches: lateral **(A and B)**, three point **(B and C)**, and thumb to index-finger tip **(C and D)**.

can be safely assessed once the physician has approved the initiation of progressive resistive exercise.

MMT provides the means for monitoring recovery from a nerve injury (Kendall et al., 2005). As the nerve reinnervates muscles, patients present with higher muscle grades (0 to 5). This change in status alters the therapy and orthotic intervention plans. For example, the orthosis must be modified for a patient with radial nerve palsy once the wrist extensors become innervated. Because the orthosis no longer needs to incorporate the wrist, the therapist should choose a hand-based MCP extension mobilization orthosis to allow the newly innervated wrist extensors to function while regaining strength.

Exercise orthoses can be fabricated to provide resistance to movement through the use of graded rubber bands, wrapped elastic cord, elastic thread, graded springs, and TheraBand® or TheraTubing® products. The patient can use the orthosis for frequent daily exercise sessions to improve strength in the targeted muscle group(s). When treating patients with adherent tendon repairs, adding resistance may aid in improving tendon glide through scar tissue.

Special Testing

Special testing depends on the specific diagnosis (Rayan & Ackelman, 2011) (Fig. 6–13). Not all testing needs to be completed on each and every patient. The previous parts of the examination, as well as the diagnosis they were referred with, will help guide the therapist regarding which special tests should be completed. For

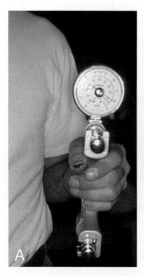
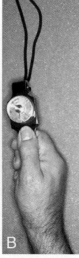

FIGURE 6–11 Grip **(A)** and pinch **(B)** dynamometers.

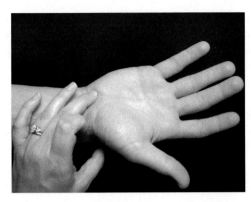

FIGURE 6–13 Phalen's test for carpal tunnel syndrome is positive when the tapping over the median nerve causes distal tingling in the median nerve distribution.

example, with a patient referred with a diagnosis of carpal tunnel syndrome, the examination should include the Phalen's test (wrist flexed position for 60 seconds), Tinel test (tapping over volar wrist to elicit distal symptoms), and Durkan compression test (direct pressure over the volar wrist) (Rayan & Ackelman, 2011). To be thorough, the proximal regions, shoulder and neck, should be screened as well to check for any contributory factors.

Problem Solving and Goal Setting

From the findings of the examination and the information gathered from the patient interview, the therapist is able to establish treatment goals. Therapists must appreciate

that orthotic intervention is only one way problems can be addressed. The therapist must first define a list of problems. Table 6–1 outlines the problems and corresponding goals for a patient at 1 week postsurgery for carpal tunnel release.

Note that for each problem, there is a short- and long-term goal. Although this is a relatively simple example, this method of creating an appropriate treatment plan is applicable to all patients. The critical thinking process allows the therapist to organize the findings of the examination and begin to plan the therapy intervention. The therapist must then prioritize the problems. It can be overwhelming to treat a patient with multiple injuries; setting priorities is mandatory (although sometimes difficult to do). All treatment problems and interventions are interrelated. For example, when edema has been successfully addressed, ROM is usually also improved.

After the problems are defined, the therapist should establish short- and long-term goals. For example, when applying a mobilization orthosis, the therapist should set reasonable short-term ROM goals that can be reached in 1 week; this encourages the patient to follow the wearing schedule and therapy program. Each time the patient reaches a goal, a new goal should be established. As mentioned previously, the patient's own goals should be integrated within the therapy goals (when appropriate).

Therapy intervention is a dynamic process, limited only by the lack of imagination on the part of the therapist. The therapist needs to take the time to interpret the evaluative findings and appreciate that as the patient progresses, the problems and priorities also change, as should the treatment goals. Ideally, all problems should be addressed. But it is unrealistic to think that one treatment modality is going to satisfy all the deficits. A comprehensive treatment plan should be

TABLE 6–1

Approach to Goal Setting

Therapy Problems	Short-term Goals (2–3 Weeks)	Long-term Goals (1–2 Months)
Healing incision	Healed incision	Soft, mobile scar
Moderate edema in hand	Minimal edema in order to be able to hold a water bottle to drink	No edema in hand or wrist to allow unimpeded use of hand while washing and blow drying hair.
Pain level: 2[a]	Pain level: 1	Pain level: 0
Decreased ROM of wrist and digits	Increase ROM of digits to normal and of wrist to 75% in order to use a pen to pay bill and be financially independent.	Normal ROM to return to work as a computer programmer.
Decreased grip and pinch strength	Increase grip to 5 lb and pinch to 2 lb for the ability to cut meat and feed self	Strength 75% of normal for lifting groceries out of car and transporting to home in order to feed family
Impaired ability to complete ADLs[b]	Independent with minimal modifications for self care activities and driving a car in order to return to work safely.	Full functional independence for all household tasks inclusive of cleaning and heavier cooking in order to care for self and family without risk of re-injury.

[a]On a scale of 0 to 10.
[b]Includes self-care, driving, cooking, and cleaning.

instituted, of which orthotic usage may or may not be a part. Therapists must use critical reasoning skills, based on knowledge and experience, to devise the best treatment regime, taking into account the patient's individual needs. Each time a patient returns to the clinic, he or she should be reevaluated to determine if changes in therapy management must be made. Integrating clinical experience and **evidence-based practice** is crucial when forming a comprehensive treatment plan. Decisions regarding intervention techniques should be based on the best systematic research whenever possible to justify services. Box 6–1 offers an overview of evidence-based practice as it relates to orthotic intervention.

In relation to the practice of occupational therapy, **frames of reference** provide the link between theory and practice. Orthotic intervention within the specialty of hand therapy would include the biomechanical and rehabilitative

BOX 6–1

Evidence-Based Practice and Orthotic Intervention

Contribution by Gary P. Austin, PT, PhD
Associate Professor of Physical Therapy
Director, Orthopaedic Physical Therapy Residency Program
    and Certificate Program in Advanced Orthopaedic
    Physical Therapy
Sacred Heart University, Fairfield, CT
Physical Therapist
Sacred Heart University Sports Medicine & Rehabilitation
    Center, Fairfield, CT

Evidence-based practice (EBP) has become an important concept in the health-care industry and currently is the dominant clinical decision-making paradigm. Unfortunately, this term has been subject to overuse, misuse, and misunderstanding. It is important that health-care providers and consumers understand both what EBP is and is not. Research has shown that "intuition, unsystematic clinical experience, and pathophysiologic rationale are insufficient grounds for clinical decision-making" (Guyatt & Rennie, 2002). EBP is classically defined as "the conscientious, explicit and judicious use of current best evidence in making decisions about the care of the individual patient. It means integrating individual clinical expertise with the best available external clinical evidence from systematic research" (Sackett, Rosenberg, Gray, Haynes, & Richardson, 1996). Contrary to popular belief, EBP is neither prescriptive, restrictive, inefficient, nor idealistic but rather guided by clinical practice and expertise; individualized/patient-specific; lifelong/career-long; self-directed; problem-based; cost-effective; and time-efficient.

The three pillars of EBP are (1) individual patient values, preferences, and expectations; (2) individual clinical expertise; and (3) clinical evidence. Evidence-based clinical decision making requires the clinician to evaluate the relevance and significance of all information and subsequent decisions within the context of each patient's unique values, preferences, and expectations. Collaborative decision making has been demonstrated to positively impact the patient and clinician (Elwyn et al., 2004; Towie, Godolphin, Grams, & Lamarre, 2006), adherence (Wilson et al., 2010), and outcomes (Godolphin, 2009; Mulley, Trimble, & Elwyn, 2012; Stiggelbout et al., 2012). Clinical expertise can be defined as the acquisition of clinical proficiency and judgment through experience and practice and is demonstrated, in part, "by effective and efficient diagnosis and in the more thoughtful identification and compassionate use of individual patients' predicaments, rights, and preferences in making clinical decisions about their care" (Sackett et al., 1996). Clinical experts are able to determine if the available evidence is relevant, and if so, how to best incorporate this information into the decision making based on the individual patient values and preferences. Clinical evidence is simply relevant and useful information that enlightens and enhances the clinician's understanding of the individual patient scenario. Evidence comes from various sources, in multiple forms, and variable strength. Clinicians must strive to be aware of and incorporate information based on the well-designed, high quality studies (e.g., randomized controlled trials). We must take caution not to dismiss weaker forms of evidence because they often provide the best available evidence. When clinicians rely on weak evidence, they acknowledge the risk of administering useless or even harmful interventions. Furthermore, clinicians must be aware of higher quality studies that provide stronger evidence as it is available and subsequently replace the weaker evidence with the higher quality information. Clinical evidence, in all its forms, can serve to both invalidate previously accepted diagnostic tests and interventions and inform the innovation and adoption of new and more powerful, more accurate, more efficacious, and safer techniques (Sackett et al., 1996). Although clinical evidence informs and is informed by clinical practice and expertise, it is not a substitute for individual clinical expertise. Ultimately, clinical practice guidelines are the best source of evidence for clinicians. Although there are numerous clinical practice guidelines available for hand therapists, few are evidence based and much work is needed to summarize and integrate the best available information related to hand therapy and upper extremity orthoses (MacDermid, 2004; Szabo & MacDermid, 2009).

The patient-centered clinical expert effectively integrates the best available clinical information with the unique patient values, such that each patient receives not similar care but uniquely individual care reflective of the vast variability among individual values and presentations. Evidence is necessary, but wholly insufficient, for the efficient and effective management of the individual patient.

The authors have integrated their clinical expertise and the best available and most contemporary evidence into this text. Readers are strongly encouraged to remain abreast of the most current and best available evidence to both inform their developing clinical expertise and to supplement the work of the authors of this text.

frames (Radomski & Trombley, 2013). These theoretical frames help guide practice in the field of hand therapy and subsequent orthotic intervention, providing therapists with reasons for their treatment based on theory. The profession of occupational therapy applies these approaches of intervention with the goal of returning the patient to their maximal functional ability. The biomechanical approach involves the principles of physics as it relates to human movement, forces, and posture, addressing deficits in ROM, strength, and endurance. The **rehabilitative approach** focuses on getting the patient back to being as independent as possible involving environmental changes and physical adaptations. Box 6–2 provides a more detailed description of this theoretical approach to treatment.

A skilled therapist would never approach two patients in the same way. Therapists need to be responsive to the specific and changing needs of their patients, altering the therapy treatment in response to changes in tissue status. For example, when considering the stage of healing of a particular tissue, therapists must apply the most appropriate orthosis for that stage. An orthosis that is appropriate for a patient for 1 week may not be the best choice a month or even a week later. In general, immobilization orthoses is appropriate for resting an acutely injured body part; this is followed by a more aggressive approach, such as mobilization orthoses, during the later stages of healing. Refer to Chapter 3 for a more detailed discussion. Taking a client-centered **bio-occupational approach** to orthotic fabrication, described by McKee and Rivard (2011b), involves the appreciation of the patient's unique needs as well as the specific biologic requirements of the involved tissues. This approach results in a functionally relevant orthosis allowing for occupational performance that maximizes the patient's functional use yet provides the affected tissues with the appropriate environment for healing. Box 6–3 provides a clinical example highlighting the main concepts of this unique approach to orthotic fabrication.

Patient Education and Precautions

Educating the patient is essential for deriving the greatest benefit from the use of an orthosis. A sample patient education handout is given in Box 6–4. An opportune time to educate the patient is during a trial wearing of the orthosis (20 to 30 minutes) in the clinic to check for any immediate problems. Patients must understand the purpose of the orthosis, which relates to understanding the diagnosis and treatment approach. The patient and caregiver should be made aware of how to don and doff the orthosis, what to expect and what to look out for while wearing the device, and when and how long to wear it. Taking photos of the orthosis properly in place with cell phones can be very helpful for the patient to have something to refer to later at home. Instructions should be clear regarding what the patient is permitted to do

in terms of activities with the orthosis on and off. Teach the patient to monitor for adverse reactions such as skin redness and irritation, circulatory compromise, and nerve compression. Educating the caregivers is mandatory, especially when dispensing an orthosis to a child or an older individual with cognitive or physical impairments.

Proper care of the orthosis is necessary for hygiene and to ensure greatest function. Patients need to wash the orthosis with warm water and soap or rubbing alcohol and replace the liners and strapping when needed. If the orthosis is exposed to heat sources, it may soften and distort; thus, the patient must keep the device away from stoves, radiators, fireplaces, and direct sunlight (e.g., the car dashboard) (Fig. 6–14). Therapists must give the patient and caregiver written instructions along with a means to contact the clinic if any problems or questions arise.

Ideally, schedule the patient for a follow-up visit to check orthosis tolerance and to review the instructions. If patients are not scheduled to return to the clinic, they often do not report problems of discomfort or ineffectiveness. There is nothing worse than getting a phone call from a physician about a patient who has not worn an orthosis because it wasn't comfortable or, worse yet, was harmful to the patient in some way. If the patient is unable to return to the clinic for follow-up because he or she lives far away, the therapist should attempt to call the patient to obtain verbal feedback and/or to offer a referral to a facility closer to his or her home, if appropriate.

Orthosis Pricing and Insurance Reimbursement

Reimbursement for orthotic fabrication depends on the specific insurance carrier and the contracts with the individual facility. Patients should be made aware of their coverage and encouraged to contact their insurance customer service representative for clarification of benefits. The pricing of orthoses depends on the facility and their individual reimbursement policy; there is no universally accepted system. Each facility determines its reimbursement schedule based on several factors. The cost of an orthosis should include fabrication time, thermoplastic materials, strapping, lining and padding, stockinettes, and components.

Cost constraints have forced therapists to be more judicious with orthotic intervention. Less costly options that do not compromise appropriate treatment standards should be offered to patients. For example, perhaps a prefabricated orthosis purchased at a medical-supply store or local pharmacy could serve the same purpose as a custom-fabricated wrist orthosis. Casting may be a less costly option when compared to the price of thermoplastic materials. Homemade outriggers from wire and scrap thermoplastic material may be less expensive than the commercially available component kits. The Clinical Pearls included in Section II note ways to

BOX 6-2

Orthotic Intervention and Occupational Therapy: A Theoretical Framework

Contribution by Gail Daddio, MHSc, OTR/L, CHT, CLT
Hand Therapist
The Orthopaedic Group, Milford CT
Adjunct Professor
Department of Occupational Therapy
Quinnipiac University, Hamden CT

When considering orthotic intervention in the rehabilitative approach, the client's occupational needs should be considered. Occupations are the actions that people take to occupy their time that are meaningful and have purpose for the individuals. Occupations encompass "the active process of living: from the beginning to the end of life, our occupations are all the active processes of looking after ourselves and others, enjoying life, and being socially and economically productive over the lifespan" (Boyt Schell, Gillen, Scaffa, & Cohn, 2013, p. 3). In occupational therapy practice, there are eight areas that define occupations, including the following:

- ADLs
- Instrumental ADLs
- Education
- Work
- Play
- Leisure
- Social participation
- Sleep

Understanding what the clients do with their time, what occupations they engage in, as well as their impact on society can aid the therapist in formulating an intervention plan that can incorporate a useful/functional orthosis with the clients. In addition, when treating a client with hand injury, the rehabilitative approach can also be combined with the occupational performance approach. The occupational performance, or the **Person, Environment, Occupation (PEO) Model**, is a theoretical frame of reference that can assist the therapist in understanding the clients' functional level, their occupation, and the environment in which they engage in at a certain time in their life span (Strong et al., 1999). The overlap of these three subsets in this model is critical in relation to the fabrication of an orthosis. The PEO model supports the hand therapist in determining how the orthosis may change the clients' functional abilities, affect their occupations, and, ultimately the overall impact the orthosis may have on their occupational performance in their environment. This systematic approach in analyzing these factors aids the therapist in assessing the therapeutic value of the orthosis as well as assisting in the determination of the specifics of the orthosis. For example, a laborer with an occupation of work returning to his job with a healing wrist fracture can benefit from a custom-fabricated wrist orthosis used for support and protection while working, as compared to the elderly woman with a mild case of osteoarthritis who is engaging in her occupation of leisure, who can benefit from a prefabricated thumb orthosis for support while performing her knitting activities.

The application of the combined rehabilitative and PEO approaches to occupational therapy practice, including the fitting of an orthosis, enables the interrelationship between the therapist and the client in determining a successful outcome to which one can engage in a meaningful occupation in a chosen environment

(Strong et al., 1999). This collaborative or client-centered approach involves the experience and knowledge of the client to facilitate set therapeutic goals with the treating therapist as it relates to the fitting and training of the orthosis (Boyt Schell et al., 2013). "Effective therapy is only as good as the quality of the relationship between the therapist and the consumer" (Boyt Schell et al., 2013, p. 133).

When assessing a client for an orthosis, not only should identification of the client's areas of occupation be determined but also his or her performance skills. This may include assessment of the client's sensory, motor, cognitive, and communication skills, all of which are imperative for compliance with an orthosis. In addition, evaluation of the demands of an activity as it relates to a specific orthosis should be determined to allow full functional mobility of the hand/upper extremity while the client is performing the desired task. Client factors such as his or her values and spiritual beliefs should be respected when assessing for an appropriate orthosis. Because therapists provide holistic interventions, identifying underlying factors that may influence a client's motivation to engage in occupations with an orthosis should be considered (American Occupational Therapy Association [AOTA], 2008).

The "Occupational Therapy Practice Framework: Domain and Process" identifies performance patterns that may affect a client's rehabilitation (AOTA, 2008). Performance patterns such as habits, routines, roles, and rituals may influence the use of an orthosis. For example, the role of a mother with child rearing can be disrupted or altered with an injury or disability; therefore, assessment of a role change as it relates to the fitting and training of an orthosis should be considered when determining the appropriate orthosis by the hand therapist (Boyt Schell et al., 2013).

Contextual influences are also part of the "Occupational Therapy Practice Framework." Contexts are interrelated conditions that surround the client that may affect the client's performance (AOTA, 2008). Some of these influences include cultural, personal, temporal, physical, virtual, and social. To elaborate on cultural influence, for example, the inability to shake hands during an introduction when wearing an orthosis may alter a client culturally. An example of a personal influence can be a client's inability to return to work while wearing an orthosis. This can affect one's socioeconomic status, thus changing the compliance of the orthosis wearing schedule. The virtual context is another example of an influence that can be affected by the application of an orthosis. In today's environment with a large emphasis on social media such as texting, the inability to communicate because of an orthosis on a client's hand can influence a person contextually.

The fabrication of an orthosis includes evaluation, intervention, and outcomes. Identification of the clients' occupational profile including their diagnosis, concerns, and performance of their occupations should be addressed (AOTA, 2008). An intervention plan regarding the wearing regimen, precautions, and care should be agreed upon prior to implementation of the orthosis. The successful use of an orthosis can support the client's overall health and participation in all of life tasks (AOTA, 2008).

BOX 6–3

Bio-Occupational Orthotic Approach

Contribution by Pat McKee, M.Sc., OT Reg. (Ont.), OT(C)
Associate Professor
Department of Occupational Science and Occupational
Therapy
University of Toronto, Toronto Canada

Susie, a 29-year-old graduate university student, "always had hand joint problems." She had right (dominant) carpometacarpal (CMC) joint pain that radiated into the first web space, thenar eminence, and second metacarpal and had difficulty with tasks such keyboarding, driving, jar opening, grasping a subway pole, and pen writing.

She was fitted with a custom-molded neoprene-lined thermoplastic, thumb CMC, MP stabilizing orthosis with IP extension block. It was secured with a stretchy hook-receptive neoprene strap that permitted some CMC and MP mobility while ensuring sufficient stabilization to relieve pain. (Fig. Box 6–3A–C). Upon donning the orthosis, she immediately noticed she could pick up and grip her laptop computer, with the affected hand only, without pain.

Initially, Susie's gross grasp was 32 kg and 28 kg with and without the orthosis, respectively, whereas her unaffected hand was 38 kg. After 4 months, gross grasp had increased to 37 kg without the orthosis. Lateral pinch strength was initially 7.5 kg with and without the orthosis and rose to 8.5 kg without the orthosis after 4 months. Susie's worst pain rating decreased from 5/10 to 1/10 and pain frequency reduced from 6.5/10 to .25/10 4 months after initiation of orthotic intervention.

Susie wore the orthosis often for about a month, then gradually decreased its use and eventually only wore it for weight-bearing activities such as push-ups. By 4 months, she did not need the orthosis at all, even for weight bearing through her hand, because of increased hand strength and reduced pain. In addition, she reported little or no difficulty with any tasks. What was most notable was the impact on her mood, sense of control over her life, and ability to engage in physical activities.

In her own words, at 4 months after orthotic fitting, "Orthoses can immediately give a person back much of their function. I didn't realize how much of my life I had abandoned because I wanted to avoid the pain. Much of the activities were leisure based like badminton, basketball, yoga, and Pilates. Since getting the orthosis, I have now lost 35 lb and counting. Having the range of activities to choose from again has been so motivating and provided more chances for successful life changes."

Susie's favorable outcomes were achieved using the client-centered *bio-occupational orthotic approach* (Mckee & Rivard, 2011b), which addresses (1) the person's biologic (anatomical and physiologic) needs and (2) factors that enable participation in activities that are important and meaningful to the person. This approach begins with understanding that an orthosis is "a prefabricated or custom-made device applied to biological structures to optimize *body function and structures*—considering nutrition, length, strength, mobility, and stability—to ultimately promote current or future *activities and participation* in roles important to the individual" (McKee & Rivard, 2011b, p. 1569).

"Body functions and structures" and "activities and participation" are key concepts influencing health, as described in the *International Classification of Functioning, Disability and Health* (ICF) published by the World Health Organization (2002). Sixteen guiding principles, described in the following text, make explicit the professional reasoning of the bio-occupational orthotic approach (Mckee & Rivard, 2011a, 2011b) (see Table 1).

Promote client-centeredness: Susie's therapist worked collaboratively with her using a holistic perspective that considered her unique personal attributes, including age; cognition; affect; physical attributes; and unique context including environment, activity demands, and culture. The therapist engaged Susie the person throughout the assessment, individualized intervention, and monitoring/modification processes.

Consider psychosocial factors: As a child, Susie had been provided with a custom-fitted hand orthosis that she had found too inconvenient and cumbersome to use. Her therapist needed to consider that when Susie came to her hand therapy appointment, negative past experiences could have posed an emotional barrier.

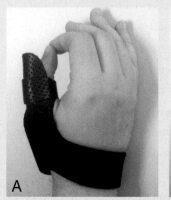 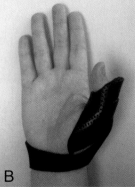 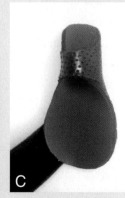

BOX 6–3 FIGURE Thumb MP-stabilizing, IP-extension-blocking orthosis made from ¹⁄₁₆" thick thermoplastic bonded to ¹⁄₁₆" neoprene with hook-receptive neoprene strap. Note unrestricted thumb IP flexion. **A**, Dorsal view, **(B)** volar view, and **(C)** palmar view of orthosis showing neoprene lining.

(continued)

BOX 6–3

Bio-Occupational Orthotic Approach (*Continued*)

Optimize body function and structures: This goal relates to the ICF's *body function and structures*, acknowledging that orthoses attend to the biologic (physical) causes of impaired function. Susie's orthosis stabilized her thumb CMC and MP joint, thus promoting resorption of lax periarticular structures. In turn, reduced pain, sustained joint stability, and enhanced hand strength and function were achieved.

Enable activity and participation: This goal relates to the ICF's *activity and participation*. For Susie, hand pain and reduced grip/pinch strength had caused difficulty with many tasks. With the orthosis, she was immediately able to perform tasks without fear of pain and over time returned to valued leisure and health-enhancing activities.

Consider environmental factors: For Susie, consideration of *environmental factors*, another key construct of the ICF, included her physical and social environments.

Well engineered: Sound design and fabrication features of Susie's orthosis included unrestricted mobility of the wrist joint and thumb interphalangeal joint flexion, secure bonding of the neoprene to the thermoplastic and incorporating a stretchy, conforming neoprene strap.

Monitor and modify: Monitoring involves ongoing evaluation and collaboration with the client/caregiver to determine whether the orthosis is meeting biologic and functional/occupational goals. It assists the therapist to identify whether or not the person is wearing the orthosis and, if warranted, to explore reasons for nonuse. Monitoring of Susie's orthotic use revealed that she was experiencing numbness in her ring and small fingers and pain over her pisiform bone. She was advised to fasten the strap more loosely and to reposition the strap to avoid pisiform pressure.

Optimize usability: To enhance the likelihood of orthotic use, ask the question, "Is this orthosis useful to this individual?" A collaborative approach optimized the usability of Susie's orthosis, ensuring that perceived benefits were more compelling than any inconvenience, discomfort, or embarrassment imposed by it. Also, it was easy to don and doff and clean.

Provide choice: Individuals feel included and respected when they are provided with choices. Choices offered to Susie included color of thermoplastic and neoprene and inclusion/exclusion of neoprene lining.

Optimize comfort: Uncomfortable orthoses are unlikely to be used, thus comfort enhances usability. The neoprene lining and stretchy neoprene strap optimized the comfort of Susie's orthosis.

Minimize harm: The orthotic intervention process should ultimately make some positive contribution to the individual's life. If the orthosis fails to achieve its intended outcome, at the very least, it should minimize biologic harm. To be specific, biologic structures must not be compromised by, among other things, pressure points that result in skin breakdown, diminished circulation, or nerve compression. For Susie, monitoring averted biologic harm from excessive compression and inappropriate positioning of the neoprene strap.

Optimize cosmesis: An orthosis becomes a part of the person's personal environment and, like clothing, is seen by others. Furthermore, it is a product of our therapeutic intervention that will be on display, representing our profession and us individually and, as such, should reflect exemplary standards. For Susie "How it looked made a huge difference for me," thus enhancing usability. Efforts to optimize cosmesis should not be viewed as time consuming and unimportant. If not putting in the required time results in the client not wearing the orthosis, then the time used to fabricate it is truly wasted.

TABLE 1

Guiding Principles of Bio-Occupational Orthotic Approach

1. Promote client-centeredness	9. Provide choice
2. Consider psychosocial factors	10. Optimize comfort
3. Optimize body function and structures	11. Minimize harm
4. Enable activity and participation	12. Optimize cosmesis
5. Consider environmental factors	13. Optimize convenience
6. Well engineered	14. Use a less-is-more approach
7. Monitor and modify	15. Provide comprehensive client/caregiver education
8. Optimize usability	16. Evaluate outcomes

From McKee, P., & Rivard, A. (2011a). Biopsychosocial approach to orthotic intervention. *Journal of Hand Therapy*, 24(2), 155–163; McKee, P., & Rivard, A. (2011b). Foundations of orthotic intervention. In T. Skirven, L. E. Osterman, J. Fedorczyk, & P. Amadio (Eds.), *Rehabilitation of the hand and upper extremity* (6th ed., pp. 1565–1580). Philadelphia, PA: Elsevier.

BOX 6-3
Bio-Occupational Orthotic Approach *(Continued)*

Optimize convenience: For Susie, the orthotic solution was optimally convenient—easy to use and clean, secure adherence of hook Velcro®, and secure bonding of neoprene lining.

Use a less-is-more approach: Minimalism in the design of Susie's orthosis included use of thin thermoplastic and neoprene (both ⅟₁₆″/1.6 mm thick), a narrow wrist strap, and no unnecessary restriction of joint mobility.

Provide comprehensive client/caregiver education: To optimize usability, the client and/or caregiver should clearly understand the rationale for the orthosis, when to wear it, how to put it on and make adjustments, how to care for it, when and how to contact the therapist, and assurance that client feedback and inquiries are welcome. For Susie, written instructions were provided. She was trained in how to don and doff the orthosis and how to use the strap.

Evaluate outcomes: Evaluation of outcomes (1) fulfills the therapist's basic professional responsibility to assess the orthotic process for the purpose of continuous program improvement and (2) identifies the extent to which biologic and functional goals have been achieved. Susie's therapist evaluated changes in grip and pinch strength, pain, and degree of difficulty with activities.

Orthoses should be comfortable, fabricated from appropriate materials, aesthetically pleasing, and convenient to use. Comfort, cosmesis, and convenience and, thus, usability, are enhanced by applying the guiding principle of less is more. Monitoring and modifying and evaluating outcomes are essential stages in a process that ensures usability of the orthosis while providing evidence of orthotic efficacy and the continuous improvement of practice guidelines.

Orthoses that are thoughtfully designed with client input can make a difference in a person's life by relieving pain, providing joint stabilization, protecting vulnerable tissues, and enabling valued activities and participation. This in turn promotes physical and emotional well-being.

BOX 6-4
Patient Education Handout

Care and Use of Your Custom Orthosis

The orthosis was custom made for you by: _____

The purpose of the orthosis is to: _____

The orthosis should be worn: _____
_____

- Notify your therapist if you notice the following:
  - Increase in pain
  - Change in swelling: generalized or between straps
  - Discoloration or temperature changes in the fingers
  - Local redness from pressure (at edges or over bony areas)
  - Numbness or tingling in hand or fingers
  - Areas of skin irritation (rash, itching, blotching)
- Do not wear the straps too tight. They should be firm but not tight or causing pain/swelling. They may require adjustments during the day.
- Wear the stockinette beneath the orthosis to help manage perspiration.

MOST IMPORTANTLY: FOLLOW THE WEARING SCHEDULE PRESCRIBED BY YOUR THERAPIST AND PHYSICIAN.

If you are allowed to remove the orthosis during the day, please remember the following:

- Keep your orthosis away from sources of heat (radiators, ovens, direct sunlight in a car).
- Your orthosis may be cleaned with soap/warm water or rubbing alcohol/disinfecting wipes. Be sure to rinse and dry the orthosis well before wearing.
- Straps and sleeves may be washed by hand and allowed to air dry.
- Do not make any adjustments to the orthosis yourself.

If you have any questions or concerns, please call the therapist who made your orthosis. If not available, please ask for the supervisor.

Therapist: _____   Phone: _____

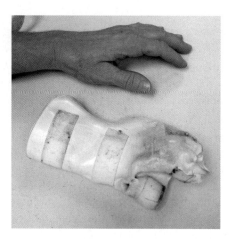

FIGURE 6–14 Flattened orthosis resulting from being left in hot car for a few hours.

decrease the costs of these devices offering cost-saving ideas to many situations. Therapists should take a proactive role in their state organizations by educating insurance companies to promote and maximize reimbursement of therapy services. Refer to Chapter 1 for additional information.

Orthotic Fabrication Process

The chapters in Section II are organized first by purpose (immobilization, mobilization, and restriction) and then by the body part of origin (digit, hand, forearm, arm). For example, a static wrist support (wrist immobilization orthosis) is described under immobilization (Chapter 7) and then within the section that focuses on forearm-based orthoses. The description of each orthosis includes common names, alternative options, primary functions, additional functions, and common diagnoses and optimal positions. Positions are suggested as only a guide; the therapist must always be sure to contact the referring physician to determine positioning. Finally, the fabrication process is detailed for each orthosis, using the "PROCESS" concept.

PROCESS

The PROCESS format, used throughout Section II, provides a highly organized, systematic approach to orthotic fabrication. The PROCESS acronym is defined as follows:

    P—Pattern creation
    R—Refine pattern
    O—Options for materials
    C—Cut and heat
    E—Evaluate fit while molding
    S—Strapping and components
    S—Survey completed orthosis

The steps for the fabrication of each orthosis are organized in this manner. Each step consists of a list of information

unique to the specific orthosis discussed. The basic principles applicable to all orthoses and a summary are included in the pull-out sleeve at the back of the book. Use the pull-out sleeve as a bookmark when fabricating orthoses and refer to these universal points when fabricating each device. Keep the book open to the appropriate page for handy reference during the fabrication process. Section II has been conveniently designed so that the photographs and pattern can be viewed simultaneously to improve comprehension and promote usability.

Clinical and Pattern Pearls are scattered throughout Section II. These include helpful hints regarding the fabrication process and creative modifications of specific orthoses that the authors have found extremely effective in clinical practice. These tricks of the trade allow the reader to create truly customized orthoses. There is no cookbook method that can be used with every patient. Therapists must individualize their approach according to the specific needs of each patient.

When applying an orthosis on a patient with an injury that does not allow optimal positioning for pattern tracing or molding, the therapist must make modifications. For example, positioning the hand flat on a table is contraindicated for patients recovering from flexor tendon repairs because this position puts the repaired structures at risk for attenuation or rupture. As an appropriate alternative, trace the pattern on the uninvolved extremity. When checking the fit of the pattern, use the uninvolved side, if needed, to eliminate unnecessary movement of the injured extremity. Other positioning techniques include laying a patient on a plinth, using foam arm supports, and getting assistance from another therapist.

The following sections introduce the general instructions for fabricating orthoses.

Pattern Creation (Fig. 6–15A)

- Obtain referral with specific custom orthosis information from physician.
- Perform upper extremity examination.
- Determine specific needs and decide on type of orthosis to fabricate.
- Trace pattern on paper towel per orthosis diagram and cut it out. Use anatomical landmarks highlighted on pattern to aid in accurate pattern creation.

Refine Pattern

- Check fit of paper pattern by trying it on patient's extremity (or on unaffected extremity if warranted).
- Mark any areas that need adjustment (i.e., add or delete material).

Options for Material

- Decide on type of thermoplastic and strapping material.
- Transfer pattern to thermoplastic material using wax pencil or pen.

Cut and Heat (Fig. 6–15B,C)

- Partially heat thermoplastic material until soft enough to cut pattern accordingly.

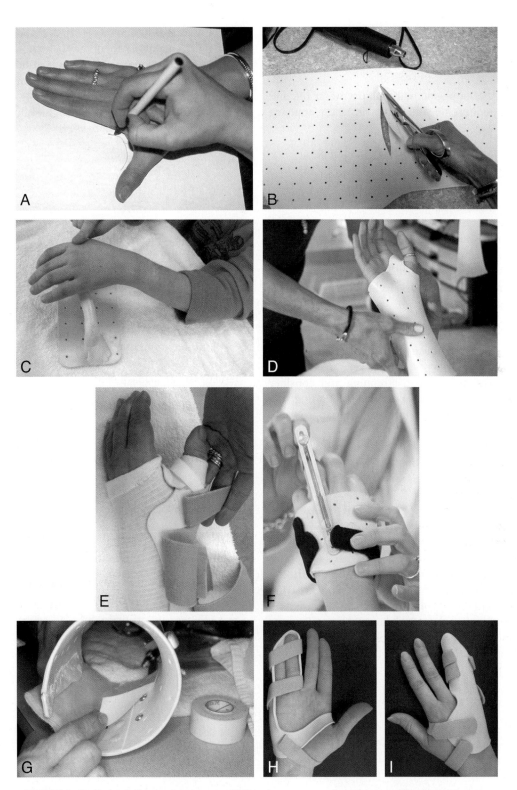

FIGURE 6–15 Orthotic fabrication process: **A,** Drawing pattern onto paper towel. **B,** Cutting pattern out of thermoplastic material. **C,** Positioning patient in a gravity-assisted position. **D,** Molding thermoplastic while visualizing creases to allow for distal mobility. **E,** Application of appropriate strapping system including padding for comfort. **F,** Adjusting component system in this mobilization orthosis. **G,** Covering the underside of screws with adhesive tape in this mobilization orthosis. **H and I,** Volar and dorsal views of a completed orthosis, checking for adjacent joint mobility and optimal strap placement.

- Place patient's extremity in desired position and heat thermoplastic material to appropriate temperature.
- Apply any padding to high-risk bony areas before molding.
- Fully heat thermoplastic material, dry water off, and check temperature on your own skin before applying to patient.

Evaluate Fit while Molding (Fig. 6–15D)

- Mold orthosis to patient, and remember to
  - Use gravity to assist whenever possible.
  - Incorporate arches.
  - Provide adequate length and width.
  - Evenly distribute pressure while molding.
  - Handle thermoplastic material gently.
- Mark areas to be trimmed with fingernail edge or pen and carefully remove orthosis from patient.
- Trim designated areas.

Strapping and Components (Fig. 6–15E–G)

- Determine optimal means of securing orthosis to extremity.
- Provide adequate width in strapping and consider foam for key straps to obtain optimal positioning.
- Place orthosis on patient's limb and apply appropriate strapping.
- Affix specific components, such as hinges or outriggers, per pattern instructions.

Survey Completed Orthosis (Fig. 6–15H,I)

- Flare edges and round sharp corners of orthosis. This is best completed by selectively dipping 1 to 2 mm of material's edge into warm water.
- Round corners of strapping.
- Provide patient with written handouts describing purpose, precautions, proper care, and wearing schedule.
- Instruct in functional use and diagnosis-specific exercise within the orthosis if appropriate.

- Check that patient is able to don and doff the orthosis independently. Patient may benefit from digital photographs of proper orthosis application.
- Provide information on replacements for stockinette, straps, or other items.
- Schedule follow-up visit to reevaluate and modify orthosis as appropriate.

Conclusion

This chapter provides an overview of the orthotic intervention process: from obtaining the physician referral to dispensing the completed orthosis. A comprehensive examination is necessary to gather the information required to make sound clinical decisions regarding specific treatment interventions. The therapist must appreciate the phases of tissue healing and how therapy and orthotic intervention are applied appropriately in order to do no harm. Effective communication with the patient and physician helps maximize the patient's final outcome.

Chapter Review Questions

1. What, ideally, needs to be included in a physician referral?

2. Why is it important to take a medical history?

3. How can pain be measured?

4. What is evidence-based practice and how does it relate to orthotic intervention?

5. Describe the "PROCESS" of orthotic fabrication as described in this chapter.

Orthotic Fabrication

MaryLynn Jacobs, MS, OTR/L, CHT
Noelle M. Austin, MS, PT, CHT

This section contains the instructions for orthotic fabrication. The orthoses have been organized into four chapters according to the type of orthosis: immobilization (Chapter 7), mobilization (Chapter 8), restriction (Chapter 9), and nonarticular (Chapter 10). Before delving into orthotic fabrication, it is important to note that the patterns given here should not be approached as if they were a recipe from a cookbook, blindly used for every patient. The patterns are a collection of frequently used designs intended to be modified to meet each specific patient's needs and diagnosis requirements. Therapists must tailor their approaches to orthotic fabrication according to the unique needs of each patient. Again, these patterns are to be used as *basic guidelines only*. More detailed information about orthotic fabrication for specific patient populations and diagnoses can be found in Section IV.

To be consistent when naming orthoses, this text will continue to support and integrate historical nomenclature; however, the language set forth by the Centers for Medicare & Medicaid Services (CMS) takes precedence and will be fully described and incorporated into naming all orthoses. The authors of Chapter 1 have taken the modified ASHT Splint Classification System (1992) and the current CMS L-Code orthotic descriptions and created a modified, streamlined classification system that will be used for the primary name of each orthosis described in this book. The fabrication instructions for each orthosis will also include the common names of each orthosis design, which will allow the reader to cross-reference and use the terms preferred in a specific clinical setting.

Included is a list of common names that are used by the majority of practitioners caring for the patient with a hand injury. Under the heading "Alternative Orthosis Options," other orthoses are noted that may be used as a substitute or alternative if for some reason the described orthosis is not appropriate because of the specific circumstances of the patient or diagnosis.

The patterns for the orthoses also include the most common reason for application, primary function, and other uses listed under the heading "Additional Functions." The reader may use the cross-reference index (found in the back of the book) to locate a specific pattern. Also, when reading through each chapter, there may be a photo of an orthosis that is of interest to the reader. All the orthoses found in the chapters will have a reference under the photo as to where in the pattern section (Section II) the instructions to fabricate that specific orthosis can be found.

"Common Diagnoses and General Optimal Positions" are outlined for each orthosis. As noted, these lists are intended to be general guidelines. For example, only the most common diagnoses for each orthosis are noted. The fabrication method of each orthosis follows the PROCESS acronym, which is described in detail in Chapter 6 as well as on the foldout book mark.

The PROCESS acronym is defined as follows: (Table 7–1)

P — **Pattern creation**
R — **Refine pattern**
O — **Options for material**
C — **Cut and heat**
E — **Evaluate fit while molding**
S — **Strapping and components**
S — **Survey completed orthosis**

This updated edition includes Pattern Pearls that are alterations/modifications made to the pattern. These alterations in the pattern may include ways to accommodate for use with different materials or modify the existing pattern to meet the specific needs of the patient.

Clinical Pearls are found throughout Section II. Clinical Pearls can be "tricks of the trade" and/or "clinical tips" that stimulate *clinician creativity, critical thinking,* and *problem solving* when attempting to fabricate the best option for the patient and the circumstances surrounding the diagnosis. Many of the Clinical Pearls shown throughout Section II can be applied to various orthoses/conditions and not just to the orthosis they are located adjacent to in the text. See the list of Clinical Pearls at the beginning of the book to locate a specific "pearl" of interest.

In this revised text, both the clinical and pattern pearls are numerous and well detailed via accompanying photographs. These photographs and additional instructions further highlight how the fabricator should consider modifying the specific orthosis to meet the patient's unique orthotic requirements. The Clinical Pearl photographs are of true patients gathered from the authors and their colleague's years of clinical practice. Many of these pearls are not "perfect" in construction/design; however, the authors felt they are wonderful teaching tools as is. These imperfections reflect what happens in daily practice given the shortage of time, materials, and perhaps lack of experience. On the appropriate orthoses, the authors have noted the problematic areas with suggestions for improvements.

Most of the orthoses shown in Section II (except for many of the Pattern and Pearls) were fabricated using TailorSplint™ thermoplastic material (Patterson Medical, Warrenville, IL). A nonperforated material was used for the photographed orthoses to minimize distractions and improve visualization of details. The therapist is encouraged to use the most appropriate material for the diagnosis and patient; more information may be found under the heading "Options for Materials" and in Chapter 5.

TABLE 7–1		
P-R-O-C-E-S-S of Orthotic Fabrication		
P	Pattern creation	• Obtain referral with specific custom orthosis information from physician.
		• Perform upper extremity examination.
		• Determine specific needs and decide on type of orthosis to fabricate.
		• Trace pattern on paper towel per orthosis diagram and cut it out. Use anatomical landmarks highlighted on pattern to aid in accurate pattern creation.
R	Refine pattern	• Check fit of paper pattern by trying it on patient's extremity (or on unaffected extremity if warranted).
		• Mark any areas that need adjustment (i.e., add or delete material).
O	Options for materials	• Decide on type of thermoplastic and strapping material.
		• Transfer pattern to thermoplastic material using wax pencil or pen.
C	Cut and heat	• Partially heat thermoplastic material until soft enough to cut pattern accordingly.
		• Place patient's extremity in desired position and heat thermoplastic material to appropriate temperature.
		• Apply any padding to high-risk bony areas prior to molding.
		• Fully heat thermoplastic material, dry water off, and check temperature on your own skin before applying to patient.
E	Evaluate fit while molding	• Mold orthosis to patient, and remember to
		• Use gravity to assist whenever possible.
		• Incorporate arches.
		• Provide adequate length and width.
		• Evenly distribute pressure while molding.
		• Handle thermoplastic material gently.
		• Mark areas to be trimmed with fingernail edge or pen, and carefully remove orthosis from patient.
		• Trim designated areas.
S	Strapping and components	• Determine optimal means of securing orthosis to extremity.
		• Provide adequate width in strapping and consider foam for key straps to obtain optimal positioning.
		• Place orthosis on patient's limb and apply appropriate strapping.
		• Affix specific components—such as hinges or outriggers—per pattern instructions.
S	Survey completed orthosis	• Flare edges and round sharp corners of orthosis. This is best completed by selectively dipping 1–2 mm of material's edge into warm water.
		• Round corners of strapping.
		• Provide patient with written handouts describing the orthosis' purpose, precautions, proper care, and wearing schedule.
		• Instruct in functional use and diagnosis-specific exercises within the orthosis if appropriate.
		• Check that patient is able to don and doff the orthosis independently. Patients may benefit from digital photographs of proper orthosis application.
		• Provide information on replacements for stockinette, straps, or other items.
		• Consider taking digital photographs of completed custom-fabricated orthosis for patient records and to verify accurate accounting and billing to payers.
		• Schedule follow-up visit to reevaluate and modify orthosis as appropriate.

CHAPTER 7

7   Immobilization Orthoses

General Clinical Pearls Related to Immobilization Orthoses

Pattern Creation/Refine Pattern

CLINICAL PEARL 7-X1.
Transferring Pattern to Material

There are many ways to transfer the paper towel pattern to the thermoplastic material. The main goal is to avoid an unsightly orthosis with pen markings along the edges. Here are some techniques: Allow the paper towel to adhere to the wet material during the cutting process (**left**), use a wax pencil to outline the design (**right**), or scratch the thermoplastic material with an awl to draw the pattern.

CLINICAL PEARL 7-X2.
Pattern Considerations for Border Digits

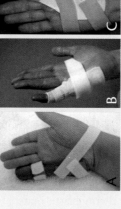
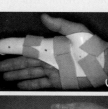

To provide for better stability of the orthosis on the hand and to achieve increased purchase of distal joints, include a portion of the metacarpal (and overlying thenar and hypothenar eminences) within the orthosis. This is especially helpful when applying orthoses on small hands.

CLINICAL PEARL 7-X3.
Pin Care Window

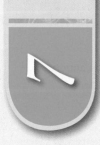

For patients with complicated injuries that require pin care during the immobilization period, consider fabricating a removable window for easy access to the pins. This technique eliminates the need to remove the entire orthosis when inspecting pin sites. While molding the material over the pin(s), use a piece of gauze or cotton batting to prevent the thermoplastic material from adhering to the pins; this also provides a protective bubble to ensure the material will not place undue pressure directly over the area.

CLINICAL PEARL 7-X4.
Orthoses for Use during Therapy Session

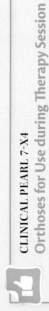
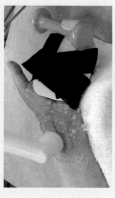

A thermoplastic volar hand piece with an integrated hook can hold a weight to apply a passive stretch during a therapeutic intervention technique such as shown with ultrasound

Options For Materials

CLINICAL PEARL 7-X5.
Elastic-Based Materials Allow for Remolding

Consider an elastic-based material when fabricating an orthosis on an edematous extremity or when it is known that an orthosis will need to be modified during the rehabilitation because of diagnosis-specific issues. When reheated, the memory characteristic in these materials allows the material to closely return to its original shape.

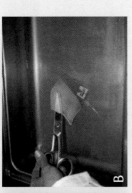

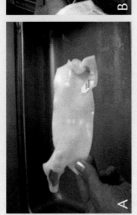

CLINICAL PEARL 7-X7.
Reusing Old Orthoses

To save money, reuse old orthoses to fabricate new ones when appropriate. For example, during the initial phases of healing after a UCL injury, the patient may require a thumb immobilization orthosis for protection (**A**). Once the fracture has healed, the patient may experience joint stiffness at the thumb MP and/or IP joints that requires mobilization. The original immobilization orthosis can be remolded into a mobilization orthosis by simply trimming the thumb region and attaching components (**B**).

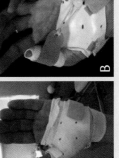
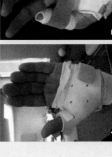

CLINICAL PEARL 7-X6.
Using Scrap Thermoplastic Material

Scrap pieces of thermoplastic material come in handy for many different situations. For example, material can be molded around a writing utensil or tools to build up the handle. Also, scraps can be used for the fabrication of small digit orthoses and for securing mobilization components onto bases.

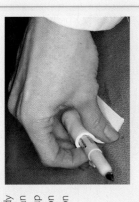

CLINICAL PEARL 7-X8.
Cutting a Slit into Thermoplastic

A spot heater can be used when it is too cumbersome to partially heat a thermoplastic material to make either a hole or a slit as shown here. This is particularly true when working with a large piece of material. Shown is the use of a spot heater to warm the middle section of the pattern in order to create the "slit" used in this dorsal volar forearm immobilization orthosis. Once warmed, sharp scissors are able to cut through the material without creating jagged edges.

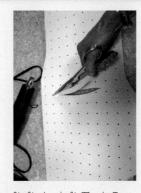

CLINICAL PEARL 7-X9.
Use of a Dremel

A, A Dremel is a helpful tool to have in the clinic. This can be used to perforate solid material in a specific area to prevent skin issues (**B**), make holes in areas not reachable with a hole punch, and cut slits in material for creative strapping techniques (**C**).

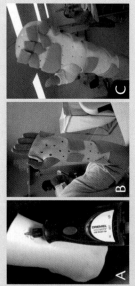

Cut and Heat

CLINICAL PEARL 7-X10.
Quality Scissors

Not all scissors are appropriate for every task. Having various types of scissors on hand can make the fabrication process a lot easier. **A,** Gingher Super Shears are best used for cutting out orthosis patterns on warm thermoplastic material and may not be effective for small detailed cutting. **B,** Unlimited Scissors are an excellent alternative for detailed cutting in small areas. **C,** When serial static finger orthoses are fabricated using a circumferential method of application, small Serial Cast Cutter Scissors are extremely useful for easy removal; the blunt nose prevents any risk of injury for the patient. **D,** Fiskars® Non-Stick Scissors are ideal for cutting adhesive products because of the protective coating. **E,** Pinking Shears can be an excellent addition to a utility drawer. Using these scissors to cut stockinette off a roll can prevent and/or prolong the fraying of this material. (All available through Patterson Medical.)

CLINICAL PEARL 7-X11.
Caring for Scissors

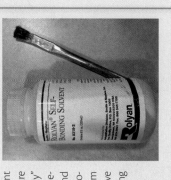

First, investing in quality scissors is a must for the frequent orthotic maker. Proper care of the scissors is crucial to ensure their effective use. Designating scissors "thermoplastic only" and "strapping only" prevents the strapping material's adhesive from sticking to the thermoplastic when cutting and trimming warm material. Use solvent, adhesive remover, alcohol wipes, or nail polish remover to clean the adhesive from scissors. Furthermore, sharpen the scissors often to achieve smooth edges when cutting materials (Rolyan® Self-Bonding Solvent; Patterson Medical).

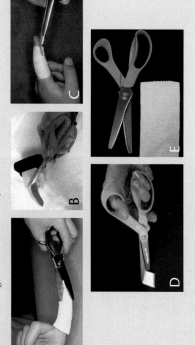

Heating Materials

CLINICAL PEARL 7-X12.
Tips for Heating Thermoplastic Materials

Use a designated heating device such as a commercially available heat pan or skillet. The addition of pan netting as well as a spatula can prevent thermoplastics from sticking to the bottom of the unit. Empty and clean the unit regularly. Adding a small amount of liquid soap to the water can help "soften" any potentially hard water, making thermoplastics less sticky and easier to handle. Avoid using a hot pack unit to heat the materials; they are not hygienic or heat controlled. Also, be sure to partially heat material for approximately 30 seconds prior to cutting out the pattern to save your own thumbs from the potential wear and tear of the repetitive forceful cutting of hard thermoplastics.

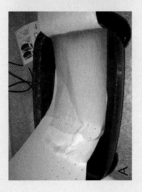
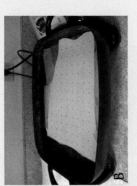

CLINICAL PEARL 7-X14.
Handling Warm Thermoplastic Material

The surface used to dry off warmed thermoplastic material after removal from the heat pan can cause unsightly ridges or markings, especially with materials that are very contouring. Lift the heated material out of the heating pan with a spatula or lift with netting to prevent overstretching. To prevent towel markings, place the warm material on a pillowcase before molding it onto the patient's extremity.

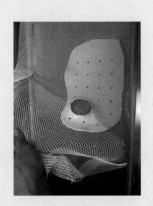

CLINICAL PEARL 7-X13.
Heating Large Piece of Material Evenly

Warm a section of material that will fit into the heating pan, making sure that there is netting on the bottom of the heating pan. Once it begins to soften, cover the section that is in the water completely with a paper towel. Then gently allow the remaining section to fold over the paper towel into the water. Pull the entire folded piece out of the water using the netting. Gently unfold and apply to patient.

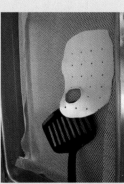
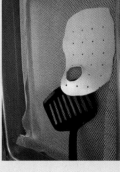

Evaluate Fit while Molding

CLINICAL PEARL 7-X15.
Using a Wrap or Stockinette Sleeve to Aid Fabrication

An elasticized wrap (Ace™), prewrap, or stockinette can aid in the fabrication and setting of a forearm-based orthosis, especially when positioning the joints is a challenge or when there is no assistant available to help with positioning. Use the wrap proximally to allow for hands-on positioning distally. Be sure to watch for compression forces at the forearm borders of the orthosis; just before the orthosis sets up, remove the wrap/sleeve and gently flare the borders away from the skin.

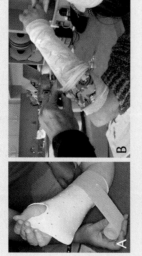

CLINICAL PEARL 7-X16.
Fabricating an Orthosis over Edema Management Products and Wound Dressings

During orthosis fabrication, the thermoplastic material can inadvertently adhere to the edema products (Coban™) and/or wound dressing. The dressing could potentially be pulled off the healing tissue. To avoid that risk, place a piece of stockinette over the wrap or dressing before molding the orthosis to the area. Once the orthosis is completely set, simply cut off the stockinette and remove the orthosis.

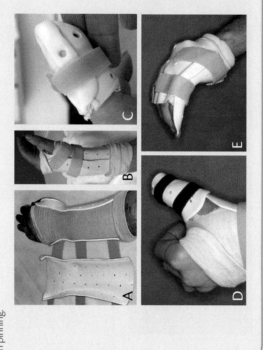

CLINICAL PEARL 7-X17.
Techniques for Adding Clamshell Piece

Many orthoses can be modified by molding an additional piece of thermoplastic material dorsally to create a "clamshell" orthosis commonly used with wrist and wrist/thumb immobilization orthoses **(A and B)**. This modification can provide additional protection and more rigid immobilization of the region. First, fabricate the volar orthosis per the instructions, but do not apply the strapping. Next, create the pattern for the dorsal piece, allowing approximately ½" of overlap of the dorsal piece over the molded volar segment. Prepad any bony prominences such as the ulnar styloid process to help prevent irritation. Use a coated material if possible to prevent unwanted adherence of the two pieces. If uncoated material is the only choice, use a stockinette or a wet paper towel over the volar segment while molding the dorsal piece. Other examples of dorsal protection provided for **(C)** distal phalanx crush injury, **(D)** thumb proximal phalanx pinning, and **(E)** multiple metacarpal fractures with pinning.

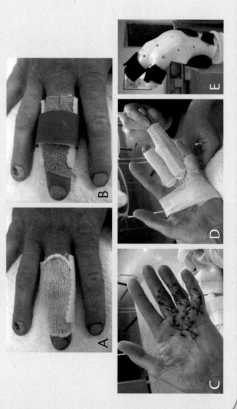

CLINICAL PEARL 7-X18.
Flaring versus Rolling of Edges

A flaring force should be gently applied to the warmed edge (approximately ¼") by the therapist's thenar and hypothenar regions. When deciding how to finish the edges, consider the advantages of flaring and the disadvantages of rolling. Rolling does not allow for simple modifications, such as widening the opening for the thumb or shortening the distal border to allow unimpeded MCP joint motion. Rolling back of a previously rolled region may lead to a bulky, unsightly orthosis. Flaring provides for easy adjustments and a neater looking orthosis.

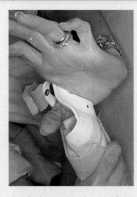

CLINICAL PEARL 7-X19.
Overstretching of Material

Caution should be taken when intending to overlap material for a closure technique. If not enough material is estimated, then overstretching and material breakdown will occur.

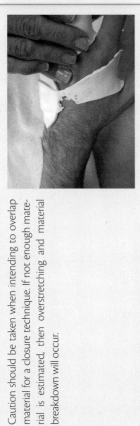

Strapping and Components

CLINICAL PEARL 7-X20.
Strapping Material Choices

Strapping comes in different colors, widths, and properties. The majority of orthoses can be secured using standard hook-and-loop closure, which is the most economical choice. Instead of buying various widths, purchase multiple colors of 2" loop and cut these down to fit the needs of the orthosis, keeping the scraps for later use. Using 1" adhesive hook allows for securing of both 1" and 2" loop without any extra trimming of the adhesive necessary. In certain circumstances, providing specialty straps may be indicated, such as the use of soft strapping for the arthritic patient (**A**), thin strapping for between digits (**B**), and elasticized loop for functional orthoses, allowing for muscle movement beneath the straps (**C**).

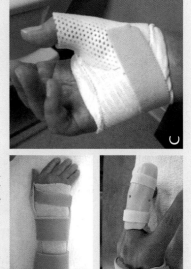

CLINICAL PEARL 7-X21.
Cutting Straps to Avoid Pressure on "At-Risk" Sites

Careful trimming of soft straps to avoid pressure on sensitive areas can greatly assist in orthosis compliance. **A**, This neoprene strap avoids pressure on the pin site. **B and C**, These 2" foam straps have been cut strategically to pass from volar to dorsal, allowing gentle radial deviation pressure on the proximal phalanges without irritating the digital web spaces. Both these materials tend to not fray.

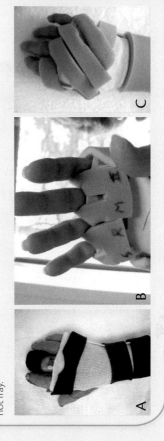

CLINICAL PEARL 7-X22.
Foam beneath Strapping

Application of strategically placed foam can be extremely helpful in obtaining the desired joint positions. **A,** Note the foam on the distal strap encouraging PIP joint extension as the pressure is applied volarly in this dorsal orthosis for a patient after Dupuytren release. **B,** In this volar design, the dorsal corrective pressure is applied over the PIP joint. **C,** Note the addition of foam under the distal phalanx volarly as well as the PIP joint dorsally to obtain full PIP extension. **D,** With volar forearm-based orthoses, the strap just proximal to the wrist crease is the most important, and the addition of foam will further encourage the wrist in the desired position, preventing wrist flexion within the orthosis. **E,** Slits cut into rectangle of 2″ foam strapping and slid onto 1″ strapping material can help improve pressure distribution as well as provide softer material against the skin.

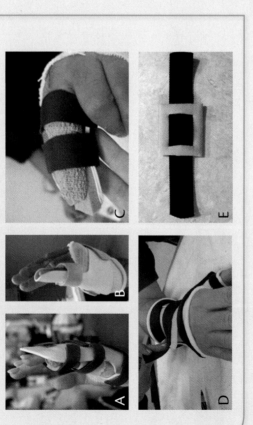

CLINICAL PEARL 7-X23.
Rotating Rivet for Flexibility in Strap Orientation

A thin piece of adhesive-backed Moleskin, adhesive loop, or similar material can be applied to both sides of a strap where the rivet is to be placed. A hole punch is then used to create a hole through the layers of strap, Moleskin and thermoplastic material. The rivet stem and cap is then closed with the blunt-nosed pliers; however, caution is taken to set the rivet with a gentle force. The rivet should be able to allow the strap to swivel in various directions as shown.

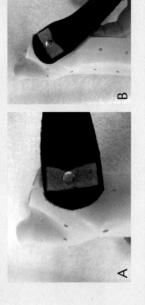

CLINICAL PEARL 7-X24.
Various Stockinette/Liner Choices

Several choices are available that add a layer of protection between the skin and the material. These liners help absorb perspiration and prevent any skin irritation that can occur at the skin–material interface. They can be removed multiple times a day and washed. The choices include materials such as cotton, elastic (for edema-reducing compression properties), polyester, and/or a combination of these. Removable liners offer a more hygienic option compared to semipermanent adhesive liners that need to be removed frequently if soiled. For long-term use, consider using a men's silk sock by cutting the end off and adding a hole for the thumb.

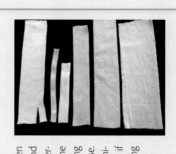

CHAPTER 7

CLINICAL PEARL 7-X25.
Edging Thermoplastic Material

A, One method is to use ⅟₁₆″ material to line the orthosis border. This works particularly well with perforated material because the edges of the cut holes can irritate the skin. Cut ⅟₁₆″ material in 1½″ to 2″ wide strips by the length required to go around the periphery of the orthosis. Apply solvent to the orthosis base to remove the protective coating and allow adherence of the strip. Once the strip is thoroughly heated, gently stretch (to disrupt the coating) and quickly place it along the orthosis border. The strip must be gently stretched and pinched over the edges to flatten out. This application must be done quickly and accurately because thin materials set readily. **B,** Other methods include (from left to right) Rolyan® Polycushion® Padding, Microfoam™ tape, and elastic therapeutic tape (Kinesio® Tex Tape, Patterson Medical) to line the borders. These methods work well for "quick fixes." **C,** Microfoam™ tape also can be used for smaller areas to provide relief from irritating edges as commonly seen in the first web space.

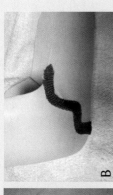

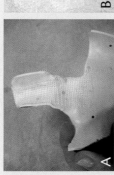

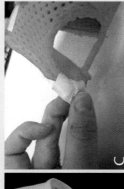

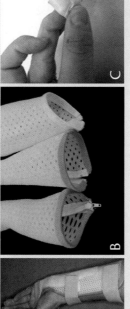

A   B   C

CLINICAL PEARL 7-X26.
Casting Tapes as Reinforcement Strips

Heated casting materials such as QuickCast 2 **(A)** or Orficast™ (Patterson Medical) can be used to add additional reinforcement to a weak area or an area that has been "thinned out" by overzealous stretching/molding.

A   B

CLINICAL PEARL 7-X27.
Elastomer Scar Molds Integrated into Orthosis

Scar management products such as Rolyan® 50/50 Mix™ Elastomer Putty (Patterson Medical) can be integrated into orthotic designs. Perforated thermoplastics allow for the material to set within the holes, securing the elastomer in place during the setting process. When using nonperforated materials, mold around one or more borders to assist in holding the product in the correct position.

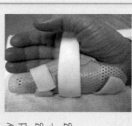

Survey Completed Orthosis

CLINICAL PEARL 7-X28.
Forearm Trough Height

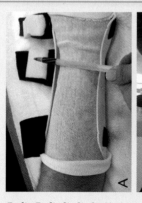
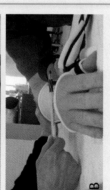

A
B

The forearm trough borders should be high enough to completely support and stabilize forearm. The deeper this trough, the more rigid the orthosis design and the more comfortable for the patient. Use the 45° angle technique (Clinical Pearl 7-44) to estimate two-thirds the circumference of the forearm. Once applied, be sure the borders are not too high; the straps should not "float" on top of the forearm but should sit flush against this area to secure the orthosis on the extremity. The addition of foam beneath the straps can help secure the position. Inspect the borders with the orthosis off the patient as well by looking down the shaft of the orthosis, proximal to distal, checking for symmetry and matching heights.

CLINICAL PEARL 7-X29.
Color Stain Test

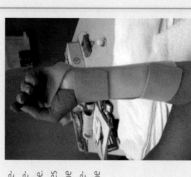

When a patient complains of irritation from an orthosis, have him or her mark the area on the skin using a washable marker or lipstick then put the orthosis back. When it is removed again, the color can be seen on the thermoplastic and the therapist can visualize the specific part that needs to be adjusted.

CLINICAL PEARL 7-X30.
Final Strap Check

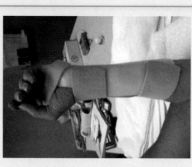

With the orthosis on the patient, check that all hook material on the orthosis is fully covered by the loop. This will prevent the hook from sticking to clothing, bedding, and the like. Make sure all hook-and-loop material is rounded on the edges to prevent areas from lifting off the orthosis. Finally, assess the mechanics of the orthosis; the straps should be placed strategically throughout, taking full advantage of the length of the orthosis as shown here.

CLINICAL PEARL 7-X31.
Keeping Orthosis Dry

With some specific diagnoses, an orthosis may have to be worn 24 hours a day, including during bathing. It can be challenging for the patient to keep the area completely dry. For finger-based designs, options include using a glove **(A)** or finger cot (available at local drugstores); for longer orthoses, try long bags, including newspaper or umbrella sleeves or protective wraps such as Saran™ or Glad® ClingWrap **(B)**. An elastic or adhesive tape proximally will help prevent area from getting wet. Patient should be told to remove wrap after bathing and alert the therapy office if the area/orthosis gets wet; this will need to be addressed in a timely manner to prevent any issues of maceration and potential skin breakdown.

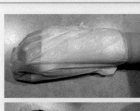
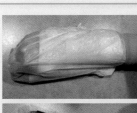
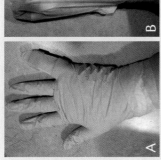

A   B

CLINICAL PEARL 7-X32.
Cleaning of an Orthosis

Adhesive removers (Goo Gone), rubbing alcohol, soft nonabrasive cleansers (Soft Scrub), and specialized scrubbers called Mr. Clean Magic Eraser can all be used to clean marks and remove adhesives off an orthosis. Antibacterial wipes such as Lysol® Disinfecting Wipes can also be used as a quick way to cleanse the inside of an orthosis to remove any sweat or remove odors.

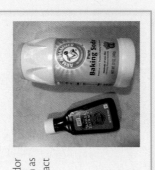

CLINICAL PEARL 7-X33.
Removing Odors from an Orthosis

Various products such as Febreze can be used to control odor from an orthosis. Other techniques have been described such as soaking the device in a solution of 50% water and vanilla extract or water and baking soda.

1 Digit- and Thumb-Based Orthoses

Distal Interphalangeal (DIP) Immobilization Orthosis (FO) (Fig. 7–1)

Common Names
- DIP extension splint
- DIP resting splint
- Static DIP extension splint
- Mallet finger splint

Alternative Options
- Aluminum padded splint
- Stax finger splint
- Finger cast
- Ring design splints

Primary Functions
- Immobilize DIP joint to allow healing of involved structure(s).

- Rest a painful and/or inflamed DIP joint.

Additional Functions
- Promote gliding of flexor digitorum superficialis (FDS) tendon by restricting movement of DIP joint during active flexion exercises.
- Statically position DIP joint flexion contracture at maximum extension to facilitate lengthening of tissue (mobilization).
- Restrict proximal interphalangeal (PIP) hyperextension.

Common Diagnoses and General Optimal Positions	
Zone I extensor tendon injury and/or repair (mallet finger)	0 to +10° hyperextension
Distal phalanx fracture	Tolerable ext
Partial fingertip amputation	Tolerable ext
Crush injury to distal phalanx	Tolerable ext
Nail bed injury and repair	Tolerable ext
DIP jt osteoarthritis	Position of comfort

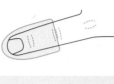

FIGURE 7-2

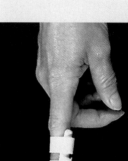
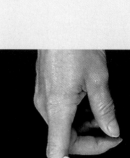

FIGURE 7-1

Fabrication Process

Pattern Creation (Fig. 7-2)

- Mark for proximal border just distal to middle digital crease.
- Allow extra ¼" to ½" of material around borders, depending on digit circumference.

Refine Pattern

- Proximal border should allow nearly full PIP joint motion.
- Lateral borders should encompass two-thirds circumference of digit to prevent undue compressive stress from straps and maximize rigidity. If borders are too generous, there may be too much digit mobility allowed within orthosis.

Options for Material

- Consider nonremovable circumferential design or cast for young children or questionably compliant patients.
- Perforated thermoplastics may prevent skin maceration; consider using them for patients who require full-time use.

- Use thinnest material possible that provides necessary strength to decrease bulk (¹⁄₁₆").
- Materials that can be reheated and remolded several times are a good option if ongoing modifications become necessary to accommodate for fluctuations in edema or changes in desired joint position.

Cut and Heat

- Position patient's forearm supinated (volar design) and pronated (dorsal design) for gravity-assisted molding. If using elasticized edema wraps or dressings under orthosis, apply to digit before heating material. (Use layer of tubular gauze over any dressing to prevent adherence.)

Evaluate Fit while Molding

DORSAL DESIGN

- Place material on dorsal aspect of digit just distal to PIP joint. Maximizing length of orthosis will improve stability and leverage.

- Avoid applying direct pressure over dorsum of DIP joint while molding, which may cause pressure areas. Incorporate thin padding if necessary.

VOLAR DESIGN

- Place material on volar aspect of digit just distal to PIP joint crease.
- Apply slight DIP joint extension force (patient may aid in extending tip by using his or her other hand to gently position tip via fingernail).
- Pinch together excess material distally then trim to shape of fingertip, aiding to further protect a sensitive or painful tip.

Strapping and Components

- Use two ½" straps or one 1" strap to secure over DIP joint.
- Extra-thin ½" strapping material can help decrease bulk between digits.
- May consider various tapes (such as paper tape or Microfoam™ tape, Patterson Medical) to secure the orthosis because these work very well.

DORSAL DESIGN

- Place straps at proximal border and over distal phalanx.

VOLAR DESIGN

- Place straps at proximal border and directly over DIP joint.
- Thin padding under distal strap may reduce migration and improve comfort.

Survey Completed Orthosis

- Smooth material borders; avoid rolling and flaring, which may irritate adjacent soft tissues or interfere with PIP joint movement.
- Check for mobility of uninvolved joints.

🖐 PATTERN PEARL 7-1 to 7-10.

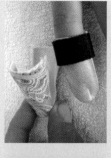

PP7-1

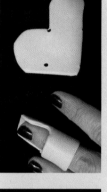

B

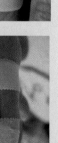

PP7-2

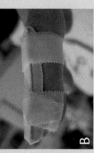

PP7-3

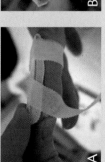

PP7-4

A and B, Dorsal AlumaFoam® with tape; note angle of distal tape to contour at tip.   Stax-type splint.   L pattern.   Bivalve design.

PATTERN PEARL 7-1 to 7-10. *continued*

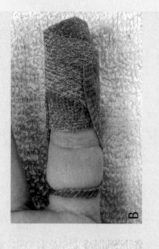

PP7-5

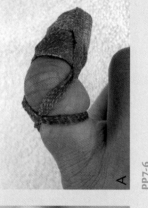

A and B, Incorporating postsurgical pin.

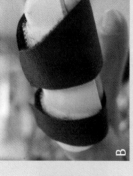

PP7-6

A and B, Circumferential with proximal anchor strip.

CLINICAL PEARL 7-1.
Management of Mallet Finger

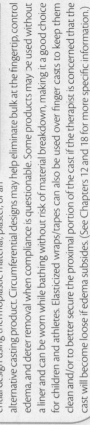

When treating a mallet finger, the DIP joint should be positioned in neutral to slight hyperextension uninterrupted for approximately 6–8 weeks during the healing process. Preventing skin breakdown on the dorsum of the DIP joint is imperative. If using a removable design, reliable patients may be instructed to carefully remove for hygiene and skin inspection while maintaining DIP extension; all other patients should be seen regularly by the therapist for skin inspection. Consider a circumferential design using thermoplastic material, plaster, or an alternative casting product. Circumferential designs may help eliminate bulk at the fingertip, control edema, and deter removal when compliance is questionable. Some products may be used without a liner and can be worn while bathing without risk of material breakdown, making it a good choice for children and athletes. Elasticized wraps/tapes can also be used over finger casts to keep them clean and/or to better secure the proximal portion of the cast if the therapist is concerned that the cast will become loose if edema subsides. (See Chapters 12 and 18 for more specific information.)

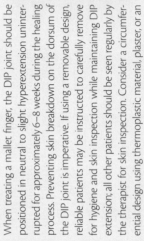

PP7-7

Nail bed protector.

PP7-8

Clamshell design.

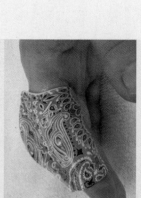

PP7-9

U pattern.

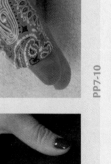

PP7-10

Dorsal edge to ease removal.

CLINICAL PEARL 7-3.
Securing Circumferential DIP Orthoses

Elasticized tapes, adhesive or nonadhesive (such as Coban™ or Microfoam™ tape, Patterson Medical), can be used to secure a circumferential DIP orthosis.

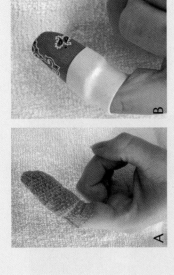

CLINICAL PEARL 7-2.
Protective Fingertip Caps

Create a contour at tip of digit by pinching the excess distal material together while warm, then cut to the shape of the tip, forming a protective cap (**A and B**). Carefully smooth the seam while the material is warm to prevent separation. May need to use solvent and heat gun to be sure area stays adhered. This closed design protects the area after crush, nail bed injury, or amputations (**C and D**).

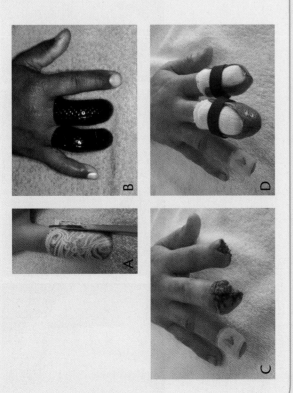

PIP Immobilization Orthosis (FO) (Fig. 7–3)

Common Names

- Finger splint
- PIP resting splint
- Static PIP extension splint
- Finger gutter splint

Alternative Options

- Aluminum padded splint
- Finger cast
- Ring design splints

Primary Functions

- Immobilize PIP joint to allow healing of involved structure(s).
- Rest a painful and/or inflamed PIP joint.

Additional Functions

- Promote gliding of flexor digitorum profundus (FDP) tendon by restricting movement of PIP joint during active flexion exercises.
- Statically position PIP joint flexion contracture at maximum extension to facilitate lengthening of tissue (mobilization).
- Restrict specific amount of extension (e.g., dorsal dislocation of PIP joint) or flexion (e.g., zones II and III extensor tendon injury) to protect healing structures (restriction).

Common Diagnoses and General Optimal Positions

Zones III and IV extensor tendon injury	0°
Boutonniere deformity	0°
PIP jt sprain	0°
PIP jt intra-articular fracture	0°
PIP jt arthritis	Position of comfort
PIP jt arthroplasty	0°

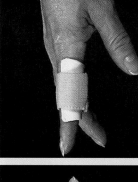
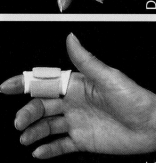
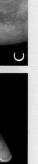

FIGURE 7-3

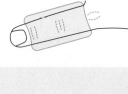

FIGURE 7-4

Fabrication Process

Pattern Creation (Fig. 7-4)

- Mark for proximal border at proximal digital crease and distal border at distal digital crease.
- Appreciate the proximal oblique angle of the border digits (index and small) because this angle should be incorporated into the pattern to allow increased stability via a longer lever arm and better strap placement
- Proximal border should be oblique, providing for long lever to maximize mechanical advantage.
- Allow extra ¼" to ½" of material around borders, depending on digit circumference.
- Consider including DIP joint if digit is small (children, small adults) to improve ability of orthosis to secure desired PIP joint position or mobilize PIP joint to improve leverage.

Refine Pattern

- Proximal border should allow unrestricted MCP joint motion.
- Distal border should allow unrestricted DIP joint motion.
- Lateral borders should encompass two-thirds circumference of digit to prevent undue compressive stress from straps and maximize rigidity. If borders are too generous, there may be too much digit mobility allowed within orthosis.
- Web space areas should have adequate rooms to allow unrestricted motion of adjacent digits.
- May extend pattern distally to include DIP joint.

Options for Materials

- Consider using ³⁄₃₂" thermoplastic material (perforated or nonperforated); it is light and thin but still provides stability to PIP joint.
- Perforated thermoplastics may prevent skin maceration; consider using them for patients who require full-time use.
- Materials that can be reheated and remolded several times are a good option if ongoing modifications become necessary to accommodate for fluctuations in edema or changes in desired joint position.
- A circumferential design fabricated with plaster, digit casting products, or thermoplastic material can help when addressing the small finger PIP joint. Small surface area can make it difficult for the traditional design to obtain adequate purchase.

Cut and Heat

- Position patient's forearm supinated (volar design) and pronated (dorsal design) for gravity-assisted molding.
- If using elasticized edema wrap or dressings under orthosis, apply to digit before heating material. (Use layer of tubular gauze to prevent adherence.)
- Thin padding over PIP joint may be incorporated into dorsal design if necessary; apply before heating material.

Evaluate Fit while Molding

DORSAL DESIGN

- Place material on dorsal aspect of digit just proximal to dorsal DIP joint skin folds and distal to MCP joint. Maximizing length of orthosis will improve stability and leverage.
- Allow gravity to form lateral borders. Avoid grabbing or wrapping material around digit.
- Avoid applying direct pressure over dorsum of PIP joint while molding, which may cause pressure areas.

VOLAR DESIGN

- Place material on volar aspect of digit, just clearing DIP joint crease and slightly distal to MCP joint crease.
- Allow gravity to form lateral borders; avoid grabbing or wrapping material around digit.
- If used to address flexion contracture, carefully mold with even, gentle pressure throughout length of orthosis in direction of extension.
- Important to note: With PIP flexion contractures, the clinician will need to incorporate the longest lever arm possible; therefore, including the DIP (especially true with short digits) and proximal edge of the proximal phalanx is critical. When including the DIP, positioning in gentle flexion is preferable in order to prevent hyperextension forces at the PIP joint.

Strapping and Components

- Use two ½" straps or one 1" strap to secure orthosis directly over PIP joint.
- Proximal strap should have slight oblique orientation.
- Extra-thin ½" strapping material can help decrease bulk between digits.

DORSAL DESIGN

- Place straps at proximal border and over middle phalanx.

VOLAR DESIGN

- Place straps over proximal and middle phalanx.
- Place one strap with piece of foam directly over PIP joint if maintaining PIP extension is a priority.
- Thin padding under distal strap may reduce migration and improve comfort.
- Proximal straps for border digits will have a slight oblique orientation.

Survey Completed Orthosis

- Smooth material borders; avoid rolling or flaring, which may irritate adjacent soft tissues and web spaces or interfere with MCP and/or DIP joint movement.
- Check for mobility of uninvolved joints.

PATTERN PEARL 7-11 to 7-18.

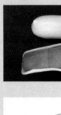
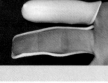
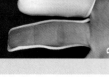
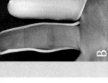

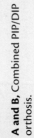
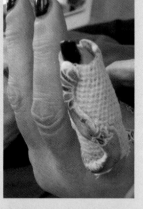

PP7-11

A and B, Combined PIP/DIP orthosis.

PP7-12

QuickCast 2 (Patterson Medical) with thermoplastic strip for reinforcement.

PP7-13

Plaster of paris PIP cast.

PP7-14

Dorsal extension restriction orthosis for volar plate injury.

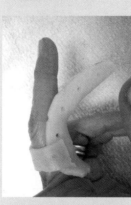
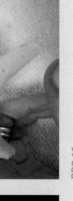

PP7-15

Volar flexion restriction orthosis for extensor tendon injury.

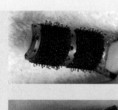

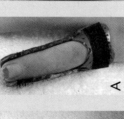
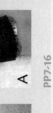

PP7-16

A and B, Dorsal/volar digit orthosis PIP.

PP7-17

Silver Ring™ Splint to restrict extension for swan-neck deformity.

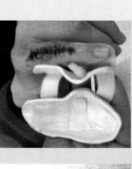
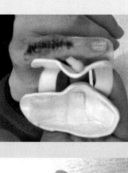

PP7-18

Bivalve design to protect pins.

CLINICAL PEARL 7-5.
Small Finger PIP Orthoses

With short fifth digits, the clinician may find it helpful to incorporate a portion of the fifth metacarpal. This provides a longer lever arm and increases the stability and position of the orthosis onto the hand. Shown is **(A)** QuickCast 2 (Patterson Medical) material, **(B)** a night orthosis for a child with camptodactyly; notice foam on the dorsum of the PIP strap to encourage PIP extension.

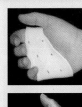
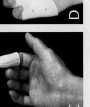
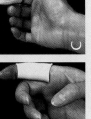

CLINICAL PEARL 7-4.
Digit Exercise Orthoses

An orthosis that immobilizes all the PIP and DIP joints in extension can aid in directing the forces of flexion to the MCP joints during active flexion exercises **(A)**. This can be used as an exercise tool to increase active MCP flexion, which is often lacking after MCP joint arthroplasty. An orthosis that immobilizes the PIP joint in extension can aid in directing the force of flexion to the DIP joint during active flexion exercises **(B)**. This can be used as an exercise tool to increase active DIP flexion, to maximize FDP tendon glide, and/or to stretch tight oblique retinacular ligaments. An orthosis that immobilizes the DIP joint in extension can aid in directing the force of flexion to the PIP joint during active exercises. This can be used as an exercise tool to increase active PIP flexion and/or maximize FDS tendon glide **(C)**. Finally, an orthosis that immobilizes the MCP joints in extension can encourage differential flexor tendon gliding as well as actively stretch the intrinsic muscles in the hand **(D)**.

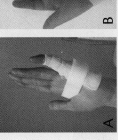
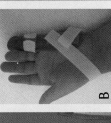
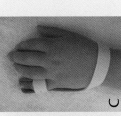

CLINICAL PEARL 7-7.
Strapping Alternatives for PIP Orthoses

A and B, As shown, split strap designs can be used to increase the surface area for attachment of the loop material onto the hook. **C,** To prevent migration of digit-based orthoses, elasticized wraps can be used to secure the orthosis to the hand.

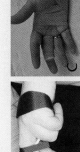
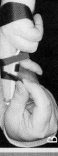
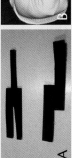

CLINICAL PEARL 7-6.
Spiral Design with "Cling Wrap" for Edema

A spiral design orthosis fabricated with ⅟₁₆" Orfit® (North Coast Medical, Morgan Hill, CA) material was used to allow limited IP motion 8 weeks after PIP joint arthroplasty. The plastic wrap was used under the orthosis to control edema and prevent orthosis migration.

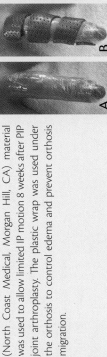
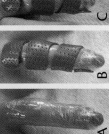

Thumb Interphalangeal (IP) Immobilization Orthosis (FO) (Fig. 7-5)

Common Names
- Thumb IP extension splint
- Static thumb splint

Alternative Options
- Aluminum padded splint
- Stax splint
- Thumb cast
- Ring design orthosis

Primary Functions
- Immobilize thumb IP joint to allow healing of involved structure(s).

- Rest a painful and/or inflamed thumb IP joint.

Additional Functions
- Statically position IP joint flexion contracture at maximum extension to facilitate lengthening of tissue (mobilization).
- Restrict IP hyperextension.

Common Diagnoses and General Optimal Positions

Zone TI extensor tendon injury (mallet)	+5 to +15° hyperextension
Distal phalanx fracture	0 to +15° hyperextension (depends on flexor pollicis longus [FPL] status)
Crush injury to distal phalanx	0° to slight hyperextension
Nail bed injury and repair	0°
Partial tip amputation	Tolerable ext
IP jt sprain	0° to slight hyperextension
IP jt arthritis	Position of comfort

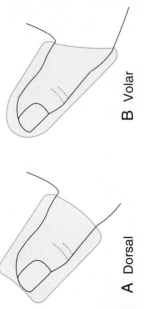
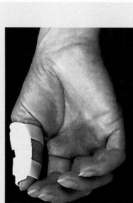
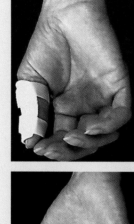

FIGURE 7-5

A Dorsal   B Volar

FIGURE 7-6

Fabrication Process

Pattern Creation (Fig. 7–6)

- Mark for proximal border at proximal thumb crease.
- Proximal border has an oblique angle and should be incorporated into orthosis, providing for long lever to maximize mechanical advantage.
- Allow extra ¼" to ½" of material around borders, depending on thumb circumference.
- Dorsal design may improve function of thumb by providing partial sensory input.

Refine Pattern

DORSAL DESIGN

- Extend proximal border to middle of dorsal MP joint skinfolds.
- Lateral borders should encompass two-thirds circumference of digit to prevent undue compressive stress from straps and maximize rigidity. If borders are too generous, there may be too much digit mobility allowed within orthosis.
- Taper lateral borders slightly volar and distal to avoid irritation at first web space.
- Proximal border has an oblique angle and should be incorporated into orthosis.

VOLAR DESIGN

- Extend proximal border just distal to volar MP joint crease.
- Taper lateral borders slightly dorsal and proximal to form oblique border.

Options for Materials

- Consider nonremovable circumferential orthosis or cast for young children or questionably compliant patients.
- Perforated thermoplastics may prevent skin maceration; consider using them for patients who require full-time use.
- Use thinnest material possible that provides necessary strength to decrease bulk (⅟₁₆" or ³⁄₃₂").
- Materials that can be reheated and remolded several times are a good option if ongoing modifications become necessary to accommodate for fluctuations in edema or changes in desired joint position.

Cut and Heat

- Position patient's forearm supinated (volar design) and pronated (dorsal design) for gravity-assisted molding.
- IP joint position depends on diagnosis.

- If using elasticized edema wrap or dressings under orthosis, apply to thumb before heating material. (Use layer of tubular gauze to prevent adherence.)

Evaluate Fit while Molding

DORSAL DESIGN

- Place material on dorsal aspect of thumb to middle of dorsal MP joint skinfolds. Maximizing length of orthosis will improve stability and leverage.
- Avoid applying direct pressure over dorsum of IP joint while molding, which may create pressure spots. Thin padding may be incorporated if necessary.
- Allow gravity to form lateral borders; avoid grabbing or wrapping material around digit.
- Slightly flare material about the MP joint.

VOLAR DESIGN

- Place material on volar aspect of thumb, just clearing volar MP joint crease.
- Apply slight IP extension pressure (patient may aid in extending tip by using his or her other hand to gently lift tip via fingernail).

Strapping and Components

- Use two ½" straps or one 1" strap to secure over DIP joint.
- Proximal strap should have slight oblique orientation.
- Extra-thin ½" strapping material can help decrease bulk between digits.
- May consider paper tape to secure as well.

DORSAL DESIGN

- Place straps at proximal border (as close to MP flexion crease as possible without interfering with MP joint flexion) and over distal phalanx.

VOLAR DESIGN

- Place straps at proximal border and directly over IP joint.
- Thin padding under distal strap may reduce migration and improve comfort.

Survey Completed Orthosis

- Smooth material borders; avoid rolling and flaring, which may irritate adjacent soft tissues or interfere with MP joint movement.
- Check for mobility of uninvolved joints.

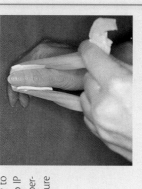

CLINICAL PEARL 7-8.
TheraBand®-Assisted Molding

TheraBand® (Patterson Medical) can be applied volarly to the distal phalanx while molding a volar DIP or thumb IP orthosis. This technique aids in positioning the DIP in hyperextension and precludes the need to apply direct pressure dorsally at the DIP joint.

PATTERN PEARL 7-19 to 7-25.

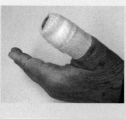

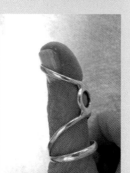

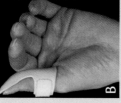

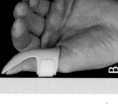

PP7-19

PP7-20

PP7-21

A and B, Thumb IP orthosis with tab.

Silver Ring™ Splint (Silver Ring Splint Company, Charlottesville VA) to prevent IP joint deviation with pinch.

Thumb IP cast using QuickCast 2.

PP7-22

PP7-23

Cast with volar free for sensation.

U pattern.

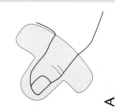

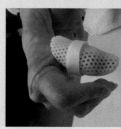

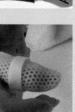

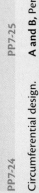

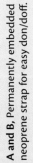

PP7-24

PP7-25

Circumferential design.

A and B, Permanently embedded neoprene strap for easy don/doff.

Notes

② **Hand-Based Orthoses**

Dorsal MCP/PIP/DIP Immobilization Orthosis (HFO) (Fig. 7–7)

Common Names

- Hand-based digit extension splint
- Hand-based digit resting splint
- Static finger splint
- Dorsal hand splint

Primary Functions

- Immobilize the MCP, PIP, and/or DIP joint(s) to allow healing or rest of the involved structure(s).

Additional Functions

- Restrict specific amount of extension (e.g., after digital nerve repair) to protect healing structures.

Common Diagnoses and General Optimal Positions

Intra-articular fracture of PIP/DIP jt	MCP: 60° flex; PIP/DIP: 0°
Dupuytren's surgical and nonsurgical	All jts maximal ext; 3 to 6+ months: maximum ext at night only
Trigger finger	MCP: 0°; PIP/DIP: free
Tenosynovitis	Position of comfort, intrinsic plus
Infection	Position of comfort, intrinsic plus
MCP/PIP jt volar plate injury	MCP/PIP: 20 to 30° flex

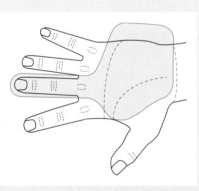

A   B

FIGURE 7-7

FIGURE 7-8

Fabrication Process

Pattern Creation (Fig. 7–8)

- Consider dorsal design if patient presents with volar wound/incision to allow for air circulation.
- Mark for proximal border at dorsal wrist crease.
- Allow extra ¼" to ½" of material around borders, depending on digit circumference.
- Be sure the proximal portion of the orthosis has adequate surface area for strap application.
- For small finger (SF), consider including ring finger (RF) to provide greater protection, better stabilization, and improved comfort.
- If MCP is to be flexed, allow extra material distally to accommodate for flexion angle. If material must be stretched over MCP joint, a weakened and unstable orthosis may result.
- Draw pattern with fingers slightly abducted. Be sure to provide enough surface area to accommodate all immobilized digits. Remember, material can always be trimmed away after initial molding is completed.

Refine Pattern

- Proximal border should allow full wrist motion and clearance of ulnar styloid.

- Lateral borders should encompass two-thirds circumference of digit to prevent undue compressive stress from straps and maximize rigidity. If borders are too generous, there may be too much digit mobility allowed within orthosis.
- Allow adequate room in digit web space areas to allow unrestricted motion of unaffected digits.

Options for Materials

- Use drapable material to achieve intimate fit over MCP joints to prevent migration and improve comfort.
- Coated material will allow for overlapped ulnar border to pop apart after setting fully.
- Perforated thermoplastics may help prevent skin maceration; consider using them for patients who require full-time use of orthosis.
- Materials that can be reheated and remolded several times are a good option if ongoing modifications become necessary to accommodate for fluctuations in edema, changes in motion, or bulk of dressings.

Cut and Heat

- Position patient's forearm pronated for gravity-assisted molding.

- If using elasticized wrap or dressings under orthosis, apply to digit before heating material.
- To prevent adherence to dressings, consider the following:
  - A layer of tubular gauze or stockinette over dressings that can be removed with the orthosis when set
  - Lightly and evenly spread a thin layer of lotion over dressings
- Thin padding may be incorporated dorsally across MCP joint(s) if necessary; apply before heating material.

Evaluate Fit while Molding

- Place material over dorsum of hand and gently pull tab through first web space and temporarily adhere to ulnar border, being sure to place material just proximal to distal palmar crease (DPC).
- Lateral borders of the digit should form a deep trough (instead of a flat pan), which will act to strengthen and support the molded orthosis.
- Contour dorsal MCP area well.
- Avoid applying direct pressure over dorsum of MCP and PIP joints while molding.

- Consider light rolling of the material edges about the dorsum of the MCP joints when using thin material. This is especially applicable when the orthosis is fabricated to include only one digit.

Strapping and Components

- Apply straps at DIP joint, around proximal phalanx, at overlapped ulnar border, and about wrist to prevent migration.
- Watch for radial sensory nerve irritation that may occur with a tight wrist strap
- If applying a stiff loop material through the web space, consider "fringing" the edges to increase contour of the strap as it traverses through the web space.
- Consider using rivets to secure one end of proximal strap to minimize space needed for hook material.

Survey Completed Orthosis

- Smooth material borders; avoid rolling or flaring, which may irritate adjacent soft tissues and web spaces or interfere with unaffected/adjacent joint movement.
- Check mobility of uninvolved joints.

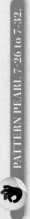

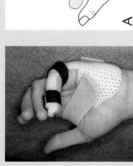

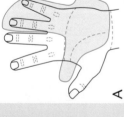

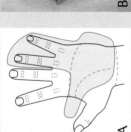

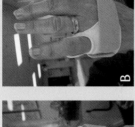

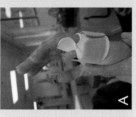

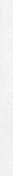

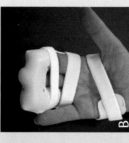

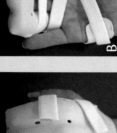

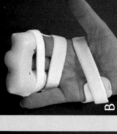

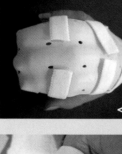

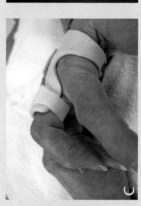

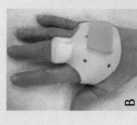

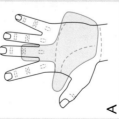

PP7-26

PP7-27

Digit extension restriction orthosis.

A and B, RF/SF orthosis used post-Dupuytren release.

PP7-28

RF/SF and thumb orthosis used post-Dupuytren release.

PP7-29

Volar/dorsal MCP joint orthosis for trigger finger.

PP7-30

A and B, Volar/dorsal MCP joint orthosis for trigger finger.

PP7-31

A–C, Dorsal MCP joint orthosis.

PP7-32

A and B, Dorsal-based tip protector.

CLINICAL PEARL 7-9.
Strapping through Web Spaces

Trim strapping material to contour through the web spaces to prevent the borders from irritating these sensitive areas (**A**) may be helpful to cover the edge with a thin lining material to decrease likelihood of soft tissue irritation (**B**). Note that many elasticized strapping materials may fray if trimmed. Another specialty strap is a thin material to decrease bulk between the digits (**C**). Neoprene is an alternative strapping material that contours nicely and can be trimmed without risk of fraying (**D**). Trim soft foam straps by "feathering" the edges to prevent skin irritation (**E**).

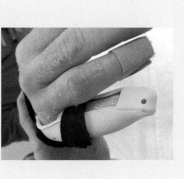
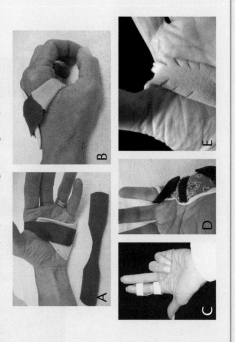

CLINICAL PEARL 7-10.
Flaring for Dorsal MCP Joint

When applying material dorsally across MCP joints, be sure to flare material away from bony prominences. Note: In this orthosis, the material over the DIP protects a distal tip injury.

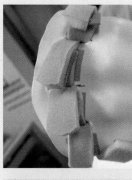
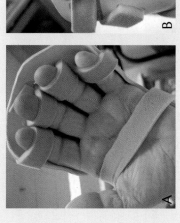

CLINICAL PEARL 7-11.
Strap Alternative for Dorsal Hand Immobilization

This "split" strap is cut from neoprene material and conforms well as it traverses through the first web and base of the thumb.

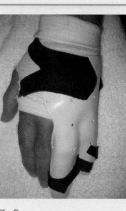

CLINICAL PEARL 7-12.
Dorsal Weave for Strap Application

Slits can be made in a dorsal hand orthosis to direct straps into extension. This is especially helpful when digits vary in degrees of contracture.

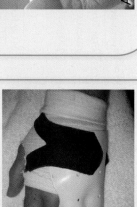

Volar MCP/PIP/DIP Immobilization Orthosis (HFO)   (Fig. 7-9)

Common Names

- Hand-based digit extension splint
- Hand-based digit resting splint
- Static finger splint
- Volar resting splint
- Volar hand splint
- Finger gutter splint

Primary Functions

- Immobilize the MCP, PIP, and/or DIP joint(s) to allow healing or rest of the involved structure(s).

Additional Functions

- Statically position MCP joint contracture at maximum flexion or extension to facilitate lengthening of tissue (mobilization).
- Restrict specific amount of flexion (e.g., after zone IV extensor tendon repair) to protect healing structures (restriction).

Common Diagnoses and General Optimal Positions

Intra-articular fracture of PIP or DIP jt	MCP: 60° flex;PIP/DIP: 0°
Fracture of proximal and/or middle phalanx	MCP: slight flex; PIP/DIP: 0°
Dupuytren's surgical and nonsurgical	All jts maximal ext; 3 to 6+ months: maximum ext at night only
MCP jt sprain	MCP: 60 to 80° flex; PIP/DIP: 0°
Trigger finger release	MCP: 0°; PIP/DIP: free
Tenosynovitis	Position of comfort, intrinsic plus
Infection	Position of comfort, intrinsic plus
Crush injury	MCP: 60 to 80° flex; PIP/DIP: 0°
Zone IV extensor tendon injury	MCP/PIP/DIP: 0°
Sagittal band injury and repair	MCP: 0° with slight deviation to side of injury or repair; PIP/DIP: free
Ulnar nerve injury	PM use: MCP: 60 to 80° flex; PIP/DIP: 0°

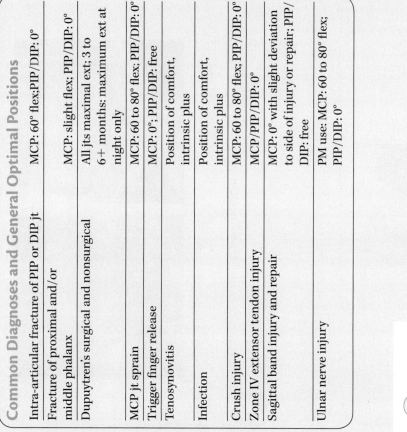

FIGURE 7-10

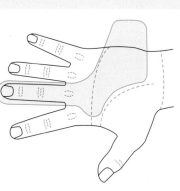

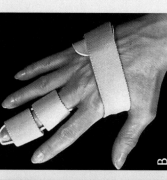

A   B

FIGURE 7-9

Fabrication Process

Pattern Creation (Fig. 7–10)

- Consider volar design if patient has dorsal wound/incision or extruding pins to allow for air circulation.
- Mark for proximal border at volar wrist crease.
- Allow extra ¼" to ½" of material around borders, depending on digit circumference.
- Be sure proximal portion of the orthosis has adequate surface area for strap application.
- For SF, consider including RF to provide greater protection, better stabilization, and improved comfort.
- Draw pattern with fingers slightly abducted. Be sure to provide enough surface area to accommodate all immobilized digits. Remember, material can always be trimmed away after initial molding is completed.

Refine Pattern

- Proximal border should allow full wrist motion.
- Radial border should allow nearly full thumb motion.

Cut and Heat

- Lateral borders of the involved digit(s) should encompass two-thirds circumference of digit to prevent undue compressive stress from straps and maximize rigidity. If borders are too generous, there may be too much digit mobility allowed within orthosis.
- Allow adequate room in digit web space areas to allow unrestricted motion of unaffected digits.
- May modify pattern to exclude PIP and/or DIP joints if necessary.

Options for Materials

- Coated material will allow for over-lapped ulnar border to pop apart after setting fully.
- Perforated thermoplastics may prevent skin maceration; consider using them for patients who require full-time orthosis use.
- Materials that can be reheated and remolded several times are a good option if ongoing modifications become necessary to accommodate for fluctuations in edema, changes in motion, or bulk of dressings.

Cut and Heat

- Position patient's forearm supinated for gravity-assisted molding.
- If using elasticized wrap or dressings under orthosis, apply to digit before heating material. (Use layer of tubular gauze or stockinette to prevent adherence.)

Evaluate Fit while Molding

- Lateral borders of the digit should form a deep trough (instead of a flat pan), which will act to strengthen and support the molded orthosis.
- Remember that when addressing index finger (IF), thumb mobility is somewhat hindered because of necessary contouring about thumb web to obtain proper stabilization.

Strapping and Components

- Apply straps at DIP joint, over PIP joint proximal phalanx, at over-lapped ulnar border, and about wrist to prevent migration.
- Consider using rivets to secure one end of proximal strap to minimize space needed for hook material.

- Padding under proximal phalanx strap may reduce migration and rotation, maintain MCP joint position, and improve comfort.

Survey Completed Orthosis

- Smooth material borders; avoid rolling or flaring, which may irritate adjacent soft tissues and web spaces or interfere with unaffected/adjacent joint movement.
- Check mobility of uninvolved joints.

PATTERN PEARL 7-33 to 7-39.

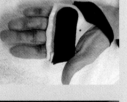

PP7-33

A and B, Volar MCP joint orthosis for trigger finger.

PP7-34

A and B, "Ring" design for trigger finger.

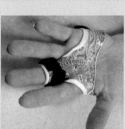

PP7-35

All MCP joints included for active intrinsic stretching.

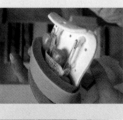

PP7-36

A–C, IF/MF thumbhole design; **D,** IF only.

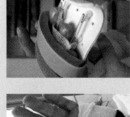

PP7-37

Protecting pins with distal edge.

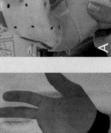

PP7-38

A and B, Volar/dorsal design.

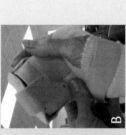

PP7-39

A and B, Clamshell design for additional protection.

CLINICAL PEARL 7-13.
Thermoplastic Strap through Web Space

Orthotic material can be used as an alternative method for securing both volar and dorsal hand-based orthoses. This is especially useful in the thenar web space because it eliminates the need for loop traversing through this potentially sensitive region as well as decreasing the amount of hook needed on the orthosis itself. The material can be lightly stretched to "thin" it out. Be sure to keep a narrow width in order to not impede IF MCP flexion.

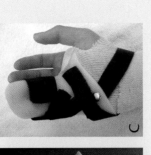
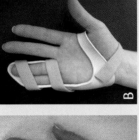
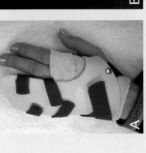

CLINICAL PEARL 7-14.
Strapping around Wrist to Prevent Migration

An elasticized wrist strap such as neoprene or elasticized loop can be used to secure a hand-based orthosis onto the hand. Rivets can be helpful to anchor the strap onto the base because surface area may be limited. Rivets also aid in maintaining orientation of the strap.

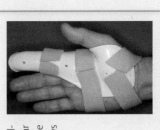

CLINICAL PEARL 7-15.
Rolling Material through Web Spaces

Avoid cutting material to accommodate for web space areas. This may significantly alter the rigidity. Instead, carefully roll and flatten a small border of the warm material back onto itself, just enough to clear for mobility of the adjacent digits.

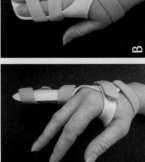
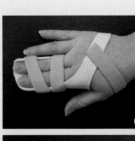

CLINICAL PEARL 7-16.
Contouring around Thumb to Increase IF Stability

Allowing unimpeded thumb mobility when immobilizing the IF is challenging; because to adequately stabilize this digit, a portion of the thenar eminence must be included in the orthosis. The contouring technique shown provides good stability along the radial volar aspect yet allows functional thumb mobility.

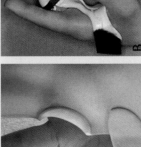
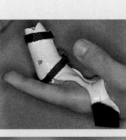
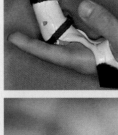

Ulnar MCP/PIP/DIP Immobilization Orthosis (HFO) (Fig. 7-11)

Common Names

- Hand-based ulnar gutter splint
- Hand-based ulnar fracture brace
- Metacarpal fracture brace
- Clamdigger splint

Alternative Options

- Plaster cast

Primary Functions

- Immobilize proximal phalanxes and metacarpals of RF and SF to allow healing and/or protection of involved structure(s).

Additional Functions

- Restrict MCP joint extension secondary to low ulnar nerve injury (restriction).

Common Diagnoses and General Optimal Positions

Metacarpal head or neck fracture	MCP: 60 to 90° flex (may include PIP/DIP: 0°)
Proximal phalanx fracture	MCP: 60 to 90° flex; PIP/DIP: 0°
Complicated middle phalanx fracture	MCP: 60 to 90° flex; PIP/DIP: 0°
MCP capsulectomy	MCP: 60 to 90° flex; PIP/DIP: 0°
Digital ulnar nerve injury	MCP: 60 to 90° flex; PIP/DIP free (include fourth and fifth metacarpals)

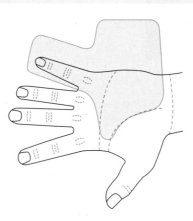

FIGURE 7-11

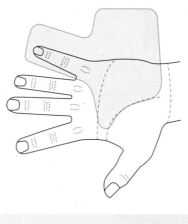

FIGURE 7-12

Fabrication Process

Pattern Creation (Fig. 7–12)

- Mark for proximal border at wrist crease, clearing ulnar styloid.
- Allow extra ½″ to 1″ of material distally to accommodate for flexion angle at MCP joints.

Refine Pattern

- Proximal border should allow full wrist motion.
- Radial border should allow full thumb, IF, and middle finger (MF) motion.
- Make sure pattern encompasses third metacarpal proximal to MCP joint. Remember, fourth and fifth metacarpals are relatively mobile compared to the radial side; thus, if goal is to immobilize a metacarpal fracture, orthosis must be anchored to stable third metacarpal.
- Allow unimpeded motion of MF by keeping pattern accurate.

Options for Materials

- Use drapable material to achieve intimate fit about MCP joints to prevent migration and improve comfort.

- Perforated thermoplastics may prevent skin maceration; consider using them for patients who require full-time use of orthosis.
- Materials that can be reheated and remolded several times are a good option if ongoing modifications become necessary to accommodate for fluctuations in edema and changes in MCP joint motion.

Cut and Heat

- Position patient's extremity with shoulder and elbow flexed with forearm pronation to achieve gravity-assisted position (ulnar border of hand should face upward).
- Place MCP joint in appropriate amount of flexion.
- If included, position PIP and/or DIP joints as per diagnosis.
- If using thin padding dorsally across MCP joints, apply to the area before heating material.

Evaluate Fit while Molding

- Place material on ulnar aspect of hand just distal to wrist.

- Gently stretch dorsal material over MCP joints while maintaining arches of hand.
- Allow gravity to assist while gently contouring and encompassing digits and MCP joints proximally.
- Incorporate natural descent of fifth MCP below fourth MCP.
- Be sure to maintain desired joint positions as material sets.
- Avoid applying direct pressure over dorsum of MCP and PIP joints while molding.
- Do not seal off distally; allow for ability to check for vascular compromise and provide some air exchange.
- Amount of MCP flexion requested may be difficult to achieve initially because of pain, stiffness, and/or dorsal edema; serial positioning into flexion may be necessary.

Strapping and Components

- Soft or elasticized straps work well around wrist to prevent migration.
- Consider a customized soft foam strap through first web space to

improve comfort and prevent skin irritation caused by friction from traditional loop material.
- Consider using rivets to secure one end of proximal strap to minimize space needed for hook material.
- Traditional straps will suffice to secure digits; be sure to trim straps between digit web spaces to prevent skin irritation.

Survey Completed Orthosis

- Smooth material borders, making sure there are no sharp edges, especially at ulnar styloid.
- If PIP and DIP joints are included, trim excess material from distal end to allow for visualization of fingertips.
- Check clearance of wrist and MF, making sure there is no abutment with material.

PATTERN PEARL 7-40 to 7-42.

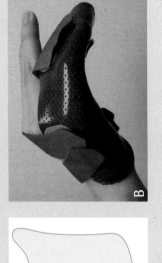

PP7-40

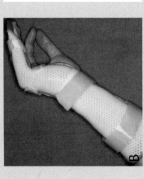

PP7-41

A and B, Including the wrist in pattern.

A and B, Including RF AND SF.

CLINICAL PEARL 7-17.
Accommodation for Dorsal Pins

Using therapy putty (medium resistance) and sterile petroleum-impregnated gauze can be a way to safely make room and provide cover for dorsal protruding pins. Place gauze over pins. Then form a small ball of putty, partially flatten out, and gently rest over the pin(s), making sure to fully cover the pin and immediate surface area. Next, either place an additional piece of gauze over the putty prior to thermoplastic application or add a thin layer of lotion. This step is to prevent the thermoplastic material from "sticking" to the putty. Once molded and set, remove the thermoplastic material carefully from the hand. It should slide right off the putty without fear of pin extraction. The putty and gauze can then be removed from the orthosis. The patient now has a well-molded orthosis with "bubbles" that protect the pin from external forces.

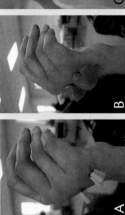

A   B   C   D

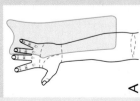

B   C

PP7-42

A–C, IP joints free.

Radial MCP/PIP/DIP Immobilization Orthosis (HFO) (Fig. 7–13)

Common Names

- Hand-based radial gutter splint
- Hand-based radial fracture brace
- Metacarpal fracture brace
- Clamdigger splint

Alternative Options

- Plaster cast

Primary Functions

- Immobilize proximal phalanxes and metacarpals of IF and MF to allow healing and/or protection of involved structure(s).

Common Diagnoses and General Optimal Positions

Metacarpal head or neck fracture	MCP: 60 to 90° flex (may include PIP/DIP: 0°)
Proximal phalanx fracture	MCP: 60 to 90° flex; PIP/DIP: 0°
Complicated middle phalanx fracture	MCP: 60 to 90° flex; PIP/DIP: 0°
MCP capsulectomy	MCP: 60 to 90° flex; PIP/DIP: 0°
Sagittal band injury or repair	MCP: 0° with slight deviation to affected side; PIP/DIP: free

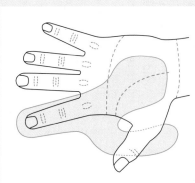

FIGURE 7-14

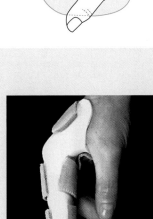

A B

FIGURE 7-13

Fabrication Process

Pattern Creation (Fig. 7-14)

- Mark for proximal border at wrist crease.
- Allow extra ½" to 1" of material distally to accommodate for flexion angle at MCP joints.

Refine Pattern

- Proximal border should allow full wrist motion.
- Ulnar border should allow full MF motion.
- Make sure pattern encompasses third metacarpal dorsally for improved stability.

Options for Materials

- Perforated thermoplastics may prevent skin maceration; consider using them for patients who require full-time use of orthosis.
- Materials that can be reheated and remolded several times are a good option if ongoing modifications become necessary to accommodate for fluctuations in edema and changes in MCP joint motion.
- Use drapable material to achieve intimate fit about MCP joints to prevent migration and improve comfort.

Evaluate Fit while Molding

- Place material on radial aspect of hand just distal to wrist.
- Gently stretch dorsal material over MCP joint while maintaining arches of hand.
- Allow gravity to assist while gently contouring and encompassing IF/MF and MCP joints proximally.
- Be sure to maintain desired joint positions as material sets.
- Avoid applying direct pressure over dorsum of MCP and PIP joints while molding.
- Do not seal off distally; allow for ability to check for vascular compromise and provide some air exchange.
- Amount of MCP flexion requested may be difficult to achieve initially because of pain, dorsal edema, or stiffness; serial static positioning into flexion may be necessary.

Cut and Heat

- Position patient's forearm in neutral rotation to achieve gravity-assisted position.
- Place MCP joints in appropriate amount of flexion.
- Position PIP and DIP joints as per diagnosis; place thumb in palmar abduction and opposition.
- If using thin padding dorsally across MCP joints, apply to area before heating material.

Strapping and Components

- Soft or elasticized straps work well around wrist to prevent migration.
- Consider using rivets to secure one end of proximal strap to minimize space needed for hook material.
- Traditional straps suffice to secure digits; be sure to trim straps in between digit web spaces to prevent skin irritation.

Survey Completed Orthosis

- Smooth material borders, making sure there are no sharp edges, especially with thumb motion.
- If PIP and DIP joints are included, trim excess material distally to allow for visualization of fingertips.
- Check clearance of wrist and MF, making sure there is no abutment with material.

PATTERN PEARL 7-43 to 7-46.

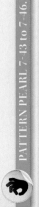
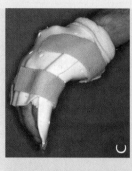

PP7-43

A and B, Forearm based with IP joints free.

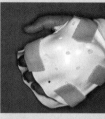

PP7-44

A and B, IP joints free.

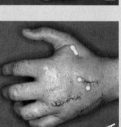
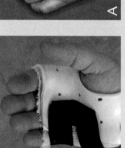
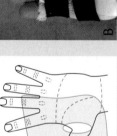
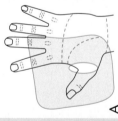
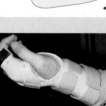
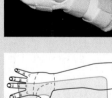

PP7-45

A–C, Clamshell design to cover pins.

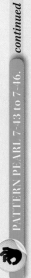

PATTERN PEARL 7-13 to 7-46. *continued*

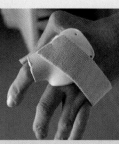

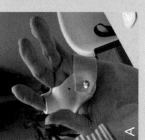

PP7-46

A and B, IF MCP joint only.

CLINICAL PEARL 7-18.
Pinch and Trim to Seal Distal Border

When an injury necessitates complete coverage of the distal digit(s), consider pinching excess material together and trimming with quality scissors. The trimming should be done when the material is still warm in order to form a seal. The material may still pop apart upon removal; however, hook-and-loop closures can be added.

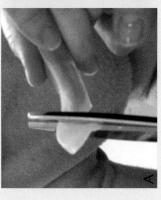

CLINICAL PEARL 7-19.
Clearing Thenar Region for Unrestricted Mobility

Careful attention should be taken when making an orthosis for the radial digits; the thumb is often left free. Material should be carefully molded about the thenar, leaving room for thumb mobility. Note: In this orthosis, the strapping system incorporates volar and dorsal adhesive hook in order to maximize surface area of strap application.

CLINICAL PEARL 7-20.
MCP Flexion (Antideformity) Positioning

When molding about the MCP joints of the hand, meticulous attention should be given to proper angle measurements of not only the MCP but the IP joints as well. This orthosis holds the hand in the antideformity position. Note the clearance of the thumb.

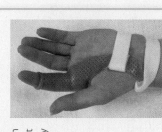

Thumb MP Immobilization Orthosis (HFO) (Fig. 7–15)

Common Names

- Short opponens splint
- MP splint
- Basal joint splint
- First CMC splint
- Mickey Stanley (Detroit) splint
- Gamekeeper's thumb splint

Alternative Options

- Prefabricated thumb supports
- Neoprene thumb and wrist wraps
- Ring design splints

Primary Functions

- Immobilize thumb MP joint to allow for healing of involved structure(s).
- Rest painful and/or inflamed MP joint.

Additional Functions

- Promote gliding of FPL tendon by restricting movement of MP joint during active thumb flexion exercises.

Common Diagnoses and General Optimal Positions

Ulnar collateral ligament (UCL) injury (grades 1 to 3)	Slight MP flex with UD
Radial collateral ligament (RCL) injury (grades 1 to 3)	Slight MP flex with RD
Trapeziometacarpal (TM or carpometacarpal [CMC]) jt arthritis	MP: slight flex; CMC: neutral
MP jt arthritis	Position of comfort
MP jt arthroplasty	Near full ext
MP jt dorsal dislocation	20 to 30° MP flex

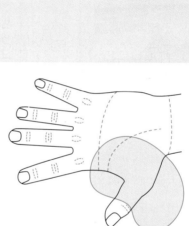
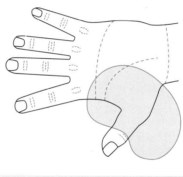

FIGURE 7-16

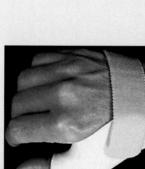

FIGURE 7-15

Fabrication Process

Pattern Creation (Fig. 7–16)

- Mark for proximal border just distal to wrist crease and distal border at IP joint.
- Mark for ulnar border at third metacarpal, which approximates the thenar crease.
- Pattern will resemble a symmetrical kidney bean with the dip in the bean at the IP joint.

Refine Pattern

- Proximal border should allow full wrist motion.
- Remember to allow unimpeded motion of wrist, IF MCP, and thumb IP joints by keeping pattern accurate.
- Volar ulnar border should allow full mobility of hypothenar area ending at thenar crease.
- May extend pattern distally to include IP joint if necessary.

Options for Materials

- Use drapable material to achieve intimate fit at MP joint, prevent migration, and improve comfort.
- Consider using coated material so circumferential thumb piece can be popped open without permanent bonding, providing an intimate contour at MP joint and proximal phalanx.
- Use thinnest material possible that provides necessary strength to decrease bulk.
- Remember that elastic materials tend to shrink around proximal phalanx of thumb (making it difficult to don and doff); do not remove until completely set.

Cut and Heat

- Position patient's forearm in slight supination for gravity-assisted molding.
- Place thumb in midpalmar–radial abduction and MP joint in slight flexion.

- Consider placing light layer of lotion on thumb before molding to ease removal.

Evaluate Fit while Molding

- Distally, place "dip of the bean" just proximal to IP joint on radial side of proximal phalanx.
- Mold material volarly to thenar crease and dorsally about proximal phalanx, being sure to extend to IP joint.
- Carefully tug and wrap material through first web space from volar to dorsal, overlap material onto itself by approximately 1".
- After overlapping through thumb web space, have patient gently oppose to IF, which helps maintain desired thumb CMC and MP joint positions as material sets.
- Avoid applying direct pressure over dorsum of MP joint while molding.

Strapping and Components

- One 1" strap around wrist provides secure fit. Place strap at base of hypothenar eminence to prevent migration.
- Elasticized straps are preferred to allow mobility of hypothenar muscles.
- If circumferential portion of orthosis needs to be popped apart for donning and doffing over IP joint, a small strap must be applied at this opening.

Survey Completed Orthosis

- Smooth distal and proximal borders.
- Gently flare proximal to thumb IP joint.
- Check clearance of wrist, thumb IP, and IF MCP joints, making sure there is no abutment with thermoplastic material.

PATTERN PEARL 7-17 to 7-53

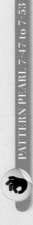
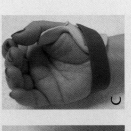

PP7-47

A and B, MP joint left free.

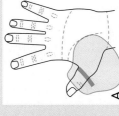

PP7-48

Volar/dorsal design: IP included.

PP7-49

A–C, Volar/dorsal design: IP free for trigger thumb.

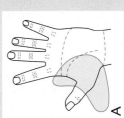

CHAPTER 7

PATTERN PEARL 7-47 to 7-53. *continued*

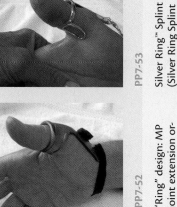

PP7-50

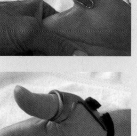

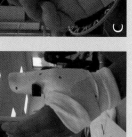

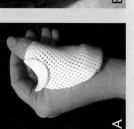

B

C

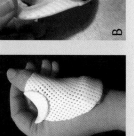

PP7-51

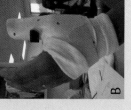

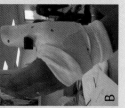

A

B

PP7-52

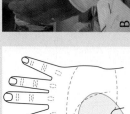

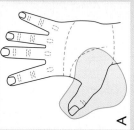

PP7-53

A, IP joint included applied **(B)** dorsal and **(C)** volar.

A and B, Incorporated beneath orthosis at CMC region.

"Ring" design: MP joint extension orthosis.

Silver Ring™ Splint (Silver Ring Splint Company) to block MP joint motion.

CLINICAL PEARL 7-21.
Easing Circumferential Thumb Orthosis Removal

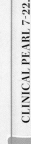

If thumb orthosis needs to come off for exercise sessions, make sure the patient can indeed remove the orthosis. Often, the circumference of the IP joint is larger than that of the proximal phalanx, making removal difficult or impossible. Wrapping tape or Coban™ around the proximal phalanx before molding can help to relatively build up the circumference of the phalanx region equaling the IP joint. One disadvantage is that this technique may cause some looseness in fit. Another method involves applying a thin layer of lotion to the thumb area before molding to ease removal. Consider using the trap door method as described elsewhere in this text.

CLINICAL PEARL 7-22.
Thumb Exercise Orthoses

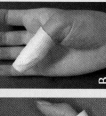

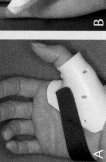

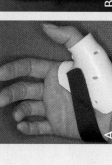

A

B

A, An orthosis that immobilizes the thumb MP joint in extension can help direct the force of flexion to the IP joint during active exercises. This can be used as an exercise tool tc increase active IP flexion and/or maximize FPL tendon glide. Note that the position of the MP joint should be in extension to increase tension on the FPL. **B,** A circumferential IP extension orthosis or cast can be used to isolate MP joint motion. Make sure that the orthosis has the longest proximal lever arm without interfering with volar MP flexion.

Thumb CMC Immobilization Orthosis (HFO) (Fig. 7–17)

Common Names

- CMC palmar abduction splint
- Short thumb spica splint
- Short opponens splint
- MP splint

Alternative Options

- Prefabricated thumb support
- Comfort Cool® splint
- Push CMC brace
- Neoprene thumb and wrist wrap
- Plaster cast

Primary Functions

- Immobilize thumb CMC and MP joints to allow healing, rest, and/or protection of involved structure(s).

Additional Functions

- Improve functional use by positioning thumb in functional opposition.
- Promote gliding of FPL or extensor pollicis longus (EPL) tendon by restricting movement of MP and CMC joint during active flexion and extension exercises.

Common Diagnoses and General Optimal Positions

TM jt arthritis	Slight MP flex with palm abd and th opp
Lax or mildly subluxed TM jt	Slight MP flex with palm abd and th opp
UCL injury (grades 1 to 3)	Slight MP flex with UD
RCL injury (grades 1 to 3)	Slight MP flex with RD
Low median nerve injury	Slight MP flex with palm abd and th opp

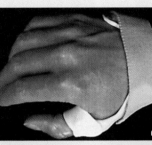
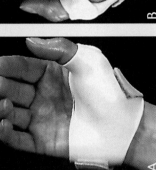

FIGURE 7-17

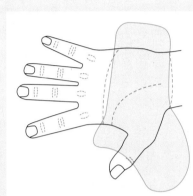

FIGURE 7-18

CLINICAL PEARL 7-23.
Trap Door for Circumferential Thumb Orthoses

To ease donning and doffing of a circumferential thumb orthosis, use a coated material (which will not adhere onto itself). Once the material is completely cool, pop apart the overlapped segment to create a trap door. Use a thin piece of loop material to "close" the door. This technique helps when there is an enlarged joint or potential fluctuating edema about the thumb MP or IP joint but still allows for complete immobilization of the MP joint. Permanently bonding this area may require enlarging the thumbhole to allow for donning/doffing, which can then allow MP motion, leading to possible areas of excess pressure.

Fabrication Process

Pattern Creation (Fig. 7–18)

- Mark for proximal border just distal to wrist crease.
- Mark for distal border at thumb IP flexion crease and DPC.

Refine Pattern

- Allow unimpeded motion of wrist, thumb IP, and digit MCP joints by keeping pattern accurate.
- Provide ample material within web space to support palmar abduction position adequately.
- Allow enough material to mold around ulnar border without overlapping dorsally.
- May extend pattern distally to include IP joint or trim pattern to omit MP joint if necessary.

Options for Materials

- Use drapable material to achieve intimate fit about CMC and MP joints

to prevent migration and improve comfort.
- Use coated material so circumferential thumb piece can be popped open without permanent sealing.
- Use thinnest material possible that provides necessary strength to minimize bulk.
- Remember that elastic materials tend to shrink around thumb (making it difficult to don and doff); do not remove until completely set.

Cut and Heat

- Position patient's forearm in slight supination to achieve gravity-assisted position.
- Place thumb MP joint in appropriate amount of flexion and CMC joint in desired amount of palmar abduction and opposition.
- Consider placing light layer of lotion on thumb before molding to ease removal.

Evaluate Fit while Molding

- Place material on volar aspect of hand and thumb while maintaining desired joint positions; at the same time, gently contour palmar arches.
- Carefully tug and wrap material through first web space from volar to dorsal; overlap material onto itself by approximately 1".
- After overlapping through thumb web space, have patient gently oppose to IF, which helps maintain desired thumb CMC and MP joint positions as material sets.
- Avoid applying direct pressure over dorsum of MP joint while molding.
- Proximally, mold well around base of CMC joint.
- Ulnarly, wrap material around ulnar border to fourth metacarpal dorsally.
- Clear IP joint flexion crease

- Avoid rolling material just proximal to the IP flexion crease (circumferentially) unless using a very thin material where light rolling may aid in strengthening this area.

Strapping and Components

- One 1" strap attached dorsally to radial and ulnar segments suffices.
- Consider using rivets to secure dorsal strap.
- If circumferential portion needs to be popped apart for donning and doffing over IP joint, small strap must be applied at this opening.

Survey Completed Orthosis

- Smooth distal and proximal borders.
- Gently flare proximal to thumb IP joint.
- Check for clearance of wrist, thumb IP, and digit MCP joints. Make sure there is no abutment with thermoplastic material.

PATTERN PEARL 7-54 to 7-61.

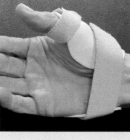

PP7-54

A–C, IP joint included.

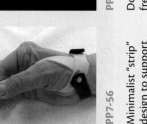

B

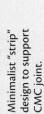

PP7-55

IP joint included, molded dorsally.

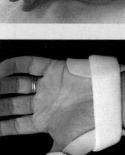

PP7-56

Minimalist "strip" design to support CMC joint.

PP7-57

Dorsal-based IP joint free.

CLINICAL PEARL 7-24.
IF MCP Joint Border

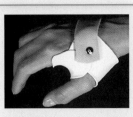

It is imperative when applying an orthosis around the first web space to be sure the index border is not too high. The orthosis shown here has an overgenerous border that impedes IF MCP joint motion; this may cause tissue irritation.

CLINICAL PEARL 7-25.
Thumb Positioning

Always check thumb position before, during, and after the molding process. When positioning the thumb for function, the CMC joint should be placed midway between palmar (**A**) and radial (**B**) abduction, and the MP joint should be in slight flexion (20 to 30°) (**C**). This allows for effective pinch to the index and MFs. If the therapist is not careful, as the patient relaxes his or her hand during the molding process, the wrist will tend to flex, which promotes thumb extension and radial abduction. This places the thumb in a poor position for function.

In this exaggerated example, note the adduction posture of the first metacarpal and the hyperextension of the thumb MP joint (**D**). Because the thumb was passively correctable, a custom orthosis was able to position the thumb to allow light opposition for daily activity (**E**)

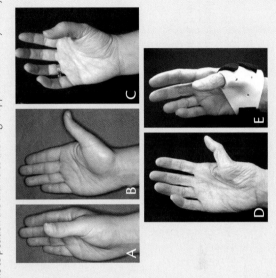

PATTERN PEARL 7-54 to 7-61. *continued*

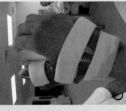
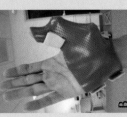
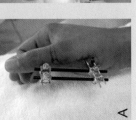

PP7-58

A–C, Accommodation of external fixator.

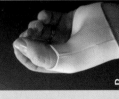
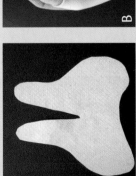

PP7-59

A and B, "Gauntlet" design.

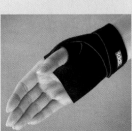
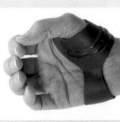
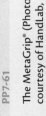

PP7-60

3pp® ThumbSling® NP prefabricated (Photo courtesy of 3-Point Products, Stevensville, MD).

PP7-61

The MetaGrip® (Photo courtesy of HandLab, Raleigh, NC).

Thumb Abduction Immobilization Orthosis (HFO) (Fig. 7-19)

Common Names

- CMC splint
- Web stretcher
- C-bar splint

Alternative Options

- Plaster cast

Primary Functions

- Prevent soft tissue contracture of first web space as result of median nerve injury or disease.

Additional Functions

- Statically position first web space contracture at maximum palmar abduction to facilitate lengthening of tissue (mobilization).

Common Diagnoses and General Optimal Positions

Median nerve injury	Maximum palm and rad abd
Postoperative contracture release	Maximum palm and rad abd

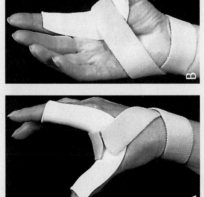

FIGURE 7-19

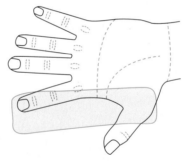

FIGURE 7-20

Fabrication Process

Pattern Creation (Fig. 7-20)

- Pattern is rectangular.
- Width is two-thirds circumference of the thumb.
- Length is measured from IF DIP joint to tip of thumb.

Refine Pattern

- Allow enough material to encompass two-thirds of thumb circumference ulnarly and two-thirds of IF radially.
- Provide ample material within web space to support palmar and radial abduction position adequately and to allow enough surface area for strap application.

Options for Materials

- Use ⅛″ thermoplastic material to provide rigidity needed to maintain position of tissue.
- Use highly drapable material to achieve intimate fit through web space to prevent migration and improve comfort.
- Consider perforated material when orthosis will be used in conjunction with scar management products such as elastomer or silicone gel.
- Materials that can be reheated and remolded several times are a good option if ongoing modifications become necessary to accommodate for changes in motion (a common issue because it is difficult to achieve desired joint position initially).

Cut and Heat

- Position patient with elbow resting on table and forearm in slight supination to achieve gravity-assisted position.
- Place thumb in appropriate amount of palmar and radial abduction.

Evaluate Fit while Molding

- Place warm material along thumb and IF while maintaining desired position.
- Mold with even pressure throughout length of orthosis, focusing on gentle abduction pressure to distal portions of first and second metacarpals. Avoid applying pressure at thumb distally, which can actually place undue tension on UCL, not first web space.
- Flare around thumb and IF MCP joints.
- Maintain desired thumb position as material sets.

Strapping and Components

- Apply one 1″ elasticized strap directed from volar web space around wrist 1½ times and attach to dorsal aspect.

Survey Completed Orthosis

- Smooth distal and proximal borders.
- Define consistent wearing schedule for patient. Many therapists suggest patients wear these orthoses at night only, allowing functional use during day.

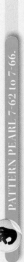

PATTERN PEARL 7-62 to 7-66.

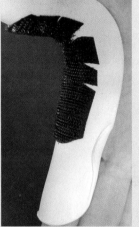

PP7-62

Foam with strapping.

PP7-63

Using ribbon as way to secure orthosis (Photo courtesy of Jill Peck-Murray).

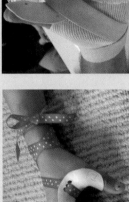

PP7-64

Including full length of IF for better purchase; notice Figure-8 strap around wrist.

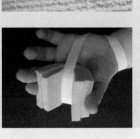

PP7-65

Feathered hook in web space area to allow full contact.

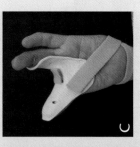

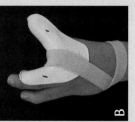

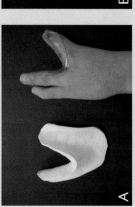

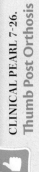

PP7-66

PATTERN PEARL 7-62 to 7-66. *continued*

A–C, Gel beneath orthosis used after web space reconstruction procedure. Note the widened middle portion of this pattern to achieve better purchase and stability on the hand.

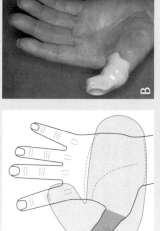

CLINICAL PEARL 7-27.
Incorrect Pressure Application to Address First Web Tightness

If pressure is applied distal to the MP joint, stress is placed on the UCL instead of the intended first web space (as shown here). This force may eventually disrupt the UCL. Make sure pressure is applied to the most proximal ulnar portion of the first metacarpal and avoid applying pressure distal to the MP joint.

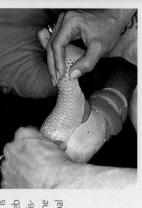

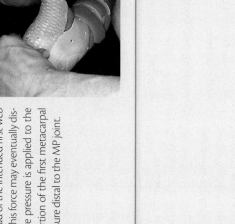

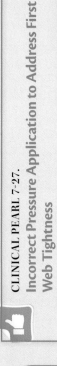

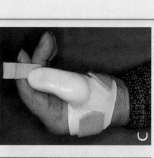

CLINICAL PEARL 7-26.
Thumb Post Orthosis

For patients without a thumb (congenital or traumatic), this design provides a functional pinch for light activities of daily living (ADLs) or may act as a temporary mold (preprosthesis) to allow the patient to adjust to the use of a prosthetic. This temporary mold may help determine the optimal length and position of a permanent prosthetic. The pattern depends on the level of the amputation or congenital anomaly **(A)**. Products such as elastomer or prosthetic foam instead of thermoplastic material can be used to fabricate the internal spacer **(B)**. The length and width of the post are determined by the amount of amputated thumb—use the unaffected side as a guide. Use ⅛" material that has maximal rigidity and durability. Remember that this is a functional orthosis and must be able to withstand the rigors of ADLs **(C)**. While molding, maintain the desired thumb post position as the material sets to allow for effective three-point pinch. Because the prosthetic thumb has no sensation, tell the patient to use vision with all thumb activities.

CLINICAL PEARL 7-28.
Improving Pressure Distribution beneath First Web Immobilization Orthosis

Gel products or open cell foams can be used under the orthosis for reducing scar sensitivity and improving pressure distribution (**A**). Elastomer-type products can also be used to achieve better pressure distribution in such areas. Here, a previously molded $\frac{3}{32}''$ perforated material is being applied over soft, curing elastomer (**B**). Such curing materials can be made to seep through the holes in a perforated material, providing a way to secure the product onto the thermoplastic (**C**). These products work well for patients who have undergone a first web space surgical release by incorporating the known benefits of scar management and maintaining the desired range of motion.

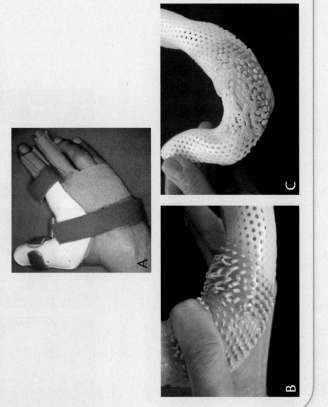

CLINICAL PEARL 7-29.
First Web Space "Handshake Hold" Molding Technique

A great technique to maintain maximal stretch of the first web space while molding is to use a "handshake" hold (web space to web space) while applying the material.

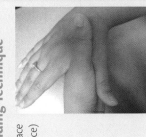

3   Forearm-Based Orthoses

Dorsal Wrist Immobilization Orthosis (WHO)   (Fig. 7–21)

Common Names

- Dorsal wrist cock-up splint
- Dorsal wrist support
- Wrist extension splint
- Static wrist splint
- Radial bar wrist splint

Alternative Options

- Prefabricated wrist orthosis
- Cast
- Zipper design orthosis

Primary Functions

- Immobilize wrist joint to allow healing, rest, or protection of involved structures(s).

Additional Functions

- Substitute for weak or absent wrist extensor muscle function.
- Improve functional grasp and pinch by positioning wrist in extension and maximizing mechanical advantage of finger flexors.
- Provide base for outrigger attachment when fabricating digit extension mobilization orthoses.

Common Diagnoses and General Optimal Positions

Carpal tunnel syndrome	0°
Median and/or ulnar nerve repair	0 to 15° flex
Radial nerve palsy	20 to 35° ext

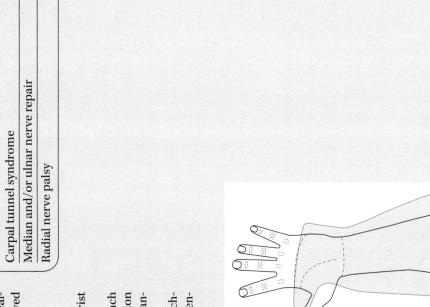

FIGURE 7-22

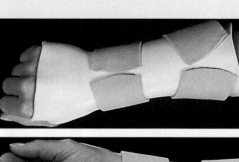
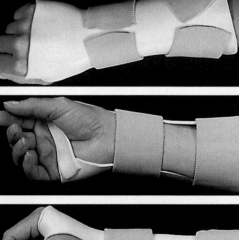

FIGURE 7-21

Fabrication Process

Pattern Creation (Fig. 7–22)

- Consider dorsal design for patients who are not comfortable in volar design.
- Dorsal design allows for better sensory input to palm than does volar design.
- Good design for patients with volar skin grafts, wounds, pins, or hypersensitive scars.
- Remember that this design may not provide necessary strength to immobilize wrist completely; volar thumbhole design is better option for maximizing wrist immobilization.
- Mark for proximal border two-thirds length of forearm.
- Mark distal border just proximal to MCP joints.
- Distal radial tab (palmar bar) should be long enough (approximately 3″) to traverse through palm and secure on distal ulnar border.
- Tab should incorporate oblique angle from index to SF metacarpal heads.
- Mark thumb clearance by making arc from thumb MP to base of first CMC joint.
- Allow enough material to encompass two-thirds circumference of forearm, remembering that forearm tapers distally.

Refine Pattern

- Proximal border should allow full elbow motion.
- Distal border should allow unimpeded motion of digital MCP and thumb joints.
- Provide appropriate amount of material within palmar surface to support arches adequately.

Cut and Heat

- Position patient with elbow resting on table and forearm pronated for gravity-assisted molding. Position thumb in palmar abduction.
- Prepad ulnar styloid with adhesive-backed foam, putty, cotton ball, or silicone gel.

Evaluate Fit while Molding

- Position material on dorsum of involved hand and wrist just proximal to MCP joints.
- Place radial bar through thumb web and guide rest of bar along palmar surface just proximal to DPC, overlapping and securing on distal ulnar border (pull material if needed for increased length).
- Carefully incorporate arches of hand by using smooth, even strokes and constantly redirecting material into arches. Continual molding over volar bar is mandatory to prevent negative effects of gravity.
- Do not grab proximal region or try to secure with tight circumferential bandage. This may cause borders to irritate skin. Instead, allow gravity to assist in forming forearm trough. Make sure desired wrist position is maintained. Some patients tend to flex and deviate wrist while orthosis is being formed.

Options for Materials

- Consider 1/8″ thermoplastic material to provide needed rigidity to maintain wrist position.
- If patient has difficulty maintaining wrist extension (e.g., secondary to radial nerve injury), consider uncoated materials or those that are slightly tacky to help prevent material from slipping and to make it easier to position patient and mold the orthosis.
- Gel- or foam-lined materials help provide dorsal wrist scar compression, decrease distal migration, and increase comfort.
- Consider perforated material when orthosis will be used during activity or in conjunction with scar-management products such as elastomer. Scar products seep through perforations, which helps anchor them into the orthosis.

Strapping and Components

- Distal strap: 1″ strap connecting radial bar to distal ulnar border.
- Middle strap: (Key Strap!) 2″ strap just proximal to dorsal wrist crease; use piece of adhesive foam to further stabilize wrist and prevent migration. Foam should not overlap edges.
- Proximal strap: 2″ soft or elasticized strap is good choice, especially if patient will use orthosis for functional purposes. Such straps can better accommodate changes in forearm bulk during movement than traditional loop strap.

Survey Completed Orthosis

- Smooth and slightly flare borders.
- Gently flare around dorsal thumb region; avoid rolling, which can make future modifications difficult.
- Check clearance of elbow, radial and ulnar styloid processes, thumb, and MCP joints.
- Pay careful attention to index metacarpal, which frequently abuts radial tab as it traverses through first web space.
- Check for compression over radial and ulnar sensory nerve branches.

PATTERN PEARL 7-67 to 7-70

PP7-67

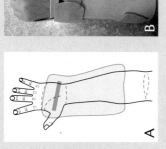

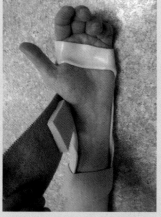

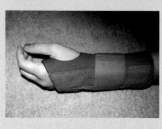

A and B, Incorporating thumb into the dorsal design.

PP7-68

Prefabricated wrist orthosis with dorsal stay as an alternative (Grip-Fit™ Splint by Alimed, Dedham, MA).

PP7-69

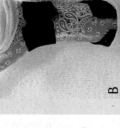

Soft foam can assist in securing wrist position.

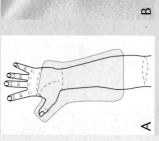

PP7-70

A–C, A volar/dorsal design.

CLINICAL PEARL 7-30.
Prepadding of the Ulnar Styloid

Adhesive foam can be used to prepad the ulnar styloid process before an orthosis is applied (**A**). Dab the adhesive side of the foam a few times on a towel to decrease the tackiness and make removal more comfortable for the patient. Apply and gently mold the orthosis. Once the thermoplastic material has cooled, remove the padding from the skin and invert back onto the orthosis (**B**).

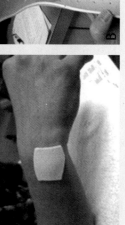

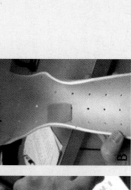

CLINICAL PEARL 7-31.
Proximal Forearm Strap Applied on an Oblique Angle

To apply a strap appropriately around the proximal forearm, the therapist must appreciate the tapered shape of this region. Straps should be applied with a slight angle to avoid shear stress (**A**) on the forearm tissue and achieve contour about the musculature. Soft or elasticized straps may contour and accommodate for forearm bulk better than more rigid straps (**B**).

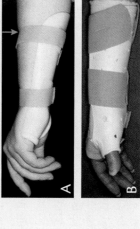

Volar Wrist Immobilization Orthosis (WHO) (Fig. 7–23)

Common Names

- Wrist cock-up splint
- Thumbhole wrist splint
- Wrist gauntlet splint
- Palmar wrist cock-up splint
- Static wrist splint
- Wrist drop splint

Alternative Options

- Prefabricated wrist orthosis
- Cast
- Zipper design orthosis

Primary Functions

- Immobilize wrist joint to allow healing, rest, and/or protection of involved structures(s).

Additional Functions

- Statically position wrist flexion contracture at maximum extension to facilitate lengthening of tissue (mobilization).
- Substitute for weak or absent wrist extensor muscle function.
- Improve functional grasp and pinch by positioning wrist in extension and maximizing mechanical advantage of finger flexors.
- Provide base for outrigger attachment when fabricating mobilization orthoses.

Common Diagnoses and General Optimal Positions

Diagnosis	Position
Carpal tunnel syndrome	0°
Carpal tunnel release	20 to 35° ext
Wr tenosynovitis and post-tenosynovectomy	Flexors: 0°; extensor: 20 to 40° ext
Rheumatoid arthritis or osteoarthritis	Position of comfort
Wr arthroplasty	0°
Wr arthrodesis	Dictated by fusion
Ganglion excision	20 to 35° ext
Wr sprain or instability	Dictated by structures involved
Distal radius and/or ulna fracture (post cast)	Maximal ext
Carpal fracture	Dictated by structures involved
Metacarpal fracture or dislocation (base)	Slight ext
Epicondylitis	Medial: 0°; lateral: 20 to 35° ext
Radial nerve palsy	20 to 35° ext

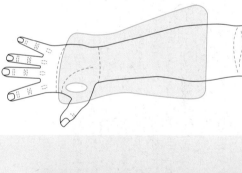

FIGURE 7-24

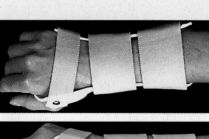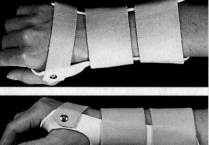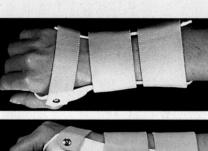

FIGURE 7-23

Fabrication Process

Pattern Creation (Fig. 7-24)

- Mark for proximal border two-thirds length of forearm.
- Mark for distal border at palmar crease.
- Incorporate oblique angle that traverses from index to small metacarpal heads.
- Allow enough material to encompass two-thirds circumference of forearm, remembering that forearm tapers distally.

Refine Pattern

- Proximal border should allow full elbow motion.
- To maximize leverage, distal border should end at DPC and thenar region should be cleared enough to allow opposition to index and MFs, clearing approximately two-thirds of the-nar region.
- For average adult, thumbhole should be about the size of elongated half dollar. When measuring pattern on patient, hole should lie approximately over thumb MP joint.
- Provide appropriate width of material within first web space to support thumb position and provide adequate surface area for strap application dorsally.

Options for Materials

- Material selection depends on orthotic requirements.
- Consider ⅛″ thermoplastic material to provide needed rigidity to support an unstable ligamentous injury or postoperative repair.
- Consider ³⁄₃₂″ material for immobilizing wrist that does not require rigid support or for patients who will not place high demands on the orthosis (e.g., patient with arthritis).
- Materials that can be reheated and remolded several times are a good option if ongoing modifications become necessary to accommodate for fluctuations in edema or changes in desired joint position.
- Gel- or foam-lined materials help provide volar wrist scar compression, decrease distal migration, and increase comfort.
- Consider perforated material when orthosis will be used during activity or in conjunction with scar management products such as elastomer. Scar products seep through perforations, which helps anchor them into orthosis.

Cut and Heat

- Position patient with elbow resting on table and forearm supinated for gravity-assisted molding. Position thumb in gentle palmar abduction and opposition.

- If patient has difficulty supinating forearm (e.g., distal radius fractures after cast immobilization), have patient flex elbow on table and adduct shoulder toward midline or lie patient supine with shoulder abducted and externally rotated 90° with elbow flexed.
- Fully heat distal/radial corner separately first to cut out thumbhole. Either make series of holes with hole punch before heating or by carefully piercing the warm material with sharp scissors.

Evaluate Fit while Molding

- Heat full pattern and lay warm material on towel, positioning thumbhole on correct side of material as if material were to be placed on supinated forearm.
- Using IFs, gently open hole, slightly enlarging and elongating it (making it egg shaped); avoid rolling. Use borders of thenar crease as landmarks for length and width of hole.
- Place thumbhole over thumb and guide rest of material evenly along volar wrist and forearm, keeping distal edge just proximal to DPC.
- Gravity tends to pull material away from hand dorsally (elongating thumbhole); continually reposition material as needed.

- Do not grab proximally or try to secure with tight circumferential bandage. This may cause borders to irritate skin. Instead, allow gravity to assist in forming forearm trough.
- Carefully incorporate arches of hand by using smooth, even strokes and constantly redirecting material into arches. Avoid strongly molding into arches, which may cause significant discomfort in palm once material has set.
- Rotate forearm into pronated position at end of molding to check for clearance of ulnar and radial styloid processes; flare about styloids as necessary.
- Make sure desired wrist position is maintained. Some patients tend to flex and ulnarly deviate wrist while orthosis is being formed.
- Caution should be taken when moving the forearm in order to correctly position the wrist. Occasionally, the forearm trough can get "twisted" through the distal molding process.

Strapping and Components

- Distal strap: 1″ strap directed from radial dorsal web area to distal ulnar border. Strip of adhesive foam can be used under strap to further stabilize metacarpals.

(Continued)

Fabrication Process

(Continued)

- Middle strap: (Key Strap!) 2″ strap just proximal to dorsal wrist crease; use piece of adhesive foam to further stabilize wrist and prevent migration. Foam should lie directly over ulnar styloid and should not overlap edges.

- Proximal strap: Depending on size of forearm, 1″ or 2″ strap may suffice; strap should have slight volar to dorsal angle.

Survey Completed Orthosis

- Smooth and slightly flare distal and proximal borders.
- Gently flare around thenar hole; avoid rolling, which can make future modifications difficult.
- Check clearance of elbow, radial and ulnar styloid processes, thumb, and finger MCP joints.
- Pay careful attention to index metacarpal, which frequently abuts radial portion as it traverses through first web space.

PATTERN PEARL 7-71 to 7-74

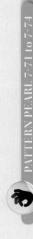

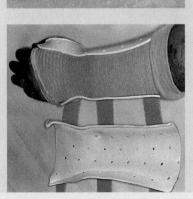

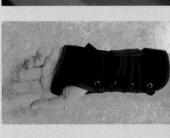

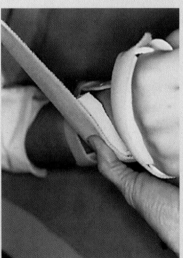

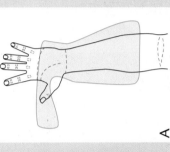

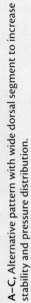

PP7-71

Clamshell design: dorsal material applied to simulate a circumferential orthosis or cast.

PP7-72

Prefabricated wrist orthosis with hard stay (Suede Wrist Lacer Splint shown by Corflex, Manchester, NH).

PP7-73

Soft padding over the middle strap can assist in stabilization of wrist position.

PP7-74

A–C, Alternative pattern with wide dorsal segment to increase stability and pressure distribution.

CHAPTER 7

CLINICAL PEARL 7-32.
Alternative Methods for Securing Straps

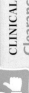

A, Riveting straps helps secure and maintain the strap position and prevent the strap from falling off, especially in small areas where it may be difficult to adhere hook material. Always apply a thin lining material, such as moleskin, on the underside of the rivet to avoid skin irritation (see Clinical Pearl 7-40 for further instruction). **B and C,** Alternatively, a strap can be riveted with the strapping material resting against the skin side. For many patients, this can be advantageous, imparting additional light force over the tissue as shown with this deviated rheumatoid wrist. **D and E,** Another method is to apply adhesive hook volar and dorsal on the radial web thumbhole segment. Direct the strap from the volar hook to the dorsal hook and then over to the ulnar border and rest the strap down. This method allows the clinician to use the full surface area about the thumbhole, which can often be challenging. Soft strapping material is recommended. **F,** A homemade rivet can also be made to secure strap. Fabricate out of thermoplastic material by heating a scrap piece of thermoplastic and forming into a small ball the size of a pea, then hyperheat this over a heat gun. Prepare the attachment site surface for bonding by scratching the area and/or brushing with solvent to remove any coating. Make a hole through the strap and apply the warm ball through the hole and onto the orthosis. Be careful to correctly position and align the strap because once the material hardens, it is not easily adjusted.

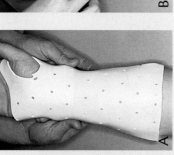

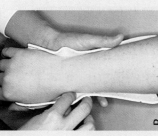

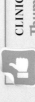

CLINICAL PEARL 7-33.
Clearance of Radial and Ulnar Styloid Processes

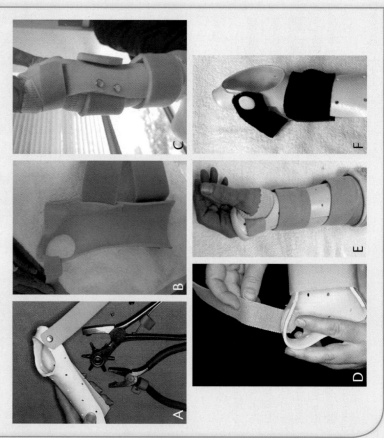

Near the end of the molding process of an orthosis that includes the forearm, place the arm in both a pronated and supinated positions to check for clearance of the styloid processes. Note that the forearm muscle bulk orientation changes as the forearm rotates. Using IFs, gently reach under the slightly warm material and pull out or lift along the styloids. When using elastic materials, constant redirecting or reminding the material is necessary. For plastic materials, one gentle adjustment is all that is needed. For more rigid rubber materials, a stronger lift is necessary to achieve the desired clearance.

CLINICAL PEARL 7-34.
Thumbhole Preparation Prior to Application

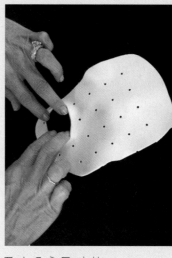

As soon as the material is removed from the water, place on smooth surface and gently elongate the hole in an oval shape oriented longitudinally (not in a circle, which is not the ideal shape to fit about the thenar region). The therapist must take caution not to overstretch the material.

CLINICAL PEARL 7-35.
Light Tip Pinch to Incorporate Palmar Arches

To improve incorporating the arches of the hand within an orthosis, have the patient very lightly hold a piece of cotton or like material between the thumb and IF. This technique can be used with many volar and circumferential orthoses to help achieve an intimate fit in the hand, improving comfort and maximizing functional use. Do not let patient pinch too hard because this may exaggerate thumb opposition, especially with thumb orthoses, because the "firing" of thenar muscles will make the orthosis too loose when the muscles are then relaxed.

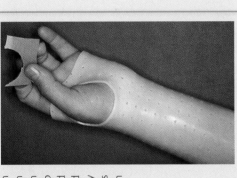

CLINICAL PEARL 7-37.
Reinforcing Volar Portion of the Orthosis

A strip of thermoplastic material or cast tape can be used to reinforce potential areas of weakness within an orthosis. To reinforce an orthosis fabricated with a coated thermoplastic material, the therapist must first remove the coating with solvent or by vigorously scratching the surface.

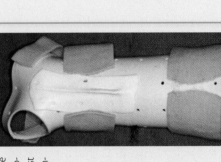

CLINICAL PEARL 7-36.
Preventing Buckling of Material about the Thumb

To prevent buckling of material dorsally when fabricating the thumbhole wrist orthosis, consider the following points: (1) Do not overheat the thermoplastic material; (2) do not make the thumbhole too big; (3) when placing the heated material on the hand, think "distal and ulnar" and do not position the thumbhole too far radially (the hole should allow visualization of approximately two-thirds of thenar eminence); and (4) during the molding process, gently and continually reposition the dorsal piece against the skin to counteract the effects of gravity.

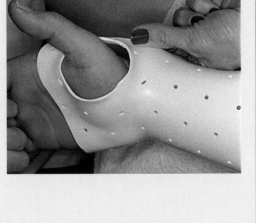

Ulnar Wrist Immobilization Orthosis (WHO) (Fig. 7-25)

Common Names
- Ulnar gutter splint

Alternative Options
- Prefabricated wrist orthosis
- Cast

Primary Functions
- Immobilize wrist joint to allow healing of involved structure(s).

Additional Functions
- Maximize radial hand function while immobilizing ulnar side of hand.

Common Diagnoses and General Optimal Positions

RF or SF metacarpal fracture (base)	Wr: 0 to 20° ext; RD and UD: 0°
Lunate, triquetrum, or hamate instability or fracture	Wr: 0 to 20° ext; RD and UD: 0°
Triangular fibrocartilage complex (TFCC) injury or repair	Wr: 0°; RD and UD: 0°
Extensor carpi ulnaris tenosynovitis	Wr: 0 to 20° ext with slight UD
Flexor carpi ulnaris tenosynovitis	Wr: 0° with slight UD
Ulnar nerve compression at Guyon's canal	Wr: 0° with slight UD

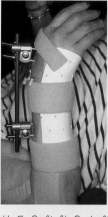

CLINICAL PEARL 7-38.
Ulnar Wrist Immobilization Orthosis for External Fixator

Commonly, patients are referred for a wrist orthosis to be worn in conjunction with an external fixator to provide added support to the wrist, improve comfort, and protect the arm from inadvertent external forces. Because the patient is unable to rotate the arm freely to achieve a gravity-assisted position, the therapist must use an alternative approach. Lay the patient supine with the elbow and shoulder flexed to achieve the desired gravity-assisted position for molding. (see Clinical Pearl 7-39 for further instruction). Straps should be applied carefully and thoughtfully. Avoid strap contact with the pin sites, which can be sensitive and prone to skin irritation and infection. Be meticulous when trimming the straps to obtain a comfortable fit. As an alternative, circumferential wraps can be used to secure the orthosis on the arm; this is especially beneficial if edema is an issue.

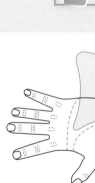

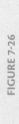

FIGURE 7-26

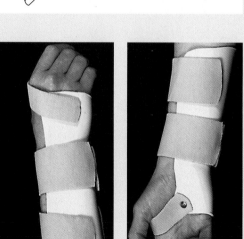

FIGURE 7-25

Fabrication Process

Pattern Creation (Fig. 7-26)

- Mark for proximal border two-thirds length of forearm.
- Mark distal border at DPC of MF to SF.
- Incorporate oblique angle that traverses from index to small metacarpal heads.
- Mark for thenar crease from MP flexion crease between IF and MF and base of CMC joint.
- Allow enough material to encompass two-thirds circumference of forearm, remembering that forearm tapers distally.

Refine Pattern

- Proximal border should allow full elbow motion.
- Distal border should allow unimpeded motion of MCP joints and full thumb mobility.

Options for Materials

- Consider ⅛" thermoplastic material to provide needed rigidity to support unstable ligamentous injury or healing fracture.
- If patient has difficulty achieving gravity-assisted position, consider uncoated materials or those that are slightly tacky to help prevent material from slipping and to make it easier to position patient and mold orthosis.
- Gel- or foam-lined materials may help with molding over ulnar styloid and bony dorsum, decrease distal migration, and increase comfort.

Cut and Heat

- While material is heating, prepad ulnar styloid using self-adhesive padding or silicone gel.

- Position extremity with patient supine with shoulder and elbow flexed to 90° (ulnar aspect of hand facing ceiling) or with patient sitting with shoulder flexed to 90° and elbow flexed fully; radial side of hand (thumb) should be pointing toward floor.

Evaluate Fit while Molding

- Drape warm material centrally over ulnar border of forearm and hand, making sure palmar material lies along thenar crease and just proximal to DPC.
- Gently flare material along distal borders.
- If addressing RF or SF proximal metacarpal fracture, completely incorporate MF metacarpal to anchor orthosis and prevent mobility of ulnar two metacarpals.
- Do not grab proximally or try to secure with tight circumferential bandage. This may cause borders to irritate skin. Instead, allow gravity to assist in forming forearm trough.
- Carefully incorporate arches of hand by using smooth, even strokes and constantly redirecting material into arches.
- When material is almost set, gently rotate forearm to check for clearance of ulnar styloid. Styloid becomes more

prominent with forearm rotation; if space is not incorporated when molding, ulnar styloid irritation may occur during functional use. If patient complains of abutment, carefully push out material, forming small bubble.
- Make sure desired wrist position is maintained. Some patients tend to flex and deviate wrist while orthosis is being formed.

Strapping and Components

- Distal strap: 1" strap, trimmed to contour around first web space, is directed from volar radial to dorsal radial border. Consider riveting strap on volar surface to secure strap firmly and decrease bulk within palm.
- Middle strap: 2" strap just proximal to dorsal wrist crease; use piece of adhesive foam to further stabilize wrist and prevent migration (avoid excessive compression over radial sensory nerve).
- Proximal strap: Depending on size of forearm, 1" or 2" strap may suffice; strap should have slight volar to dorsal angle.

Survey Completed Orthosis

- Smooth and slightly flare all borders.
- Check clearance of elbow, thumb, and MCP joints.

PATTERN PEARL 7-75 to 7-76.

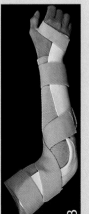

PP7-75

A and B, Elbow included in ulnar-based wrist orthosis.

CLINICAL PEARL 7-40.
Rivet Setting Techniques

A, Small or medium sized rivets can be used to secure straps onto an orthosis. The following techniques can help prevent the loop material from pulling off the rivet once set. **B and C,** A small piece of adhesive hook can be adhered on the area where the strap will be placed. This additional step of adding a piece of material between the strap and the thermoplastic prevents the material from eventually stretching over the rivet and separating from the strap. Place the strap over this area and, with a quality hole punch, make a hole through all three pieces (thermoplastic, hook material, and strap), creating a clean small hole. Place the stem of the rivet on the skin side of the orthosis and push through all three layers. Apply the rivet cap and close together using blunt-nosed pliers. Remember to cover the surface of the rivet that contacts the skin with a thin adhesive lined material (such as Moleskin) to prevent skin irritation. **D,** Another technique to prevent the loop from pulling off includes using a homemade washer made out of thin thermoplastic material. This is placed between the rivet cap and the loop material as shown.

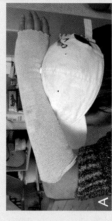

B

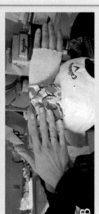

A

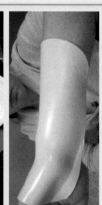

C

D

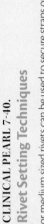

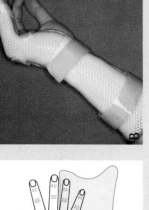

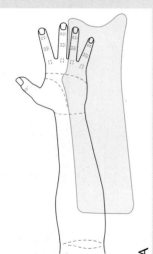

PP7-76

A

B

A and B, RF and SF included in ulnar-based wrist orthosis.

CLINICAL PEARL 7-39.
Gravity-Assisted Molding with Ulnar-Based Orthoses

When fabricating an ulnar-based orthosis, it can be quite helpful to have the patient place the arm in a gravity-assisted position with the ulnar side of the forearm facing upward parallel to the floor. This position can be achieved in several ways, but commonly it includes either a sitting or supine position. The patient or assistant can hold or rest the radial side of the forearm above or on the head, or the patient can be instructed to support the radial side of the arm out in front of him or her (**A and B**). Whatever position is chosen when using gravity as an assist, the clinician must be acutely aware of not letting the wrist drop into too much radial deviation (with gravity) as the orthosis is being fabricated (**C**).

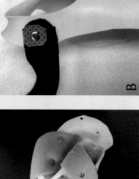

A

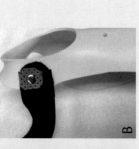

B

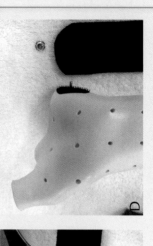

C

Circumferential Wrist Immobilization Orthosis (WHO) (Fig. 7–27)

Common Names

- Wrist fracture brace
- Circumferential wrist splint
- Circumferential wrist cock-up splint
- Circumferential thumbhole wrist splint
- Wrist gauntlet splint

Alternative Options

- Clamshell wrist orthosis
- Cast
- Prefabricated orthosis

Primary Functions

- Immobilize wrist joint to allow healing, rest, and/or protection of involved structure(s).

Additional Functions

- Statically position wrist flexion or extension contracture at maximum length to facilitate lengthening of tissue (mobilization).
- Substitute for weak or absent wrist extensor muscle function.

- Improve functional grasp and pinch by positioning wrist in extension and maximizing mechanical advantage of finger flexors.
- Provide base for outrigger attachment when fabricating digital mobilization orthoses.

Common Diagnoses and General Optimal Positions

Wr sprain or instability	Dictated by structures involved
Distal radius and/or ulna fracture (post cast)	Maximal ext
Carpal fracture	Dictated by structures involved
Metacarpal fracture or dislocation (base)	Slight ext

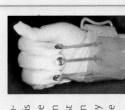

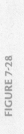

CLINICAL PEARL 7-41.
Circumferential Orthosis as a Base for Mobilization Components

Circumferential designs provide a stable base for attaching mobilization components to address distal issues. Because of the intimate fit provided with this all-encompassing design, migration can be minimized. Here, a flexion glove was used over the Rolyan® AquaForm™ Zippered Wrist Splint (Patterson Medical) to provide a flexion mobilization force to the digits while the wrist remains stabilized in extension. This prevents the common compensation problem of the wrist flexing to reduce the stretch on tight digits caused by the flexion glove's corrective force. Component systems, both homemade and commercially available, can also be attached directly to this orthosis.

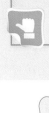

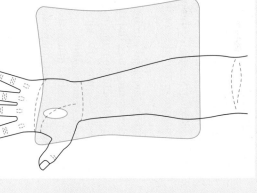

FIGURE 7-28

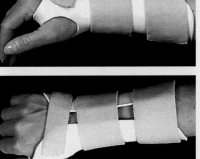

FIGURE 7-27

Fabrication Process

Pattern Creation (Fig. 7–28)

- Alternative to clamshell wrist immobilization orthosis.
- Mark for proximal border two-thirds length of forearm.
- Mark for distal border just proximal to DPC.
- Widen pattern proximally, remembering that forearm tapers distally.
- Incorporate oblique angle that traverses from index to small metacarpal heads.
- Mark for thumbhole, located distally and approximately two-thirds from ulnar border; position hole down 1″ from this point.

Refine Pattern

- Proximal border should allow full elbow motion.
- Distal border should allow unimpeded motion of MCP joints and nearly full thumb mobility.
- For average adult, thumbhole should be about the size of elongated half dollar. When measuring pattern on patient, hole should lie approximately over thumb MP joint.

Options for Materials

- Elastic materials are an excellent choice because they tend to stretch easily when heated and provide an intimate fit. Remember that elastic materials tend to shrink around the body part; do not remove until it is completely set.
- Use 3∕32″ material, which is adequate for stabilizing forearm; circumferential nature of this design makes it rigid.
- Although 1∕8″ material can be used, its thickness increases the rigidity, making it difficult to remove.
- May use 1∕16″ material for young children and older adults.
- Lightly perforated materials allow air exchange and increase flexibility, making donning and doffing easier.

Cut and Heat

- Position patient with elbow resting on table and forearm supinated for gravity-assisted molding. Position thumb in palmar abduction and opposition.
- If patient has difficulty supinating forearm, have patient flex elbow on table and adduct shoulder toward midline or lay patient supine with shoulder abducted and externally rotated 90° with elbow flexed.
- Cut out thumbhole in material either by making a series of holes with hole punch before heating or by carefully piercing the slightly warm material with sharp scissors.
- Prepad ulnar styloid (and radial styloid, if necessary) with adhesive-backed padding or gel.

Evaluate Fit while Molding

- Lay warm material on towel, positioning thumbhole on correct side of material as if it were to be placed on forearm.
- Using IFs, gently open hole, slightly enlarging and elongating it.
- Place thumbhole over thumb (using thenar crease as guide) and gently stretch and guide rest of material evenly.
- Do not grab proximal portion or try to secure with tight circumferential bandage.
- Gently redirect dorsal surface by applying smooth strokes over area.
- Carefully incorporate arches of hand by using smooth, even strokes and constantly redirecting material into arches. Avoid strongly molding into arches, which may cause significant discomfort in palm once material has set.
- Rotate forearm into pronated position at end of molding to check for clearance of ulnar and radial styloid processes.
- Make sure desired wrist position is maintained. Some patients tend to flex and deviate wrist while orthosis is being formed.

Strapping and Components

- Self-adhesive D-ring straps: 1″ strap distally and 2″ straps proximally work well, because they allow firm and easy closure. Patient can make adjustments according to comfort.

Survey Completed Orthosis

- Smooth and slightly flare distal and proximal borders as well as thenar hole.
- Check clearance of elbow, radial and ulnar styloid processes, thumb, and finger MCP joints.
- Pay careful attention to index metacarpal, which frequently abuts radial portion as it traverses through first web space.

PATTERN PEARL 7-77 to 7-79.

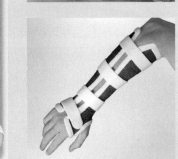

PP7-77

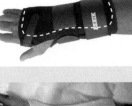
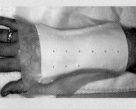
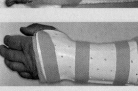

PP7-78

A simple "clamshell" design.

PP7-79

Prefabricated wrist orthosis with moldable thermoplastic stay (W-310 Wrist Support shown. Photo courtesy of Benik Corp., Silverdale, WA).

Delta-Cast® (BSN medical, Inc., Charlotte, NC) material used as an alternative.

CLINICAL PEARL 7-42.
Zippered Circumferential Wrist Orthosis

A, The Rolyan® AquaForm™ Zippered Wrist Splint (Patterson Medical) provides another option for a circumferential design. Choose the appropriate size per catalog instructions, keeping in mind that these tend to run large; so, when in doubt, opt for the smaller size because this elastic material stretches. Position the patient with the elbow resting on a table and forearm in neutral. Fully heat and apply the warmed orthosis (material should be completely clear or opaque) with the zippered edge along the dorsal ulnar border, zip it down while keeping the distal border at the DPC—this can be challenging to get the zipper started so if the material starts to set, immediately remove and reheat fully. Because this is elastic material, it will shrink back to the original shape. The distal edge needs to stay as distal as possible, allowing full MCP motion, but do not overclear for the DPC, which can affect the mechanical advantage and allow for wrist motion within the final orthosis. Once zippered, gently place the wrist in desired position by having patient assume a gently opposed posture to capture the arches in the hand. Remember to use the stretch in this material to your advantage; the "shrinking" will provide for a well-contoured final product. While the material sets, gently rotate the forearm from midpronation to midsupination to allow for a small hollowed area to form for the ulnar styloid process. This orthosis is an excellent option for patients who require continued immobilization (eg, fractures, wrist fusion) yet need to remove the orthosis for protected exercises and hygiene. This is not appropriate for patients presenting with significant or fluctuating edema because of potential circulation issues. This can be tricky to don and doff; be sure to educate the patient and or caregiver on how best to apply. If required, this device can be remolded as needed by reheating the whole orthosis fully; avoid partially heating a small area because the elasticized nature of this material will cause localized shrinkage and possible fit issues.
B–D, The length can be cut down as needed and a homemade zipper stop fabricated from scrap thermoplastic to prevent the zipper from falling off. Be sure to prepare the proximal on the orthosis with solvent and heat briefly with heat gun to ensure a strong bond.

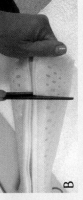
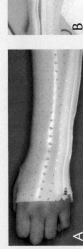

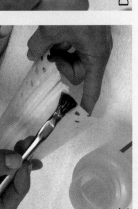
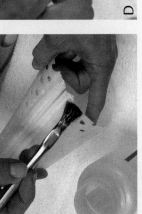
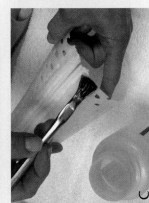

A

B

C

D

CLINICAL PEARL 7-43.
Material with Memory: Using Stretch, Pinch, and Cut Technique

Thin perforated materials with memory and a protective coating have minimal resistance to stretch and can be used for making lightweight circumferential orthoses. Most of these materials can be reheated as often as needed to achieve optimal positioning. Once the material is heated and applied to the hand/forearm, the therapist can gently stretch and pinch the borders together. Once sealed but still warm, the material can be trimmed to form a seam. The therapist can leave this sealed or can snap the borders apart (once the material has cooled) and apply straps for closure. If straps are applied, the borders may be lined with a material such as Moleskin or a stockinette can be applied prior to orthosis application.

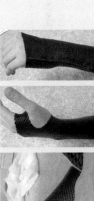
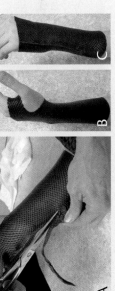

A

B

C

Radial Wrist/Thumb Immobilization Orthosis (WHFO) (Fig. 7–29)

Common Names

- Radial gutter splint
- Radial gutter thumb spica splint
- Thumb gauntlet splint
- Radial wrist support
- Long opponens splint

Alternative Options

- Prefabricated wrist and thumb orthosis
- Cast

Primary Functions

- Immobilize wrist and thumb joint(s) to allow healing, rest, and/or protection of involved structure(s).

Additional Functions

- Improve functional pinch by positioning wrist and thumb in optimal positions.

Common Diagnoses and General Optimal Positions

deQuervain's tenosynovitis	Wr: 20° ext; th CMC: between rad and palm abd; MP: slight flex; IP: included or free, depending on severity
Th UCL reconstruction	Wr: 20° ext; th CMC: palm abd; MP: 5° flex and slight UD
Th RCL reconstruction	Wr: 20° ext; th CMC: palm abd; MP: 5° flex and slight RD
Th scaphotrapeziotrapezoid (STT) or CMC jt arthritis	Wr: 0 to 20° ext; th CMC: between rad and palm abd; MP: 5 to 10° flex
EPL repair	Wr: 25 to 30° ext; th CMC: rad abd; MP: ext; IP: slight hyperextension
Tendon transfers for th ext	Wr: 25 to 30° ext; th CMC: rad abd; IP: slight hyperextension

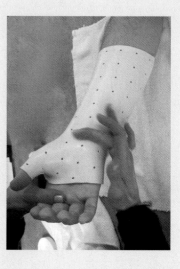

CLINICAL PEARL 7-44.
Contouring about Wrist

Gentle contouring about the pisiform/ulnar wrist will assist in better orthosis purchase and assist in decreasing distal migration. Choosing a material that drapes well and being sure to heat it fully is key to successfully obtaining this desired contour.

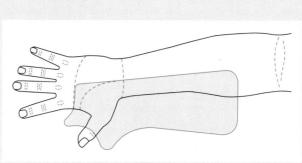

FIGURE 7-30

FIGURE 7-29

Fabrication Process

Pattern Creation (Fig. 7–30)

- Mark proximal border two-thirds length of forearm.
- Mark distal border at IF and MF proximal palmar crease.
- Mark ulnar and radial sides of thumb IP joint.
- Allow enough material to encompass one-half circumference of forearm, remembering that forearm tapers distally.

Refine Pattern

- Proximal border should allow full elbow motion.
- Distal border should allow unimpeded motion of MCP joints and thumb IP flexion.

- Circumferential thumb portion should allow enough material to overlap ½" to 1".
- Provide an appropriate amount of material within and dorsal to web space to support thumb position adequately and provide surface area for strap application dorsally.

- Use ¹⁄₁₆" or ³⁄₃₂" material for immobilizing patients with arthritis; this makes for lightweight orthosis with adequate rigidity.
- Gel- or foam-lined materials may help provide radial styloid scar compression, decrease distal migration, and increase comfort.

Cut and Heat

- While material is heating, prepad (with soft adhesive foam, silicone gels) at first dorsal compartment if tender.
- Consider placing light layer of lotion on thumb before molding to ease removal.
- Position patient with elbow resting on table with forearm slightly supinated for gravity-assisted molding. Thumb should be positioned per diagnosis. Commonly, position of function is palmar abduction and opposition.

Options for Materials

- Remember that materials with memory tend to shrink around proximal phalanx; do not remove until completely set.
- Use coated material so material will pop apart once completely cooled, forming trap door to allow for easy donning and doffing.

- Avoid direct pressure over radial styloid, STT joint, and dorsal MP joint.
- Do not grab proximally or try to secure with tight circumferential bandage. This may cause borders to irritate skin. Instead, allow gravity to assist in forming forearm trough.
- Carefully incorporate arches of hand by using smooth, even strokes and constantly redirecting material into arches.
- Make sure desired wrist position is maintained. Some patients tend to flex and deviate wrist while orthosis is being formed.

Strapping and Components

- Distal strap: 1" strap directed from dorsal web area to volar ulnar border.
- Middle strap: 2" strap just proximal to dorsal wrist crease; use piece of adhesive foam to further stabilize wrist and prevent migration. Foam should lie directly over ulnar styloid and should not overlap edges.
- Proximal strap: Depending on size of forearm, 1" or 2" strap may suffice; strap should have slight volar to dorsal angle.

Survey Completed Orthosis

- Smooth and slightly flare all borders and around thumb opening.
- Check clearance of elbow, thumb IP joint, and IF MCP joint flexion.

Evaluate Fit while Molding

- Place thumb portion of material on radial proximal phalanx and guide rest of material evenly along radial forearm.
- Carefully contour dorsal section of distal thumb material through web space.
- Gently pull and overlap dorsal thumb material through web space to support proximal phalanx and lightly overlap onto volar piece.

PATTERN PEARL 7-80 to 7-82.

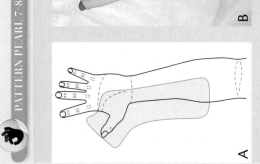

PP7-80   A and B, IP joint included.

CLINICAL PEARL 7-46.
Accommodating Sensitive Areas with Gel and Foam Padding

A thin layer of silicone gel can be placed directly over (**A**) or around (**B**) the radial sensory nerve to prevent pressure on a hypersensitive area/scar either postinjury or surgery. This collegiate volleyball player had a custom orthosis fabricated that incorporated the silicone gel (over the radial sensory nerve) and foam padding (over the ulnar styloid) to protect her during play (**B and C**). Strapping systems can also be modified by cutting out a protective "donut" with adhesive padding to improve comfort as they traverse bony and sensitive areas. Shown is a patient with a hypersensitive scar post-open reduction internal fixation (ORIF) for a distal ulnar fracture (**D**). As another alternative, therapy putty can be used to create a "bubble" over the sensitive area or bony prominence. To prevent the putty from sticking to the thermoplastic, apply a thin layer of lotion prior to molding. After the orthosis has set, remove the putty to form the protective bubble.

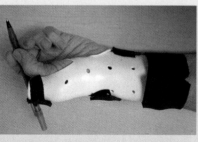
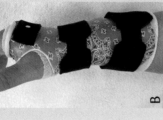
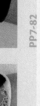
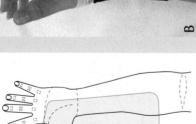
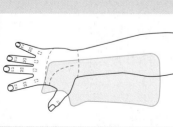

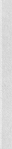

PATTERN PEARL 7-80 to 7-82.   *continued*

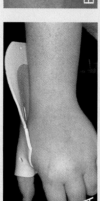

PP7-81

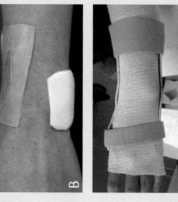
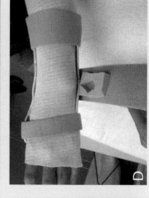

PP7-82

A and B, MP joint free.

Thumb MP and IP joints can be released for light functional use.

CLINICAL PEARL 7-45.
Estimating Material Required to Obtaining Two-Thirds Forearm Circumference

Including two-thirds the circumference of the forearm when fabricating forearm-based orthoses not only provides for maximal pressure distribution but also improves the rigidity of the final orthosis. This generally results in a more comfortable fit for the patient. To estimate the amount of material needed while drawing the pattern, angle the pen at 45° on the dorsal forearm and draw both side of the forearm to the wrist level. The resulting pattern should have more material proximally because of the tapered nature of the musculature, covering approximately two-thirds of the forearm.

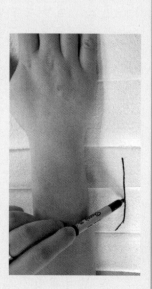

Volar Wrist/Thumb Immobilization Orthosis (WHFO) (Fig. 7-31)

Common Names

- Thumb spica splint
- Long opponens splint

Alternative Options

- Prefabricated wrist and thumb orthosis
- Zipper design thumb and wrist orthosis
- Cast
- Silicone rubber orthosis

Primary Functions

- Immobilize wrist and thumb joint(s) to allow healing, rest, and/or protection of involved structure(s).

Additional Functions

- Improve functional pinch by positioning wrist and thumb in optimal positions.

Common Diagnoses and General Optimal Positions

Diagnosis	Position
Scaphoid fracture (after cast immobilization)	Wr: 0 to 20° ext; RD and UD: 0°; th: between rad and palm abd; MP: 10° flex; IP: free
Bennett fracture (after cast immobilization)	Wr: 0 to 20° ext; RD: 5°; th: 45° rad abd; MP: 5 to 10° flex
deQuervain's tenosynovitis	Wr: 20° ext; th CMC: between rad and palm abd; MP: slight flex; IP: included or free (depends on severity)
Intersection syndrome	Wr: 20° ext; RD and UD: 0°; th CMC: rad abd; MP: 5 to 10° flex
Th STT or CMC jt arthritis	Wr: 0 to 20° ext; th CMC: between rad and palm abd; MP: 5 to 10° flex
STT or CMC/TM arthroplasty	Wr: 20° ext; RD and UD: 0°; th: between rad and palm abd; MP: 5 to 10° flex
Lax or mildly subluxed STT jt	Wr: 0 to 20° ext; th CMC: medium palm abd; MP: slight flex
EPL repair (th CMC: slight rad abd)	20 to 40° ext; MP: 0°; IP: 0 to 5° ext
Extensor pollicis brevis (EPB) or abductor pollicis longus (APL) repair	Wr: 20 to 40° ext; th CMC: slight rad abd; MP: 0°
Tendon transfers (opponensplasty)	Wr: 0°; th CMC: medium palm abd; MP: 5 to 10° flex
Th UCL reconstruction	Wr: 20° ext; th CMC: palm abd; MP: 5° flexion with slight UD
Th RCL reconstruction palm	Wr: 20° ext; th CMC: abd; MP: 5° flex with slight RD

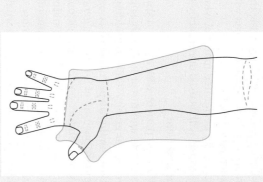

FIGURE 7-32

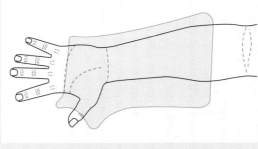

FIGURE 7-31

Fabrication Process

Pattern Creation (Fig. 7-32)

- Mark proximal border two-thirds length of forearm.
- Mark distal border at thumb IP flexion crease and DPC.
- Allow enough material to encompass one-half to two-thirds circumference of forearm, remembering that forearm tapers distally.

Refine Pattern

- Proximal border should allow full elbow motion.
- Distal border should allow unimpeded motion of IF to SF MCP and thumb IP joint.
- Provide an appropriate amount of material within and dorsal to web space to support thumb position adequately and provide surface area for strap application dorsally.

Options for Materials

- Use drapable material to achieve intimate fit about thumb STT and MP joints to prevent migration and improve comfort.
- Remember that elastic materials tend to shrink around proximal phalanx; do not remove until orthosis is completely set.
- Consider placing light layer of lotion on thumb before molding to ease removal.

- Use coated material to allow material to pop apart once completely cool. This forms trap door for easy donning and doffing.
- Use $\frac{1}{16}$" or $\frac{3}{32}$" material for immobilizing patients with arthritis; this makes for lightweight orthosis with adequate rigidity.
- Consider perforated material when orthosis will be used during activity.

Cut and Heat

- Position patient with elbow resting on table and forearm slightly supinated for gravity-assisted molding.
- Position thumb per diagnosis. Commonly, position of function is gentle palmar abduction and opposition.
- If patient has difficulty supinating forearm (e.g., after cast immobilization), have patient flex elbow on table and adduct and externally rotate shoulder toward midline.
- Consider prepadding of radial or ulnar styloid if prominent.

Evaluate Fit while Molding

- Lay warm material on towel, positioning thumb portion on correct side of material as if it were going to be placed on supinated forearm.
- Place thumb portion centrally over thumb and guide rest of material evenly along arm.

- Gently pull and overlap volar thumb material through web space to support proximal phalanx and lightly overlap onto dorsal piece. It is important for material to mold through web space to radial side of second metacarpal to provide adequate rigidity.
- Avoid direct pressure over radial styloid, STT joint, and dorsal MP joint.
- Do not grab proximally or try to secure with tight circumferential bandage. This may cause borders to irritate skin. Instead, allow gravity to assist in forming forearm trough. While molding, place thumb joints in appropriate position. Have patient gently oppose to IF during the molding process.
- Carefully incorporate arches of hand by using smooth, even strokes and constantly redirecting material into arches.
- Make sure desired wrist position is maintained. Some patients tend to flex and deviate wrist while orthosis is being formed.
- Clear for radial and ulnar styloid, avoiding pressure over radial sensory nerve.
- Once material has cooled completely, pop apart overlapped thumb piece if concerned about doffing difficulty.

Strapping and Components

- Distal strap: 1" strap directed from radial dorsal web area to volar ulnar border. Use piece of adhesive foam under strap to further stabilize metacarpals if needed.
- Middle strap: 2" strap just proximal to dorsal wrist crease; use piece of adhesive foam to further stabilize wrist and prevent migration. Foam should lie directly over ulnar styloid and should not overlap edges.
- Proximal strap: Depending on size of forearm, 1" or 2" strap may suffice; strap should have slight volar to dorsal angle.
- Apply small $\frac{1}{2}$" strap across trap door.

Survey Completed Orthosis

- Smooth and slightly flare all borders.
- Check for clearance of radial and ulnar styloids, elbow, thumb IP joint, and finger MCP joints.
- Pay careful attention to IF MCP, which frequently abuts radial portion as it traverses through first web space. If orthosis is to be functional, check that patient can at least touch thumb to index fingertip.
- Make sure that patient does not experience pinching under overlapped thumb portion.

PATTERN PEARL 7-83 to 7-86.

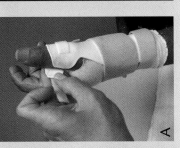

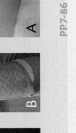

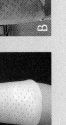

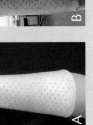

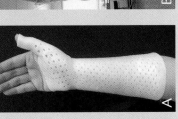

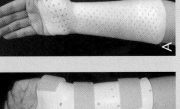

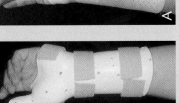

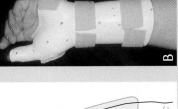

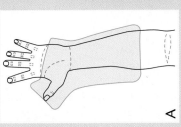

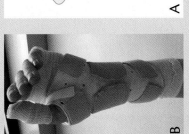

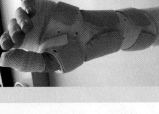

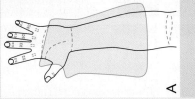

PP7-83

A and B, Thumb MP joint free, often used post-scaphoid fracture (note IP cast used for concomitant distal phalanx fracture).

PP7-84

A and B, IP joint included.

PP7-85

Rolyan® AquaForm™ Zippered Wrist and Thumb Splint Zipper with IP included (**A**) and free (**B**) (Patterson Medical).

PP7-86

A, Trap door for easy donning/doffing and (**B**) optional "open" design to accommodate for edema or healing wounds.

CLINICAL PEARL 7-48.
Gentle Traction on Thumb during Molding Process

Applying gentle traction distally in the desired direction/position of the thumb will assist in proper molding and minimize undesired "excessive" thumb MP flexion.

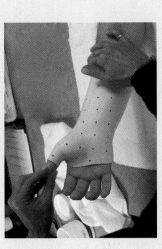

CLINICAL PEARL 7-47.
Neoprene Strap for Sensitive Thumb MP Joint

Commonly, there can be irritation of the skin at the thermoplastic distal MP joint border. Alternatively, a soft neoprene volar sling can be fabricated to substitute for a circumferential "hard" thermoplastic support about the thumb column. Neoprene will adhere to warm thermoplastic material so the therapist can be creative in designing a comfortable thumbhole, which the patient can slip on and off with ease and use functionally without irritation. (See Chapter 14 on "Neoprene Orthosis" for more information.)

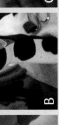

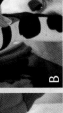

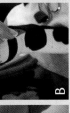

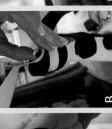

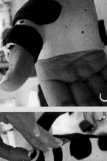

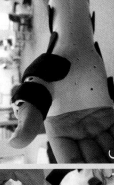

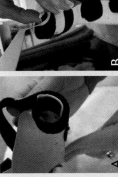

Dorsal Wrist/Hand (Optional Thumb) Immobilization Orthosis (WHFO)   (Fig. 7–33)

Common Names

- Dorsal protective splint
- Dorsal blocking splint
- Extension block splint
- Dorsal shell

Primary Functions

- Immobilize wrist, MCP, PIP, and DIP joints in flexion to allow healing of involved structure(s).

Additional Functions

- Promote early protected active and/or passive motion of repaired tendons to facilitate healing and prevent adherence to surrounding structures (mobilization or restriction).

Alternative Options

- Cast

Common Diagnoses and General Optimal Positions

Optimal positions for tendon and nerve injuries depend on the severity of the injury, the integrity of repaired structures (tendon, nerve, vascular structures, pulleys, and bone), and the physician's rehabilitation protocol. Chapter 18 provides details.

FDS or FDP tendon repair	Wr: 0 to 45° flex; MCP: 30 to 60° flex; IP: 0 to 30° ext (depending on nerve status)
FPL tendon repair	Wr: 0 to 45° flex; th CMC: 0 to 45° palm abd; MP: 20 to 40° flex; IP: 0 to 20°

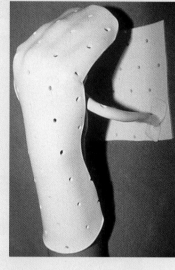

🖐 **CLINICAL PEARL 7-49.**
Use of Hand Rest for Joint Positioning

A rest for the palmar surface of the hand can aid considerably when fabricating a dorsal wrist and hand immobilization orthosis. This device, consisting of a platform and rolled palmar support, can be constructed from thermoplastic material. The raised palmar support should be oblique in form to support distal transverse arch. The rest should also be high enough to allow the fingers and thumb to drape over it without touching the table and keeping the wrist in the desired amount of flexion.

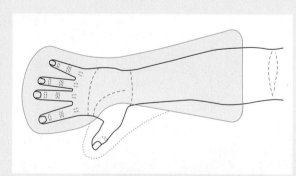

FIGURE 7-34

FIGURE 7-33

Fabrication Process

Pattern Creation (Fig. 7–34)

- Note: Because unimpeded active motion is contraindicated, draw pattern on uninjured hand if possible.
- Mark for proximal border two-thirds length of forearm.
- Mark distal border approximately 1″ distal to fingertips; this additional material is necessary to compensate for flexed position of wrist and MCP joints.
- If thumb is not involved, mark thumb clearance by making an arc from thumb MP to base of first STT joint (using thenar crease as landmark).
- If thumb is involved, mark 1″ distally and allow enough material around borders to support thumb and allow for strap application (dotted line on pattern).
- Allow enough material to encompass two-thirds circumference of forearm, remembering that forearm tapers distally.

Refine Pattern

- Proximal border should allow full elbow motion.
- Distal border should completely protect and cover fingertips (and thumb, if applicable).
- If thumb is not involved, full mobility of thumb should be available.

Options for Materials

- Use ⅛″ thermoplastic material to provide needed rigidity to maintain joint positions.

- If patient has significant pain and swelling, the fabrication process may be quite difficult. Consider uncoated materials or those that are slightly tacky and drapable to help prevent material from slipping and to make it easier to position patient and mold the orthosis.
- Materials that can be reheated and remolded several times are a good option if ongoing modifications become necessary to accommodate for fluctuations in edema or changes in desired joint position.
- Consider ⅛″ perforated material because orthosis will likely be worn continuously for several weeks.

Evaluate Fit while Molding

- Lay warm material on towel, positioning thumb cut out or thumb piece, if involved, on correct side of material as if it were going to be placed on pronated forearm.
- Position material on dorsum of involved hand, wrist, and forearm. Be sure to cover fingertips adequately. Allow gravity to aid in contouring about metacarpal heads and styloids.
- Depending on material chosen, molding around IF and SF metacarpal borders may be difficult; buckling of material may occur.
- Do not grab proximally or try to secure with tight circumferential bandage. This may cause borders to irritate skin. Instead, allow gravity to assist in forming forearm and hand trough.
- Digits often want to assume flexed posture secondary to edema, pain, and postsurgical complications, making molding of dorsal hood in 0° of IP extension a challenge. Gently lift material and approximate optimal position. Volarly applied soft strap progressively extends digits to reach dorsal hood.
- Make sure desired wrist and digit positions are maintained. It is crucial to use goniometer to ensure accurate positioning. Be careful of joint position during removal of orthosis.

Cut and Heat

- Position patient with elbow resting on table and forearm pronated for gravity-assisted molding. If involved, position thumb in gentle palmar abduction and opposition.
- If wound dressings are necessary, they must be incorporated into the design. Place stockinette over dressing to prevent thermoplastic material from sticking. This can be easily cut away when molding process is complete.
- Consider using palmar support to rest hand on; this helps control of positioning wrist and MCP joints during fabrication.
- Prepad ulnar/radial styloids and Lister tubercle with adhesive foam or silicone gel if appropriate.

Strapping and Components

- Distal strap: 2″ soft strap running slightly oblique from radial distal border to ulnar distal border. Strap should traverse and support all fingertips against dorsal hood. Use adhesive foam on straps to support digits in position.
- Volar MCP strap: 1″ to 2″ (trimmed) strap provides support volarly to MCP joints; use piece of adhesive foam to further stabilize wrist and prevent migration. Foam should not overlap edges.
- Wrist strap: 2″ soft strap with adhesive foam to further stabilize joints and prevent migration.
- Proximal strap: 2″ soft or elasticized strap.
- Thumb strap: 1″ strap traversing on oblique angle to incorporate thumb IP and proximal phalanx.

Survey Completed Orthosis

- Smooth and slightly flare all borders.
- Gently flare around dorsal thumb and lateral MP regions; do not roll, which makes future modifications difficult and unnecessarily bulky.
- Check clearance of elbow and thumb (if applicable).
- Check for compression stress at radial and ulnar styloid processes and over dorsal MCP joints.
- Check for compression over radial and ulnar sensory nerves.

PATTERN PEARL 7-87 to 7-88.

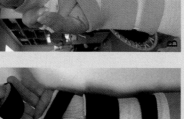
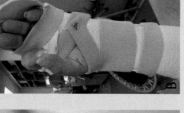

PP7-87

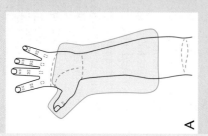
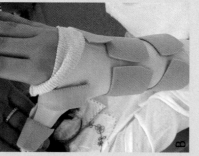
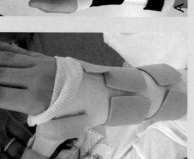

PP7-88

A and B, Thumb only.

A, Radial digits only.
B, Ulnar digits only.

CLINICAL PEARL 7-50.
Techniques for Accommodating MCP Flexion Angle

When molding material dorsally over flexed MCP joints, it can be challenging to accommodate for the flexion angle. Consider the following techniques (shown here from top to bottom): (1) Cut just enough material to support the area. If using a material with some drapability, with a small tug distally, the material will fall into place without overlapping. This is an advanced technique that takes much practice but provides the most cosmetically pleasing look. Be careful not to pull the material too much or the material will thin out and weaken the area. (2) Dog-ear the material by first snipping in approximately ½" at the MCP joints and then overlapping it. The material must be treated with solvent to remove any coating and heated with a heat gun to ensure a strong bond. This technique makes future modifications of the MCP flexion angle difficult. (3) Gently stretch and overlap the material dorsally at the MCP joints to take up the excess. Note that the material is not rolled. This technique also makes future changes a challenge. (4) Pinch the excess material together when warm and snip it off. May need to reinforce this seam with additional thermoplastic material or cast tape in order to prevent the seam from popping apart.

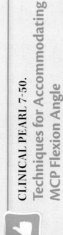

CLINICAL PEARL 7-51.
Strapping Techniques to Prevent Distal Migration

Orthoses may shift in position if not secured adequately. This can adversely alter joint angles and place the repaired or healing structures at risk for attenuation. To help prevent this occurrence, the following strapping techniques can be employed. Apply an adhesive foam to the 2" strap just proximal to the distal wrist crease **(A)**. Split the 2" strap in half at the thenar crease **(B)**. Rivet an additional 1" strap to the MCP joint strap at the midthenar crease to anchor the orthosis about the base of the thumb **(C)**. Mold a thermoplastic palmar bar from the radial dorsal aspect of the IF MCP area and guide ulnarly through the thumb web along the palmar surface just proximal to the DPC, overlapping and securing on the distal ulnar SF MCP border (pull the material if needed for increased length) **(D)**. Carefully incorporate the arches of the hand by using smooth, even strokes, constantly redirecting the material into the arches.

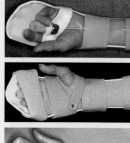
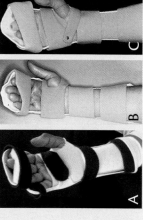

Volar Wrist/Hand (Optional Thumb) Immobilization Orthosis (Fig. 7–35)

Common Names

- Resting hand splint
- Resting pan splint

Alternative Orthosis Options

- Prefabricated orthosis
- Cast

Primary Functions

- Immobilize wrist and hand (and thumb) joints to allow healing or rest of involved structure(s).

Additional Functions

- Statically position tight flexor tendons at maximum extension to facilitate lengthening of tissue (mobilization orthosis).
- Prevent or minimize joint contractures of wrist, fingers, and thumb.
- Prevent overstretching of weak or absent wrist and digit muscle–tendon units.
- Aid in reducing muscle tone in wrist and digits.

Common Diagnoses and General Optimal Positions

Burn injury	Wr: 30° ext (volar or circumferential burns), 0° (dorsal burns); MCP: 60 to 90° flex; IP: 0°; th: between palm abd and th opp
Rheumatoid	Wr: 30° ext; MCP: slight arthritis flex; IP: comfortable flex; th: abd and th opp (Note: If patient has carpal tunnel symptoms, decrease wr ext.)
Crush injuries	Wr: 30° ext; MCP: 60° flex; IP: 0°; th: palm abd
Tendon transfers	Dictated by structures involved
Extensor tendon repairs (zones V to VI)	Wr: 40 to 45° ext; MCP: 0 to 20° flex; IP: 0°
Radial nerve injury or repair	Wr: 30° ext; MCP: 30 to 40° flex; PIP: 40° flex; DIP: 20° flex; th: rad abd
Infection or cellulitis	Functional position or intrinsic plus position; include one jt higher than infection
Replantation or transplantation	Dictated by structures involved
MCP capsulectomy	Wr: 10 to 30° ext; MCP: 75 to 90° flex; IP: 0°
Abnormal tone	Depends on therapist and physician rationale

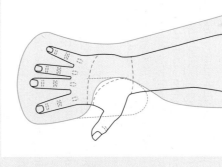

FIGURE 7-36

FIGURE 7-35

Fabrication Process

Pattern Creation (Fig. 7-36)

- Mark for proximal border two-thirds length of forearm.
- Allow enough material to encompass one-half to two-thirds circumference of forearm, remembering that forearm tapers distally.
- Mark width of hand plus 1/4" to 1/2" on each side to allow for hand trough.
- Mark distal border, approximately 1" distal to fingertips.
- Mark for thumb only if included in orthosis.
- Radial aspect of thumb: From distal border (approximately 1" radial to index fingertip), draw line through center of thumb IP joint proximally toward thumb MP joint, ending just proximal to CMC joint.
- Proximal and medial aspect: Curve proximal and medial to CMC joint along palmar edge of thenar eminence. Curved thumb pattern should end at midthenar mass (along thenar crease), in line with third metacarpals.

Refine Pattern

- Proximal border should allow full elbow motion.
- If thumb is free, check for nearly full motion.
- If thumb is included, thumb piece should be wide and deep enough to encompass thumb.

Options for Materials

- Material selection depends on requirements.
- Consider 1/8" thermoplastic material to provide needed rigidity to maintain stretch on tight tissue or support painful edematous hand.
- Materials with moderate stretch properties can be difficult to handle when fabricating this orthosis, especially if patient has increased tone.
- If patient has difficulty achieving supinated gravity-assisted position, consider uncoated materials or those that are slightly tacky to help prevent material from slipping and to make it easier to position patient and mold orthosis.
- Materials that can be reheated and remolded several times are a good option if ongoing orthosis modifications become necessary to accommodate for fluctuations in edema or changes in desired joint position. Gel- or foam-lined materials help provide volar wrist scar compression, decrease distal migration, and increase comfort.
- Consider perforated material when orthosis will be worn continually or in conjunction with scar management products such as elastomer. Scar products seep through perforations, which helps anchor them into orthosis.

Cut and Heat

- Position patient with elbow resting on table with forearm supinated for gravity-assisted molding.
- Position thumb or leave free per diagnosis.
- If patient has difficulty supinating forearm (e.g., pain extremity), have patient flex elbow on table and adduct shoulder toward midline or lie supine with shoulder abducted and externally rotated 90° with elbow flexed.
- When cutting thumb area of orthosis, leave small space (make notch) between proximal thumb piece and radial forearm trough to keep material ends from touching and adhering during molding process.

Evaluate Fit while Molding

- Lay warm material on towel, positioning thumb piece on correct side of material as if it were going to be placed on supinated forearm.
- Position material on volar aspect of involved hand and wrist, with thumb component applied within index and thumb web space (commonly referred to as C-bar). Material must be stretched slightly to achieve even contouring along dorsal web and within palm.
- Lift thumb trough and place it centrally over thumb's medial/ulnar border. Once positioned, carefully stretch outer border to form C shape. Medial portion (snipped section) should adequately cover wrist and partially cover thenar eminence. Pay close attention to thumb joint positions.
- Use palmar aspect of hand to help support volar arches and first web space, simulating handshake hold.
- Position digits in slight abduction with MCP, PIP, and DIP joints positioned per diagnosis.
- Guide rest of material evenly along arm.
- Borders of orthosis should be curved to form hand trough (1/4" to 1/2" at hand and thumb). These curved sides keep fingers from falling off orthosis border.
- Gravity tends to pull material away from thumb and toward IF; continually reposition material as needed.
- Do not grab proximal orthosis or try to secure with tight circumferential bandage. This may cause borders of orthosis to irritate skin. Instead, allow gravity to assist in forming forearm trough.
- Check for pressure areas at ulnar aspect of thumb MP and IF and SF MCP joints.
- Check for compression of dorsal sensory branches of radial and ulnar nerves.
- Rotate forearm into pronated position at end of molding to check for clearance of ulnar and radial styloid processes; flare around styloids as necessary.
- Make sure desired wrist position is maintained. Some patients tend to flex and deviate wrist while orthosis is being formed. May use goniometer to ensure correct positioning; this is especially important for diagnoses requiring specific positioning (e.g., tendon repairs and transfers).
- Do not stress UCL of thumb MP joint when attempting to palmarly abduct thumb.

(Continued)

Chapter 7 • Immobilization Orthoses 199

Fabrication Process

(Continued)

- When fabricating an orthosis for increased tone or for use with serial static designs, it may be necessary to reinforce wrist portion with another strip of thermoplastic material or consider different design, such as a dorsally based orthosis.

Strapping and Components

- Distal strap: 1" to 2" strap directed from radial border of proximal IF to ulnar border of proximal SF. Strip of adhesive foam can be used under

strap to stabilize and contour about proximal phalanxes.
- Metacarpal strap: 1" strap directed from radial web space to midulnar border.
- Wrist strap: 2" strap just proximal to dorsal wrist crease; use piece of adhesive foam to further stabilize wrist in orthosis and prevent migration. Foam should lie directly over ulnar styloid and should not overlap orthosis edges.
- Proximal strap: Depending on size of forearm, 1" or 2" strap may

suffice; strap should have slight volar to dorsal angle.
- Thumb strap: 1" strap across proximal phalanx.
- In some cases (eg, with severe edema), traditional strapping may not be appropriate; cotton wrap or elasticized bandage may be better option.
- Some conditions of arthritis may require straps or finger separators to aid in positioning deviating joints.
- Patients with an increase in tone may need additional straps to maintain joint position.

Survey Completed Orthosis

- Smooth and slightly flare distal and proximal borders.
- Gently flare around thenar segment; avoid rolling, which makes future orthosis modifications difficult and leads to unnecessarily bulky orthosis.
- Check clearance of elbow, styloid processes, thumb, and IF to SF joints.

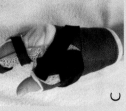

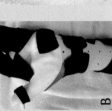

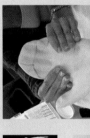

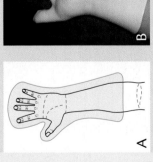

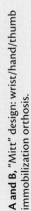

PP7-89   PP7-90   PP7-91   PP7-92

PATTERN PEARL 7-89 to 7-92.

A and B, "Mitt" design: wrist/hand/thumb immobilization orthosis.

A, Position of function.
B, Antideformity position.

A–C, Addition of material to create a volar wrist/hand orthosis. Volar hand segment added over cast for finger positioning.

Digit IP joints free to promote tendon gliding.

CHAPTER 7

CLINICAL PEARL 7-52.
Dacron Batting to Absorb Perspiration

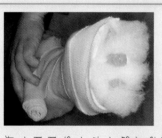

Patients who have to wear an orthosis for extended periods of time (e.g. after surgery), especially in warmer months, tend to perspire within the orthosis, which may lead to skin maceration and an unpleasant odor. Polyester batting (used for quilting), applied between the digits and lightly about the hand and forearm, wicks away moisture from the skin, promoting a dry environment. The batting, readily available at most fabric stores, should be changed daily. Note the bias cut material used to secure the orthosis. This nonelastic wrap applies gentle circumferential pressure to aid in reducing edema. It is applied with gentle tension in much the same manner as an elasticized wrap. This technique of securing the orthosis can be used temporarily during the initial days postinjury/surgery followed by a transition to traditional strapping.

CLINICAL PEARL 7-53.
Finger Separators

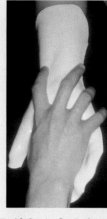

There are several creative ways to position deviating (or potentially deviating) joints of patients with rheumatoid arthritis. Finger spacers are often necessary for correct positioning and comfort (**A and B**). Thermoplastic separators can be formed using scissors, bandage applicator, or pencil. When designing the pattern, allow extra material at the hand width. While the material is still warm, gently take the edge of a pair of closed scissors (tip pointing into the web) or another similarly shaped object and apply pressure volar to dorsal to create a trough for each digit that is approximately ½" deep. Lightly pinch together and move on to the next digit. Foam finger separators can be constructed using an adhesive-backed product such as ⅜" Rolyan® Temper® Foam (Patterson Medical) (**C**) or ¼" Rolyan® Polycushion® Padding (Patterson Medical) (**D**). These do not need to extend completely into the web to provide slight abduction. **E,** Another option is to use Rolyan® 50/50 Mix™ Elastomer Putty (Patterson Medical) to create an insert for the hand to rest within. They are very comfortable and easy to apply. For patients with dense scar between the digits, a mold can be used to aid in scar remodeling. **F,** Fabricate soft strap separators from about 12" strip of 2" soft strapping. Apply adhesive hook to the volar portion of the orthosis and form gullies or troughs with the soft strap. This technique works well for patients with arthritis or fragile skin.

CLINICAL PEARL 7-54.
Strap Placement to Facilitate Digit Joint Alignment

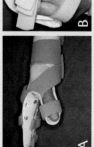

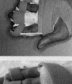

Strapping techniques can be the key to improving positioning of the distal joints. **A,** Riveting the radial end of the MCP strap within the orthosis can help guide the IF metacarpal head ulnarward while the distal straps can be directed radially. **B,** The placement of the distal strap can aid in aligning the proximal structures as well. **C,** Post-extensor tendon realignment: The distally placed straps help prevent recurrent ulnar deviation and maintain neutral alignment of the digits. **D and E,** Strap weaving techniques work well to encourage proper digit alignment. Soft straps can be incorporated into a night resting orthosis for maintaining and correcting the digit position for diagnoses such as rheumatoid arthritis and Dupuytren release. The slits can be made with a hole punch, drill (Dremel), or heated awl. Adhesive hook is applied to the surface of the orthosis material corresponding to each involved digit. The loop material for each finger attaches first to the hook and then is directed about the digit and through the appropriate web space slit, terminating back on the hook.

CLINICAL PEARL 7-55.
Hints for Molding First Web Space

The "handshake hold" technique helps control the thermoplastic material while maintaining the first web space. Use a light grasp distally while working proximally. Stretch and contour the material between the IF and thumb to create a "C" (similar to a thumb abduction orthosis) for the thumb and IF to rest in. Be careful not to dig the fingertips into the warm material, creating a potential pressure area.

Volar/Dorsal Wrist/Hand Immobilization Orthosis (WHFO) (Fig. 7-37)

Common Names

- Antispasticity splint
- Bisurfaced forearm-based static wrist hand orthosis
- Dorsal platform splint
- Dorsal resting splint

Alternative Orthosis Options

- Cast
- Prefabricated antispasticity orthosis
- SaeboStretch® orthosis

Primary Functions

- Immobilize wrist and hand joints to allow healing, rest, or proper positioning of involved structures(s).

Additional Functions

- Statically position tight flexor tendons at maximum extension to facilitate lengthening of tissue and lessen joint contractures (mobilization orthosis).
- Aid in reducing muscle tone in wrist and digits.

Common Diagnoses and General Optimal Positions

General hand trauma	Wr: 30° ext; MCP: 60° flex; IP: 0°
Burn injuries	Wr: 30° ext; MCP: 60 to 90° flex; IP: 0°
Rheumatoid arthritis	Wr: 30° ext; MCP: slight flex; IP: comfortable flex; (Note: If patient has carpal tunnel symptoms, decrease wr ext.)
Abnormal tone	Depends on therapist and physician rationale

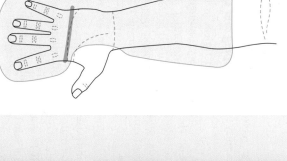

FIGURE 7-38

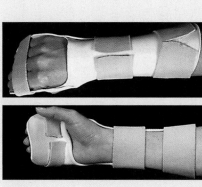
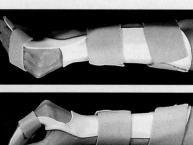

FIGURE 7-37

Fabrication Process

Pattern Creation (Fig. 7–38)

- Can be an alternative pattern to volar or dorsal wrist and hand immobilization orthosis; may be used when it is necessary to avoid fabricating an orthosis over fragile or grafted dorsal or volar surfaces (burns, skin grafts, pins, open wounds).
- Positions depend on injury and structures involved.
- Mark for proximal border two-thirds length of forearm.
- Allow enough material to encompass one-half to two-thirds circumference of forearm, remembering that forearm tapers distally.
- Mark distal border approximately 1" distal to fingertips; this additional material may be necessary to compensate for material consumed by positions of joints.
- Mark thumb clearance by making an arc from thumb MP to base of first CMC joint.
- Opening for digits should be marked at mid-IF MCP joint and run slightly oblique to SF MCP joint.

Refine Pattern

- Proximal border should allow full elbow motion.
- Distal border should protect finger-tips.
- Make sure that opening for digits is wide enough to accommodate width of MCPs, allowing approximately ½" material on sides.
- To aid in tone inhibition, incorporate finger separators into volar pan.

Options for Materials

- Use ⅛" material because strength and rigidity are important characteristics for this device, especially because of potentially weak and narrow area at junction of MCPs.
- Materials with high resistance to stretch may offer more control for therapist; highly conforming materials may be difficult to control against gravity.
- Increase strength at borders of slotted piece by overlapping edges.
- If patient has significant pain and swelling, fabricating an orthosis with this design may be quite awkward and difficult; consider materials that are slightly tacky and drapable to help prevent material from slipping and to make it easier to position patient and mold orthosis.

Cut and Heat

- Before fabrication, use a technique to reduce tone in extremity if needed (see Chapter 21).
- Ideally, position forearm and hand in pronation; forearm can rest on elevated platform with MCPs over edge.
- Prepad ulnar/radial styloids and Lister tubercle with adhesive foam or silicone gel if appropriate.

Evaluate Fit while Molding

- Lay warm material on towel and position MCP slot on correct side of material as if it were going to be placed on pronated forearm. (The MCP slot should be more distal on radial side.)
- Slide digits through slot, then carefully lay proximal portion on dorsal forearm and allow gravity to assist.
- One hand should simultaneously support volar piece at MCPs and digits, incorporating arches.
- Fold MCP flaps over onto material and flatten out to add strength to this potentially weak section.
- Do not grab proximal orthosis or try to secure with tight circumferential bandage. This may cause borders of orthosis to irritate skin. Instead, allow gravity to assist in forming forearm trough.

- Make sure desired wrist and digit positions are maintained.

Strapping and Components

- If orthosis is to be used for burn injury management, consider circumferential bandages to avoid localized pressure caused by straps on fragile healing skin or grafts.
- Distal strap: 1" or 2" strap to traverse across PIP joints. May use foam to improve extension positioning of digits.
- Wrist and proximal strap: 2" strap of soft, elasticized, or traditional loop.
- If adhesive foam is used to pad ulnar styloid during fabrication, carefully lift it off patient's skin and place it back into orthosis.

Survey Completed Orthosis

- Check that opening for digits is wide enough for easy donning and doffing of orthosis.
- Make sure that sides of IF and SF MCPs are strong enough to support weight of digits. If not, an additional strip of thermoplastic material may be added for support.
- May need to apply piece of thermoplastic material volarly to reinforce wrist position.

PATTERN PEARL 7-93 to 7-97.

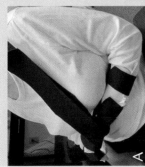
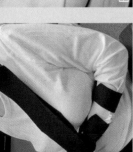
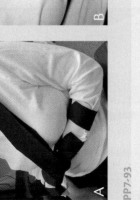

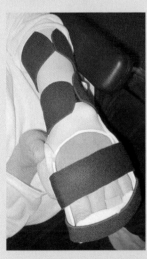

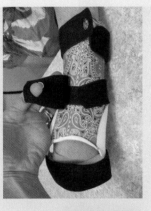

PP7-93

A and B, Application of shoulder strap to control elbow flexion and forearm rotation.

PP7-94

Adhesive foam on distal straps can assist in positioning digits in extension to manage flexion contractures.

PP7-95

Loops incorporated into strapping system can make application and removal easier for specific patient populations.

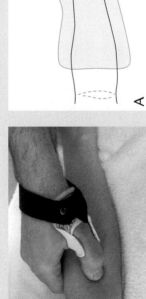
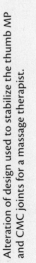

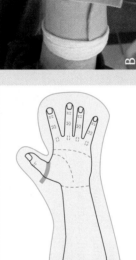

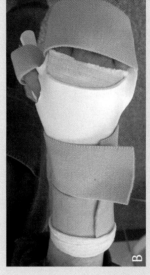

PP7-96

Alteration of design used to stabilize the thumb MP and CMC joints for a massage therapist.

PP7-97

A and B, Addition of thumb into design.

Antispasticity Cone Orthosis   (Fig. 7–39)

Common Names

- Antispasticity splint
- Forearm-based ulnar cone-style splint

Alternative Orthosis Options

- Cast
- SaeboStretch° orthosis
- Prefabricated antispasticity orthosis

Primary Functions

- Immobilize wrist, digits, and thumb for individuals with moderate to severe spasticity.
- Help decrease tone and reduce risk of joint and soft tissue contracture.

Additional Functions

- Statically position tight flexor tendons at maximum extension to facilitate lengthening of tissue and reduce or prevent contractures (mobilization orthosis).

Common Diagnoses and General Optimal Positions

Abnormal tone	Depends on therapist and physician rationale
Jt contractures and muscle shortening	Functional position

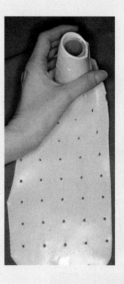

CLINICAL PEARL 7-56.
Therapy Cone to Aid Fabrication of Antispasticity Orthoses

Using a therapy cone when fabricating the central portion of this orthosis can be extremely helpful. If an appropriately sized cone is not available, fabricate one out of scrap thermoplastic material. If there is a chance that the materials may stick to each other during the fabrication process, simply wrap the cone with a wet paper towel, layer with lotion, or cover with a stockinette.

FIGURE 7-40

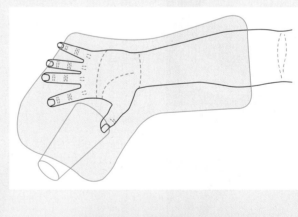

FIGURE 7-39

Fabrication Process

Pattern Creation (Fig. 7–40)

- Note: Because of increased tone, positioning extremity for creating this pattern may be quite difficult; draw pattern on contralateral extremity or estimate size.
- Mark for proximal border two-thirds length of forearm.
- Allow enough material to encompass one-half of forearm circumference of forearm, remembering that forearm tapers distally.
- Mark distal border using pattern illustration for an example. Material distally follows contour of digits.
- From MF distal phalanx tip radially, pattern extends beyond thumb approximately 2".
- Pattern follows contour of thumb proximally, leaving 1½" to 2" border radially. At this point, pattern comes in toward proximal thumb MP 1" then continues proximally.

Refine Pattern

- Proximal border should allow full elbow motion.
- Distal border should protect digits.
- To prevent adherence, line cone (fabricated from thermoplastic or commercial) with light layer of lotion before placing on material.
- Make sure that pattern material for cone portion is generous and wide

enough to accommodate hand size. Patients with tight, contracted hands may need to start with smaller cone that can be progressively enlarged as tissue elongates.

Options for Materials

- Use ⅛" material because strength and rigidity are important characteristics for this orthosis.
- Consider perforated materials, which allow air exchange between skin and orthosis, especially for patients who are cognitively impaired or who lack full sensation.
- Skin breakdown and maceration can become problems under these orthoses. Do not line orthosis with moleskin or similar padding because they tend to absorb moisture and are difficult to clean. Closed cell foam that can be readily washed may work well.
- If patient has significant tone, fabricating an orthosis with this design may be quite awkward and difficult. Consider materials that are less conforming and more rigid to make it easier to position patient and mold orthosis.

Cut and Heat

- Before fabrication, use a technique to reduce tone in extremity (see Chapter 21).

- While material is heating, prepad ulnar styloid using self-adhesive padding or silicone gel.
- Ideally, position extremity with shoulder and elbow flexed and forearm neutral to achieve gravity-assisted position.
- Make sure desired position is maintained.

Evaluate Fit while Molding

- Note: The fabrication of this orthosis may warrant an "extra set of hands" to assist during the molding process.
- Lay warm material on towel, positioning large radial section on correct side of material as if it were going to be placed on extremity.
- Place warm material on proximal forearm and allow gravity to hold it in place.
- Working distally, lay material into palm and place cone on material. Wide end of cone is on ulnar border pointing through web space.
- Wrap thumb portion over cone, then bring distal straight border over this material to forming cone. (While this occurs, ulnar aspect of orthosis should form an ulnar trough for digits to rest in.)
- Keep redirecting wrist into appropriate position. If there is considerable tone in hand, then orthosis can

be made in sections. After molding forearm and wrist portions, cone section can be made while the orthosis is off patient.
- Do not grab proximal portion of the orthosis or try to secure with tight circumferential bandage. This may cause borders of the orthosis to irritate skin. Instead, allow gravity to assist in forming forearm trough.

Strapping and Components

- Digits: often not necessary.
- Cone straps: Straps originating from top of cone can be quite effective for keeping hand correctly positioned. Soft 1" straps traversing just proximal to MCP, PIP, DIP, thumb MP, and IP joint(s) are appropriate.
- Wrist and proximal strap: 2" strap of soft, elasticized, or traditional loop.
- If ⅜" adhesive foam or silicone was used to pad ulnar styloid during fabrication, carefully lift it off patient's skin and place it back into orthosis to cushion styloid.

Survey Completed Orthosis

- Smooth and slightly flare borders.
- Check that cone is of adequate width to position digits properly.
- Check clearance of elbow.

Antispasticity Ball Orthosis (WHFO) (Fig. 7–41)

Common Names
- Antispasticity splint

Alternative Orthosis Options
- Prefabricated antispasticity orthosis
- SaeboStretch® orthosis

Primary Functions
- Immobilize wrist, digits, and thumb for individuals with moderate to severe spasticity.

- Aid in decreasing tone and reducing risk of tissue contracture.

Additional Functions
- Statically position tight flexor tendons at maximum extension to facilitate lengthening of tissue and to reduce or prevent contractures (mobilization orthosis).

Common Diagnoses and General Optimal Positions

Abnormal tone	Depends on therapist and physician rationale
Joint contractures and muscle shortening	Functional position

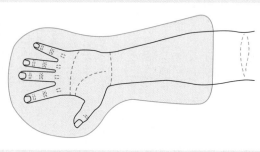

FIGURE 7-42

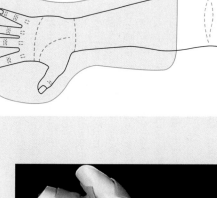

FIGURE 7-41

Fabrication Process

Pattern Creation (Fig. 7-42)

- Note: Because of increased tone, positioning extremity for creating this pattern may be quite difficult; draw pattern on contralateral extremity or estimate size.
- Mark for proximal border two-thirds length of forearm.
- Allow enough material to encompass one-half to two-thirds circumference of forearm, remembering that forearm tapers distally.
- Mark distal border, approximately 1" beyond fingertips, using pattern illustration for an example.
- Radially, follow contour of first web space along distal and radial thumb borders, meeting at thumb base. Allow ½" distally and 1" radially for sufficient troughing and strap application.

Refine Pattern

- Proximal border should allow full elbow motion.
- Distal border should extend just distal to fingertips.
- Make sure that digit and thumb material is generous and wide enough to accommodate web spacers.

Options for Materials

- Use ⅛" material because strength and rigidity are important characteristics for this orthosis.
- Consider perforated materials, which allow air exchange between skin and orthosis, especially for patients who are cognitively impaired or who lack full sensation.
- Skin breakdown and maceration can become problems under these devices. Do not line orthosis with moleskin or similar padding because they tend to absorb moisture and are difficult to clean.

- Consider material with no memory, because maintenance of web spacers after material has been stretched is key to this design.
- If patient has significant tone, fabricating an orthosis with this design may be quite awkward and difficult. Consider materials that are less conforming and more rigid to make it easier to position patient and mold orthosis.

Cut and Heat

- Before fabrication, use a technique to reduce tone in extremity (see Chapter 21 for specific information).
- Consider placing light layer of lotion on ball before molding to prevent thermoplastic from adhering.
- Consider fabricating forearm trough first and then making hand component as described in the following text. This will allow more control over an already hard-to-control extremity. Prepare to pronate hand on medium-sized ball (large enough to encompass entire hand).

Evaluate Fit while Molding

Note: The fabrication of this orthosis may warrant an "extra set of hands" to assist during the molding process.

- To simplify fabrication process, warm forearm section first and carefully mold to achieve good fit.

- Next, place warmed distal section on ball and rest patient's hand over it.
- Make sure that digits and thumb are fully abducted.
- Use pair of closed scissors, small dowel, or bandage applicator to pull material up between fingers and thumb (see Clinical Pearl 7-53).
- During this process, it helps to have an assistant maintain wrist and forearm position.

Strapping and Components

- Digits and thumb: 2" soft strap just distal to MCP joints is sufficient. Some patients with severe flexor tone need straps threaded over proximal and distal phalanges.
- To prevent digits from lifting off palmar piece, 1" soft foam strap can be woven through web spacers.
- Wrist and proximal strap: 2" strap of soft, elasticized, or traditional hook can be used.

Survey Completed Orthosis

- Smooth and slightly flare borders.
- Check that palmar section is of adequate width to properly position digits and allow easy donning and doffing of orthosis.
- Check clearance of elbow.

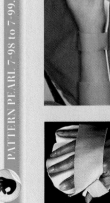
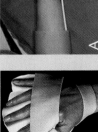
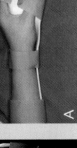

PP7-98   PP7-99

PATTERN PEARL 7-98 to 7-99.

Hand-based design   **A,** Rolyan® Preformed Neutral Position Splint. **B,** Hand-based design (Patterson Medical).

4 Arm-Based Orthoses

Posterior Elbow Immobilization Orthosis (EO) (Fig. 7–43)

Common Names
- Posterior elbow splint

Alternative Orthosis Options
- Cast
- Prefabricated orthosis

Primary Functions
- Immobilize elbow joint and surrounding soft tissues to allow healing, rest, and/or protection of involved structures(s).

Additional Functions
- Limit or prevent forearm rotation.
- Statically position an elbow extension contracture at maximum flexion to

facilitate lengthening of tissue (mobilization orthosis).
- Restrict specific degree of elbow extension (restriction orthosis).

Common Diagnoses and General Optimal Positions

	Position of comfort
Rheumatoid arthritis	Position of comfort
Elb arthroplasty	Dictated by structures involved
Ulnar nerve compression at cubital tunnel	Elb: 30 to 45° flex; FArm: neutral
Ulnar nerve transposition:	Elb: 70 to 90° flex; FArm: neutral to 30° pro; wr: 0°
Nerve repairs (high lesions)	Elb: 30 to 45° flex (depends on repair); FArm: neutral; wr: 0° to slight ext; digits free
Tendon transfers for wr and digit extensors	Elb: 90°; FArm: pro; wr: 30 to 45° ext; MCP and th: ext
Biceps tendon repair	Depends on physician and status of tendon repair; generally start elb 45° active ext to 90° passive flex
Posterior or anterior dislocation	Elb: 90°; FArm: neutral
Collateral ligament repair (medial or lateral)	Elb: 90°; FArm: sup with 10° deviation to side of repair
Proximal radius dislocation	Elb: 90°; FArm: sup
Medial epicondyle fracture	Elb: 90 to 110°; FArm: pro
Lateral epicondyle fracture	Elb: 90 to 110°; FArm: sup
Olecranon fracture	Elb: 20 to 35° flex; FArm: neutral
Acute lateral epicondylitis	Elb: 90°; FArm: neutral; wr: 30 to 45° ext
Acute medial epicondylitis	Elb: 90°; FArm: neutral; wr: 0°

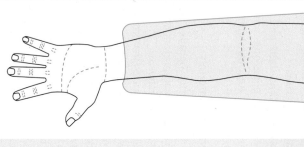

FIGURE 7-44

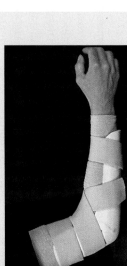

FIGURE 7-43

Fabrication Process

Pattern Creation (Fig. 7–44)

- Posterior design is better for positioning elbow at greater than 45° of flexion. Volar design is more appropriate for positioning elbow at less than 45°.
- Mark for proximal border two-thirds length of humerus.
- Mark for distal border just proximal to ulnar styloid.
- Allow enough material to encompass one-half to two-thirds circumference of upper arm and forearm.
- Remember that the longer and wider the orthosis, the more comfortable it is to wear.

Refine Pattern

- Proximal border should allow unimpeded shoulder motion and not irritate axillary region with arm positioned at side of body.
- Distal border should allow full wrist motion.
- Note that pattern should be wider proximally because circumference of upper arm is greater than that of forearm.

- Make sure there is enough material to encompass elbow posteriorly. Insufficient material in this area requires stretching of material, which weakens the orthosis' support.

Options for Materials

- Use ⅛" material because strength is necessary for this orthosis.
- Consider rubber-based material to have more control and to minimize stretching.
- Gel- or foam-lined materials help provide scar compression, decrease distal migration, and increase comfort.
- Consider perforated thermoplastics for patients who require full-time orthosis use.

Cut and Heat

- While material is heating, consider prepadding medial and lateral epicondyles and olecranon process.
- Position patient to allow for gravity-assisted molding: prone with shoulder neutral; supine with shoulder flexed 90°; or standing while leaning on table, forward flexed at waist, and shoulder extended (upper arm parallel to floor).

- If possible, have an assistant help support proper elbow and forearm positions.

Evaluate Fit while Molding

- Drape warm material centrally over posterior aspect of upper arm and forearm, allowing gravity to assist. Be sure to position material proximal enough to support upper arm.
- Gently stretch and flare material around epicondyles and distal and proximal borders.
- Depending on desired degree of elbow flexion, excess material at elbow flexion crease may require attention.
- Techniques such as pinching, snipping, and folding material over to make the complete corner may be useful.
- Do not grab the orthosis or try to secure with tight circumferential bandage. This may cause borders of orthosis to irritate skin. Instead, allow gravity to assist in forming upper arm and forearm troughs.
- Check for clearance of ulnar styloid distally.

- Make sure desired elbow flexion and forearm rotation positions are maintained. Some patients tend to flex their elbows excessively while orthosis is being formed.

Strapping and Components

- Use stockinette or elasticized sleeve (if edema is present) to eliminate pinching of skin against orthosis borders once straps are applied.
- Proximal strap: 2" soft strap applied at most proximal portion of orthosis to anchor orthosis adequately to upper arm.
- Middle straps: Crisscross design directly over anterior elbow to maintain elbow position.
- Distal strap: 1" or 2" soft strap.
- Consider securing orthosis with elasticized wrap if edema is problematic.

Survey Completed Orthosis

- Smooth and slightly flare all distal and proximal borders.
- Check for clearance and/or irritation at axilla, ulnar styloid, epicondyles, and olecranon process.
- Check for compression of ulnar nerve at cubital tunnel area and of superficial sensory branch of radial nerve.

PP7-100

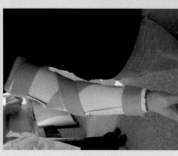

Crossing straps on anteriorly to increase purchase.

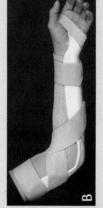

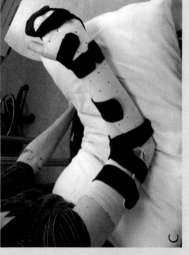

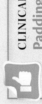

PP7-101

A and B, Posterior elbow orthosis including wrist, commonly with forearm in neutral rotation.

C, Including dorsal wrist and hand for concomitant flexor tendon injury.

CLINICAL PEARL 7-57.
Padding over Bony Prominences

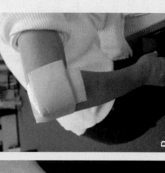

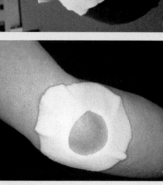

With a posterior elbow design, the olecranon process and/or epicondyles may rub against the orthosis. To prevent this, apply a small adhesive donut-shaped pad directly over the at-risk bony prominence(s) *prior* to molding the orthosis. Once the orthosis is set, the padding can be removed from the skin and inverted back onto the orthosis. Avoid padding *after* the molding process is complete because this may actually shift the excess pressure to another region of the orthosis.

PP7-102

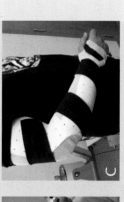

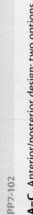

A–C, Anterior/posterior design: two options.

CLINICAL PEARL 7-58.
Techniques to Accommodate Elbow Flexion Angle

A common problem occurs when fabricating an orthosis for the elbow in a flexed position (similar to molding over the flexed MCP joints dorsally): managing the excess material at the elbow flexion crease. There are several techniques that can be used to accommodate for this angle.

- **A,** Carefully take up material medially and laterally and then overlap it onto itself, as shown. Make sure not to inadvertently apply excess pressure onto the bony areas. This technique adds strength and support to the curved area of the orthosis. However, making adjustments later may be difficult.

- **B,** Gently stretch and contour the material to provide a seamless, streamlined trough. This can be challenging for less experienced therapists and works best for angles of flexion that are less than 90°, as shown.

- **C and D,** The excess material can be pinched together rather aggressively (to ensure the material coating has been disrupted) and then cut to form a seam. This technique is the most cosmetically appealing and readily allows for orthosis adjustments. However, the orthosis is less stable and more susceptible to breaking at this seam. Treat the seam with solvent, cut a strip of scrap thermoplastic, and heat both regions until tacky. Attach strip onto seam to prevent area from cracking open.

- **E,** Take the excess material, pinch it, and then overlap it onto itself. This method is simple but can be bulky and future modifications are difficult.

- **F,** Make small transverse snips medially and laterally and dog-ear the material onto itself. Use solvent and a heat gun to create a strong bond between the two surfaces. This method makes future orthosis adjustments difficult, and the orthosis may look bulky and thick.

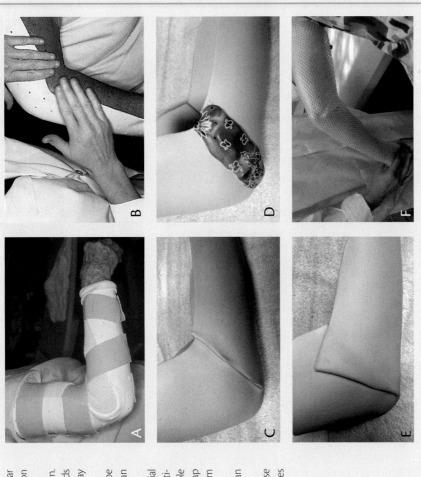

Anterior Elbow Immobilization Orthosis (EO) (Fig. 7–45)

Common Names
- Anterior elbow splint

Alternative Orthosis Options
- Cast
- Prefabricated orthosis

Primary Functions
- Immobilize elbow joint and surrounding soft tissues to allow healing of involved structures(s).

Additional Functions
- Limit or prevent forearm rotation.
- Statically position elbow flexion contracture at maximum extension to facilitate lengthening of tissue (mobilization orthosis).
- Restrict specific degree of elbow flexion (restriction orthosis).

Common Diagnoses and General Optimal Positions

	Position of comfort
Rheumatoid arthritis	Elb: 30 to 45° flex; FArm: neutral
Ulnar nerve compression at cubital tunnel	Elb: 30 to 45° flex (depends on repair); FArm: neutral; wr: 0° to slight ext; digits free
Nerve repairs (high lesions)	
Olecranon fracture	Elb 20 to 35° flex; FArm: neutral

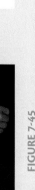
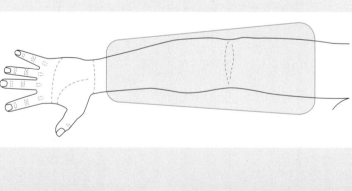

FIGURE 7-45

FIGURE 7-46

CLINICAL PEARL 7-59.
Stretch, Pinch, and Pop Technique for Elbow Orthoses

This technique can be helpful in situations when the patient is unable to assume a gravity-assisted position or when the therapist is challenged managing this large pattern of orthotic material. Use ⅛" or ³⁄₃₂" coated elastic material (such as Aquaplast®; Patterson Medical). When the material is stretched, the coating is disrupted partially to allow a temporary bond where pieces are gently pinched together. Keep in mind that the farther the material has to stretch around the body part, the thinner the material will become, possibly weakening the overall orthosis. Position the patient sitting, with the elbow flexed and forearm rotated in the desired position. After heating fully, the material can be applied to the volar or dorsal surface and stretched in the around the region. As shown here, the material is placed on the anterior surface of the elbow and then quickly stretched and pinched segmentally along the posterior surface **(A)**. Be sure to maintain the desired elbow and forearm positions while the material cools. Once the orthosis is *completely* set, pop the seams apart. Neatly trim and smooth any rough edges **(B)**. This technique can also be used to fabricate nonarticular arm (humerus) or forearm orthoses.

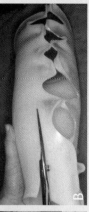
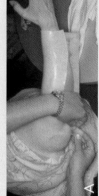
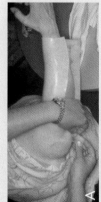

Fabrication Process

Pattern Creation (Fig. 7–46)

- Anterior design is best used for positioning elbow in less than 45° of flexion. Posterior design is more appropriate for positioning elbow greater than 45°.
- Mark for proximal border two-thirds length of humerus.
- Mark for distal border just proximal to ulnar styloid.
- Allow enough material to encompass one-half to two-thirds circumference of upper arm and lower forearm.
- Remember that the longer and wider the orthosis, the more comfortable it is to wear.

Refine Pattern

- Proximal border should allow unimpeded shoulder motion and not irritate axillary region with arm positioned at side of body.
- Distal border should allow full wrist motion.
- Note that pattern should be wider proximally because circumference of upper arm is greater than that of forearm.

- Make sure there is enough material to encompass elbow posteriorly. Insufficient material in this area requires stretching of material, which weakens orthosis' support.

Options for Materials

- Use either ³⁄₃₂″ or ⅛″ thermoplastic material, depending on patient's arm size and desired orthosis strength.
- Gel- or foam-lined materials help provide scar compression, decrease distal migration, and increase comfort.
- Consider perforated thermoplastics for patients who require full-time orthosis use and when air exchange is necessary.

Cut and Heat

- While material is heating, consider prepadding medial and lateral epicondyles if needed; remember that a well-formed orthosis does not require padding.
- Position patient to allow for gravity-assisted molding: supine with shoulder neutral or seated with elbow resting on table.

Evaluate Fit while Molding

- Drape warm material centrally over volar aspect of upper arm and forearm, allowing gravity to assist. Be sure to position material proximal enough to support upper arm.
- Gently flare material around epicondyles, distal, and proximal borders.
- Do not grab orthosis or try to secure with tight circumferential bandage. This may cause borders of orthosis to irritate skin. Instead, allow gravity to assist in forming upper arm and forearm troughs.
- Check for clearance of wrist distally.
- Make sure desired elbow extension and forearm rotation positions are maintained. Some patients tend to flex their elbows excessively while orthosis is being formed. Gently support patient's arm in correct position by supporting at wrist.

Strapping and Components

- Use stockinette or elasticized sleeve if edema is present to eliminate pinching of skin against orthosis borders once straps are applied.
- Proximal strap: 2″ soft strap applied at most proximal portion of orthosis to anchor orthosis adequately to upper arm and to prevent rocking.
- Middle straps: 2″ straps to hold elbow adequately in orthosis.
- Distal strap: 1″ or 2″ soft strap.
- Consider securing orthosis with elasticized wrap if edema is problematic.

Survey Completed Orthosis

- Smooth and slightly flare all distal and proximal borders.
- Check for clearance and/or irritation at axilla and epicondyles.
- Check for compression of ulnar nerve at cubital tunnel area and of superficial sensory branch of radial nerve.

PP7-103

Crossing straps on posteriorly to increase purchase.

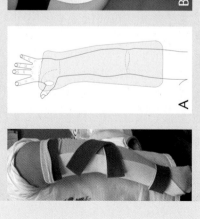

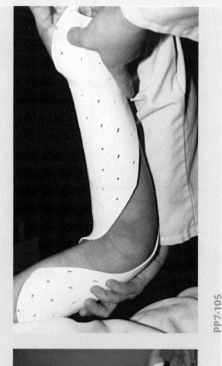

PP7-104

A and B, Anterior elbow orthosis including wrist, commonly with forearm in neutral to full supination.

PP7-105

Spiral design to avoid pressure on sensitive scar area medially.

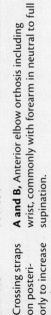

PP7-106

A and B, Anterior elbow orthosis with seam to accommodate for 90° flexion angle.

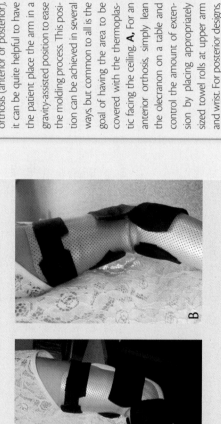

CLINICAL PEARL 7-60.
Gravity-Assisted Positioning for Elbow Orthoses

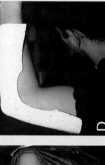

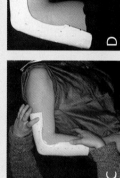

When fabricating an elbow orthosis (anterior or posterior), it can be quite helpful to have the patient place the arm in a gravity-assisted position to ease the molding process. This position can be achieved in several ways, but common to all is the goal of having the area to be covered with the thermoplastic facing the ceiling. **A,** For an anterior orthosis, simply lean the olecranon on a table and control the amount of extension by placing appropriately sized towel rolls at upper arm and wrist. For posterior designs, the patient or assistant can hold the various positions as shown: **(B)** prone on plinth, **(C)** flexed at hips with upper arm parallel to floor (good position to control amount of forearm rotation distally), and **(D)** shoulder abducted with hand resting on head. Whatever position is chosen when using gravity as an assist, the clinician must be acutely aware of not letting the elbow drop into too much flexion with posterior orthoses or too much extension (with anterior designs) as the orthosis is being fabricated.

Shoulder Abduction (or Adduction) Immobilization Orthosis (SO/SEO) (Fig. 7–47)

Common Names

- Gunslinger splint
- Airplane splint

Alternative Orthosis Options

- Prefabricated orthosis

Primary Functions

- Immobilize shoulder joint to allow healing of involved structure(s).

Common Diagnoses and Optimal Positions

Brachial plexus injury	Sh: 30° abd, 30 to 45° flex, slight ER; elb: 90° flex; FArm: neutral rotation
Tendon transfers for plexus injury	Sh: add, 30 to 45° flex, slight ER; elb: 90° flex; FArm: neutral rotation
Sh and humeral arthroplasty	Sh: 30° abd and flex; 15° ER; elb: 90° flex; FArm: neutral rotation

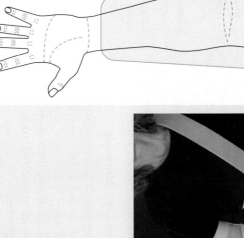

Bar

Diskette

Center of hip

FIGURE 7-48

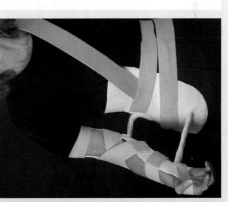
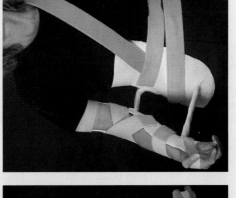

FIGURE 7-47

Fabrication Process

Pattern Creation (Fig. 7–48)

- Correct positions of shoulder and elbow depend on injury and/or surgical procedure. Communicate with physician before orthosis application.
- Pattern should be made with patient's clothing on. If possible, fabricate trunk orthosis before surgical procedure; posterior elbow orthosis may also be fabricated before surgery. But remember that postoperative edema may alter fit, and accommodation may be needed.
- Posterior elbow component
  - Follow directions for posterior elbow immobilization orthosis, making certain that there is adequate troughing to accommodate connector bars.
- Trunk component
  - Take measurements on affected side with patient standing.
  - Mark distal border from midsternum to vertebral border dorsally.
  - Mark proximal border from naval to vertebral border dorsally.
  - Connect to form lateral borders (should somewhat rectangular).
- Connector component
  - Length of connector bars determined by desired shoulder position: the more elevation, the longer the bars.
  - Measure 1½" to 2" for width. This material will be rolled onto itself for added strength.

- Four 2" in diameter disks of thermoplastic material help secure connector bars onto trunk and elbow portions.

Refine Pattern

- Wrist inclusion is optional, depending on diagnosis and patient comfort. After determining length of connector bars, allow extra 1" on each end for application onto trunk orthosis.
- To provide added strength, include ³⁄₃₂" aluminum wire within thermoplastic roll. This is especially helpful for maintaining shoulder elevation, owing to potential high force delivered to connector bars.

Options for Materials

- Use uncoated thermoplastic material to aid in bonding of connector bars. If uncoated materials are not available, then disrupt coating on all connected surfaces before adhering.
- Posterior elbow component: use ⅛" uncoated perforated plastic or elastic-based material. Choose elastic material if patient has pain and/or cannot assist in shoulder positioning because tackiness may aid during molding process.
- Trunk component: consider ⅛" solid, rubber-based, uncoated material for its strength and stability.
- Connector component: use ⅛" solid, rubber-based, uncoated material for bars and disks.

Cut and Heat

- Use plinth where there is full access to involved extremity to increase ease of molding process. Have assistant support arm in appropriate position.
- Position patient side lying with affected extremity superior to achieve gravity assistance.
- If necessary, prepad bony prominences: iliac crest, epicondyles, olecranon process, and ulnar styloid.

Evaluate Fit while Molding

Note: The fabrication of this orthosis may warrant an "extra set of hands" to assist during the molding process.

- Posterior elbow component
  - Carefully mold as described for posterior elbow immobilization orthosis.
  - Allow enough material for connector bar application.
- Trunk component
  - Remove warm material from heating pan and support with both hands. Carefully place along trunk, as shown.
  - Mold well about waist and over iliac crest to prevent orthosis from sliding off hip.
- Connector component
  - Remove warm material, place on flat surface. Position wire in center of material and roll onto itself, forming thick bar. Repeat process for other bar.

- Apply strapping before adhering components together.

Strapping and Components

- Posterior elbow component
  - Use stockinette or elasticized sleeve if edema is present before orthosis application to eliminate pinching of skin once straps are applied.
  - Apply 2" soft straps to proximal and distal portions of orthosis.
  - Proximal strap should be wide and applied at most proximal portion of orthosis to prevent rocking.
  - Crisscross design directly over anterior elbow helps maintain elbow securely in orthosis.
  - Consider using an Ace™ wrap or 3" Coban™ to secure if edema is an issue.
- Trunk component
  - Apply one 3" to 6" soft strap or two 2" straps with D-ring closure about waist (width and number of straps depend on patient's trunk size).
  - Apply 2" soft strap directed from sternum, across uninvolved shoulder, to posterior vertebral border. D-ring attachment is recommended for ease of adjustment.
  - Pad portion of strap that traverses opposite shoulder to maximize comfort.

(Continued)

Fabrication Process

(Continued)

- Connector components
  - Disks act as reinforcements and should be applied once bars are attached.
  - While an assistant maintains desired position of shoulder, apply trunk and elbow orthosis.
  - Mark for upper and lower bar placements on both orthosis components.
  - Prepare all surfaces for bonding.

- Heat 1″ of both ends of two connector bars and secure to premarked areas.
  - Throughout process, check that correct shoulder position is maintained; making adjustments can be difficult.
  - Heat disk thoroughly; make slit halfway through disk; open; and wrap about bar and orthosis base, molding firmly into place.

Survey Completed Orthosis

- Trunk orthosis can be lined with Microfoam™ tape or padding material (gel or foam) to help prevent migration and rotation.
- Smooth and slightly flare all distal and proximal borders.
- Check for clearance and/or irritation of trunk, axilla, ulnar styloid, epicondyles, and olecranon process (thumb and MCP joints, if wrist included).
- Check for compression of ulnar nerve at cubital tunnel area and of superficial sensory branch of radial nerve.

Discussion Points Questions

1. What types of injuries are most appropriate for an Immobilization orthosis?

2. What stage of wound healing is most often treated with immobilization?

3. Give two examples of immobilization orthosis for a wrist fracture. Include;
   - the proper positioning of the joints involved
   - proper placement of straps and foam
   - what are the most important considerations during fabrication?

4. Give an example of an immobilization orthosis that would allow increased functional use of the hand.

CHAPTER 7

8 Mobilization Orthoses

General Clinical Pearls Related to Mobilization Orthoses

CLINICAL PEARL 8-X1.
Fingernail Attachments

A, Hook material. A small piece of hook strapping material (size should accommodate the length and width of the nail) can be glued to the fingernail using a gel-based glue. Once set, a strip of ½" loop (preferably soft material such as Rolyan® SoftStrap®, Patterson Medical) can be added to the hook with the line attached and pulling proximally. This technique may work well for patients who have a large nail surface area.

B, Dress hooks. A dress hook can be glued to the nail using a gel-based glue. Bend the hook slightly to provide optimal contour with the nail (contoured hooks can be purchased). Take care to place the hook as proximal on the nail as possible. If the hook is placed too far distally, the force may apply undue pressure on the nail bed. The line is either applied directly to the hook or attached first to a small piece of loop that has been attached to the dress hook. Some clinicians prefer this loop method because it prevents the line from digging into the skin as it traverses over the fingertip.

C, Commercially available devices. Prefabricated devices are available lines with nonskid material to prevent slippage. 3pp® Finger Trapper™ (IF) and Rolyan® Wrap-On™ Finger Hooks offer an alternative to using glue on the nail (both available through Patterson Medical).

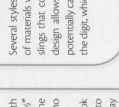
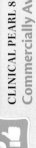

CLINICAL PEARL 8-X2.
Commercially Available Digit Slings

Several styles of slings are commercially available in a multitude of materials with various thicknesses. Care should be taken with slings that converge into one line (also known as a loop). This design allows little accommodation for fluctuations in edema, potentially causing compressive forces about the lateral aspects of the digit, which may lead to neurovascular compromise.

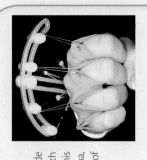

CLINICAL PEARL 8-X3.
Finger Sling Combined with Thermoplastic Material

Mold ⅟₁₆" material to the volar (**A**) or dorsal (**B**) aspect of a digit to function as a sling. The material should extend the full length of the segment being mobilized (clearing the creases) and encompass half to two-thirds the circumference of the segment. The thermoplastic sling maximally distributes pressure and prevents excessive compressive forces, which are sometimes caused by constrictive soft slings (refer to Chapter 4 for greater detail). A small strip of adhesive hook is placed on the mid-dorsal or volar portion of the sling. The midpoint of a 1" by 3" strip of loop material is placed over the adhesive hook. One hole is punched on both distal ends of the loop material. Monofilament line or elastic force is then attached at both ends of the loop and fed through the line guide and pulley to the proximal attachment device (**A and B**). A thin layer of foam can be added beneath the thermoplastic sling to increase comfort, if necessary. Another option is using neoprene or foam material on the digit, then forming a more rigid sling over the material with a casting tape such as QuickCast 2 shown (Patterson Medical) (**C**).

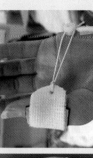
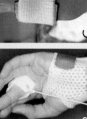
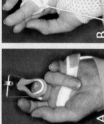
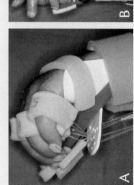
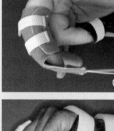

CLINICAL PEARL 8-X4.
Line Guides

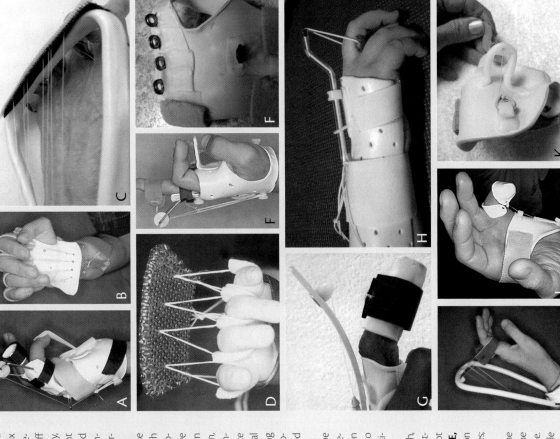

A, Safety pin. A safety pin is a cost-effective way to provide a smooth and simple guide for a monofilament line. Shown is a combination PIP extension (dynamic via rubber band and Phoenix Outrigger System; Patterson Medical) and PIP flexion (static progressive via hook-and-loop material) mobilization orthosis. Note how the placement of the safety pin lifts the monofilament line off the dorsum of the MCP joint, preventing the line from dragging across the orthosis base. To apply, bend and flatten the wide end of the safety pin. Scratch the application surface and use solvent over this area. Next, holding the "eye" end of the safety pin with flat nose pliers, heat the flattened end with a heat gun and embed it into the desired area of the orthosis. This step should be completed with the orthosis off the patient's hand. Secure the safety pin by adding a scrap piece of thermoplastic material over the union. Allow the area to set before feeding the line through the hole.

B and C, Thermoplastic. Scrap pieces of thermoplastic material can be used to create a line guide in many orthoses. **B,** In this case, an MCP flexion mobilization orthosis. The length and width of the line guide depends on the location and severity of the contracture(s). Secure the thermoplastic line guide to the orthosis base by scraping the attachment site and using solvent to remove any protective coating. Heat the section of material that will be attached, dry off water, and then embed that section into the prepared base. Hold the nonheated section in a perpendicular fashion, maintaining a 90° angle with the segment that is to be mobilized (in this case, the proximal phalanges). Once set, use a hole punch to create holes at the appropriate area to form a 90° angle of force application. As ROM increases, create a new hole to maintain the optimal angle of pull; the material can also be cut down. Highly perforated material provides many holes to choose from, eliminating the need for a hole punch. **C,** For an MCP extension mobilization orthosis, a scrap piece of thermoplastic material can be rolled and formed into an outrigger. Adhesive hook material can be applied dorsally to guide the lines. Use a strip of loop on top to keep lines in place.

D, Custom bent outrigger and perforated thermoplastic material. An outrigger can be created by bending 3/32″ aluminum wire to form a dorsal segment. Cover it with perforated material, slightly overlap the material at the wire's edge, then pinch and seal it. The slings are placed on the digits, and the line is threaded through the appropriate hole in the thermoplastic material to produce a 90° angle of pull. The elastic force is then attached to the line and directed to the proximal attachment device.

E–H, Commercially available devices. Commercially available guides are simple to attach, remove, and reuse. However, some of these devices do not provide the extended length and adjustability many orthoses require to maintain the desired 90° angle of force application. If the angle is not close to 90°, the line may drag through an edge of the line guide, creating increased frictional force. **E,** The Phoenix single digit outrigger (Patterson Medical); **F,** Rolyan® Individual Line Guides (Patterson Medical); **G,** Base 2″ Outrigger System (North Coast Medical) and commercially available line guides; and **H,** Orfitube™ System (North Coast Medical) with cap ends to prevent elastic from fraying.

I–K, Aquatubes®. Used as line guides, Aquatubes® (Patterson Medical) can prevent the lines from getting caught on an adjacent digit's line or on clothing and bed linens. **I,** Cut the Aquatubes® into 1/4″ disks, spot heat, and attach to a thermoplastic outrigger to create a line guide. **J,** Aquatubes® can be cut into small tubes (1″ to 2″) and the pieces used to create a low-profile design. **K,** The Aquatubes® was heated and formed into this line guide to maintain optimal line of force application.

CLINICAL PEARL 8-X5.
Line Stops

A line stop can be placed on the monofilament line to limit motion, as required with some extensor tendon and early mobilization protocols (Phoenix Outrigger System; Patterson Medical). This provides the therapist a way to restrict joint flexion to a specific degree. The patient is allowed to flex the joints actively within the range permitted by the stop bead; the dynamic component passively brings the digits back into extension. Stop beads (or line stops) can be purchased commercially or simply fabricated by using tape (although not as aesthetically pleasing). Commercial line stops can be repositioned to allow for a progressive increase in motion as healing allows. Most recently, ROM-Stops™ (North Coast Medical) were introduced; they involve the use of plastic rods of various lengths used to restrict a specific ROM.

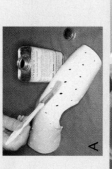

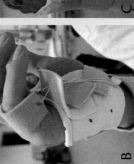

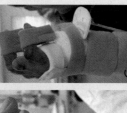

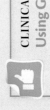

CLINICAL PEARL 8-X6.
Preparing Coated Materials for Bonding

When using thermoplastic material with a protective coating, the surfaces must be prepared if bonding of two pieces is necessary. This is especially true if the bonded piece will be used as a line guide where forces will be place upon or generated through this bonded piece (**B and C**). To prepare the surfaces, use solvent to eliminate the coating on the material's surface or scratch and score the material's surface to disrupt the coating. To ensure a strong bond, press the materials firmly together. Use a heat gun to hyperheat the material, which helps make it tacky and more likely to adhere.

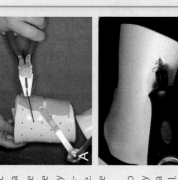

CLINICAL PEARL 8-X7.
Forming Holes in Thermoplastic Material

A, Heated wire technique. To form holes in thermoplastic material in regions where a hole punch cannot reach, heat a ³⁄₃₂″ piece of wire over a heat gun using flat-nose pliers. Pierce the hot end of the wire onto the premarked area. Move the heated wire around, forming a small hole, and immediately position the rubber band post or rivet in place. As an alternative, heat the end of an Allen wrench or awl instead of a wire. Note that this procedure should always be done with the orthosis off the patient.

B, Dremel. A small hand drill can be a handy tool to keep in a clinic, because it provides a quick and easy way to make holes in difficult-to-reach areas. When available, a Dremel can be used to form a hole in thermoplastic material. Caution should be taken to ensure the surface area that abuts the skin does not have residual sharp ridges/edges from the drilling process.

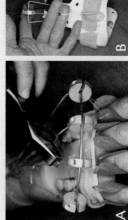

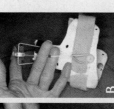

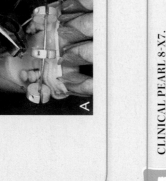

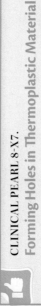

CLINICAL PEARL 8-X8.
Using Goniometer to Determine 90° Line of Force Application

A goniometer ensures that a 90° line of application has been achieved (Rolyan® Outrigger; Patterson Medical). This maximizes the effectiveness of the force application. Orthoses may need to be readjusted frequently, depending on the responsiveness of the tissue to the mobilization force. Another useful method includes holding an Allen wrench (perpendicular bend in metal) to the side of the segment mobilized to help visualize the 90° angle.

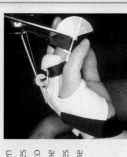
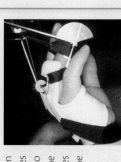

CLINICAL PEARL 8-X9.
Mobilization Forces

A, Elastic cord. Wrapped elastic cord is a quick and commonly used method for providing a mobilization force for dynamic orthoses. The wrapped elastic can be directly fastened from the sling to the proximal attachment device. Be aware that if the cord traverses through line guides, the friction (or drag) may alter the force placed on the intended structures. Because the elastic cord is wrapped with cotton, it is less elastic and forgiving than rubber bands and should not be treated in the same way. Doubling the resting length of the cord will generate a much greater tension than doubling the length of a rubber band. This combination custom MCP flexion mobilization orthosis includes a Phoenix Outrigger (Patterson Medical) for PIP extension mobilization.

B, Rubber bands. Rubber bands are the most commonly used component for generating tension in mobilization orthoses. They are readily available, inexpensive, easy to apply and adjust, and come in various lengths and widths. Be aware that the tension generated is directly related to the rubber band's length and width. Thinner rubber bands provide less tension and are more susceptible to fatigue and breaking; thus, they need to be replaced more often. The orthosis shown is a homemade PIP flexion mobilization device.

C, Spring coils. Graded spring coils offer a consistent way to control force accurately in a dynamic mobilization orthosis. Springs generate a given force based on their overall length and width, coil

tightness, and the distance they have to travel from the proximal to distal attachment. Springs have been shown to be more durable and to last longer than rubber bands. However, they are more expensive than rubber bands and elastic cord. A clinic should have various springs on hand to address a potential range of needs, although this may not always be feasible. The PIP dynamic traction orthosis shown includes a Base 2" Outrigger (North Coast Medical).

D, TheraBand® or TheraTubing® (Patterson Medical). These work especially well with larger designs such as wrist, forearm, and elbow mobilization orthoses. The force delivered to the tissue depends on the tension property of the band. A custom wrist and digit extension mobilization orthosis is shown.

E, Tape. Microfoam™ tape (Patterson Medical) can be used to quickly fabricate a mobilization orthosis. The tape can be adjusted easily and be effectively reused several times. A custom PIP flexion mobilization orthosis is shown.

F, Neoprene. Neoprene material, because of its elastic nature, can be used effectively for a cost-saving way to provide a mobilization force. Refer to Chapter 14 for further instruction. Shown here is a wrist, thumb, and digit extension mobilization orthosis applied to a radial nerve injured hand.

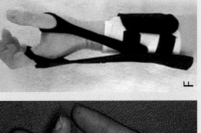

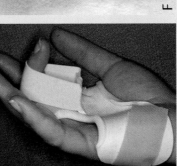

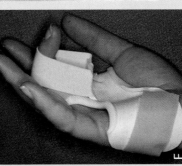

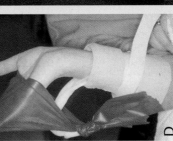

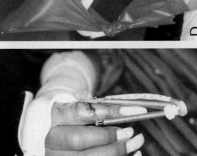

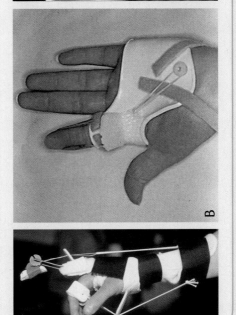

A   B   C   D   E   F

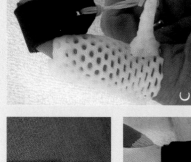

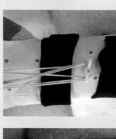
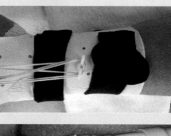
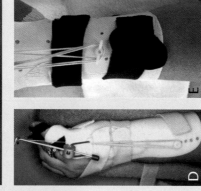

CLINICAL PEARL 8-X10.
Proximal Attachment Devices

A, Aquatubes®. An orthosis being used as a mobilization device during the scar-remodeling phase of wound healing for a patient who sustained a severe crush injury. Rehabilitation focused on increasing digit ROM. Note the creative use of applying mobilization forces to the tissue. Static progressive stretch is applied to the MF via thin strapping material attached by hook on the nail and to the adhesive hook on the orthosis base proximally. The RF and SF are placed in PIP/DIP flexion mobilization straps. The SF has an additional sling that applies flexion force to the MP joint, creating a composite stretch to that digit. Note the Aquatubes® (Patterson Medical) used as the custom-made proximal attachment device; as an alternative, a scrap piece of thermoplastic can be fashioned into a hook as well.

B, Various. Paper clips and dress hooks can be bent, heated, and applied to the thermoplastic material **(far right)**. Rubber band posts and thumb nuts are also easy devices to apply to an orthosis for attaching mobilization components **(middle)**. Another technique is to heat the small section where the proximal attachment device should be placed; then pierce through the material with scissors, lifting up from the orthosis base with a pencil (or similar object) to form an elongated hole that is approximately ⅕". This forms a raised area where rubber bands can be attached **(far left)**.

C, Thermoplastic. Shown is a homemade line guide and proximal attachment device for a DIP mobilization orthosis.

D and E, Commercially available devices. These provide a quick and easy way to attach mobilization components. They can be easily reused and/or adjusted. The orthosis shown has several holes for the rubber band post to allow for quick adjustment as ROM improves **(D)** (Rolyan® Outrigger System; Patterson Medical). Note that more than one proximal attachment device may be needed, depending on the number of rubber bands to be attached. Wing nuts or similar devices can also be used as shown here **(E)**.

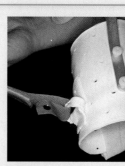
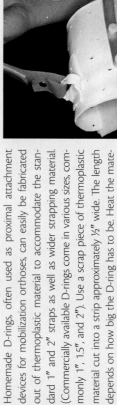

CLINICAL PEARL 8-X11.
Homemade D-ring

Homemade D-rings, often used as proximal attachment devices for mobilization orthoses, can easily be fabricated out of thermoplastic material to accommodate the standard 1" and 2" straps as well as wider strapping material. (Commercially available D-rings come in various sizes, commonly 1", 1.5", and 2"). Use a scrap piece of thermoplastic material cut into a strip approximately ½" wide. The length depends on how big the D-ring has to be. Heat the material, roll it onto itself for rigidity, overlap the ends, and pinch together firmly. Use your IFs to maintain the shape until the material is set. Be sure to prepare the surfaces of the material for bonding to ensure a strong attachment. Shown here is a homemade D-ring for the attachment of a static progressive strap for an elbow flexion mobilization orthosis.

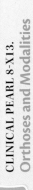

CLINICAL PEARL 8-X12.
Elbow and Shoulder Harnesses to Secure Arm Orthoses

When designing a mobilization orthosis for the upper extremity, special consideration should be taken regarding potential migration. Some degree of migration will inevitably occur when the orthosis is worn secondary to the forces that are generated in order to mobilize tissue. A therapist can consider proximal stabilization that may assist in proper positioning and security of the orthosis onto the arm.

A, A shoulder harness can be fabricated from 2" soft strapping material. The shoulder harness, which helps prevent distal migration of large arm orthoses, can be fabricated in various ways. The strapping is initiated on the posterior border of the orthosis and directed across the back and toward the opposite shoulder. It then passes across chest to attach to the anterior orthosis. An additional strap is initiated on the anterior aspect of the orthosis and traverses posteriorly to attach to the other strap. The straps can be riveted together.

B, For smaller orthoses that do not have a mobilization force yet need additional stabilization, consider a simple cross chest neoprene strap as seen in this nonarticular proximal humeral orthosis.

C, Forearm orthoses such as wrist flexion and/or extension mobilization orthoses can be anchored to the elbow to counteract the tendency for these devices to migrate distally on the forearm. When this occurs, there may be interruption of full mobility and irritation of bony prominences. There are numerous ways to secure orthoses to the proximal arm. Shown here is a simple foam strap that traverses about the posterior elbow and meets at the same proximal attachment device as the rubber bands. The elbow should be in flexion in order for this to be most effective.

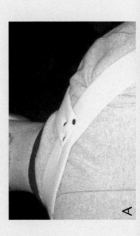

A

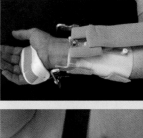

B

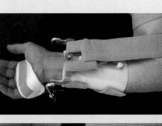

C

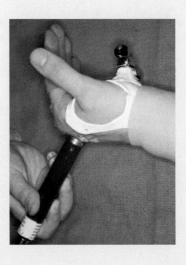

CLINICAL PEARL 8-X13.
Orthoses and Modalities

A mobilization orthosis can be used to enhance the use of therapeutic modalities. For example, a static progressive IF MCP flexion mobilization orthosis (shown here) can be applied while ultrasound is being used on the adherent extensor tendons over the dorsum of the IF. Another example is stabilizing the wrist (blocking the wrist flexors and extensors) with a wrist immobilization orthosis while applying neuromuscular stimulation to the extrinsic digital flexors and/or extensors to facilitate tendon glide. Orthoses can be worn directly over electrodes as long as the patient is instructed in proper electrode application and maintenance.

1 Digit- and Thumb-Based Orthoses

Distal Interphalangeal (DIP) Flexion Mobilization Orthosis (FO) (Fig. 8-1)

Common Names

• Dynamic DIP flexion splint

Alternative Orthosis Options

• Prefabricated orthosis
• Casting (serial static flexion)

Primary Functions

• Provide low-load, prolonged flexion mobilization force to DIP joint to facilitate lengthening of tissues.

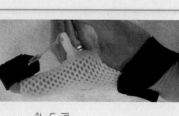

CLINICAL PEARL 8-1.
Including MCP Joint to Increase Effectiveness of DIP Stretch

To better secure the PIP joint, consider including the MCP joint in the orthosis. The additional length allows for a longer line of application, which can increase the effectiveness of this type of device. This is especially helpful when fabricating an orthosis on a small hand.

CLINICAL PEARL 8-2.
Creating 90° Angle of Application on a Digit Orthosis

It is often challenging and cumbersome to add an outrigger to a digit orthosis. When compliance and functionality are not an issue, consider a simple "homemade" thermoplastic outrigger applied to the most proximal base of the digit orthosis; this can be easily modified to obtain the optimal angle by heating and reshaping.

Common Diagnoses and General Optimal Positions

DIP jt ext contracture

Proximal interphalangeal (PIP) 0°;
DIP: terminal flexion

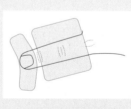
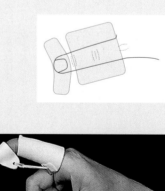

FIGURE 8-2

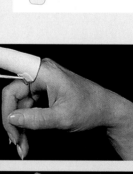

FIGURE 8-1

Fabrication Process

Pattern Creation (Fig. 8–2)

- For individuals with short digits, orthosis may need to include the metacarpophalangeal (MCP) joint to better stabilize PIP joint for optimal force application distally.
- For proximal attachment device, prepare one scrap (½" by 1") of thermoplastic material.

Refine Pattern

- Make sure that digital web spaces are cleared and that PIP joint is held in 0° extension.
- DIP flexion crease should be cleared proximally.

Options for Materials

- Use nonperforated ⅟₁₆", ⅟₃₂", or ⅛" material.
- Plastic materials conform well to contours of digit.

Cut and Heat

- Position patient with hand supinated, digits slightly abducted, resting over platform.
- Warm material.
- Prepare mobilization components: sling, line, rubber band, and proximal attachment device.

Evaluate Fit while Molding

- Fabricate PIP orthosis.
- Clear distally to allow unimpeded DIP flexion.

Strapping and Components

- Circumferential design does not require straps.
- Sling must be wide enough to distribute pressure over dorsum of DIP joint and short enough to prevent interference with line guide if used.

- Secure proximal attachment device at most proximal border of orthosis along longitudinal axis of proximal phalanx.
- Connect rubber band to sling and loop at proximal device.

Survey Completed Orthosis

- Adjust tension per patient and/or tissue tolerance; goal is low-load stretch over prolonged period of time.

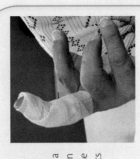

CLINICAL PEARL 8-3.
Serial Static Casting to Mobilize Stiff DIP Joint

Application of a digit cast can be an effective way to provide a low-load, prolonged flexion force (serial static) to a DIP extension contracture. Including the PIP joint and the entire length of the proximal phalanx will increase the purchase of the cast and its overall effectiveness.

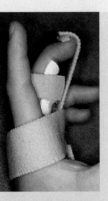

CLINICAL PEARL 8-4.
Thermoplastic Distal Phalanx Caps

Slings used to mobilize DIP joint extension contractures frequently slip during use. One solution is to fabricate a circumferential cap from ⅟₁₆" material to form a joined volar tab for the line attachment. Heat the material, and place it dorsally over the distal phalanx, quickly stretching to form a small volar tab. Pinch both ends to seal. Once set, punch a hole through the tab to serve as the attachment for the monofilament line. This can also be used when designing composite IP flexion mobilization orthoses as shown here.

PATTERN PEARL 8-1 to 8-2.

PP8-1
Circumferential stabilization of PIP joint, with Kinesio® Tex Tape (Patterson Medical) strap applying gentle flexion force to DIP joint.

PP8-2
Dynamic force via elastic strapping attached to adhesive hook on nail.

CHAPTER 8

PIP/DIP Mobilization Orthosis (FO) (Fig. 8–3)

Common Names

- PIP/DIP strap
- Interphalangeal (IP) flexion strap

Alternative Orthosis Options

- Taping in flexion
- Elasticized wrap
- Neoprene orthosis
- Flexion glove
- Prefabricated straps

Primary Functions

- Provide low-load, prolonged flexion mobilization force to DIP and PIP joints to facilitate lengthening of tissues.

Additional Functions

- Facilitate extensor digitorum communis (EDC) function and glide during exercise.

Common Diagnoses and General Optimal Positions

Intrinsic tightness	PIP/DIP terminal flex
PIP and DIP jt tightness	PIP/DIP terminal flex
Ext contracture	PIP/DIP terminal flex

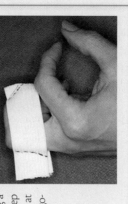

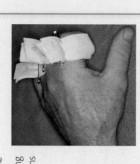

CLINICAL PEARL 8-5.
Sewing Technique for Increasing Strap Effectiveness

When DIP joint flexion is extremely limited, applying a PIP/DIP strap can be challenging. One way to help keep the strap in place and provide a more effective stretch at the DIP joint is to sew the distal end of the strap diagonally to form a "pocket" for the fingertip.

CLINICAL PEARL 8-6.
PIP/DIP Strap for Increasing EDC Glide

PIP/DIP straps can be used to position the joints in flexion during exercises to facilitate glide of the EDC tendons. Here, safety pins were used to secure the straps.

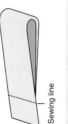

FIGURE 8-3

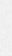

Sewing line

FIGURE 8-4

Fabrication Process

Pattern Creation (Fig. 8–4)

- Cut strip of ¾" elastic strapping (pajama elastic) to approximately 1½ times length of digit.

Refine Pattern

- Be sure width of elastic is adequate for size of digit.

Options for Materials

- ¾" elastic strap is generally appropriate for adult digits; ½" for children.

Cut and Heat

- Be sure length is adequate to secure around digit.

Evaluate Fit while Molding

- While placing center of strip along dorsal distal phalanx, have patient flex PIP and DIP joints of affected digit (claw position).

- Stretch strap ends to meet across dorsum of proximal phalanx, hold together, and adjust tension to tolerance.
- Apply strap at an oblique angle with light downward pressure to increase force in DIP flexion.
- Mark both pieces of elastic and remove slowly from digit.

Strapping and Components

- Sew straps together on sewing machine, if available.
- Use safety pin or staples for simple, quick closure technique.
- May add a piece of soft foam under portion of straps that comes in contact with nail to soften contour of elastic over this sometimes sensitive area.

Survey Completed Orthosis

- As range of motion (ROM) increases, tension in strap must be adjusted accordingly.
- Periodically check elasticity of strap; may need to be replaced with prolonged use.

- When fabricating straps for more than one digit, label them to ensure correct strap is placed on each digit.
- Adjust tension per patient and/or tissue tolerance; goal is low-load stretch over prolonged period of time.

PATTERN PEARL 8-3 to 8-5.

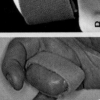

PP8-3
Use of foam over distal phalanx to dissipate pressure and provide conforming fit.

PP8-4
Rolyan® PIP/DIP Finger Flexion Strap (Patterson Medical, Warrenville, IL).

PP8-5
Final Flexion Wrap (Photo courtesy of 3-Point Products, Stevensville, MD).

CHAPTER 8

CLINICAL PEARL 8-7.
PIP/DIP Mobilization Straps

Consider using a gentle dynamic or static progressive approach for mobilizing stiff IP joints. These techniques may be helpful for patients who have difficulty donning the traditional elastic PIP/DIP straps or for those who require frequent tension adjustments. Here are three ways to achieve this type of stretch.

A, Soft nonelastic strap method. This works best with less severe contractures because the foam strapping does not contour as well as an elastic-based strap and may cause tissue irritation. Use soft ½" nonelastic foam strapping material. The severity of passive limitation determines the exact amount of strapping needed (i.e., the greater the contracture, the more material required). Use approximately two times the length of the digit. The fabrication method is the same as described for the PIP/DIP strap, except for the closure technique. A small strip of double-sided hook (adhesive hook folded onto itself) is placed on one end of the strap. Gentle tension is applied and then secured into place.

B, Neoprene (elastic type) strap. ⅛" Neoprene strapping material contours well and typically has a layer of foam sandwiched between the outer layers. Because of this, patients find neoprene comfortable to wear for longer periods of time. The fabrication principles are the same as described previously. A simple safety pin can be used for closure or if the neoprene has loop material as one of the outer layers; double-sided hook can be considered for closure.

C, Thermoplastics and straps. For this method, fabricate a thermoplastic thimble over the distal phalanx and a thermoplastic sling on the proximal phalanx. Then apply a strip of adhesive hook on the lateral aspect of each thermoplastic piece. Connect the two segments with a ¼" strip of nonelastic loop strapping material.

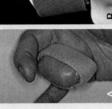

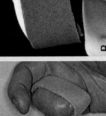

② Hand-Based Orthoses

PIP Extension Mobilization Orthosis (HFO) (Fig. 8–5)

Common Names
- Dynamic PIP extension splint

Alternative Orthosis Options
- Cast (serial static)
- Prefabricated orthosis

Primary Functions
- Provide low-load, prolonged extension mobilization force to PIP joint to facilitate lengthening of tissues.

Additional Functions
- Facilitate extensor tendon function and glide during exercise.

Common Diagnoses and General Optimal Positions

PIP flex contracture	MCP: 60°; PIP: terminal ext
Zone III or IV ext tendon repair	MCP: 0° ext; PIP: 0° ext (for complex injury)

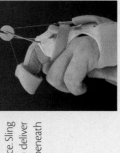

CLINICAL PEARL 8-8.
PIP Extension Mobilization Used as Exercise Orthosis

A PIP extension mobilization orthosis can be used to facilitate PIP and DIP flexion by flexing against the resistance of the dynamic force. Sling can be applied at distal phalanx or at the middle phalanx to deliver resistance to DIP or PIP joint. Note use of Kinesio® Tex Tape beneath orthosis for edema management.

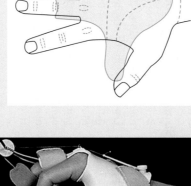

FIGURE 8-6

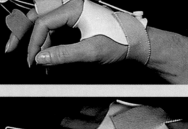

FIGURE 8-5

Fabrication Process (Using Phoenix Outrigger)

Pattern Creation (Fig. 8–6)

- Mark proximal border at wrist crease.
- If holding MCP joint at 0°, mark distal border only to mid-PIP crease. If holding MCP in flexion, mark distal border beyond PIP joint. Note: Additional material is needed to accommodate for flexion angle at MCP joint.

Refine Pattern

- Proximal border should allow wrist motion.
- Lateral borders of PIP extension bar should trough proximal phalanx, encompassing half to two-thirds of this segment.
- Ulnar aspect of hand orthosis should support hypothenar eminence.
- Make radial bar long enough to attach to volar ulnar border.

Options for Materials

- Use solid $^3/_{32}$" material, which is lightweight, yet strong enough to support MCP joint in flexion while accepting extension force.
- Plastic materials contour well, with minimal handling into arches and digital web spaces.
- If radial bar is intended to pop apart, coated material is necessary.

Strapping and Components

- Use ½" to 1" strap at proximal phalanx.
- Attach 1" strap at ulnar–radial segment interface.
- Place an elasticized or soft foam strap at wrist to prevent orthosis migration.
- Mark desired outrigger attachment; position outrigger to extend distally over midportion of middle phalanx, extending it high enough so volar sling attached to line will clear pulley.
- Remove orthosis from patient and heat outrigger's proximal ends with heat gun. Press lightly to embed outrigger into marked area.
- Use extreme care when applying heated metal onto thermoplastic material. Metal may pierce through orthosis. Always perform this process off patient.
- Treat surfaces to be bonded with orthosis solvent. Place strip of heated thermoplastic material over outrigger and adhere to orthosis base. With flat-nose pliers, bend clasp part of safety pin at 90° angle. Heat same end over heat gun and embed into orthosis base over MCP joint.
- Position eye of safety pin along longitudinal axis of involved digit; secure with thermoplastic material scrap.

Cut and Heat

- Position patient with hand over platform, digits slightly abducted, and MCP joint positioned per diagnosis.
- Heat two additional pieces of material (1" by 1") for securing outrigger and safety pin.

Evaluate Fit while Molding

- Dry and apply warm material onto hand, making sure to clear all creases, trough around involved proximal phalanx, and encompass ulnar border of hand.
- Gently pull radial bar through thumb web space and across volar MCPs to meet with ulnar segment. Pinch and seal lightly.
- Make sure radial bar crosses proximal to MCP joints and incorporates arches to help maintain proper orthosis position. Maintain MCP joint position.

- If index finger (IF) and/or small finger (SF) MCPs are enlarged or if there is degree of thenar or hypothenar atrophy, the union must be popped open to ease donning and doffing.
- Use components of choice, following manufacturer's directions for correct application.

- Attach Phoenix wheel to outrigger using appropriately sized Allen wrench.
- Affix proximal attachment device for rubber band at most proximal border.
- Attach line on both sides of sling and apply sling to middle phalanx. Thread line through pulley and safety pin.
- Loop appropriate rubber band onto end of line and connect to proximal attachment device.

Survey Completed Orthosis

- Check for clearance of thumb, wrist, and uninvolved digits.
- Material should be flared about digital web spaces to avoid irritation.
- Check for equal traction on both sides of digit and for any possible rotational force.
- Adjust angles of pull to 90° by simply loosening pulley and rotating. Securely tighten in desired position with Allen wrench.
- Align pulley with longitudinal axis of proximal phalanx. Adjust by loosening pulley and sliding it transversely along width of outrigger. Securely tighten in desired position with Allen wrench.
- Adjust tension per patient and/or tissue tolerance; goal is low-load stretch over prolonged period of time.

PATTERN PEARL 8-6 to 8-10

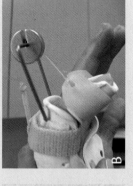
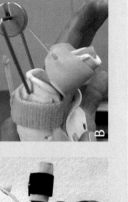

PP8-6

A–C, Rolyan® Adjustable Outrigger (Patterson Medical) using same pattern.

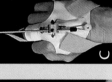

PP8-7

To further isolate PIP joint, consider immobilization of DIP for increased purchase of sling: **(A)** circumferential and **(B)** volar.

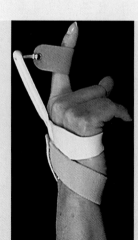

PP8-8

Digit extension mobilization orthosis using Aquatubes® (Patterson Medical) or can use rolled thermoplastic.

CLINICAL PEARL 8-9.
Serial Static Casting to Mobilize Stiff PIP Joint

Casting tapes or plaster of paris can be used to apply a low-load, prolonged stress to PIP flexion contracture. In this case, QuickCast 2 (Patterson Medical) casting tape was applied; the DIP joint was included for better purchase on this small digit.

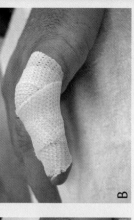
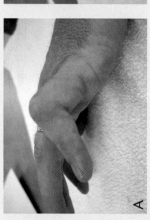

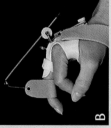

PP8-9

LMB Spring Finger Extension Assist Orthosis (North Coast Medical, Morgan Hil,l CA).

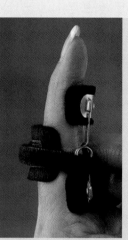
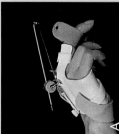

PP8-10

Bunnell™ Mini Modified Safety Pin Splint (Photo courtesy of North Coast Medical).

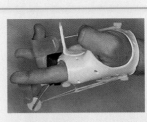

CLINICAL PEARL 8-11.
Multipurpose Orthosis: Alternating PIP Flexion/Extension Mobilization

Creating an orthosis that incorporates two functions such as PIP flexion and PIP extension mobilization can be a cost-saving measure and convenient for the patient. This hand-based orthosis addresses a stiff PIP joint with a custom outrigger for flexion mobilization and Phoenix Outrigger (Patterson Medical) for extension mobilization. The patient is effectively able to alternate between flexion and extension mobilization throughout the day using just one orthosis.

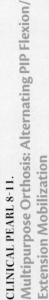

CLINICAL PEARL 8-10.
Forearm-Based PIP Extension Mobilization Orthosis

When fabricating an orthosis on a patient with multiple PIP joint flexion contractures, or a PIP flexion contracture that is greater than approximately 60°, consider a forearm-based design. The longer design may work well when addressing both MCP and PIP joint contractures within one orthosis. The pattern is similar to the hand-based PIP extension mobilization orthosis but includes the wrist. Shown is an RF–SF PIP extension mobilization orthosis. The patient had significant, longstanding PIP flexion contractures secondary to an ulnar nerve injury. She presented with a 75° flexion contracture on the RF and a 45° flexion contracture on the SF. Note the length of the outrigger on the RF to achieve a 90° line of pull. The outrigger platform for the wheel had to be custom made to incorporate the height and achieve the optimal angle of force application. The detachable extension outrigger can be positioned higher or lower, moved proximally or distally, and (to a lesser degree) slide radially and ulnarly. The more severe the contracture, the more distal and higher the rod will need to be. As the contracture resolves, the rod is retracted proximally and tightened back into place with the appropriate Allen wrench. The component shown here is the Rolyan® Adjustable Outrigger (Patterson Medical), which can be adjusted to hold single or multiple rod extenders.

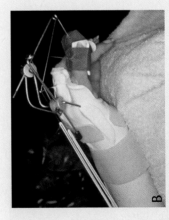

A

B

CHAPTER 8

PIP Flexion Mobilization Orthosis (HFO) (Fig. 8–7)

Common Names

- Dynamic PIP flexion splint

Alternative Orthosis Options

- Elastic wraps
- Flexion glove
- Prefabricated orthoses

Primary Functions

- Provide low-load, prolonged flexion mobilization force to PIP joint to facilitate lengthening of tissues.

Common Diagnoses and General Optimal Positions

PIP ext contracture   MCP: 0°; PIP: terminal flex

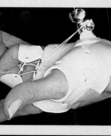
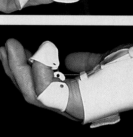
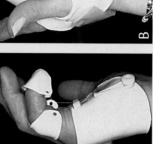

CLINICAL PEARL 8-12.

Convert Dynamic Orthosis to Static Progressive Using MERiT™ Component

These composite digit flexion orthoses have similar design characteristics as the hand-based mobilization orthoses previously described. The clinician can use creativity in "tweaking" the designs to meet particular patient needs. At times, a patient may have stiffness in all three joints (MCP, PIP, DIP), and the clinician is challenged to incorporate as many joints as possible to not burden the patient (and insurance carrier) with multiple orthoses. **(A)** SF composite flexion mobilization orthosis using a dynamic approach, which employs rubber band traction and homemade line guides (Aquatubes®; Patterson Medical) to increase SF MCP, PIP, and DIP flexion. **(B)** MF composite flexion orthosis is using a static progressive approach, incorporating eyelets of safety pins as the line guides and a MERiT™ component to provide the static progressive force. The turn screw is gradually tightened to increase the tension applied to the MF.

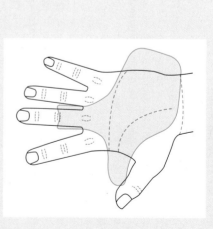

FIGURE 8-7

FIGURE 8-8

Fabrication Process

Pattern Creation (Fig. 8–8)

- Severity of contracture and number of joints involved determine whether orthosis is forearm or hand-based.
- This hand-based pattern can easily be modified to include wrist.
- Mark proximal border at distal wrist crease.
- Mark distal border at proximal PIP crease.

Refine Pattern

- Lateral borders should encompass half to two-thirds of circumference of proximal phalanx (flush with dorsal surface).
- Borders should clear uninvolved MCP joint creases and encompass hypothenar eminence.
- When fabricating an orthosis for the IF and middle finger (MF), there should be enough material molded around thenar eminence to allow for line guide attachment.
- Radial bar should traverse through thumb web space, across dorsum of hand, and attach to ulnar border.

Options for Materials

- Use solid, coated $\frac{3}{32}$" material (elastic or plastic) for this orthosis; this makes for lightweight orthosis with adequate strength to support MCP joint in extension while accepting flexion force.
- Elastic materials allow excellent visualization of creases during molding.
- Plastic materials tend to contour well, with minimal handling, into arches and about digital web spaces.
- To seal off circumference of orthosis, choose an uncoated material; however, if dorsal segment is intended to pop apart, then coated material is recommended.
- Use components of choice (custom-fabricated line guide is shown).

Cut and Heat

- Position patient with hand supinated resting over platform, digits slightly abducted, and MCP joint extended.

Evaluate Fit while Molding

- Dry and apply warm material onto hand, making sure to clear all creases; trough about involved proximal phalanx; and encompass ulnar border.
- Gently pull radial bar through thumb web space and across dorsum to meet with ulnar segment. Pinch and seal lightly, and return focus to volar aspect.
- Make sure arches are incorporated into the orthosis to maintain orthosis position properly on hand.
- MCP joint should be positioned as close to 0° as possible.

Strapping and Components

- Use ½" to 1" across proximal phalanx. If necessary, attach 1" strap dorsally at ulnar and radial segments. This area may be permanently sealed; however, if IF and SF MCPs are enlarged or if there is some degree of thenar or hypothenar atrophy, it will be difficult to doff orthosis without popping it open.
- Place elasticized or soft foam strap at wrist to prevent migration (if needed).

- Position sling over middle phalanx.
- Apply line guide at level of distal palmar crease, making sure it is extended far enough to create 90° angle of pull when force is applied to middle phalanx.
- Proximal attachment device should be attached at most proximal border of orthosis.
- Once force is applied, may need strap applied to proximal orthosis and about wrist to prevent tilt of the proximal edge of the device.

Survey Completed Orthosis

- Connect line to rubber band and loop about proximal device.
- Check for equal traction of both sides of digit and for any possible rotational force. Correct, if necessary, by adjusting monofilament line.
- Material should be flared, trimmed, and smoothed around digital web spaces to avoid irritation.
- Check that volar orthosis borders do not irritate uninvolved MCPs.
- Adjust tension per patient and/or tissue tolerance; goal is low-load stretch over prolonged period of time.

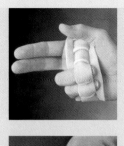

PP8-11

A and B, Phoenix Outrigger System (Patterson Medical).

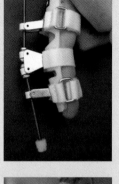

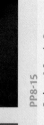

PP8-12

Static progressive approach: note height of MERiT™ (Patterson Medical) component to achieve 90° angle of pull.

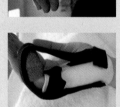

PP8-13

Neoprene applied over DIP cast to isolate stretch to PIP (Orficast™, North Coast Medical).

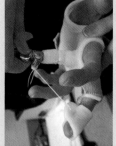

PP8-14

Microfoam™ tape used to provide gentle flexion force (Patterson Medical).

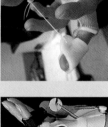

PP8-15

Rolyan® Static Progressive Finger Flexion Splint (Patterson Medical).

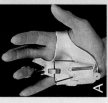

PP8-16

Norco™ Cinch Strap (Photo courtesy of North Coast Medical).

CLINICAL PEARL 8-13.
Forearm-Based PIP Flexion Mobilization Orthosis

When fabricating an orthosis on a patient with multiple PIP joint extension contractures, consider a forearm-based design. The pattern is similar to the hand-based PIP flexion mobilization orthosis but includes the wrist; the additional material provides the surface for the proximal attachments. Shown is an IF–RF PIP flexion mobilization orthosis with a homemade outrigger and with dynamic force application via spring coils.

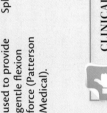
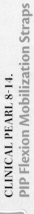

CLINICAL PEARL 8-14.
PIP Flexion Mobilization Straps

Elastic, nonelastic, or neoprene-type straps can be used to effectively mobilize a stiff PIP joint(s). **(A)** The strap is directed from the middle phalanx of the involved digit, through the thenar web space, and across the ulnar border of the hand to terminate on the dorsum of the hand as shown in this elastic-based strap. **(B)** The use of a thermoplastic cuff or foam over the middle phalanx will assist in comfort and optimal pressure distribution as noted in this foam (nonelastic strap). The tension should be gentle and adjusted appropriately to maintain the correct stretch on the joint. **(C)** Pajama elastic secured with safety pins dorsally; note isolated PIP flexion stretch on IF.

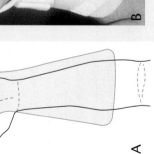
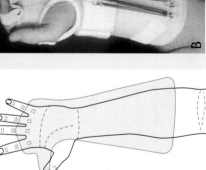
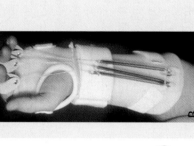
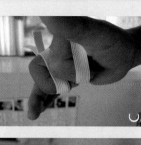
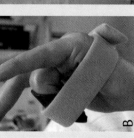
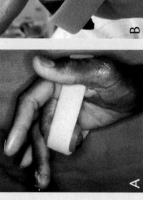

Thumb IP Flexion Mobilization Orthosis (HFO) (Fig. 8–9)

Common Names

- IP flexion splint

Alternative Orthosis Options

- Elastic wraps

Primary Functions

- Provide low-load, prolonged flexion mobilization force to thumb IP joint to facilitate lengthening of tissues.

Common Diagnoses and General Optimal Positions

Th IP jt ext contracture

MCP: 0°; (carpometacarpal [CMC]): midpalmar–rad abd; IP: terminal flex

CLINICAL PEARL 8-15.
Thumb MP/IP Flexion Mobilization Orthosis

Often after injury to the thumb, both the MP and IP joints can be stiff, requiring mobilization. Stiffness may present after cast immobilization of the ulnar collateral ligament (UCL) or radial collateral ligament (RCL) sprain or repair, scaphoid or metacarpal fracture, scaphotrapeziotrapezoid (STT) fusion, CMC joint arthroplasty, or other thumb injury. To provide flexion forces to the MP and IP joints simultaneously, fabricate an orthosis similar to the thumb IP flexion mobilization orthosis, but the thumb portion should only extend as far as the MP joint flexion crease (**A**). This allows adequate stabilization of the first metacarpal while forces are directed to the MP and IP joints. For a dynamic approach, use rubber band traction (**B**). A small piece of hook is adhered to the nail to allow for loop attachment. For a static progressive approach, use adhesive hook-and-loop strapping for the proximal attachment device (**C**). The adhesive hook is diagonally placed at the proximal border of the orthosis base, and the loop strapping is then directed to the hook and attached. This provides a gentle stretch that should be adjusted as the patient's tolerance permits.

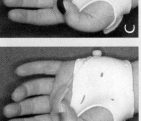

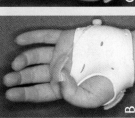

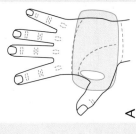

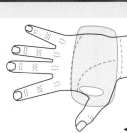

FIGURE 8-9

FIGURE 8-10

Fabrication Process (Using Splint-Tuner™; North Coast Medical for Static Progressive Force)

Pattern Creation (Fig. 8–10)

- Mark proximal border at wrist crease.
- Mark distal border proximal to thumb IP flexion crease and distal palmar crease.

Refine Pattern

- Proximal border should allow full wrist motion.
- Distal border should allow unimpeded motion of digit MCP and thumb IP flexion.
- Provide appropriate amount of material within and dorsal to web space to support thumb CMC and MP position adequately and provide surface area for strap application dorsally.

Options for Materials

- Use solid, coated, 1/16″ or 3/32″ material; this makes for lightweight orthosis with adequate strength to support CMC and MP joints while accepting flexion force to IP joint.
- Elastic materials allow excellent visualization of creases during molding.
- Plastic material contours well, with minimal handling into arches and thumb web space.
- Use components of choice (Splint-Tuner™ is shown).

Cut and Heat

- Position hand supinated over an armrest, with thumb in midpalmar and radial abduction.
- Heat an additional piece of material (1″ by 1″) to secure Splint-Tuner™ component.

Evaluate Fit while Molding

- Lay warm material on towel, positioning thumb portion on correct side of material to place it on supinated hand.
- Place thumb section centrally over thumb proximal phalanx and guide rest of material evenly along palm.
- Take dorsal section of thumb material (between IF and thumb) and carefully contour through web space.
- Gently pull proximal volar thumb material and lightly overlap onto dorsal piece.
- While molding, avoid direct pressure over CMC joint and dorsal MP joint. Be sure to maintain thumb CMC and MP joints in appropriate positions.
- Carefully incorporate arches of hand by using smooth, even strokes and constantly redirecting material.
- Once material has cooled completely, pop apart overlapped pieces if necessary; otherwise, carefully remove orthosis.

Strapping and Components

- If necessary, attach 1/2″ strap dorsally at overlapped web space area. Attach 1″ strap dorsally at ulnar and radial segments.
- To attach Splint-Tuner™ component, first treat surfaces to be bonded with solvent (orthosis base and small thermoplastic piece).
- Heat small piece of material and wrap around component stem to form cylinder.
- Reheat material over heat gun; then set at predetermined site on orthosis base.
- Firmly press component into orthosis base and gently rotate cylinder to achieve an intimate fit about grooves of stem onto orthosis base.
- Position Splint-Tuner™ component so axis of rotating cylinder is perpendicular to line.
- Apply sling to distal phalanx, then attach static orthosis line, allowing enough so that orthosis can be easily donned and doffed but not so much that it is cumbersome to tighten up each time it is loosened.
- Make sure the Splint-Tuner™ component is completely cooled and set before applying line or it will pop off the orthosis base from the force/torque being applied.
- Thread line through hole in Splint-Tuner™ and tie line back onto itself.

Survey Completed Orthosis

- Check for clearance of wrist, especially around radial and ulnar styloids.
- Smooth and slightly flare all borders and around thumb IP opening.
- Pay careful attention to IF MCP, which frequently abuts radial portion of orthosis as it traverses through first web space.
- Make sure web tissue is not pinched under overlapped pieces.
- Adjust tension by rotating turn screw per patient and/or tissue tolerance; goal is low-load stretch over prolonged period of time.

PATTERN PEARL 8-17 to 8-19.

PP8-17

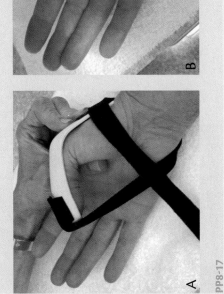

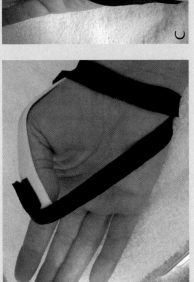

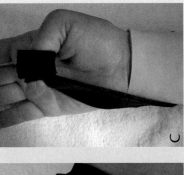

A and B, Composite thumb MP/IP flexion using a dorsal approach with neoprene. **C,** Simple IP neoprene loop directed to a wrist cuff.

PP8-18

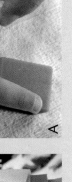

Thumb MP flexion using elastic cord and neoprene/QuickCast 2 sling (Patterson Medical).

PP8-19

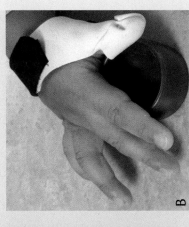
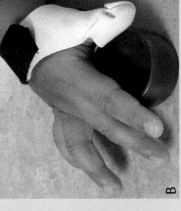
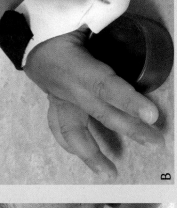

Serial static design for congenital trigger thumb **(A)** IP flexion contracture. **B,** Dorsal design promoting IP extension.

MCP Extension Mobilization Orthosis (HFO) (Fig. 8–11)

Common Names

- Zero profile splint[1]
- Posterior interosseous nerve splint

Alternative Orthosis Options

- Dynamic MCP extension orthosis
- Prefabricated orthosis

Primary Functions

- Dynamically support MCP joints in extension while allowing active digit (and thumb) flexion.

Common Diagnoses and General Optimal Positions

Returning radial nerve function	MCP: 0°; PIP: free
Posterior interosseous nerve injury	MCP: 0°; PIP: free
Weak extrinsic extensor function	MCP: 0°; PIP: free

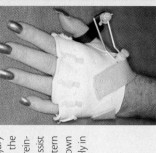

 CLINICAL PEARL 8-16.
Adding Thumb to Hand-Based MCP Extension Mobilization Orthosis

Loss of thumb extension is commonly seen after radial nerve injury and can impair functional use of the hand. To better position the thumb (out of a flexed and adducted posture) while awaiting reinnervation, consider adding a dynamic thumb MP extension assist to the MCP extension mobilization orthosis. The basic pattern does not change. A Phoenix Outrigger (Patterson Medical) shown here or similar system works well to support the thumb passively in extension while allowing active functional flexion.

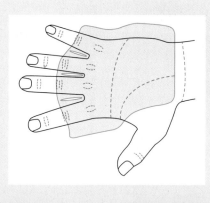

FIGURE 8-11

FIGURE 8-12

[1]Designed by Tina Steen, OTR/L, and Lois Carlson, OTR/L, CHT.

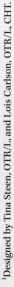

Fabrication Process

Pattern Creation (Fig. 8–12)

- Mark proximal border at wrist crease.
- Mark distal borders at middorsal PIP creases.
- Note small slits at digit web spaces for elastic to pass through.

Refine Pattern

- Radial aspect should extend enough to trough radial index and partially trough web space (just beyond proximal palmar crease); the trough should lie flush to volar surface and not interfere with digit flexion.
- Ulnar border should encompass hypothenar eminence but not interfere with MCP flexion.

Options for Materials

- Use solid ³⁄₃₂″ plastic material; this makes for a lightweight orthosis with adequate strength to support MCP joints in extension while accepting flexion forces.

- Plastic material contours well, with minimal handling about metacarpal heads and between digital web spaces.
- Cut ¼″ to ½″ elastic strapping (pajama elastic), depending on size of hand, twice width of hand (at MCP joint level); elastic should cover approximately two-thirds length of proximal phalanxes.
- Use three small pieces of scrap thermoplastic material (or Aquatubes®) to secure elastic loops dorsally.

Cut and Heat

- Heat thermoplastics, including small pieces.
- Position hand, pronated with digits slightly abducted; MCP joints should be positioned and held in extension. (Patient may need to support digits in extension with unaffected hand.)

Evaluate Fit while Molding

- Heat and apply material to dorsum of hand, carefully making sure that MCPs are extended and proximal phalanxes are precisely contoured, forming small troughs.
- Mold with care over metacarpal heads to avoid pressure areas. Wrap about hypothenar border volarly along fifth metacarpal to add stability to the orthosis.
- Radial border should be molded along radial aspect of IF and lie flush to its volar surface.

Strapping and Components

- Once set, use hole punch or hand drill to form slits that start approximately ½″ from distal orthosis border between the IF and MF; the MF and ring finger (RF), and the RF and SF. Weave elastic through slits to support each proximal phalanx.

- Tension of elastic strap should be just enough to hold proximal phalanx in extension; excessive tension can lead to neurovascular compromise.
- Prepare surface of dorsal loop areas with solvent for adhering rods.
- Place small pieces of warm thermoplastic material (rolled into rods) underneath each dorsal loop. Press rods into place, sealing elastic loop against orthosis base.
- Consider using rivets to secure radial and ulnar extensions of elastic.
- Use soft or elasticized 1″ strap through palm and at wrist crease to secure orthosis on hand.

Survey Completed Orthosis

- Check for pressure areas at dorsum of MCP joints during active flexion.
- Check tension on each proximal phalanx support, monitoring for signs of neurovascular compromise.

PATTERN PEARL 8-20 to 8-24.

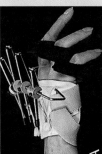

PP8-20

Using wider elastic to better support larger digits.

PP8-21

Included hypothenar within the orthosis allows better purchase during digital flexion.

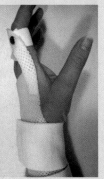

PP8-22

A and B, Neoprene material can be used to provide gentle MCP extension mobilization forces while allowing a degree of flexion for functional use.

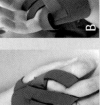

PP8-23

Forearm-based MCP extension mobilization orthosis for proximal radial nerve injury—notice cut out to relieve pressure at MCP joints.

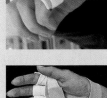

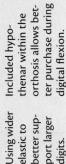

PP8-24

A and B, Rolyan® Adjustable Outrigger System (Patterson Medical).

3 Forearm-Based Orthoses

Wrist Extension Mobilization Orthosis (WHO) (Fig. 8–13)

Common Names

- Dynamic wrist extension splint
- Wrist mobilization splint

Alternative Orthosis Options

- Casting (serial static)
- Adjustable wrist hinged orthosis
- Incremental wrist hinged orthosis
- Preformed dynamic wrist orthosis
- Static progressive wrist orthosis kit

Primary Functions

- Provide low-load, prolonged extension mobilization force to wrist joint to facilitate lengthening of tissue.

Additional Functions

- Restrict specific degree of motion by blocking movement through hinge device (restriction orthosis).

Common Diagnoses and General Optimal Positions

Wr flex contracture   FArm: pronated; wr: terminal ext

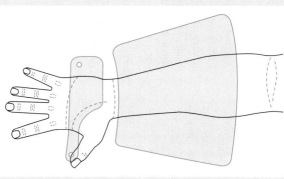

FIGURE 8-14

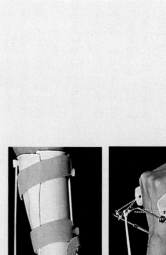
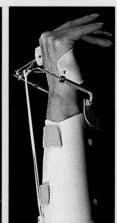
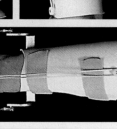
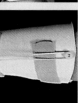
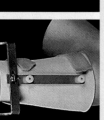

FIGURE 8-13

Fabrication Process (Using Phoenix Wrist Hinge)

Pattern Creation (Fig. 8–14)

Forearm orthosis
- Length of orthosis should be at least 5" to allow adequate attachment of outrigger.

Hand orthosis
- Width should be approximately 1½ times width of hand (at distal palmar crease).
- Length should extend ulnarly from distal palmar crease to hamate bone and radially allow enough material to contour through first web space.

Refine Pattern
- Allow adequate clearance for unimpeded wrist motion.

Options for Materials
- Use 1/16" or 3/32" material for both orthosis pieces; the thinness allows for easy removal and application.
- Use components of choice (Phoenix wrist hinge is shown).

Cut and Heat
- Heat and fabricate each piece separately.
- For forearm orthosis, position forearm in neutral rotation.
- For hand orthosis, position forearm supinated.

Evaluate Fit while Molding

Forearm orthosis
- Prepad ulnar styloid process.
- After heating material, place material on volar surface of forearm and gently wrap around onto itself.
- Opening must be either on radial or ulnar aspect of forearm; volar or dorsal opening will impede outrigger placement.
- If using coated material, lightly overlap so it will adhere to itself; if using uncoated material, place wet paper towel between overlapped layers.
- Allow orthosis to set and then snap apart.

Hand orthosis
- Place material on volar hand and mold it around to dorsal surface.
- Flare edges to clear thenar eminence and distal palmar crease.
- Mark palmar orthosis for trimming just above ulnar and radial borders on dorsal surface.
- Mark hole along ulnar and radial borders of hand orthosis for attaching nylon fasteners.
- Remove orthosis, trim as needed, and smooth edges.

Strapping and Components
- Add straps once wrist hinge placement is determined.

Forearm orthosis
- With forearm orthosis on patient, position wrist hinge volarly.
- Align long arm of wrist hinge with axis of motion.
- Mark two holes on volar orthosis to match up with holes on long arm of wrist hinge.
- Remove orthosis and punch out holes.
- Attach hinge with rubber band posts (included with Phoenix wrist hinge).
- Affix rubber band post to proximal dorsal border for attachment of mobilization component.
- Apply forearm orthosis to hand.
- Set screws on lateral bars allow proximal and distal height adjustment of 1½". Loosen set screws with Allen wrench and adjust distal bar to accommodate appropriate position; tighten screws.
- Make necessary lateral adjustments for extreme radial or ulnar deviation by using screw on T-bar. Loosen set screws with screwdriver and slide hinge radially or ulnarly to desired position.

Hand orthosis
- Punch holes on dorsal pieces.
- Thread nylon fastener through dorsal holes on hand orthosis.
- Apply hand orthosis.
- Loop nylon fasteners around outrigger bar within movable collars of wrist hinge and adjoin fasteners.
- Place wrist in maximum extension while adjusting fasteners to achieve 90° angle of pull with metacarpal bones.
- Position two movable collars on distal bar of wrist hinge so they prevent nylon loops from slipping laterally.
- Attach appropriate rubber band to distal bar, directing it to proximal attachment device.

Survey Completed Orthosis
- Add 1" to 2" strip of thin adhesive back padding (e.g., moleskin) along length of inside border to prevent skin from being pinched when orthosis is overlapped and secured. Moleskin is doubled over (with thermoplastic edge in between adhesive sides of padding) and acts as flap.
- Line length of forearm orthosis and proximal and distal borders with nonskid material to decrease orthosis migration greatly. May use Microfoam™ tape, adhesive Dycem, or adhesive silicone gel sheets.
- Check for accommodation of ulnar styloid and full elbow ROM.
- Adjust tension per patient and/or tissue tolerance; goal is low-load stretch over prolonged period of time.

CHAPTER 8

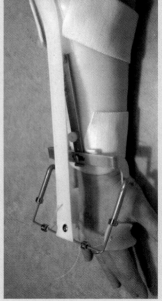

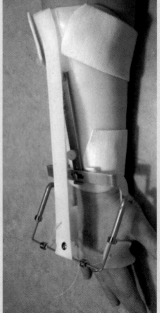

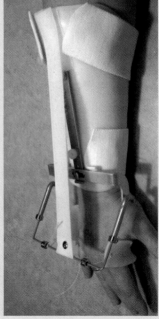

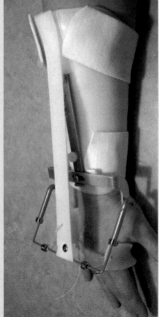

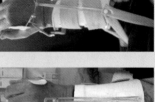

PP8-25

Hook-and-loop strapping material used as static progressive force; loop riveted to bar and directed proximally onto strip of hook.

PP8-26

Use of Microfoam™ tape at distal edge of forearm segment to prevent migration.

PP8-27

A and B, Digitec Outrigger (Patterson Medical) with neoprene adhered to distal edge for padding.

PP8-28

Use of elbow strap to prevent distal migration of forearm segment.

CLINICAL PEARL 8-17.
Rolyan® Incremental Wrist Hinge

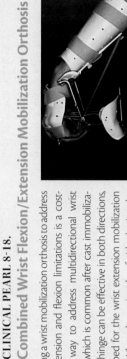

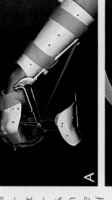

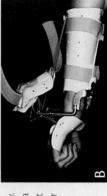

As an alternative, the Rolyan® Incremental Wrist Hinge (Patterson Medical) can be used to fabricate a wrist mobilization orthosis. The pattern differs from the Phoenix Wrist Hinge, as shown. The hinge can be locked in position for serial static positioning, and components can be added to provide the mobilization forces. Follow the manufacturer's instructions for specific outrigger application.

CLINICAL PEARL 8-18.
Combined Wrist Flexion/Extension Mobilization Orthosis

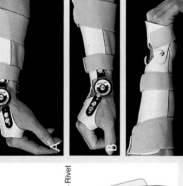

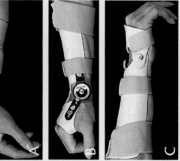

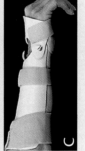

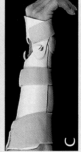

Fabricating a wrist mobilization orthosis to address both extension and flexion limitations is a cost-effective way to address multidirectional wrist stiffness, which is common after cast immobilization. The hinge can be effective in both directions, as described for the wrist extension mobilization orthosis. When the patient has finished using the extension component, the hand is taken out of the palmar cuff, and the hinge is left to drop volarly. The dorsal cuff is then applied and directed to a volar proximal attachment device **(A)**. The patient can alternate use of wrist extension and flexion per therapist's recommendations **(B)**.

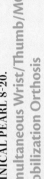

CLINICAL PEARL 8-19.
Wrist Flexion Mobilization Orthosis

The pattern and instructions for the wrist extension mobilization orthosis (forearm orthosis and hinge) can be used to create a wrist flexion mobilization orthosis with minor changes. The material for the forearm orthosis is applied so that there is no overlapping material on the volar surface. Shown here, the forearm orthosis is not overlapping and nearly meets on the dorsum of the forearm. For the dorsal hand segment, place a rectangular piece of warm material on the dorsal surface of the hand and mold it well over the bony areas. Once set, line the inner surface of the orthosis to prevent migration and improve comfort (Microfoam™ tape works well). The Splint-Tuner™ (North Coast Medical) shown here is used to provide the wrist flexion mobilization force. Note **(A)** is fabricated without an outrigger and does not have an accurate 90° angle of force application. In **(B)**, a Digitec Outrigger (Patterson Medical) is used to achieve a better angle.

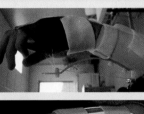
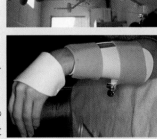

CLINICAL PEARL 8-21.
Custom Hinges

A custom hinge can be fabricated as an alternative to a commercially available device. **(A)** Scrap pieces of thermoplastic connected loosely via a rivet or carefully rolled thermoplastic can be used. **(B)** Crimped Aquatubes® (Patterson Medical) were added to this mobilization orthosis to prevent migration of proximal segment.

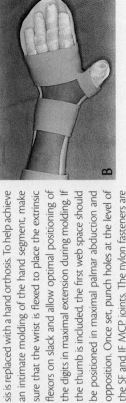
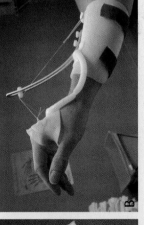

CLINICAL PEARL 8-20.
Simultaneous Wrist/Thumb/MCP/IP Extension Mobilization Orthosis

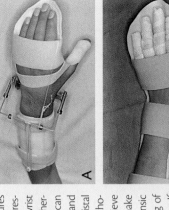
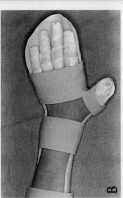

Patients who have sustained severe wrist fractures or extrinsic flexor tendon repairs occasionally present with significant limitations in passive wrist extension and/or extrinsic flexor tendon adherence. A wrist extension mobilization orthosis can be converted to mobilize wrist extension and extrinsic flexor tendons simultaneously. The distal palmar bar of a wrist extension mobilization orthosis is replaced with a hand orthosis. To help achieve an intimate molding of the hand segment, make sure that the wrist is flexed to place the extrinsic flexors on slack and allow optimal positioning of the digits in maximal extension during molding. If the thumb is included, the first web space should be positioned in maximal palmar abduction and opposition. Once set, punch holes at the level of the SF and IF MCP joints. The nylon fasteners are attached at this level and directed to the distal bar of the hinge. The mobilization force is then connected and terminated on the proximal attachment device **(A)**.

Note that if the contracture is severe, the distal bar (the side arms) may be too short to create an accurate 90° line of pull. A custom extended outrigger, fabricated from ³⁄₃₂″ aluminum wire, can be fit in the side bar of the hinge. Several nylon fasteners may need to be linked together to accommodate the outrigger's extra length.

(B) A serial static approach can address this same problem. Consider using QuickCast 2 (Patterson Medical) or Orficast™ (North Coast Medical) tapes for digit and thumb IP extension orthoses and a volar thermoplastic base (made of elastic or rubber material to allow for frequent remolding as mobility increases) to serially elongate the extrinsic flexor tendons and increase the passive wrist motion.

Wrist Extension, MCP Flexion/Wrist Flexion, MCP Extension Mobilization Orthosis (WHFO)   (Fig. 8–15)[2]

Common Names

- Radial nerve palsy splint
- Tenodesis splint

Alternative Orthosis Options

- Phoenix Extended Outrigger Kit
- Rolyan® Static Radial Nerve Orthosis
- Wrist extension immobilization orthosis

Primary Functions

- Provide passive wrist and MCP extension, allowing finger flexion, active wrist flexion, and digit and thumb extension. (Grasp and release through natural tenodesis action.)

Common Diagnoses and General Optimal Positions

Radial nerve palsy

Posterior interosseous nerve palsy

The goal is to hold the wrist and MCPs in a comfortable degree of extension, allowing functional flexion

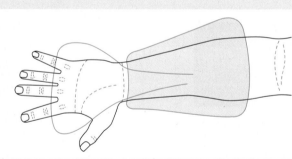

FIGURE 8-16

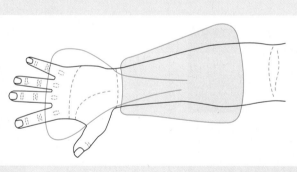

FIGURE 8-15

[2]Designed by Judy C. Colditz, OTR/CHT.

Fabrication Process

Pattern Creation (Fig. 8–16)

- Mark for dorsal forearm piece; proximal to wrist joint and 1" to 1½" distal to elbow crease.
- Consideration could be given to making the orthosis base a circumferential design (in this case, thinner material can be used as shown in wrist extension mobilization orthosis pattern).
- Circumference is half to two-thirds of forearm.

Refine Pattern

- Adjust length and width appropriately.

Options for Materials

- Use ⅛" thermoplastic material for orthosis base (unless a circumferential design is chosen where a thinner material such as a ¹⁄₁₆" material can be considered).
- Consider foam- or gel-lined materials to decrease distal orthosis migration.
- Cut three extra pieces of thermoplastic material (preferably non-coated) for
  1. Adherence of outrigger onto orthosis base (2" by 2")
  2. Formation of pulleys over distal outrigger wire (4" by 3") for individual proximal phalanx slings
  3. Creation of the proximal attachment for the nylon line

Cut and Heat

- Heat forearm piece while arm is resting pronated on table.
- Heat additional two pieces (one piece approximately 6" by 3"; the other 1" by 3")

Evaluate Fit while Molding

- Apply heated material to forearm.
- Mold radial and ulnar aspects of forearm piece so they cup slightly.

Strapping and Components

- Apply distal and proximal strap to secure forearm orthosis. Elastic-based or D-ring–type straps may help prevent distal orthosis migration.
- Per pattern, bend an outrigger of ³⁄₃₂" wire into desired shape.
- Bend outrigger at level of wrist joint at approximately 40° of wrist extension.
- Off patient, heat proximal end of outrigger and apply it to orthosis. When placed on patient's hand, outrigger should rest at middle of each proximal phalanx with fist position.
- Check location of outrigger; if correct, apply solvent to orthosis surface around outrigger.
- *Line Guide:* Adhere warm piece of thermoplastic material intimately about outrigger (use solvent before heating) to form sturdy attachment,

remembering that this area must accept weight of hand.

- Take warmed second strip of the orthosis material and apply to distal width of outrigger end, draping it over onto itself. Immediately trim to ½" to ¾" width.
- When cool, mark and punch hole over middle of each proximal phalanx.
- *Proximal Attachment:* Take third piece of warmed material; apply to center of most proximal end of orthosis (having applied solvent to this area prior); roll and press into the base, leaving half unattached and rolling back onto to form a "C" (refer to picture). Hold this "C" or hook in order for it to cool. Do not allow the piece to touch the base. Make sure enough room is provided for the nylon line to "hook" onto this segment.
- Apply slings to cover two-thirds length of proximal phalanxes. Premade leather slings work well because they are soft, comfortable, and not bulky.
- Tie long piece of nylon line to each sling.
- Place sling under each proximal phalanx and direct cord through hole punched in the orthosis material on distal outrigger.
- Hold cords while patient lifts arm off of tabletop and passively opens and closes fist.

- Adjust tension on nylon lines so that MCP joints are in 0° extension with neutral wrist and wrist is in 20 to 30° extension with full finger flexion. Adjustment process may be easier with help of assistant.
- If dorsum of patient's hand touches outrigger during finger flexion, bend outrigger into greater extension.
- Once correct line tension has been determined, ask patient to again rest full fist on tabletop so weight of hand is not on lines.
- Tie cords with firm knot and apply glue to secure it.
- Another option is to have individual lines converge at the proximal attachment.

Survey Completed Orthosis

- Flare distal edge and make sure that there is no abutment or irritation at ulnar styloid.
- If unlined material was used, consider lining orthosis with adhesive Dycem, gel, or Microfoam™ tape.

PATTERN PEARL 8-29 to 8-30

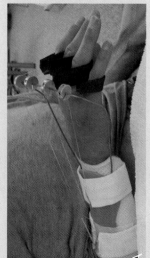
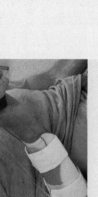

PP8-29

A and B, Custom bent wire secured with thermoplastic material, neoprene slings, and individual lines to proximal attachment device.

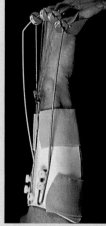
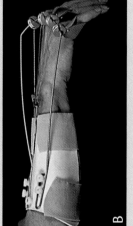
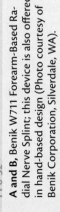

PP8-30

A–C, Phoenix Extended Outrigger Kit (Patterson Medical) includes prebent wire.

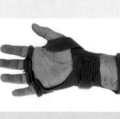
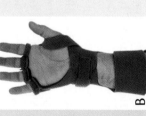
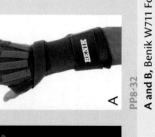
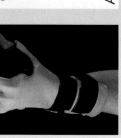
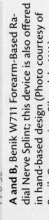

PP8-31

Robinson Forearm-Based Radial Nerve Splint (Photo courtesy of AliMed, Dedham, MA).

PP8-32

A and B, Benik W711 Forearm-Based Radial Nerve Splint; this device is also offered in hand-based design (Photo courtesy of Benik Corporation, Silverdale, WA).

Thumb CMC Palmar/Radial Abduction Mobilization Orthosis (WHFO) (Fig. 8–17)

Common Names

- CMC abduction splint
- Palmar abduction splint
- Thumb abduction splint

Alternative Orthosis Options

- Hand-based CMC abduction orthosis (serial static)
- Hand cones
- Air orthoses

Primary Functions

- Provide low-load, prolonged abduction mobilization force to first CMC joint to facilitate lengthening of tissue.

Common Diagnoses and General Optimal Positions

Th CMC add contracture   Wr: 10 to 20° ext; CMC: terminal midpalmar and rad abd

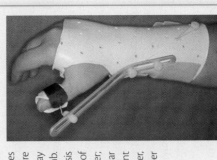

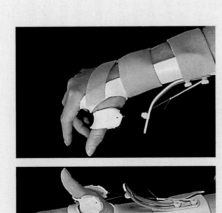

FIGURE 8-17

FIGURE 8-18

CLINICAL PEARL 8-22.

Thumb CMC Radial Abduction, MP/IP Extension Mobilization Orthosis

Thumb flexion and adduction contractures can sometimes develop after flexor pollicis longus (FPL) repair or thumb fracture immobilization. Fabricating a mobilization orthosis can be a way to stretch the volar and ulnar soft tissue structures of the thumb. The dorsal wrist immobilization pattern is used for the orthosis base. The outrigger is aligned with the dorsal longitudinal axis of the thumb column and secured to the orthosis (Digitec Outrigger; Patterson Medical). A thermoplastic sling is molded to the volar thumb surface, supporting the proximal phalanx. Monofilament line is attached, threaded through the line guide on the outrigger, and attached proximally via a rubber band. Tension is adjusted per patient's tolerance.

CHAPTER 8

Fabrication Process (Using Digitec System)

Pattern Creation (Fig. 8-18)

- Mark proximal border two-thirds length of forearm.
- Mark distal border at distal palmar crease.
- Mark for thumbhole in distal central portion of pattern, approximately 1" down and in.
- Allow enough material to encompass half to two-thirds circumference of forearm, remembering that forearm tapers distally.

Refine Pattern

- Proximal border should allow full elbow motion.
- Distal border should allow unimpeded motion of IF to MF MCP joints and full thumb mobility.

- For average adult, thumbhole should be about the size of elongated half dollar.

Options for Materials

- Consider ⅛" thermoplastic material to provide needed rigidity to withstand mobilization forces.
- Gel- or foam-lined materials may help decrease distal migration and increase comfort.
- Use components of choice (Digitec Outrigger System shown).

Cut and Heat

- Position patient with elbow resting on table and forearm supination to decrease distal migration for gravity-assisted molding; thumb should be held in gentle palmar abduction while molding.
- Cut out thumbhole in material either by making a series of holes with a hole punch before heating or by carefully piercing the slightly warm material with sharp scissors.

Evaluate Fit while Molding

- Lay warm material on towel, positioning thumbhole on correct side of material to be placed on forearm.
- Using IFs, gently open hole, making it slightly larger and more elongated (egg shaped).
- Place thumbhole over thumb and guide rest of material evenly along volar wrist and forearm.
- Carefully incorporate arches of hand by using smooth, even strokes and constantly redirecting material into arches.
- Allow for clearance at base of CMC joint; as thumb abducts in orthosis, base of thumbhole may need to be adjusted.
- Rotate forearm at end of molding to check for possible abutment of ulnar and radial styloid processes, and flare as necessary.

Strapping and Components

- Distal strap: 1" strap directed from volar to dorsal border.
- Middle strap: 2" strap applied proximal to dorsal wrist crease; use piece of adhesive foam to further stabilize wrist in orthosis and prevent migration. Foam should not overlap orthosis edges.
- Proximal strap: depending on size of forearm, 1" or 2" strap.

- Position Digitec Outrigger along radial volar aspect of orthosis base.
- Position soft sling (sling made of QuickCast 2 shown) in web space proximal to ulnar side of thumb MP (around metacarpal head). Positioning sling in this way directs forces to CMC joint, not MP joint ulnar collateral ligament.
- Check that sling and monofilament lines are directed at 90° angle from first metacarpal; attachment on outrigger may appear more proximal than anticipated.
- Next, thread monofilament line to line guide on outrigger, attach mobilization force, and secure to proximal attachment device.

Survey Completed Orthosis

- Make sure sling does not irritate web space. Fabricating wider sling may assist in distributing pressure and increasing comfort.
- Adhesive-backed Dycem or silicone gel sheet may help sling stay in place.
- Smooth and slightly flare distal and proximal borders.
- Gently flare around thenar hole, especially at base; avoid rolling, which can make future orthosis modifications difficult and can lead to an unnecessarily bulky orthosis.
- Check clearance of elbow, irritation at radial and ulnar styloid processes, and digital MCP motion. Adjust tension per patient and/or tissue tolerance; goal is low-load stretch over prolonged period of time.

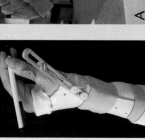
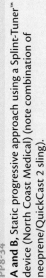
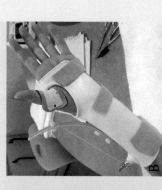

PATTERN PEARL 8-33 to 8-34.

PP8-33
Dorsal approach to obtain exact thumb placement for function.

PP8-34
A and B, Static progressive approach using a Splint-Tuner™ device (North Coast Medical) (note combination of neoprene/QuickCast 2 sling).

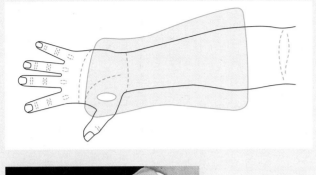

FIGURE 8-20

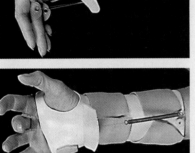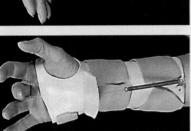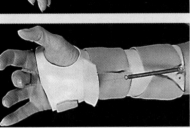

FIGURE 8-19

MCP Flexion Mobilization Orthosis (Fig. 8-19)

Common Names

- Dynamic MCP flexion splint

Alternative Orthosis Options

- Prefabricated orthosis
- Flexion glove

Primary Functions

- Provide low-load, prolonged flexion mobilization force to MCP joint to facilitate lengthening of tissue.

Common Diagnoses and General Optimal Positions

MCP ext contracture   Wr: 10 to 20° ext; MCP: terminal flexion

PATTERN PEARL 8-35 to 8-37.

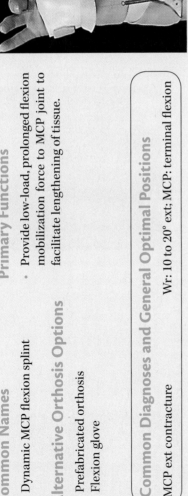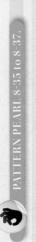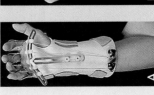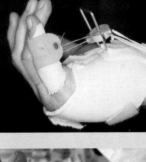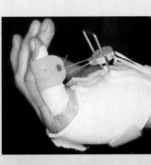

PP8-35

A and B, Base 2™ Outrigger System; note the use of a Splint-Tuner™ (North Coast Medical).

PP8-36

Hand-based design using scrap thermoplastic piece used as line guide.

PP8-37

Phoenix Outrigger (Patterson Medical) turned on side to achieve optimal angle of force application; note SF casting for improved leverage.

Fabrication Process

Pattern Creation (Fig. 8–20)

- Mark proximal border two-thirds length of forearm.
- Mark distal border at distal palmar crease.
- Mark for thumbhole in distal central portion of pattern, approximately 1" down and in.
- Allow enough material to encompass half to two-thirds circumference of forearm.

Refine Pattern

- Proximal border should allow elbow motion.
- Distal border should allow unimpeded motion of IF to MF MCP joints and full thumb mobility.
- For average adult, thumbhole should be about size of elongated half dollar.
- Distal portion of orthosis should clear proximal palmar crease to allow MCP flexion.

Options for Materials

- Use ⅛" material to provide needed rigidity to withstand mobilization forces.
- Gel- or foam-lined materials may help decrease distal migration and increase comfort.
- Custom-fabricated outrigger, made from ⅛" perforated material, acts as line guide. The best material choice for the outrigger is a material that is not coated. Solid thermoplastics can be used; however, smooth holes can be made using quality hole punch.

Cut and Heat

- Position patient with elbow resting on table and forearm supination for gravity-assisted molding.
- Cut out thumbhole in material either by making a series of holes with a hole punch before heating or by carefully piercing the slightly warm material with sharp scissors.
- Determine where outrigger should be positioned to achieve 90° angle of pull. Ideal outrigger position should allow for line of pull to scaphoid. General placement at or about wrist crease should be long enough to address degree of MCP extension contracture.
- Prepare surface with solvent and heat thermoplastic outrigger.

Evaluate Fit while Molding

- Lay warm material on towel, positioning thumbhole on correct side of material to be placed on forearm.
- Using IFs, gently open hole, making it slightly larger and more elongated. Place thumbhole over thumb and guide rest of material evenly along volar wrist and forearm.
- Carefully incorporate arches of hand by using smooth, even strokes and constantly redirecting material into arches.
- Allow for clearance at base of CMC joint. As thumb abducts in orthosis, base of thumbhole may need to be adjusted.
- Rotate forearm to check for possible abutment of ulnar and radial styloid processes, and flare as necessary.

Strapping and Components

- Distal strap: 1" strap directed from volar to dorsal border.
- Middle strap: 2" strap applied proximal to dorsal wrist crease; use piece of adhesive foam to further stabilize wrist in orthosis and prevent migration. Foam should not overlap orthosis edges.
- Proximal strap: depending on size of forearm, 1" or 2" strap.
- Affix outrigger at correct angle on base.
- Mark holes on outrigger where monofilament will be threaded to apply correct angle of pull.
- Affix proximal attachment device; several are needed if multiple digits are involved.
- Affix individual slings to proximal phalanxes, thread monofilament through predetermined holes, attach mobilization force, and attach to proximal attachment devices.
- Line of pull should be directed toward scaphoid bone, which follows natural cascade of digits.

Survey Completed Orthosis

- Make sure that sling does not irritate web space.
- Adhesive-backed Dycem or silicone gel sheet may help sling stay in place.
- Smooth and slightly flare distal and proximal borders.
- Gently flare around thenar hole, especially at base; avoid rolling, which can make future orthosis modifications difficult and can lead to an unnecessarily bulky orthosis.
- Check clearance of elbow, irritation at radial and ulnar styloid processes, and digital MCP motion.
- As MCP flexion gains are made, line of pull (changing hole in outrigger) must be adjusted, and outrigger can be cut down.
- Adjust tension per patient and/or tissue tolerance; goal is low-load stretch over prolonged period of time.

CLINICAL PEARL 8-23.
Clearance of Distal Palmar Crease

Be mindful to check for full clearance of MCP flexion to allow unrestricted mobilization. The orthoses tend to migrate distally once the force is applied; achieving good contour can help combat this tendency. Also try applying the orthosis directly on the skin or place strips of nonskid material such as Microfoam™ tape to minimize slippage. In this orthosis, the SF MCP flexion crease is blocked, limiting full flexion potential; this border needs to be cleared to the line shown.

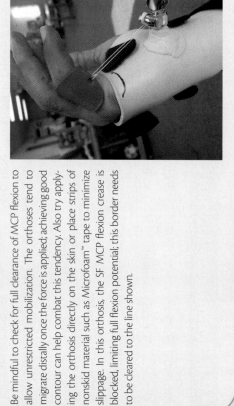

MCP/PIP/DIP Flexion Mobilization Orthosis (WHFO) (Fig. 8–21)

Common Names

- Final finger flexion splint
- Composite flexion splint

Alternative Orthosis Options

- Finger flexion glove
- Phase II composite finger flexion loop attachments
- Prefabricated orthoses
- Splint-Tuner™ Final Finger Flexion Kit
- Rolyan® Biodynamic Flexion System

Primary Functions

- Provide low-load, prolonged flexion mobilization force to MCP, PIP, and DIP joints to facilitate lengthening of tissue.

Common Diagnoses and General Optimal Positions

Extrinsic extensor tightness	Wr: 10 to 20° MCP/PIP/DIP: terminal flex
MCP, PIP, or DIP ext contractures	Wr: 10 to 20° ext; MCP/PIP/DIP: terminal flex

CLINICAL PEARL 8-24.
Forearm-Based Dorsal Design PIP/DIP Flexion Mobilization Orthosis

This dorsal design uses a simple and cost-effective static progressive approach to composite mobilization of the IP joints to address tight intrinsic muscles (monofilament line with loop material attaching proximally to adhesive hook). Note the foam-lined slings, which improve patient comfort. The slings are positioned on the distal phalanx, and the forces are dorsally directed.

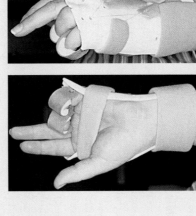

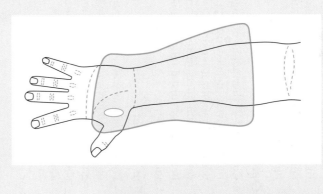

FIGURE 8-22

FIGURE 8-21

Fabrication Process

Pattern Creation (Fig. 8–22)

- Orthosis is most effective when MCP and IP joints have approximately 50% passive range of motion (PROM).
- Mark proximal border two-thirds length of forearm.
- Mark distal border at distal palmar crease.
- Mark for thumbhole in distal central portion of pattern, approximately 1" down and in.
- Allow enough material to encompass half to two-thirds circumference of forearm, remembering that forearm tapers distally.

Refine Pattern

- Proximal border should allow full elbow motion.
- Distal border should allow unimpeded motion of IF to MF MCP joints and full thumb mobility.

Options for Materials

- Consider $1/8$" thermoplastic material to provide needed rigidity to withstand mobilization forces.
- Gel- or foam-lined materials may help decrease distal migration and increase comfort.

Cut and Heat

- Position patient with elbow resting on table and forearm supination for gravity-assisted molding. Thumb should be held in gentle palmar abduction while molding.

- For average adult, thumbhole should be about size of elongated half dollar.
- Distal volar portion of orthosis should clear proximal palmar crease to allow unimpeded MCP flexion.
- Cut out thumbhole in material either by making series of holes with hole punch before heating or by carefully piercing the slightly warm material with sharp scissors.

Evaluate Fit while Molding

- Lay warm material on towel, positioning thumbhole on correct side of material to be placed on forearm.
- Using IFs, gently open hole, making it slightly larger and more elongated (egg shaped).
- Place thumbhole over thumb and guide rest of material evenly along volar wrist and forearm.
- Carefully incorporate arches of hand by using smooth, even strokes and constantly redirecting material into arches.
- Allow for clearance at base of first CMC joint. As thumb abducts in orthosis, base of thumbhole may need to be adjusted.
- Rotate forearm to check for possible abutment of ulnar and radial styloid processes, and flare as necessary.

Strapping and Components

- Distal strap: 1" strap directed from volar to dorsal border.
- Middle strap: 2" strap applied proximal to dorsal wrist crease; use piece of adhesive foam to further stabilize wrist in orthosis and prevent migration. Foam should not overlap orthosis edges.
- Proximal strap: depending on size of forearm, 1" or 2" strap.

- Apply line guides as close to the distal palmar crease as possible (approximately where digits would rest if composite fist were possible).
- Rolyan® Wrap-On Finger Hooks, used as distal attachment device, are shown.
- One or two lines guides per digit can be used. If using one line guide per digit, place in alignment with longitudinal axis of involved digit(s). If using two line guides, place in alignment with web spaces of involved digit(s).
- Line of pull should be directed to the line guide.
- Static line should be approximately triple length of hand; fold in half and guide from sling through line guides.
- Proximally, line is attached to rubber band post via springs.

Survey Completed Orthosis

- Smooth and slightly flare distal and proximal borders.
- Gently flare around thenar hole, especially at base; avoid rolling, which can make future orthosis modifications difficult and can lead to an unnecessarily bulky orthosis.
- Check clearance of elbow, irritation at radial and ulnar styloid processes, and digital MCP motion.
- Adjust tension per patient and/or tissue tolerance; goal is low-load stretch over prolonged period of time.

PATTERN PEARL 8-38 to 8-43.

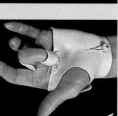

PP8-38 A and B, Hand-based design using rubber band "dynamic" approach, embedded safety pins as line guides, and $1/16$" thermoplastic slings.

PP8-39 Hand-based design using static progressive approach via the Splint-Tuner™ and thermoplastic line guides (North Coast Medical).

PATTERN PEARL 8-38 to 8-43. *continued*

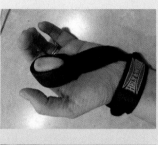

PP8-40

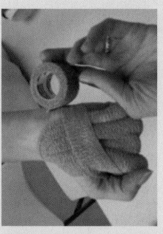
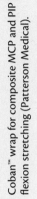

PP8-41

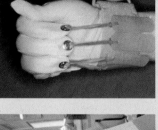
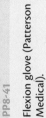

PP8-42

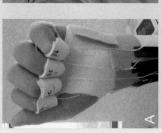

PP8-43

A and B, Hook and loop being used for a static progressive approach with each digit numbered and adjusted individually.

Flexion glove (Patterson Medical).

Coban™ wrap for composite MCP and PIP flexion stretching (Patterson Medical).

Frap Strap® (Patterson Medical) multiuse device can be used to provide composite stretch.

CLINICAL PEARL 8-25.
Simple Strapping to Address Composite Stiffness

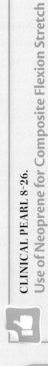

Composite MCP/PIP/DIP flexion mobilization can be initiated following an initial observation of stiffness during external fixation for a distal radium fracture. Shown here is a simple foam strapping system that the patient can apply for a gentle flexion force to tight digits. This patient is not yet a candidate for thermoplastic application.

CLINICAL PEARL 8-26.
Use of Neoprene for Composite Flexion Stretch

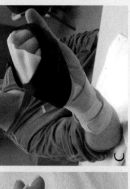

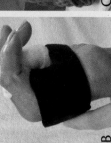

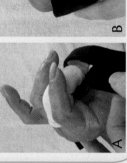

Neoprene can be used effectively to provide a gentle composite force as shown here, status post extensor tenolysis **(A and B)**. Neoprene can also be added to an orthosis base to provide a similar composite flexion stretch while the wrist is stabilized. This orthosis places the wrist in neutral and the MCP joints in maximum passive flexion. Conforming neoprene is used to encompass the distal joints and provide a gentle stretch **(C)** (see Chapter 14 for more instructive detail on the use of neoprene).

Thumb MP and IP Extension Mobilization Orthosis (WHFO) (Fig. 8–23)

Common Names
- Dynamic thumb extension splint
- Extensor pollicis longus (EPL) splint

Alternative Orthosis Options
- Casting (serial static)

Primary Functions
- Provide low-load, prolonged extension mobilization force to thumb MP and IP joints to facilitate lengthening of tissue.

Additional Functions
- Maintain thumb MP and IP joints in extension, allowing restricted flexion within predetermined range, to facilitate tendon healing, tendon glide, and prevent tendon adherence (restriction orthosis).

Common Diagnoses and General Optimal Positions
IP and MP flex contracture   Wr: 20 to 30° ext; CMC: mid rad/palmer abd; MP/IP: terminal ext

CLINICAL PEARL 8-27.
Serial Static Approach for MP and IP Extension

Oftentimes, MCP and IP stiffness is in combination with other injuries. The therapist should consider a serial static approach when faced with multiple injuries. When thumb extension is restricted because of extrinsic flexor shortening, the wrist must be included.

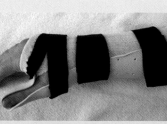
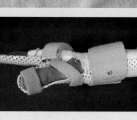

A   B

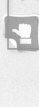

FIGURE 8-24

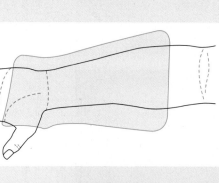

FIGURE 8-23

Fabrication Process (Using Base 2™ Outrigger System)

Pattern Creation (Fig. 8-24)

- Mark for proximal border two-thirds length of forearm.
- Mark distal border, just proximal to dorsal digit and thumb MP joint skinfolds.
- Allow enough material to encompass half to two-thirds circumference of forearm, remembering that forearm tapers distally.

Refine Pattern

- Proximal border should allow full elbow motion.
- Distal border should allow unimpeded motion of digital MCP and thumb MP and IP joints.
- Allow appropriate amount of material radially to provide surface area for component application.

Options for Materials

- Use ⅛" material to provide needed rigidity to maintain wrist joint position and accept extension mobilization force.
- Use components of choice (Base 2™ Outrigger System shown).

Cut and Heat

- Position patient with elbow resting on table and forearm pronated for gravity-assisted molding. Position thumb in abduction and opposition.
- Prepad ulnar styloid with adhesive-backed foam, putty, cotton ball, or silicone gel.

Evaluate Fit while Molding

- Position material on dorsum of involved hand and wrist just proximal to MP joints.

- Make sure desired wrist position is maintained. Some patients tend to flex and deviate wrist while orthosis is being formed.

Strapping and Components

- Thumb strap: apply volarly, allowing MP motion.
- Distal strap: 1" strap connecting distal radial and distal ulnar borders.
- Middle strap: 2" strap just proximal to dorsal wrist crease; use piece of adhesive foam to further stabilize wrist in orthosis and prevent migration. Foam should not overlap orthosis edges.
- Proximal strap: 2" soft or elasticized strap is good choice.
- Attach Base 2™ Outrigger to orthosis base using rubber band posts. Be sure outrigger aligns with thumb column and extends distally in entire length of thumb.

- Apply sling to distal phalanx. Next, thread the monofilament line through line guide on outrigger and secure the mobilization component to proximal attachment device.

Survey Completed Orthosis

- Smooth and slightly flare distal and proximal borders.
- Gently flare around dorsal thumb region; avoid rolling, which can make future orthosis modifications difficult and can lead to an unnecessarily bulky orthosis.
- Check clearance of elbow, radial and ulnar styloid processes and MCP joints.
- Adjust tension per patient and/or tissue tolerance; goal is low-load stretch over prolonged period of time.

MCP Extension Mobilization Orthosis (WHFO) (Fig. 8–25)

Common Names
- Dynamic MCP extension splint

Alternative Orthosis Options
- Preformed adjustable outrigger kits
- Prefabricated orthosis

Primary Functions
- Provide low-load, prolonged extension mobilization force to MCP joints to facilitate lengthening of tissue.
- Passively support MCP joints in extension while allowing active digital flexion.

Common Diagnoses and General Optimal Positions

MCP jt arthroplasty: Wr: 30 to 45° ext; MCP: 0 to 10° flex and slight RD

Extensor tendon repair (zones V to VII)   Wr: 30 to 45° ext; MCP: 0 to 10° flex (th zones IV to V) (if th involved: CMC ext and 45° rad abd)

Radial or posterior interosseous   Wr: 30 to 45° ext, MCP: 0° nerve injury

Extrinsic flexor tightness   Wr: 451°, IP: 0°, MCP: terminal ext

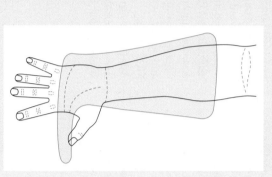

FIGURE 8-26

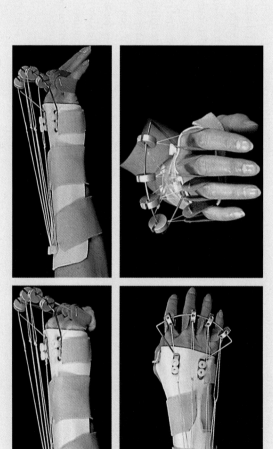

FIGURE 8-25

Fabrication Process (Using Phoenix Outrigger System)

Pattern Creation (Fig. 8–26)

- Mark for proximal border two-thirds length of forearm.
- Mark distal border just distal to dorsal digit MCP joint skinfolds.
- Make radial tab (palmar bar) long enough (approximately 3") to traverse through palm and secure on distal ulnar border.
- Allow enough material to encompass half to two-thirds circumference of forearm, remembering that forearm tapers distally.

Refine Pattern

- Proximal border should allow full elbow motion.
- Extend distal portion of orthosis to MCP head level.

Options for Materials

- Consider ⅛" thermoplastic material to provide needed rigidity to maintain wrist joint position and accept extension mobilization force.

- Use components of choice (Phoenix Outrigger System shown).

Cut and Heat

- Position patient with elbow resting on table and forearm pronated for gravity-assisted molding.
- Prepad ulnar styloid using adhesive-backed foam, putty, cotton ball, or silicone gel.

Evaluate Fit while Molding

- Position material on dorsum of involved hand and wrist just distal to MCP joints.
- Gently pull radial bar through thumb web space and across volar MCPs to meet ulnar segment. Pinch and seal lightly, and return focus to molding dorsum.
- Make sure desired wrist position is maintained. Some patients tend to flex and deviate wrist while orthosis is being formed.

Strapping and Components

- Distal strap: 1" strap connecting distal radial and distal ulnar borders (if needed).
- Middle strap: 2" strap just proximal to wrist crease; use piece of adhesive foam to further stabilize wrist in orthosis and prevent migration. Foam should not overlap orthosis edges.
- Proximal strap: 2" soft or elasticized strap.
- Mark desired outrigger attachment, positioning to extend distally over middle portion of proximal phalanx and extending high enough that when volar sling is attached to monofilament line, it clears pulley.
- Use rubber band posts to secure outrigger on orthosis.
- Attach Phoenix wheels to outrigger using Allen wrench.
- Attach line on both sides of sling, apply sling to middle phalanx, and thread line through Phoenix wheels.

- Loop appropriate rubber band onto end of monofilament line, and connect to proximal attachment device.

Survey Completed Orthosis

- Material should be flared distally to prevent irritation of MCP heads during flexion exercises; if necessary, use layer of thin padding to increase patient comfort.
- Check that mobilization force is strong enough to support and return MCP joints to desired position after active digital flexion.
- Check that mobilization force is not too strong, impeding patient's ability to flex digits in the desired amount.
- Instruct patient to monitor for signs of increased pressure over ulnar styloid and radial and ulnar sensory nerve branches.
- Consider padding of the radial styloid and Lister's tubercle, especially for patients with frail skin such as those with rheumatoid arthritis.

PATTERN PEARL 8-44 to 8-19.

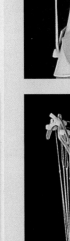
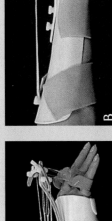
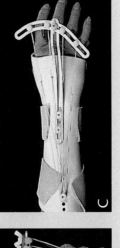
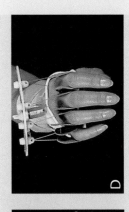

A–D, Digitec Outrigger System (Patterson Medical).

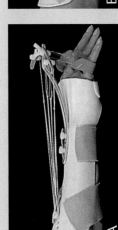

PP8-44

CHAPTER 8

PATTERN PEARL 8-14 to 8-19. *continued*

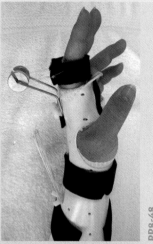

PP8-45

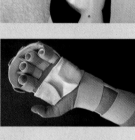

PP8-46

A

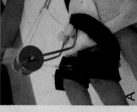

PP8-47

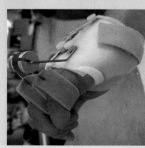

PP8-48

Hand-based design: Phoenix Outrigger System (Patterson Medical) for RF and SF.

A and B, Hand-based design: Phoenix Outrigger System (Patterson Medical) for IF and MF only. Notice slight radial deviation pull used post-MCP arthroplasty.

Static progressive approach for simultaneous MCP/PIP/DIP extension.

Volar MCP flexion block can be incorporated into the base design.

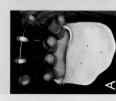

A

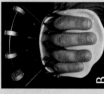
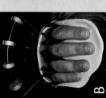

B

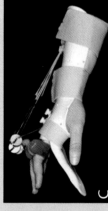

C

PP8-49

A–C, MCP flexion block secured as separate removable segment.

CLINICAL PEARL 8-28.
PIP/DIP Extension Orthoses/Cast with MCP Extension Mobilization Orthosis

A PIP/DIP extension mobilization orthosis or cast can be slipped under the slings of an MCP extension mobilization orthosis to prevent or address concurrent PIP flexion contractures. These orthoses can be worn periodically throughout the day as an exercise tool to stretch tight IP joints or to isolate/facilitate MCP flexion with exercise. Commonly, the SF can have difficulty with isolating MCP flexion; this technique of using a cast can be especially helpful with addressing this often problematic digit. Shown is QuickCast 2 (Patterson Medical).

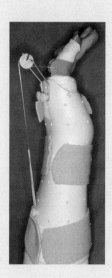

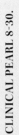

CLINICAL PEARL 8-30.
IF Radial Outrigger to Prevent Pronation and Ulnar Deviation

An IF outrigger attachment is most often found in combination with an MCP extension mobilization orthosis for patients who have undergone MCP joint arthroplasty involving reconstruction of the IF radial collateral ligament. Consider applying an ulnarly positioned dress hook (with gel-based glue) or a piece of hook material to the fingernail. If using the dress hook, attach a thin strip of loop material (via a hole) directed ulnarly, crossing the volar aspect of the fingertip. Fasten a thin rubber band to the other end and attach it to the radial outrigger. If using adhesive hook material glued to the nail, place a thin strip of loop directed as described for the dress hook. This should provide a gentle radial deviation and supination force to the IF. Note: If pronation is not an issue, a sling can be applied to the digit directed radially.

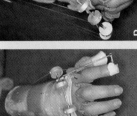
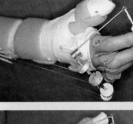

CLINICAL PEARL 8-29.
Modification of Small Finger Sling

Oftentimes, the SF sling needs to be customized for the short proximal phalanx; notice sling shown is too wide, limiting PIP flexion (**A**). Trim the width of the sling to the appropriate length, allowing for unrestricted MCP and PIP motion (**B**). The length may also need to be modified accordingly. Also, commonly when using this orthosis for exercise following an MCP joint arthroplasty, using a separate elastic of very light tension or releasing the tension completely for exercise is necessary to allow for the desired amount of MCP flexion. When the digit is at rest, the elastic must not be so tight that the MCP is held in hyperextension. (**C**) Take caution to avoid this by having the patient bring the orthosis into the clinic for therapy sessions to check these joint angles.

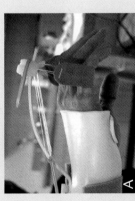
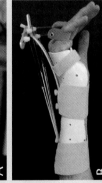
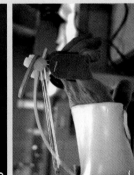
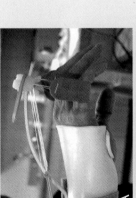
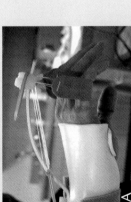
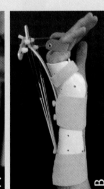
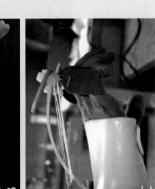

CHAPTER 8

PIP Intra-articular Mobilization Orthosis (WHFO)

Common Names

- Dynamic traction splint
- Schenck splint
- Hoop splint

Alternative Orthosis Options

- Swing Design Dynamic Traction[4]

Primary Functions

- Provide gentle, controlled distal distraction to involved PIP joint to reduce articular fragments and realign joint surfaces.

(Fig. 8–27)[3]

Common Diagnoses and General Optimal Positions

- Note: Direction of distal traction, tension on rubber band, and passive arc of flexion and extension are set by the surgeon in the operating room. Any alteration to these placements should be discussed with the surgeon. This orthosis can be modified to accommodate intra-articular MCP and thumb MP/IP joint injuries (Kearney & Brown, 1994; Schenck, 1986, 1994).
- Pilon fracture of PIP
- Fracture dislocation of PIP
- Severe fracture of grade 3 or 4; grade 2 if combined with subluxation or dislocation
- Condylar fracture
- Oblique or spiral phalangeal shaft fracture

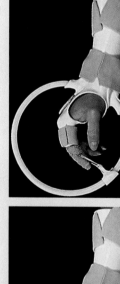

FIGURE 8-27

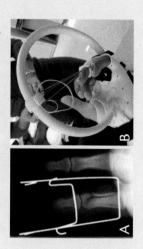

CLINICAL PEARL 8-31.
Adjusting Tension of Intra-articular Dynamic Traction Orthosis

Rubber bands play a significant role in this orthosis design for the treatment of intra-articular fractures of the digit(s). Over time, rubber bands will lose some of their elasticity when under tension. A selection of rubber bands, each of which generates slightly different degrees of tension, should be sent with the patient to each medical doctor (MD) visit **(A)**. Most often, the digit is x-rayed weekly with the rubber bands in place to confirm proper tension **(B)**. Having rubber bands accessible of varying tensions can give the MD options to correct forces, ensuring proper fracture alignment with the goal of preserving articular symmetry and space. If too much tension is generated through the fracture, the space will fill in with scar. Too little tension will be ineffective in maintaining fracture alignment.

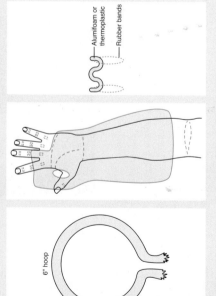

FIGURE 8-28

[3]Developed by Robert Schenck, MD; Laura Kearney, OTR/L, CHT; and Krista Brown, OTR/L, CHT. Schenck, R. R. (1986). Dynamic traction and early passive movement for fractures of the proximal interphalangeal joint. *Journal of Hand Surgery (American), 11*(6), 850–858.

[4]Designed by Griet Van Veldhoven, modified by Kadelbach, D. (2006). Swing design dynamic traction splinting for the treatment of intra-articular fractures of the digits. *Journal of Hand Therapy, 19*(1), 39–42.

Fabrication Process

Pattern Creation (Fig. 8–28)

- Orthosis should be fabricated preoperatively or in operating room as physician places wire.
- Choose appropriate base pattern for digit.
  - IF or MF (A): radial wrist extension and MCP flexion immobilization orthosis
  - RF or SF (B): ulnar wrist extension and MCP flexion immobilization orthosis
  - Thumb: wrist and thumb MP immobilization orthosis or wrist immobilization orthosis
- Fabricate 6″ hoop or partial hoop.

Refine Pattern

- Make sure wrist is extended approximately 30°, and MCP joints are flexed to approximately 60°.

- Orthosis can encompass bordering digit for maximal orthosis stabilization if necessary. Do not interfere with motion of uninvolved digits.
- Clear PIP flexion crease proximally.

Options for Materials

- Use 3/32″ or 1/8″ material.
- Hoop can be made from rolled thermoplastic material or wide Aquatubes®.

Cut and Heat

- Prepare hoop by warming material around 6″ cylindrical form (e.g., 5-lb therapy putty container), leaving about 1″ extension on each end for attachment onto orthosis base.
- Position patient with forearm in neutral and digits slightly abducted.

Evaluate Fit while Molding

- Fabricate appropriate ulnar or radial wrist extension and MCP flexion immobilization orthosis.

- Clear distally to allow unimpeded PIP flexion.

Strapping and Components

- Attach hoop to orthosis so involved joint is equidistant from hoop; align longitudinally with involved digit.
- Fabricate movable component with either thermoplastic material or AlumaFoam® (see pattern).
- Apply rubber band traction (no. 19) or spring coils to interosseous wire and measure tension so it applies approximately 300 g of force. Mark flexion and extension limits (as set by physician) on hoop with tape or marker.

- Strap orthosis base at orthosis's distal border, wrist crease, and proximal orthosis border.
- Apply 1/2″ strap about proximal phalanx.

Survey Completed Orthosis

- Carefully instruct patient on use of orthosis. Generally, patients should alternate between positions of flexion and extension. Beginning on first day of orthosis application, patient should change positions every 10 minutes while awake. When sleeping, rubber bands should be placed midway between flexion and extension. Orthosis should be worn for 6 to 8 weeks (Schenck, 1994).

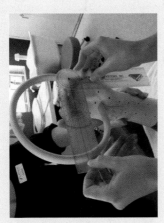

CLINICAL PEARL 8-32.
Measuring Tension of Intra-articular Dynamic Traction Orthosis

Use a goniometer or ruler to ensure equidistance from the horizontal wire on the middle phalanx to the hoop. This needs to be measured throughout the requested ROM to ensure that the traction force is applied at a constant level to the healing fracture.

PATTERN PEARL 8-50 to 8-52.

PP8-50   PP8-51   PP8-52

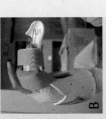

Hoop, in this case, was positioned on dorsum of the hand and volar wrist.

Creative use of Digitec Outrigger (Patterson Medical) as a lower profile option for dynamic traction.

A and B, Alternative dynamic traction treatment of an intra-articular PIP joint fracture.

4 **Arm-Based Orthoses**

Supination and Pronation Mobilization Orthosis (EWHO) (Fig. 8–29)[5]

Common Names
- Forearm rotation splint
- Static progressive or dynamic supination/pronation splint

Alternative Orthosis Options
- Dynamic supination–pronation orthosis[5]
- Cast (serial static)
- Tone and positioning (TAP) orthosis

- MERiT™ SPS forearm rotation kit
- Dynamic/static progressive orthosis
- Neoprene and thermoplastic combination orthosis (Chapter 14)

Primary Functions
- Provide low-load, prolonged rotation mobilization force to proximal and distal radioulnar joints to facilitate lengthening of tissue.

Common Diagnoses and Optimal Positions
Sup or pro contracture   Elb: 90°; wr: 0–10 degrees extension (comfortable wrist position)

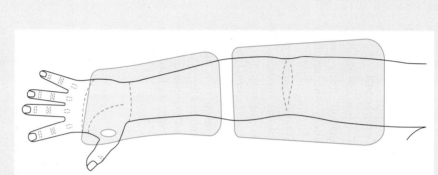

FIGURE 8-30

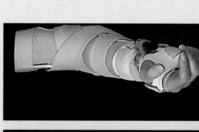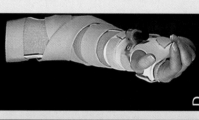
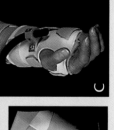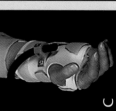
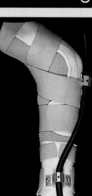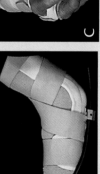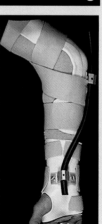

FIGURE 8-29 **A and C,** Supination. **B and D,** Pronation.

[5]Designed by Kay Collelo-Abraham.

Fabrication Process (Using Rolyan® Pronation/Supination Kit)

Pattern Creation (Fig. 8–30)

Proximal orthosis

- Fabricate orthosis per posterior elbow immobilization orthosis design.
- Orthosis should extend distally approximately 5" along ulnar border.

Distal orthosis

- Fabricate orthosis per volar wrist immobilization orthosis design.
- Orthosis should extend proximally, leaving approximately 1" of space between proximal and distal orthosis, which should not overlap.

Refine Pattern

- Be sure to allow for clearance of MCPs and thumb.
- Proximal orthosis border should allow full shoulder movement.

Options for Materials

- Use either perforated or nonperforated ⅛" materials.
- Lightweight materials may not provide rigid support necessary for length and width of this orthosis.

Cut and Heat

- Position each orthosis as described for the individual orthosis.
- Heat and cut materials accordingly.

Evaluate Fit while Molding

- Mold dorsal elbow orthosis in 90° of elbow flexion and as close to neutral forearm rotation as possible.
- Check for clearance of medial and lateral epicondyles.
- Fabricate volar wrist immobilization orthosis, making sure to clear ulnar and radial styloids.

Strapping and Components

- Mark for housing units as described here; then apply straps so they do not interfere with cable.
- Using screws, apply two metal housing components, oriented transversely, on midportion of posterior elbow orthosis (just below olecranon) and on midportion of wrist orthosis.
- Large cable is set into proximal and distal housing units; distal end of tube is set in with Allen wrench and secured.
- For supination, cable is run from volar aspect of wrist around radial border to lateral elbow area and terminates in proximal housing unit on elbow orthosis (A and B).
- For pronation, cable is run from volar wrist around ulnar aspect of forearm to medial aspect of elbow and terminates on proximal housing unit of elbow orthosis (C and D).

- Twisting cable in opposite direction of desired motion controls force.
- Cut excess cable.
- Instruct patient in wearing schedule, donning and doffing techniques, and self-adjustments.
- Adjust tension as tissue accommodates.

Survey Completed Orthosis

- Line length of proximal and distal orthosis as well as proximal and distal borders with nonskid material; this greatly decreases orthosis migration. Consider Microfoam™ tape, adhesive Dycem, or adhesive silicone gel sheets.
- Check for clearance of ulnar styloid and epicondyles.
- Check for pressure on radial sensory nerve with supination design; cable may apply pressure directly over this area.

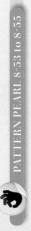

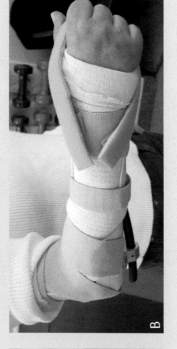

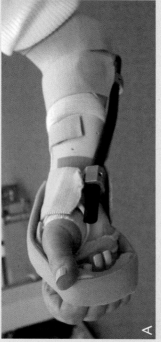

PP8-53

A and B, Additional soft strap applied for gentle digital flexion stretch.

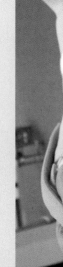

PP8-54

Comfort Cool® Spiral Arm Splint (Photo courtesy of North Coast Medical).

CLINICAL PEARL 8-33.
Combination Neoprene and Thermoplastic Forearm Rotation Orthosis

Distal wrist stabilization with addition of a neoprene wrap can provide a "dynamic" rotation mobilization force. **A,** Wrist immobilization with neoprene strapping wrapped in the direction of pronation. **B,** Wrist and thumb immobilization with a supination mobilizing force.

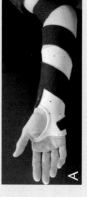
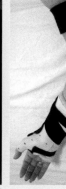
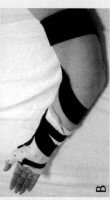

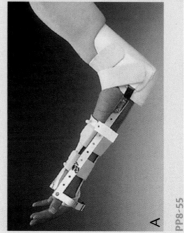

PP8-55

A and B, MERiT™ Static Progressive Forearm Rotation Orthosis Kit (Patterson Medical).

Elbow Flexion Mobilization Orthosis (EO) (Fig. 8-31)

Common Names

- Dynamic elbow flexion splint
- Static progressive elbow splint

Alternative Orthosis Options

- Prefabricated elbow flexion/extension kits
- Dynamic/static progressive orthoses

Primary Functions

- Provide low-load, prolonged flexion mobilization force to elbow joint to facilitate lengthening of tissue.

Additional Functions

- Restrict full elbow extension or flexion.
- Restrict or prevent forearm rotation.
- Minimize medial or lateral stress at elbow.

Common Diagnoses and General Optimal Positions

Elb ext contracture   Terminal elb flexion

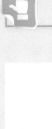

CLINICAL PEARL 8-34.
Clearance of Elbow Flexion Crease

During the fitting process, be sure to clear for unrestricted elbow flexion; note the pinching of soft tissue when flexion is attempted here. Simply trimming the volar edges of the two segments can fix this issue. Also, be sure to minimize orthosis migration by taking advantage of friction force: placing proximal cuff directly against the skin or apply strips of Microfoam™ tape within this segment.

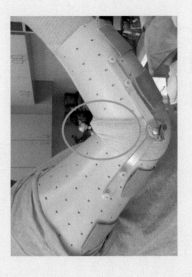

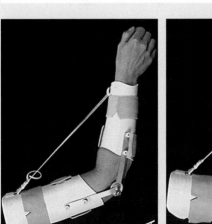

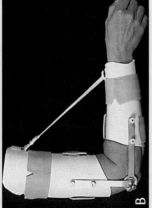

FIGURE 8-31

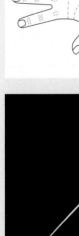

FIGURE 8-32

Fabrication Process (Using Phoenix Elbow Hinge)

Pattern Creation (Fig. 8–32)

- Proximal orthosis
  - Fabricate nonarticular humerus orthosis.
- Distal orthosis
  - Fabricate nonarticular forearm orthosis.
  - If hand is extremely edematous, painful, arthritic, or weak, consider incorporating wrist in forearm orthosis.
  - If forearm rotation needs to be controlled, include wrist in forearm design.

Refine Pattern

- Proximal orthosis borders should allow full shoulder motion and unimpeded elbow motion.
- Distal orthosis borders should allow unimpeded elbow and wrist motion.
- Check for irritation at epicondyles, olecranon, axilla, ulnar nerve (cubital tunnel), median nerve (wrist), ulnar styloid, and radial sensory nerve.

Options for Materials

- Use coated material so circumferential overlapped section can be popped open without permanent sealing.
- Remember that elastic materials tend to shrink around orthosis part; do not remove until orthosis is completely set.
- Use material that has some degree of flexibility when set (slightly perforated ⅛″ and ³⁄₃₂″ materials); important because orthoses need to give slightly when removed for hygiene and guarded exercise (if appropriate).

Cut and Heat

- When molding distal orthosis, make certain that forearm is in desired amount of forearm rotation.

Evaluate Fit while Molding

- Once both orthoses are formed, mark for hinge placement; align center (axis) of hinge with axis of rotation at elbow joint.
- Line inside of orthosis opening with moleskin as described in orthosis pattern; consider using lining over border of axilla region for comfort.

Strapping and Components

- Plan and attach hinge before securing straps.
- D-ring straps work well because of ease of application.
- Direct straps so they secure on medial aspect of arm; may be applied over hinge arms.
- With both orthoses on and forearm in desired amount of rotation and elbow in flexion, line up axis of hinge with elbow joint and mark specific placement of hinge arms.
- Remove orthoses and attach hinge to proximal and distal orthoses using rubber band posts.
- Form hook with scrap material and attach to distal third of distal orthosis.
- Attach D-ring to proximal third of proximal orthosis.
- Apply elastic cord to attachment devices.

Survey Completed Orthosis

- Consider a trial use in clinic because adjustments are frequently necessary.
- Make certain that lines of pull are appropriate for diagnosis (e.g., supina-

tion and flexion common for biceps repair, not pronation and flexion).
- Check for unwanted stress on collateral ligaments of elbow.
- Make sure orthosis allows clearance at elbow; there may be potential for abutment of distal and proximal orthosis segments as flexion increases, causing compression of skin in flexion crease and possible pressure areas. May need to trim distal border of proximal orthosis as flexion increases.
- Proximal portion of orthosis may migrate distally as tension is applied. Consider lining orthosis with adhesive Dycem, adhesive silicone gel, Microfoam™ tape, or foam. If this does not help, application of shoulder harness may be necessary. Adjust tension per patient and/or tissue tolerance; goal is low-load stretch over prolonged period of time.

Discussion Points Questions

1. What are the three types of mobilization orthoses?

2. Give an example of each type of mobilization orthosis including the rationale for use.

3. Explain what the appropriate angle of application should be and why this is important. Include the harmful effects if application is not correct.

4. Given the diagnosis of a PIP flexion contracture; what are the choices for mobilization? Why would you choose one over the other?

5. Name a minimum of three types of;
   - proximal attachments devices
   - elastic force applications
   - slings
   - line guides

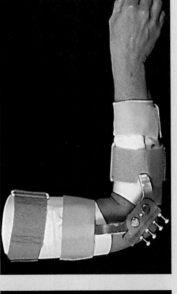

PP8-56

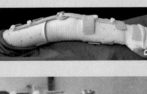

B

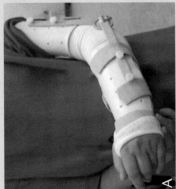

A

A and B, Modification of design to protect collateral ligament(s) of elbow; use of radial wrist orthosis to restrict forearm rotation

PP8-57   Rolyan® Adjustable Hinge (Patterson Medical).

CLINICAL PEARL 8-35.
Neoprene for Creative Wrist and Elbow Mobilization

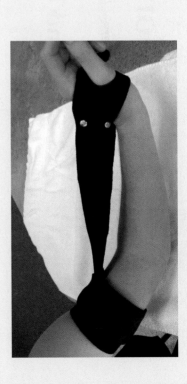

Neoprene was used in this orthosis as a creative alternative for combined elbow and wrist stiffness. The soft contouring nature of the neoprene material joined with the gentle "dynamic" force it generates when stretched offers the therapist a versatile option. See Chapter 14 for additional information on using neoprene.

CLINICAL PEARL 8-36.
Proper Hinge Placement

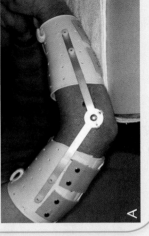

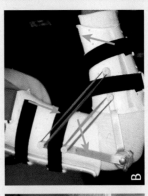

B

A

Center of elbow hinge must be placed at elbow's axis of rotation **(A).** Improper placement of hinge can lead to abnormal forces on the joint and shifting of the thermoplastic material on the body segment as noted here **(B).**

CHAPTER 8

Restriction Orthoses

9

1 Digit- and Thumb-Based Orthoses

Proximal Interphalangeal (PIP) Extension Restriction Orthosis (FO) (Fig. 9–1)

Common Names
- Anti–swan-neck splint
- Figure-8 splint
- PIP hyperextension block splint

Alternative Orthosis Options
- Buttonhole orthosis
- Ring-designed orthoses
- Taping

Primary Functions
- Maximize functional use of digit by preventing PIP joint hyperextension while allowing PIP flexion.

Common Diagnoses and General Optimal Positions

Swan-neck deformity	PIP: slight flex
PIP volar plate injury	PIP: 10 to 30° flex
PIP dorsal dislocation	PIP: 15 to 30° flex (depends on severity)

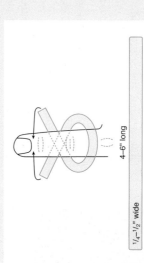

1/4–1/2" wide   4–6" long

FIGURE 9-2

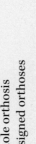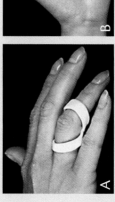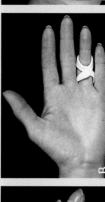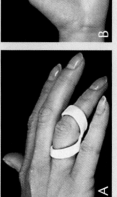

A   B   C

FIGURE 9-1

Fabrication Process

Pattern Creation (Fig. 9–2)

- Thermoplastic material for this orthosis should be approximately 4" long and ¼" to ½" wide when folded.

Refine Pattern

- The width of the material should be judged by the size of the digit; the larger the digit, the wider the strip of material.

Options for Materials

- Use thin (³⁄₃₂" or ¹⁄₁₆") elastic-based material; the memory characteristic allows for excellent contouring and intimate fit.

- Plan to overlap and/or roll material to increase strength.
- Medium to thin Aquatubes® (Patterson Medical) (flattened out) provide another option; size depends on strength required and size of digit.
- The wider the dorsal segment, the more evenly distributed the pressure and the more comfortable the fit.

Cut and Heat

- Consider placing light layer of lotion on the digit before molding to ease removal of the orthosis.

Evaluate Fit while Molding

- Center strip on middle of proximal phalanx dorsally.

- Wrap both ends volarly around to PIP joint crease (clearing the flexion crease), returning dorsally onto the middle phalanx, ending dorsally.
- Cut and pinch ends so they overlap; smooth.
- While material is setting, position PIP joint in desired amount of flexion by gently providing pressure over volar crossed segment; make sure two dorsal ring pieces are contoured well around phalanges.
- Position dorsal segments close to metacarpophalangeal (MP) and distal interphalangeal (DIP) joints to maximize leverage and improve orthosis effectiveness.

Strapping and Components

- No strapping required.

Survey Completed Orthosis

- Remove orthosis from patient and prepare overlapped pieces with solvent, spot heat and bend.
- Carefully spot heat volar crossed segment with heat gun to secure adherence and smooth edges.
- If DIP or PIP joints are enlarged owing to trauma or arthritis, gently flare rings laterally to allow extra space for removal.

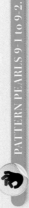

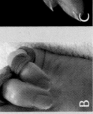
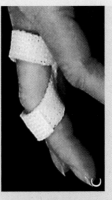
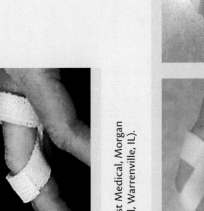

PATTERN PEARLS 9-1 to 9-2.

PP9-1

Casting tapes: **A and B,** Orficast™ (North Coast Medical, Morgan Hill, CA) or **(C)** QuickCast (Patterson Medical, Warrenville, IL).

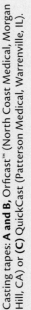
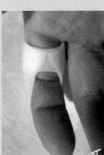
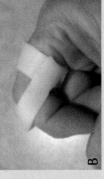
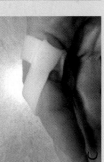
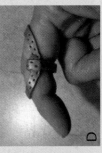
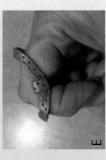

PP9-2

A–C, Ring around proximal phalanx with dorsal block. **D and E,** Lateral ring with volar strip support.

PATTERN PEARL 9-2 to 9-5. *continued*

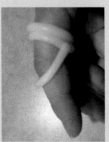

PP9-3

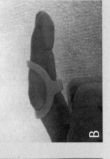

A

PP9-4

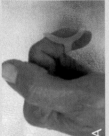

B

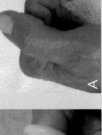

C

PP9-5

Rolyan® Aquatubes® (Patterson Medical).

A–C, Oval-8® Finger Splints (3-Point Products, Stevensville, MD).

Silver Ring™ Splints (Silver Ring Splint Company, Charlottesville, VA).

CLINICAL PEARL 9-1.
Buttonhole PIP Extension Restriction Orthosis

The buttonhole design is another option for the PIP extension restriction orthosis. This design can be more challenging to fabricate than the Figure-8 design. Remember that the degree of restriction for PIP extension depends on the diagnosis.

Use thin (³⁄₃₂″ or ¹⁄₁₆″) elastic material because its memory characteristic allows for a contoured intimate fit. Cut out the pattern on a scrap piece of thermoplastic material (approximately 2″ by 1″ piece). Prior to heating, make the slits with the widest setting on a hole punch. Once material is heated, be careful not to overstretch; gently feed the material onto finger through both holes, orienting the proximal orthosis border on the dorsum of the proximal phalanx, the middle section volar, and the distal orthosis border on the dorsal surface of the middle phalanx.

Position the PIP joint in the desired amount of flexion and fold the lateral orthosis pieces onto themselves to minimize bulk in this area. Overlap any excess volar material onto the volar PIP piece to allow PIP joint flexion. Once set, remove the orthosis from the finger and smooth the edges, especially at the volar portion of the orthosis.

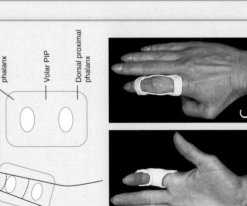

Dorsal middle phalanx

Volar PIP

Dorsal proximal phalanx

A

B

C

D

CLINICAL PEARL 9-2.
Thumb MP Extension Restriction Orthosis

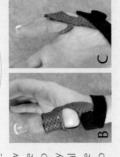

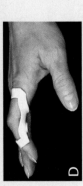

A

B

C

This orthosis is extremely effective for managing instability of the thumb MP joint and a tendency to posture in MP hyperextension while writing or engaging in activities requiring opposition. If left untreated, over time, the CMC joint may become unstable, resulting in pain and metacarpal subluxation. To fabricate this orthosis, use a ¹⁄₁₆″ material, measuring the length from the crease of the dorsal thumb interphalangeal (IP) to just distal to the radial wrist crease. Allow the width to be approximately ¼″ wider on each side of the thumb metacarpal and phalanx (see pattern). Create two slits horizontally in the center of the material approximately ¼″ to ½″ apart, leaving the ¼″ on each side. The material between the slits will form a "sling" that will rest across the volar thumb MP crease, supporting the 1st metacarpal into gentle extension.

Heat material, then, working quickly, begin to feed the widest piece onto the dorsum of the metacarpal followed by gently pulling down on the material between the two slits that have formed the sling and feeding it directly under the most distal portion of the metacarpal head (volar MP crease). The distal portion will rest on the dorsum of the proximal phalanx. Once the material is fully set, position the MP joint in the desired amount of flexion, making sure that there is adequate counter pressure on the first metacarpal (dorsal-oriented pressure from the volar sling and volar-directed pressure from both the proximal and distal dorsal segments).

CLINICAL PEARL 9-3.
Thumb MP and IP Extension Restriction Orthosis

The pattern for the thumb MP extension restriction orthosis can be modified slightly to include flexion of the IP joint for added stability. The pattern just needs to be lengthened approximately 1" distally.

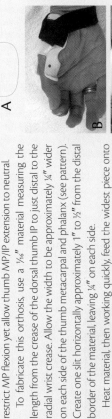

CLINICAL PEARL 9-5.
Dorsal PIP Extension Restriction Orthosis

Restriction of full PIP joint extension may be required to allow adequate healing of structures such as the volar plate. The dorsal orthosis is fabricated in much the same way as the dorsal PIP immobilization orthosis (see Chapter 7), except for positioning the PIP joint in the desired amount of flexion. Once the proximal strap is secured, the distal strap can be periodically removed to allow active-restricted (to the limit of the dorsal block) flexion and extension exercises of the PIP joint if appropriate. Early motion can help prevent capsular tightness and allow tendon gliding.

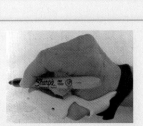

A

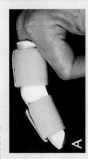

B

CLINICAL PEARL 9-7.
Spiral Design for Digit Extension/Flexion Restriction Orthosis

This spiral design is fabricated with a strip of 1⁄16" material. In this case, the design is used intermittently for lateral stabilization and guarded motion post-PIP joint arthroplasty (6 weeks). Note the use of plastic wrap for edema control and as an orthosis liner.

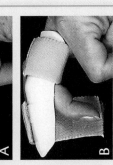

A

B

CLINICAL PEARL 9-4.
Thumb MP Flexion Restriction Orthosis

Chronic thumb MP flexion can lead to a boutonniere-type deformity with progressing pain along the thumb column. This is often seen in massage therapists and in individuals who use their thumbs in daily work tasks. This small design can be used during work to restrict MP flexion yet allow thumb MP/IP extension to neutral.

To fabricate this orthosis, use a 1⁄16" material measuring the length from the crease of the dorsal thumb IP to just distal to the radial wrist crease. Allow the width to be approximately 1⁄4" wider on each side of the thumb metacarpal and phalanx (see pattern). Create one slit horizontally approximately 1" to 1⁄2" from the distal border of the material, leaving 1⁄4" on each side.

Heat material, then working quickly, feed the widest piece onto the dorsum of the metacarpal followed by gently pulling down on the slit to form a volar "pan" for the proximal phalanx to rest in. Once the material is set in place, place the MP joint in the desired amount of extension, making sure there is adequate counter pressure on the proximal phalanx (dorsal-oriented pressure) and the first metacarpal (volar-oriented pressure).

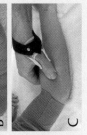

A

B

C

CLINICAL PEARL 9-6.
Volar PIP Flexion Restriction Orthosis

The volar orthosis can be used as part of a specific extensor tendon protocol to limit a particular range of PIP joint flexion when treating zones III and IV injuries. The orthosis allows early-protected motion to promote gliding of the injured or repaired extensor mechanism. The volar orthosis is fabricated in the same way as a volar PIP immobilization orthosis, except for positioning the PIP joint in the desired amount of maximum flexion (see Chapter 7). The orthosis is secured with a single proximal strap because it is generally used only for exercise sessions. The patient may flex the PIP joint to the limits of the volar block and actively extend to neutral. The orthosis can be modified weekly as the healing progresses (see Chapter 18 for further details). The patient is immobilized in PIP extension between exercise sessions. Note: This protocol requires specific patient selection and physician's approval; the therapist must have a full understanding of the theoretical basis behind any particular protocol before implementing it.

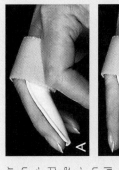

A

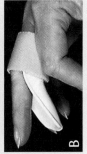

B

CHAPTER 9

2 Hand-Based Orthoses

MCP Extension Restriction Orthosis (HFO) (Fig. 9–3)

Common Names

- Lumbrical blocking splint
- Anticlaw splint
- Ulnar nerve splint
- MCP blocking splint
- Figure-8 MCP blocking splint

Alternative Orthosis Options

- Prefabricated orthoses: (spring coil, Figure-8 designs)
- Dynamic MCP flexion orthosis
- Immobilization orthosis

Primary Functions

- Maximize functional use of hand by preventing MCP joint hyperextension while allowing MCP flexion for grasp.

Additional Functions

- Prevent MCP collateral ligament tightness.
- Facilitate PIP extension.

Common Diagnoses and General Optimal Positions

Low-lesion ulnar nerve injury	ring finger (RF) and small finger (SF) MCPs: 45 to 75° flex
Combined ulnar and median nerve lesion	index finger (IF) to SF MCPs: 45 to 75° flex

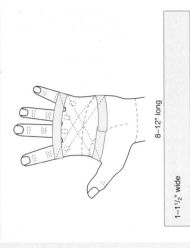

8–12" long

1–1½" wide

FIGURE 9-4

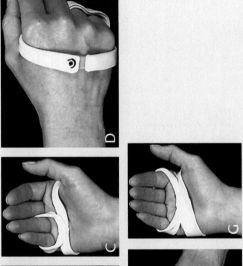

FIGURE 9-3

Fabrication Process

Pattern Creation (Fig. 9–4)

- Depending on combination of nerve injury, fabricate orthosis to include two to four MCP joints (ulnar nerve: RF and SF; median and ulnar nerves: IF to SF).
- Thermoplastic material should be 8″ to 12″ long and 1″ to 1½″ wide.

Refine Pattern

- Width of material depends on size of hand.

Options for Materials

- Use thin (3⁄32″ or 1⁄16″) elastic materials; memory characteristic allows for excellent contouring and intimate fit.
- When using elastic materials (recommended for the novice fabricator), constantly mold and redirect material over dorsum of metacarpal heads and proximal phalanges until material sets.
- If the clinician is experienced with the use of thermoplastic materials, consider the use of plastic-based materials; they tend to allow for the effective use of gravity to contour between digits, forming comfortable troughs over proximal phalanges.
- Rolled thermoplastic or Aquatubes® are not recommended; surface area in contact with skin is not wide enough to provide well-molded orthosis with adequate pressure distribution in most cases.
- Allow enough material to encompass minimum of one-third length of proximal phalanxes; the wider the dorsal segments, the more evenly distributed the pressure and the more comfortable the fit.

Cut and Heat

- Position patient with elbow resting on table, wrist extended, in an intrinsic plus position: MCPs flexed and IPs extended (patient may need to help position using unaffected hand).
- Warm material thoroughly.

Evaluate Fit while Molding

- Be sure to accommodate for natural descent of MCPs; in fist, SF MCP is lower than RF MCP, which is lower than middle finger (MF) MCP.
- Drape material centrally over middle of proximal phalanges, gently contouring material between digits; there should be an equal length of material draped on each side.
- Cross two draping pieces over each other on volar surface at distal palmar crease level.
- Press and flatten out intersection of two crossed pieces, forming less bulky bar. Constantly work material in palm to provide needed volar support for arches.
- Position remainder of pieces: one through radial web space and other over midulnar border; pinch together dorsally.
- While material is still warm, pull down and overlap excess material on ulnar SF MCP and radial RF (or IF MCP) areas to allow unimpeded MCP flexion.

Strapping and Components

- None, unless there is significant atrophy.
- Many patients with long-standing ulnar nerve injury have significant atrophy of first web space and hypothenar eminence, which may make it difficult to remove the orthosis. Pop open orthosis dorsally and apply straps to ease donning and doffing. (Orthosis shown has riveted strap.)

Survey Completed Orthosis

- Cut pinched dorsal piece, prepare surfaces with orthosis solvent, and spot heat to form permanent seal.
- If necessary, prepare surfaces and spot heat volar overlapped portion to adhere pieces together securely.
- May line dorsal bars with very thin adhesive silicone gel or wrap with Coban™ to help prevent orthosis migration during functional use and improve comfort.

PATTERN PEARL 9-6 to 9-11.

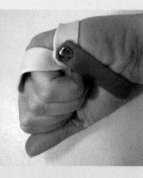
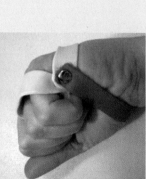

PP9-6

To accommodate hand atrophy, create dorsal opening with flap from lining material on each end to avoid "pinching" skin during closure.

PP9-7

A–D, Neoprene design for subtle clawing allows light restriction of MCP extension with full flexion.

PP9-8

Anchoring orthosis around wrist assists in preventing migration during active use.

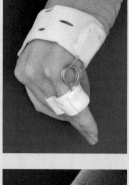

PP9-9

A–C, Rolyan® Aquatubes® (Patterson Medical).

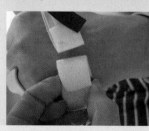
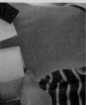
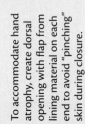

PP9-10

Knuckle Bender Splint (Patterson Medical).

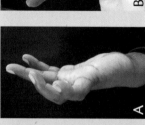
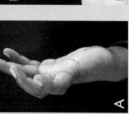

PP9-11

Spring coil design (Orfit Industries, Jericho, NY).

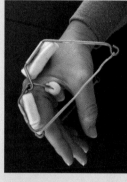

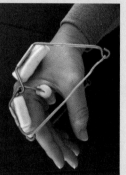

CLINICAL PEARL 9-8.
MCP Extension Restriction Orthosis with Thumb Included

With combined median and ulnar nerve injuries, the thumb is unable to abduct out of the palm because of the loss of thenar muscles, causing interference with functional use. A simple thumb abduction component can be incorporated into the MCP extension restriction orthosis to position the thumb in a functional position midway between palmar and radial abduction. The pattern is basically the same as described for the MCP extension restriction orthosis.

Heat a 12" by 1" piece of thermoplastic material. (Width depends on size of hand.) Place the thumb in the desired position (patient needs to position using unaffected hand.) Drape the material over the proximal phalanges as described, except provide the ulnar portion with 3" to 4" of additional material.

Working quickly, cross the ulnar strip radially across the palm; then guide it dorsally around the thumb MP joint, traversing back through the first web space onto the dorsum of the hand. Next, pull the radial strip ulnarward across the palm to join the strip on the ulnar dorsum of the hand. Finish as described for the MCP extension restriction orthosis. Hook and loop can be used to secure the closure and allow for easy donning and doffing. Note that the overlapped areas may need to be warmed with a heat gun to maximize adherence and minimize orthosis bulk within the first web space. This orthosis is stabilized onto the hand using a figure 8 strap closure. **(A)** Digit extension. **(B)** Digit flexion. **(C)** Volar view, note clearance of thumb MP crease.

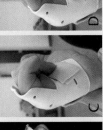
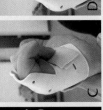
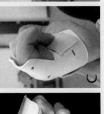
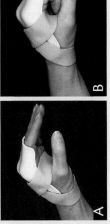

CLINICAL PEARL 9-9.
Dorsal MCP Extension Restriction Orthosis

This dorsal design provides coverage of a wider surface area maximizing pressure distribution. For some patients who have increased digital extensor tone or severe MCP extension deformity, this may be the orthosis of choice. The additional material provides greater pressure distribution, and the open volar aspect allows digital flexion. The thumb can easily be incorporated, if desired **(A and B)**. Stable proximal phalanx fractures can sometimes be managed with fabrication of a restriction orthosis as shown here **(C and D)**.

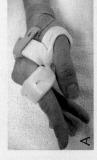
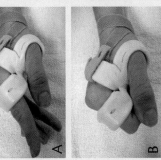
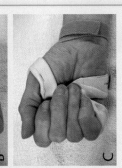
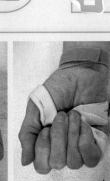

CLINICAL PEARL 9-10.
Hand-Based Digit Extension Restriction Orthosis

Restriction of full MCP, PIP, and DIP joint extension may be required to allow adequate healing of structures such as repaired digital nerves. This hand-based orthosis is fabricated in much the same way as the dorsal hand immobilization orthosis, except for positioning the MCP, PIP, and DIP joints in the desired amount of flexion (see Chapter 7). Once the proximal strap is secured, the distal straps can be periodically removed to allow active-restricted (to the limit of the dorsal block) flexion and extension exercises of the MCP, PIP, and DIP joints if appropriate. Early motion can help prevent capsular tightness and allow tendon and/or nerve gliding.

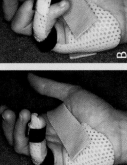
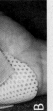
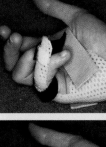

MCP Deviation Restriction Orthosis (HFO) (Fig. 9–5)

Common Names

- Ulnar deviation splint
- Protective MCP splint
- Palmar MCP stabilization splint

Alternative Orthosis Options

- Prefabricated orthoses
- Neoprene orthoses

Primary Functions

- Maintain MCP joints in alignment to protect from ulnar deviating or volar subluxation forces.

Common Diagnoses and General Optimal Positions

Arthritis of MCP jts — MCP: 0 to 25° flex with slight RD

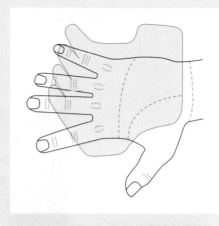

FIGURE 9-6

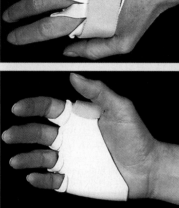
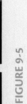
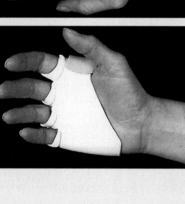

FIGURE 9-5

PATTERN PEARL 9-12 to 9-15.

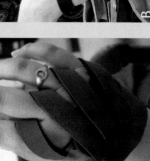
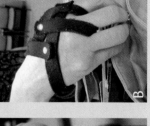
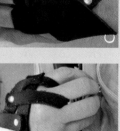
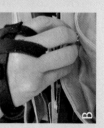
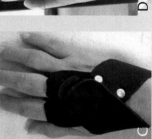
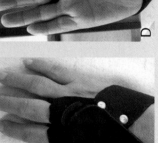
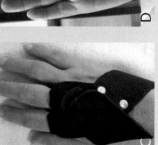
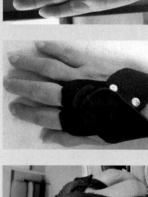

PP9-12

A–E, Various neoprene orthoses providing MCP extension restriction. Refer to Chapter 14 for further instruction.

Fabrication Process

Pattern Creation (Fig. 9–6)

- Mark just distal to each PIP joint, appreciating the difference in their heights.
- Allow approximately 1" additional material on ulnar border.
- Allow enough material radially to traverse through thumb web, contouring pattern to allow thumb mobility.
- Mark just distal to wrist crease, allowing unimpeded wrist mobility.

Refine Pattern

- Mark pattern from distal border to each digital web space, between IF and MF, MF and RF, and RF and SF.

Options for Materials

- Use thin (³⁄₃₂" or ¹⁄₁₆") elastic material; memory characteristic allows for excellent contouring and intimate fit.
- Consider ⅛" plastic material; thinner plastics may become weak as material is gently stretched about proximal phalanxes.

Cut and Heat

- Position patient with forearm supinated on table and digits slightly abducted. Digits may need to be supported in position by assistant, especially if joints are significantly deviated and/or subluxed. Warm material thoroughly.

Evaluate Fit while Molding

- Dry material quickly, and cut slits marked between digits; separate into four tabs. Each tab should be wide enough (approximately ½") to encompass proximal phalanx comfortably. Do not make this wrapped portion too narrow.
- Place material on volar aspect of hand. While working quickly, pull each tab around ulnar aspect of each proximal phalanx (onto dorsum).
- Overlap tabs onto themselves (for quick closure) or trim to form separate small cuffs.
- Constantly work material in palm to provide needed volar support for arches.
- MCPs should be supported volarly and should rest in near neutral alignment.
- Check that material traversing between digits is not thick and is free of sharp edges.

Strapping and Components

- One strap to join radial and ulnar border.
- Consider riveted strap to allow for easy donning and doffing.

Survey Completed Orthosis

- Smooth edges and between digits.
- Be sure MCP joints are supported in optimal alignment.

PATTERN PEARL 9-12 to 9-15. *continued*

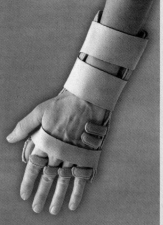

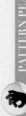

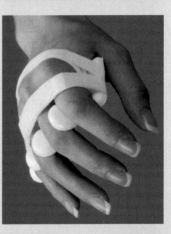

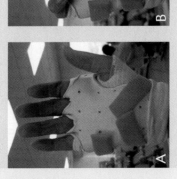

PP9-13   PP9-14   PP9-15

A and B, Wrist strap assists to secure orthosis.

LMB Soft Core Ulnar Deviation Splint (Photo courtesy of DeRoyal, Powell, TN).

Comforter™ Splint (Photo courtesy of 3-Point Products).

③ Forearm-Based Orthoses

Circumferential Wrist Flexion Restriction Orthosis (WHO) (Fig. 9–7)

Common Names

- Midcarpal instability orthosis/splint (Skirven & DeTullio, 2006)
- Ulnar boost orthosis/splint (Chinchalkar & Yong, 2004)
- Pisiform boost orthosis/splint (Garcias-Elias, 2008)
- Palmar midcarpal instability orthosis/splint

Primary Functions

- Reduction of pain and wrist "clunking."
- To provide dorsally oriented pressure on the pisiform bone with simultaneous counterpressure over the head

of the distal ulna to reduce volar sag of the carpus. This counter pressure corrects the volar flexed position of the proximal row.

- To achieve a more neutral carpal alignment by supporting the pisotriquetrial area (Chinchalkar & Yong, 2004; Garcias-Elias, 2008; Lichtman, Gaenslen, & Pollock, 1997; Skirven & DeTullio, 2006).

Additional Functions

- Allows near full wrist extension, radial deviation, and ulnar deviation and *restricts* wrist flexion.

Common Diagnoses and General Optimal Positions

*This orthosis aims to give dorsally directed pressure on the pisiform bone with simultaneous counterpressure over the head of the distal ulna to restore a neutral alignment of the ulnar wrist.

Palmar midcarpal instability/ VISI deformity (hyper volar flexion of the lunate)	Position of wrist = neutral

* The orthosis assists to eliminates the "clunk," which occurs during ulnar deviation.

* Note: This orthosis is used in most cases in combination with midcarpal stabilization exercises and with activity modifications.

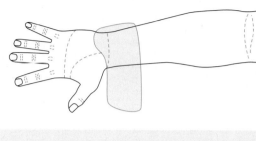

FIGURE 9-8

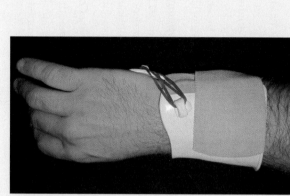

FIGURE 9-7

PP9-16

🐾 **PATTERN PEARL 9-16 to 9-20.**

A–C, Neoprene material used to create the dynamic force and rubber band posts for the attachment.

Fabrication Process

Pattern Creation (Fig. 9–8)

- Measure circumference of the wrist less than ½".
- Mark for proximal border approximately 3" proximal to the dorsal and volar wrist creases.
- The orthosis pattern is basically a rectangular piece of material with a rounded extension for application over the pisiform.
- The rounded extension measures approximately 1" wide and ¾" high. This extension varies in size depending on the individual.
- The pattern opening is on the ulnar border.

Refine Pattern

- Distal borders should allow near full wrist extension, radial deviation, and ulnar deviation but restrict flexion. The rounded extension should not extend beyond the pisiform either distally or laterally (which would cause interference with deviation motions and fully impede wrist flexion).

Options for Materials

- Use nonperforated ³⁄₃₂" or ⅛" material to achieve max stabilization. Material too thin or highly perforated may fold with attempted flexion.
- Noncoated material may be an option if homemade outrigger attachment posts are being used in the design. This would improve the adherence of the attachment device/homemade hook.

Cut and Heat

- Position patient's forearm in elbow flexion (resting on a table) and wrist in neutral.
- If using a stockinet under the orthosis, apply before heating material.

Evaluate Fit while Molding

- Starting on the ulnar volar aspect of the hand, place the extended piece over the pisiform.
- Wrap material around the radial aspect of the wrist/forearm just proximal to the wrist crease.
- Continue to guide the material over the dorsal aspect of the distal forearm ending along the ulnar lateral aspect covering the prominence of the ulnar head.
- When forming the orthosis, dorsally directed pressure is applied over the pisiform with counter pressure on the distal ulna.
- The opening is on the distal ulnar aspect of the wrist. This opening should be no wider than ½".
- Continue with this counterpressure until the orthosis has hardened.
- Avoid inadvertently applying direct pressure over the dorsal radial aspect of the distal radius to prevent radial sensory nerve irritation.

Strapping and Components

- Once material has set, apply gel or foam discs properly sized over the head of the distal ulna and pisiform bones.
- Apply low-profile outrigger attachments over the pisiform rounded extension piece and directly over the distal ulna.

- Adhere securely to the thermoplastic material.
- Place a thin padding (such as Moleskin, Kinesio® Tex Tape) along the length of both lateral borders and allow for overlap. This will prevent any "pinching" that may occur upon orthosis closure.
- Apply one 2" wide or two smaller 1" straps to secure onto the wrist.
- Using an elastic band, starting on the pisiform outrigger attachment, pull from the pisiform to the ulna and back again. This angle of application is what will reduce the ulnar volar sag. Consider using rubber band posts as outrigger attachments.

Survey Completed Orthosis

- Smooth material borders.
- Consider rolling or flaring the distal borders along the dorsal/volar wrist creases to avoid potential irritation from edges during attempted motion. Check to confirm freedom of movement in wrist extension, radial deviation, and ulnar deviation.

PATTERN PEARL 9-16 to 9-20. *continued*

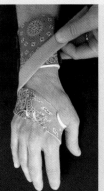

PP9-17

Counterpressure applied as orthosis is being molded.

PP9-18

Gel discs (or use foam) applied to the hardened material directly over pisiform and head of ulna.

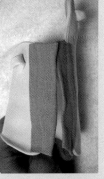

PP9-19

Overlapped 2" by 3" piece of Kinesio® Tex Tape can be used to prevent pinching of skin when orthosis is closed.

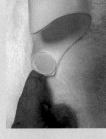

PP9-20

Original design of ulnar boost orthosis for midcarpal instability (Chinchalkar & Yong, 2004).

Wrist and IF/MF Extension Restriction Orthosis (WHFO) (Fig. 9–9)[1]

Common Names

- Tenodesis splint
- Rehabilitation Institute of Chicago (RIC) splint

Primary Function

- Maximize available grasp and release action of digits by redirecting portion of power generated during wrist extension into functional flexion arc of IF and MF against thumb (tenodesis).

Common Diagnoses and General Optimal Positions

Must have radial nerve function intact; loss of median and ulnar nerve function.

CLINICAL PEARL 9-11.
Digit Extension Restriction Strap

Some flexor tendon protocols call for the use of a restriction strap to protect the healing repairs once the dorsal orthosis has been discontinued (at 4 to 5 weeks). This strap protects the repaired structures from simultaneous wrist and digit extension. It also prevents excessive and forceful wrist extension (see Chapter 18 for details). **(A)** For the wrist strap component, use an 8" by 2" length of soft strap material (Rolyan® SoftStrap®; Patterson Medical). Secure it about the wrist with a 3" piece of adhesive hook (folded onto itself), placing the strap so that the closure is on the dorsum of the hand. Then punch a hole on the volar surface of the 2" strap. Remember that the line of pull converges toward the scaphoid bone. Make a sling from 1" by 4" length of soft strapping, and punch a hole on both ends of the sling. The overall length of the sling should be 1½" to 2". Finally, thread rubber band or elastic cord through the MCP sling and wrist strap holes. Adjust the tension so that as the wrist extends, the digit flexes; and as the wrist flexes, the digits extend. Watch for neurovascular compromise **B and C**. This orthosis was designed with neoprene for both the wrist strap and proximal phalanx sling with wrapped elastic cord as the flexion force.

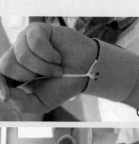
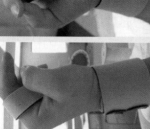
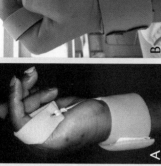

C   B   A

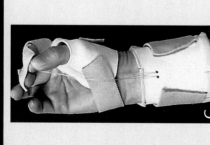

Holes for static line

Holes for static line

FIGURE 9-10

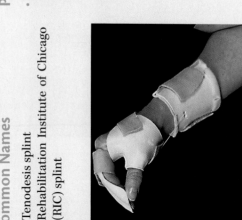
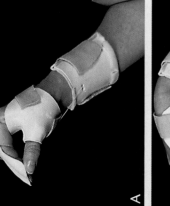

A

B

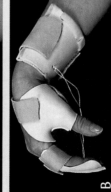

C

FIGURE 9-9

[1]Designed at the Rehabilitation Institute of Chicago.

Fabrication Process

Pattern Creation (Fig. 9-10)

- There are three separate sections of this orthosis.
- Dorsal cap for IF/MF: Orthosis should encompass both proximal phalanges and terminate at tip.
- Thumb MP orthosis: Orthosis should stabilize thumb in midpalmar abduction and opposition; thumb MP joint should be held in slight flexion.
- Thermoplastic wristband: Orthosis is fabricated to surround two-thirds circumference of wrist and is approximately 3½" wide.

Refine Pattern

- Check that lateral borders of IF and MF dorsal orthosis do not irritate radial border of RF.

Options for Materials

- Use ³⁄₃₂" or ¹⁄₁₆" material.

Cut and Heat

- Position patient with elbow resting on table, wrist extended, and MCPs flexed (tenodesis position).
- Warm material one section at a time.

Evaluate Fit while Molding

- Dorsal cap for IF/MF
  - Rest warm material over dorsum of IF and MF, making sure that PIPs are flexed to approximately 20°. There should be contouring between digits, distinguishing each one.
  - Proximal border of orthosis should extend just distal to MCPs.
- Thumb MP orthosis
  - This orthosis is fabricated per instructions for thumb carpometacarpal (CMC) immobilization orthosis.
  - Position thumb in midpalmar/radial abduction and opposition; opposition should be to middle of IF and MF. MP joint should be slightly flexed.
- Thermoplastic wristband
  - This orthosis is fabricated proximal to wrist, allowing full passive wrist flexion and active extension.
  - Place material centrally over volar wrist and wrap about radial and ulnar wrist borders. Material should terminate flush with dorsal skin.

Strapping and Components

- Thin strap of loop material secures dorsal orthosis onto digits and should be placed at proximal phalanx level.
- If needed, place optional strap distal to middle phalanx level.
- Strap thumb orthosis from volar to dorsal.
- Wrist requires 2" strap across dorsum of wrist, connecting radial and ulnar borders.
- To connect dorsal IF/MF orthosis and wristband, punch two holes along indentation of IF/MF proximal phalanx crease; punch two more holes at middle of wristband at distal border.
- Place double length of static line through holes onto dorsum of orthosis, tie securely, and feed between phalanges. Place wrist in extension and feed line through wristband holes.
- Line should have enough tension to pull MCP joints (along with dorsal orthosis) into flexion just to allow IF/MF tips to oppose thumb tip. Once proper tension is achieved, tie line through wristband holes.

Survey Completed Orthosis

- To obtain maximum benefits from this orthosis, it is crucial to achieve appropriate amount of tension.
- Line dorsal orthosis and wristband with very thin adhesive silicone gel or wrap digits and wrist with thin layer of Coban™ (or similar material) to help prevent orthosis migration during functional use and improve comfort.

4   Arm-Based Orthoses

Anterior/Posterior Elbow Extension or Flexion Restriction Orthosis (EO) (Fig. 9–11)

Common Names

- Anterior/posterior elbow splint
- Bisurfaced static elbow splint
- Elbow extension-blocking splint
- Elbow flexion-blocking splint

Alternative Orthosis Options

- Prefabricated orthosis
- Hinged elbow orthosis

Primary Functions

- Restrict specific degree of elbow extension or flexion while allowing motion in opposite direction.

Additional Functions

- Limit or prevent forearm rotation.
- Statically position elbow flexion or extension contracture at maximum length to facilitate lengthening of tissue (serial static orthosis).

Common Diagnoses and General Optimal Positions

Rheumatoid arthritis	Position of comfort and support
Ulnar nerve compression at cubital tunnel	Elb: 30 to 45° flex; FArm neutral
Posterior/anterior dislocation	Elb: 90°; FArm: neutral
Dislocation proximal radius	Elb: 90°; FArm: sup
Medial epicondyle fracture	Elb: 90 to 110°; FArm: pro
Lateral epicondyle fracture	Elb: 90 to 110°; FArm: sup
Olecranon fracture	Elb: 20 to 35° flex; FArm: neutral
Acute lateral epicondylitis	Elb: 90°; FArm: neutral; Wr: 30 to 45° ext
Acute medial epicondylitis	Elb: 90°; FArm: neutral; Wr: 0°
Elb ext contracture	Terminal flex
Elb flex contracture	Terminal ext

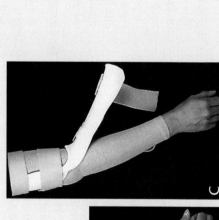
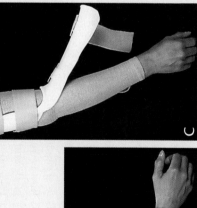

FIGURE 9-12

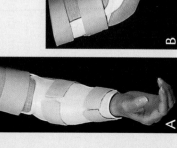
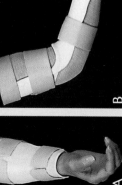

FIGURE 9-11

Fabrication Process

Pattern Creation (Fig. 9–12)

- This pattern may be alternative to anterior or posterior elbow immobilization orthosis design; consider when specific amount of flexion or extension must be restricted or when there are skin integrity issues (e.g., healing wounds or grafts).
- To restrict elbow extension: apply orthosis posteriorly on upper arm and anteriorly on forearm.
- To restrict elbow flexion: apply orthosis anteriorly on upper arm and posteriorly on forearm.
- Mark for proximal border two-thirds length of humerus.
- Mark for distal border just proximal to ulnar styloid.
- Allow enough material to encompass half to two-thirds circumference of upper arm and lower forearm, remembering that forearm tapers distally.
- Mark slit for elbow at elbow flexion crease.

Refine Pattern

- Proximal border should allow unimpeded shoulder motion and not irritate axilla region when arm is positioned at side.
- Distal border should allow full wrist motion.
- Note that pattern is wider proximally because circumference of upper arm is greater than that of forearm.
- Make sure that opening for elbow is wide enough to allow forearm and hand to pass through.

Options for Materials

- Use ⅛" material because strength is an important characteristic for this orthosis.
- Materials with high resistance to stretch (rubber) may offer more control for therapist.
- Consider material that has some degree of memory; material may stretch out as wrist and forearm pass through slotted piece.

Cut and Heat

- If patient has significant pain and swelling, consider uncoated materials or those that are slightly tacky to help prevent material from slipping, making it easier to position patient and mold orthosis.

Evaluate Fit while Molding

- Position patient seated to allow for gravity-assisted molding.
- Gravity can assist with molding only one portion of orthosis; the rest of orthosis must be attended to by therapist.
- Have an assistant help to support proper elbow and forearm positions if possible.

- Before molding orthosis, decide on which surface to apply material.
- Drape proximal piece either anterior or or posterior on upper arm, simultaneously sliding elbow carefully through slot; then place forearm portion either anterior or posterior.
- As one hand supports non–gravity-assisted piece, fold elbow flaps onto themselves to reinforce this potentially weak section.
- Do not grab proximal or distal orthosis segments or try to secure with tight circumferential bandage. This may cause borders of orthosis to dig in. Instead, allow gravity to assist in forming one trough while gently supporting the other segment.
- Check for clearance of wrist distally.

Strapping and Components

- Stockinette or elasticized sleeve (if edema is present) is recommended before orthosis application to help eliminate pinching of skin once straps are applied.
- 2" soft straps are recommended at most proximal and distal portions of orthosis.
- When used to restrict only one direction of elbow motion, forearm strap may be eliminated or released periodically to allow for exercise.

Survey Completed Orthosis

- Smooth and slightly flare all borders.
- Check for clearance and/or irritation of axilla, ulnar styloid, and epicondyles.
- Check for compression of ulnar nerve at cubital tunnel area as well as sensory branch of radial nerve.

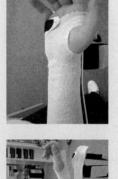

PATTERN PEARL 9-21 to 9-22.

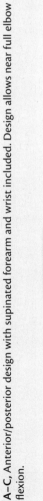

PP9-21

PP9-22

A–C, Anterior/posterior design with supinated forearm and wrist included. Design allows near full elbow flexion. Incorporating wrist will prevent distal migration and control forearm position.

Forearm Rotation/Elbow Extension Restriction Orthosis (EO) (Fig. 9–13)

Common Names

- Muenster splint
- Sarmiento elbow brace

Alternative Orthosis Options

- Sugar tong orthosis
- Cast

Primary Functions

- Restrict elbow extension and provide full flexion to allow healing of involved structure(s).

Additional Functions

- Restrict some degree of forearm rotation.
- With wrist included, restrict forearm rotation and elbow extension.

Common Diagnoses and General Optimal Positions

Proximal or distal rotation radioulnar jt injury	FArm: neutral
Interosseous membrane injury	FArm: neutral rotation
Proximal radius and ulna fracture	FArm: neutral rotation; Elb: restricted in ext (per physician's orders)
Elb dislocation	Depends on structures involved

CLINICAL PEARL 9-12.
Elbow Flexion Mobilization, Extension Restriction Orthosis

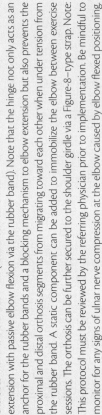

The dynamic elbow flexion orthosis with restricted elbow extension shown here is an example of the combined use of a mobilization orthosis with a restrictive component (see Chapter 8); it was designed for a patient who was referred 3 weeks after a biceps tendon repair. The orthosis segments were fabricated following instructions for the circumferential humerus and forearm orthoses. A hinge connects the segments, with the axis positioned at the elbow joint. Rubber band traction passively positions the elbow in flexion, and the hinge is set to restrict a specific amount of active elbow extension. (Similar to dynamic orthosis for digital flexor tendon injuries.) The patient periodically exercises within the orthosis limits (restricted active elbow extension with passive elbow flexion via the rubber band). Note that the hinge not only acts as an anchor for the rubber bands and a blocking mechanism to elbow extension but also prevents the proximal and distal orthosis segments from migrating toward each other when under tension from the rubber band. A static component can be added to immobilize the elbow between exercise sessions. The orthosis can be further secured to the shoulder girdle via a Figure-8–type strap. Note: This protocol must be reviewed by the referring physician prior to implementation. Be mindful to monitor for any signs of ulnar nerve compression at the elbow caused by elbow flexed positioning.

Discussion Points Questions

1. What is the purpose of a restriction orthosis?
2. Give examples of the appropriate diagnosis and functional goals for;
   - A digit extension restriction orthosis
   - A RF and SF MCP extension restriction orthosis
   - An elbow flexion restriction orthosis
3. What diagnoses would be most appropriate for a forearm rotation restriction orthosis?
4. Describe two different thumb MP restriction orthoses and the rationale for use.

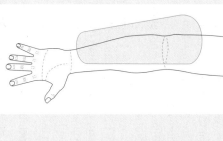

FIGURE 9-13

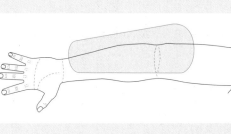

FIGURE 9-14

Fabrication Process

Pattern Creation (Fig. 9–14)

- Mark for proximal border approximately 2" above olecranon process.
- Mark for distal borders just proximal to wrist.
- Allow enough material to encompass half to two-thirds circumference of forearm, remembering that forearm tapers distally.

Refine Pattern

- Proximal border should allow limited elbow extension and unimpeded elbow flexion without irritating epicondyles or ulnar nerve.
- Distal border should allow full wrist and hand motion.

Options for Materials

- Use rubber materials (perforated or nonperforated).

- Consider elastic materials that are slightly tacky to help prevent material from slipping, making it easier to position patient and mold orthosis.

Evaluate Fit while Molding

- While supporting entire piece of warm material, place centrally along ulnar border of forearm and distal humerus.
- Proximally, bring ends together and either cut warm material to form seam or overlap material ends. This seam can be reinforced with an additional piece of material later, if necessary.

Cut and Heat

- Have patient lying supine with shoulder flexed or prone with shoulder extended to achieve gravity-assisted position. Place forearm in neutral position and elbow in desired position.
- Have patient (or assistant) maintain this position during fabrication. While material is heating, prepad olecranon process and epicondyles with self-adhesive padding or silicone gel if desired.
- Make sure desired elbow and forearm positions are maintained. Some patients may tend to flex their elbows excessively while orthosis is being formed.
- When almost set, check for clearance of ulnar styloid and epicondyles. If patient complains of abutment, simply push material out.

Strapping and Components

- Distal strap: 2" elasticized strap just proximal to wrist crease; use piece of adhesive foam to further stabilize forearm in orthosis and prevent migration. Foam should not overlap orthosis edges; avoid excessive compression over radial sensory nerve.
- Proximal strap: 2" elasticized strap placed just distal to elbow crease. Note there is no strap proximal to elbow crease—this permits elbow flexion.

Survey Completed Orthosis

- Smooth and slightly flare all edges.
- Check for complete clearance of wrist and desired elbow motion.

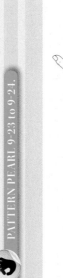
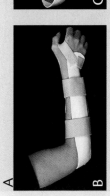

PP9-23

A–C, "Sugar tong" designed forearm restriction orthosis.

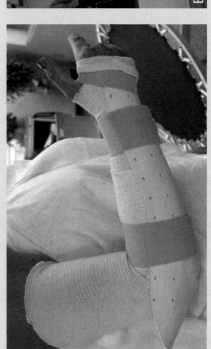

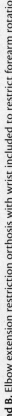
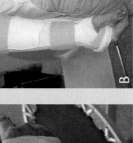

PP9-24

A and B, Elbow extension restriction orthosis with wrist included to restrict forearm rotation.

10 Nonarticular Orthoses

1 Digit- and Thumb-Based Orthoses

Proximal or Middle Phalanx Orthosis (FO) (Fig. 10–1)

Common Names
- Pulley ring

Alternative Orthosis Options
- Circumferential taping or strapping

Primary Functions
- Protect ruptured pulley.
- Protect pulley reconstruction.

Additional Functions
- Enhance tendon function (prevent bowstringing at or about A2 and A4 pulley regions) secondary to sacrificed, irreparable, or stretched out pulley mechanism.

Common Diagnoses and General Optimal Positions
Flexor tendon injury with pulley reconstruction (zones I and II)

Iatrogenic injury to pulley secondary to flexor tendon repair or tenolysis

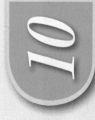
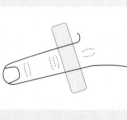

FIGURE 10-1

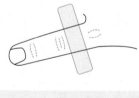

FIGURE 10-2

Fabrication Process

Pattern Creation (Fig. 10–2)

- Measure circumference of digit segment involved (e.g., proximal or middle phalanx).
- Measure width of segment involved; corresponding width of orthosis should be approximately ½" to ⅓" that of segment.
- Consider using strapping material for the dorsal component if edema or getting the ring over an enlarged joint presents as an issue.

Refine Pattern

- Accommodate for use of circumferential wrappings (Coban™, Patterson Medical, Warrenville, IL) or wound dressings beneath orthosis.

- Orthosis should allow unimpeded flexion of metacarpophalangeal (MCP), proximal interphalangeal (PIP), and/or distal interphalangeal (DIP) joints.
- Protect patient with recent flexor tendon repair in wrist/hand extension restriction orthosis (dorsal blocking orthosis) during fabrication process.

Options for Material

- Use ¹⁄₁₆" material, which provides adequate support.
- If strapping is used across dorsum of segment, consider thin strapping material.

Cut and Heat

- While material is heating, position patient with forearm supinated and digits slightly abducted.

- Allow material to completely set before removing.

Strapping and Components

- If strap is necessary, it should be approximately the same width as orthosis dorsally.
- Small metal rivet can be used to secure one end of strap.

Evaluate Fit while Molding

- Mold warm material around proximal or middle phalanx.
- For patient with no edema or with no wraps/ dressings, consider circumferential design in which ring is overlapped and/or sealed circumferentially. Otherwise, leave gap over dorsum of phalanx for orthosis removal; small strap can be applied to join ends of orthosis.
- For patients with enlarged PIP or DIP joints, be sure to leave gap over dorsum for orthosis removal.

Survey Completed Orthosis

- Smooth borders and round strap ends.
- Check for unimpeded joint motion.
- Remember that orthosis will need to be modified as edema or wound dressings worn beneath orthosis change.

PATTERN PEARL 10-1 TO 10-3.

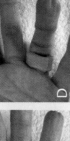

PP10-1

Modification of design used to maintain digit abduction to facilitate wound healing.

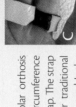

PP10-2

Orthosis used to support pulley repair status post-flexor tendon repair.

PP10-3

Orlicast™ (North Coast Medical, Morgan Hill, CA) used over elasticized wrap after A4 pulley reconstruction.

CLINICAL PEARL 10-1.
Alternative Options for Pulley Protection

A clinician might encounter an edematous digit and fear that the pulley ring will not be easily applied or removed. A patient may also have an enlarged joint, therefore making the ease of application challenging and the intimate fit required about the pulley impossible.

Consider the following:

A and B, Fabricate a volar orthosis (one-half to two-thirds the circumference of the digit) and add a small strap. The strap can either be elastic based or traditional loop material depending on the need. In the case shown, a small segment of foam was added to the dorsal strap in order to provide a snug fit.

C and D, A similar volar one-half circumference orthosis fabricated using elastic therapeutic tape for closure. The tape adheres well to the skin, keeping the pulley ring in place.

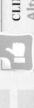
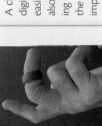

Proximal and/or Middle Phalanx Straps (FO) (Fig. 10–3)

Common Names

- Buddy straps
- Buddy splint
- Buddy taping

Alternative Orthosis Options

- Prefabricated
- Ring-designed orthoses
- Taping
- Thermoplastic material

Primary Functions

- Adjoin affected digit to border unaffected digit, minimizing lateral stress and allowing range of motion (ROM) and some function.

Additional Functions

- Facilitate passive and active ROMs of affected digit via active motion of adjacent digit.
- Use in combination with hand-based orthosis to prevent rotation of digit.

Common Diagnoses and General Optimal Positions

PIP collateral ligament injury
PIP dislocation
Volar plate injury
Stiff digit
Sagittal band injury

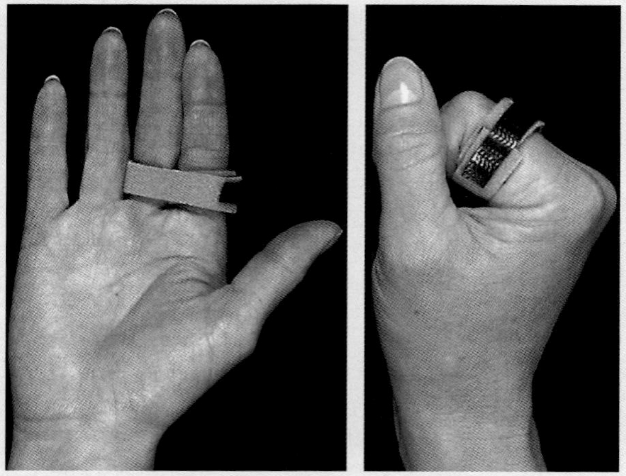

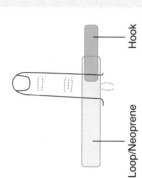

FIGURE 10-3

Loop/Neoprene — Hook

FIGURE 10-4

Fabrication Process

Pattern Creation (Fig. 10–4)

- Measure approximately 6″ of ½″ soft strapping material.
- Measure 1″ to 1½″ nonadhesive hook.

Refine Pattern

- Measure width of segment involved; corresponding width of orthosis should be one-half to one-third that of segment.
- Consider additional strap at middle phalanx for added support, depending on size of digit.

Options for Material

- Soft strapping material (Rolyan® SoftStrap®, Patterson Medical, or neoprene) works best because they are nonelastic yet soft (neoprene shown on previous page).
- Nonadhesive hook material to attach strap together.

Cut and Heat

- Trim both hook and soft strap according to digit size.

Evaluate Fit while Molding

- Position digits slightly abducted so there is adequate working room.

Strapping and Components

- From volar approach, place one end of soft strap between digits so that the end is flush with dorsum of proximal phalanx.
- Wrap other end volar to dorsal and, again, volar to dorsal, attaching to hook.

Survey Completed Orthosis

- Trim excess length and about digital web spaces if necessary.
- Consider use of gauze or polyester batting between fingers to reduce effects of perspiration.

PATTERN PEARL 10-4.

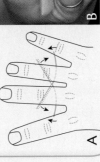

PP10-4

3pp® Buddy Loops® (Photo courtesy of 3-Point Products, Stevensville, MD).

CLINICAL PEARL 10-2.
Additional Buddy Strapping Techniques

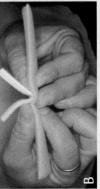

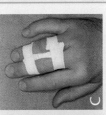

A and B, Sewing method. Lay soft strap on a flat surface, and place the center of the hook strap in the middle of the soft strap. Stitch the strap onto the hook material at the center point. Loop each side of the soft strap material completely around the digit and back to the center, completely covering the hook material. With this design, dorsal closure leaves the soft strap on the volar surface to allow for unimpeded flexion of the digits.

C, Tape. Use ½″ athletic tape to secure the digits together. Note the use of gauze between the fingers to prevent maceration.

CLINICAL PEARL 10-3.
Techniques for Buddy Strapping Small Finger (SF)

Buddy strapping the SF may pose a problem because it is much shorter than the RF, and the flexion creases of the fingers do not line up. To buddy strap these fingers effectively, allowing for PIP and DIP motion, consider the following techniques.

A–C, No-sew method. Zigzag or step-cut a piece of soft strap. Use hook to attach the loop together. The center portion of the strap should be quite narrow to decrease bulk in this area. Make sure full motion is available.

D and E, Sewing method. Fabricate two separate loops and stitch them together, off center, to the degree necessary to accommodate the digit length differential. This technique allows for a good custom fit.

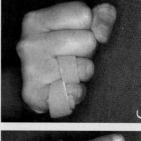

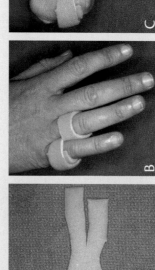

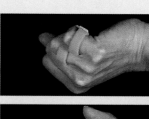

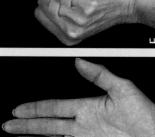

CLINICAL PEARL 10-4.
Use of Microfoam™ Tape to Prevent Migration

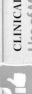

Using a strip of Microfoam™ tape (Patterson Medical) can help prevent buddy straps from falling off or slipping on digits. This low-tack tape can be replaced easily as needed. Shown is strap fabricated from neoprene with seam tape for permanent closure.

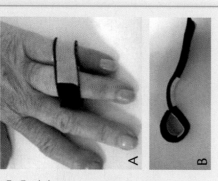

Proximal or Middle Phalanx Circumferential Orthosis (FO) (Fig. 10–5)[1]

Common Names

- Proximal phalanx fracture brace
- Middle phalanx fracture base

Alternative Orthosis Options

- Cast
- Digit immobilization orthosis

Primary Functions

- Support and protect proximal or middle phalanx during healing while allowing motion of proximal and distal joints.

Common Diagnoses and General Optimal Positions

Stable proximal phalanx fractures (not requiring internal fixation)

Unstable fractures requiring surgical fixation: pinning at 1 to 2 weeks postsurgery, depending on fracture stability; screw fixation 3 to 5 days postsurgery, depending on fracture stability

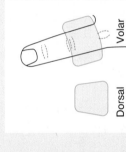

Dorsal   Volar

FIGURE 10-6

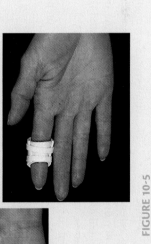

FIGURE 10-5

[1] Described by Kim Oxford, MOT, OTR, CHT, and David H. Hildreth, MD, University of Texas Health Science Center.

CHAPTER 10

Fabrication Process

Pattern Creation (Fig. 10–6)

- Mark pattern as close to digit length and circumference as possible.
- If patient cannot fully extend the involved PIP joint or is in pain, consider measuring unaffected digit.
- For more distal fractures, extend lateral supports to distal end of PIP joint.
- For more proximal fractures, extend material volarly and dorsally on MCP joint.

Refine Pattern

- Remember to accommodate for use of circumferential wrapping (Coban™) or wound dressing beneath orthosis.
- Orthosis should allow unimpeded flexion of MCP, PIP, and DIP joints.

Options for Material

- Use coated, elastic, or plastic $\frac{1}{16}$" material.

Cut and Heat

- Cut volar and dorsal pieces of material and heat.

Strapping and Components

- Use one or two $\frac{1}{4}$" to $\frac{1}{2}$" straps for optimal closure. This allows application of gentle circumferential pressure.

Survey Completed Orthosis

- Smooth borders, especially between digital web spaces.
- Check for irritation of adjacent digits and possible neurovascular compromise.

- Apply Coban™ or compression garments as necessary before orthosis application.
- Position digits slightly abducted so there is adequate working room.

Evaluate Fit while Molding

- Fabricate volar portion of orthosis and allow to set before applying dorsal piece.
- For dorsal piece, lay warmed material over proximal phalanx, slightly overlapping it onto volar piece.
- Once completely set, pop orthosis apart.

CLINICAL PEARL 10-5.
Circumferential Phalanx Orthosis

Middle or proximal phalanx nondisplaced shaft fractures can sometimes be managed with a circumferential orthosis design. Before application, examine the PIP for proximal phalanx injuries or the DIP for middle phalanx injuries to be sure that the joint is not enlarged, which would make this orthosis impossible to remove. Choose a ³⁄₃₂" or ¹⁄₁₆" material that will readily adhere to itself once the coating has been disrupted.

Cut a strip of material the full length and approximately ¼" more than the circumference of the segment being treated. Have the patient supinate the hand and slightly abduct the digits. Place the center of the warmed material over the volar proximal or middle phalanx and bring it around both the ulnar and the radial borders. Pinch the entire length of the ends together dorsally (this can also be done volarly). Carefully cut the excess material. Turn attention back to the volar aspect while still warm and check that the volar MCP/PIP or PIP/DIP creases are cleared to allow motion.

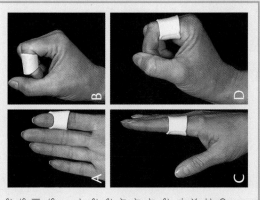

CLINICAL PEARL 10-6.
Orthosis to Facilitate Active PIP Joint Motion

Commonly, patients with stiff PIP joints compensate with excessive motion proximally at the MCP joints. The use of these ring orthoses between exercise sessions for functional use can help patient maintain gains from exercise sessions by preventing compensatory motions with activities of daily living (ADLs).

With PIP flexion deficits, they hyperflex at the MCP joints when attempting to make a fist. **(A)** The use of a Figure-8 orthosis can be an effective way to facilitate PIP joint flexion and minimize this abnormal movement pattern during functional use or exercise. This technique is most effective when addressing limitations of the MF or RF (but

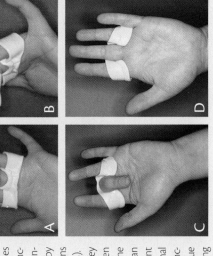

design can be modified for other digits; always include three digits in orthosis for best results). Cut a 6" by ½" strip of thermoplastic material. Thickness depends on size of hand; use thinnest possible to minimize bulk. Width should be slightly shorter than the length of the proximal phalanx. Heat, and place the central portion over the volar proximal phalanx of the involved digit. The other two ends will wrap dorsal to dorsal about the adjacent digits, forming two rings. The MCPs of the uninvolved digits are held in slight flexion while the involved digit is positioned in relative MCP extension while the orthosis sets. Check that the orthosis borders do not interfere with active movement of the involved digit. Note that the orthosis must allow unimpeded MCP and PIP motion. While the patient flexes, they should feel the gentle pressure of the material at the proximal phalanx encouraging PIP joint flexion. **(B)** Placing a DIP immobilization orthosis can further isolate PIP flexion efforts.

C and D, Similarly, with active PIP extension deficits (extension lag), an orthosis fabricated for purpose of encouraging active PIP extension can be used. For this design, once the strip of material is heated, the middle portion of the orthosis is placed dorsally on the affected digit's proximal phalanx. The other two ends will wrap volar to dorsal about the adjacent digits, forming two rings. The MCPs of the uninvolved digits are held in slight extension while the involved digit is positioned in relative MCP flexion while the orthosis sets. This is a helpful adjunct to manual PIP extension blocking exercises because the orthosis will provide blocking pressure over the proximal phalanx with active efforts, minimizing the tendency for the MCP joint to hyperextend.

2 Hand-Based Orthoses

Metacarpal Orthosis (HO) (Fig. 10–7)

Common Names
- Metacarpal fracture brace

Alternative Orthosis Options
- Cast
- Galveston fracture brace
- Prefabricated orthosis

Primary Functions
- Stabilize and protect involved metacarpal during fracture healing.

Common Diagnoses and General Optimal Positions
Stable/nondisplaced metacarpal fracture

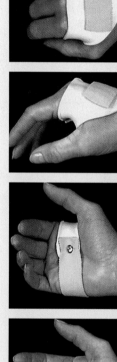
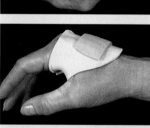
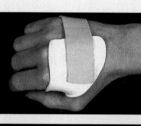

FIGURE 10-7

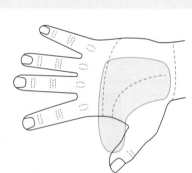
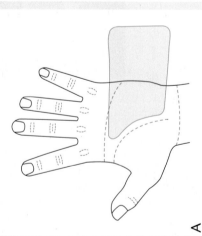
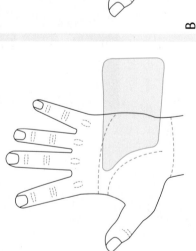

A   B

FIGURE 10-8

Fabrication Process

Pattern Creation (Fig. 10-8)

ULNAR DESIGN

- Mark proximal border at wrist crease.
- Mark just proximal to volar and dorsal borders of middle finger (MF), ring finger (RF), and small finger (SF) MCP joints.
- Volar surface should allow clearance of thenar muscles.

RADIAL DESIGN

- Mark proximal border at wrist crease.
- Mark just proximal to volar and dorsal borders of second and third metacarpals.
- Volar surface should allow for clearance of thenar muscles.

Refine Pattern

ULNAR DESIGN

- Proximal and distal borders should allow full wrist and MCP joint motion, respectively.
- Thumb should have unimpeded motion.

- Make sure pattern encompasses third metacarpal for increased orthosis stability.
- Mark just proximal to volar and dorsal borders of middle finger (MF), ring finger (RF), and small finger (SF) MCP joints.
- Volar surface should allow clearance of thenar muscles.

RADIAL DESIGN

- Proximal and distal borders should allow full wrist and MCP joint motion, respectively.
- Thumb should have unimpeded motion.

Options for Materials

- Use lightly perforated material that retains some degree of flexibility when set. Orthosis must bend slightly when set. Orthosis must bend slightly to be removed for hygiene; perforations help prevent skin maceration.
- Material should provide intimate fit about metacarpals, provide stability and protection, and prevent orthosis migration.
- Materials that can be reheated and remolded several times are a good option if ongoing orthosis modifications become necessary to accommodate for fluctuations in edema.

Cut and Heat

- For ulnar design, position extremity with shoulder forward flexed and internally rotated, elbow flexed, and forearm pronated to achieve gravity-assisted position (ulnar side of hand facing up).
- For radial design, position forearm in neutral rotation to achieve gravity-assisted position.

Evaluate Fit while Molding

ULNAR DESIGN

- Place material centrally on ulnar aspect of hand just distal to wrist.
- On volar surface, material should rest just proximal to distal palmar crease and on dorsal surface just proximal to MCP joints.
- Allow gravity to assist while gently contouring and encompassing third to fifth metacarpals.

RADIAL DESIGN

- Place material centrally on radial aspect of hand just distal to wrist.
- On volar surface, material should

rest just proximal to distal palmar crease and on dorsal surface just proximal to MCP joints.
- Allow gravity to assist while gently contouring and encompassing second to third metacarpals.

Strapping and Components

- Both ulnar and radial designs may need wrist strap to prevent migration; soft or elasticized strap works well.
- For ulnar design, use custom (trimmed) soft foam strap through first web space to maximize comfort and prevent skin irritation caused by friction (as sometimes seen with traditional loop material).
- For radial design, use elasticized strap on ulnar border to accommodate variations in muscle bulk during active hand use.

Survey Completed Orthosis

- Smooth proximal and distal borders.
- Make sure there is no irritation from strap material in first web space with thumb motion.

PATTERN PEARL 10-5 TO 10-10.

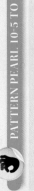

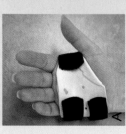

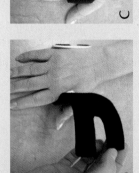

PP10-5

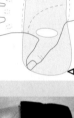

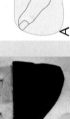

A–C, Circumferential design using thermoplastic volarly and neoprene dorsally to cushion bony anatomy.

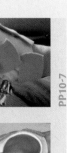
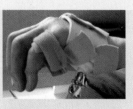
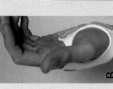
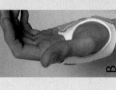
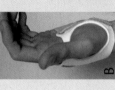
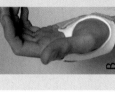
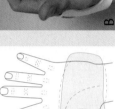
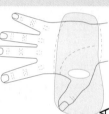
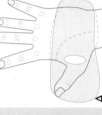
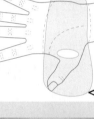
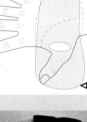
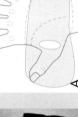
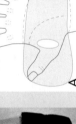
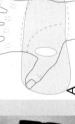
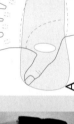
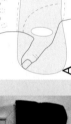
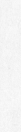

PP10-6

A and B, Thumbhole incorporated into design increasing stability.

PP10-7

Ulnar-based design used for SF MCP flexion mobilization orthosis.

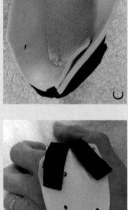

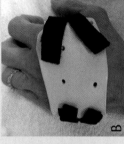
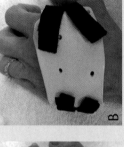

PP10-8

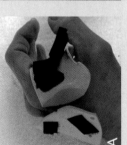
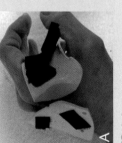
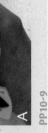

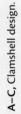

PP10-9

A and B, Orfit® Colors™ material pinched together then cut, forming a seam used to create circumferential design (Northcoast Medical).

A–C, Clamshell design.

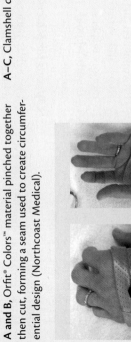

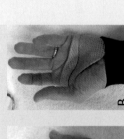

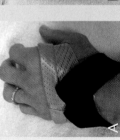
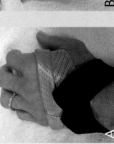

PP10-10

A and B, Elasticized strap about wrist for stabilization.

Notes

③ **Forearm-Based Orthoses**

Forearm Orthosis (WHO or EO) (Fig. 10–9)

Common Names
• Forearm fracture brace

Alternative Orthosis Options
• Cast
• Prefabricated orthosis

Primary Functions
• Stabilize and protect radius and/or ulna during fracture healing by applying gentle, circumferential compression to surrounding soft tissues.

Additional Functions
• Can be used as transitional protective device for forearm fractures after healing has occurred, when patient must return to work and/or sports.

Common Diagnoses and General Optimal Positions
Radius and ulna shaft fractures

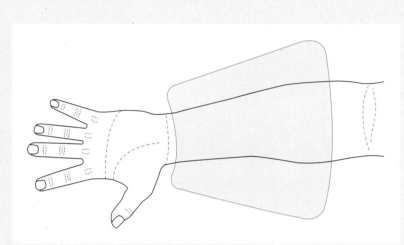

FIGURE 10-10

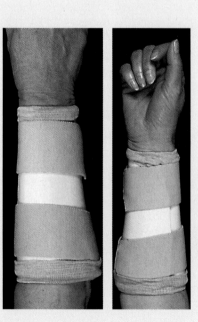

FIGURE 10-9

Fabrication Process

Pattern Creation (Fig. 10–10)

- Measure circumference of proximal border just distal to elbow flexion crease and add 1".
- Measure circumference of distal border just proximal to ulnar styloid, and add 1".
- Connect proximal to distal borders to account for length of orthosis.

Refine Pattern

- Be sure to allow enough material for approximately 1" overlap.
- In general, patients may find it easier to pull straps toward themselves rather than away; thus, overlap material on ulnar forearm from volar to dorsal.

Options for Materials

- Use coated material to avoid permanent bonding of overlapped section and to allow orthosis to pop apart.

- For adults, 3/32" material is adequate to stabilize forearm. For young children, 1/16" material can be used.
- Lightly perforated material with some degree of memory may help provide intimate fit about forearm yet allow some flexibility for ease of removal and to increase air exchange.

Cut and Heat

- Position forearm in neutral rotation to achieve gravity-assisted position.

Evaluate Fit while Molding

- Place warm material on towel; position so that wide section is applied proximally and narrow section is applied distally.
- Gently apply to forearm, keeping in mind desired overlap area.
- Begin evenly and lightly stretching material around forearm and overlapping it onto itself.

- Do not overstretch material, which may disrupt material's protective coating, causing inadvertent adherence.
- Once overlapped, apply constant moving pressure along length of orthosis until material is set.
- Remove orthosis when completely set, pop apart overlapped section, and remove from patient.

Strapping and Components

- Consider use of 1" or 2" self-adhesive D-ring straps, because they allow firm and easy closure.
- Attach D-rings so patient can tighten orthosis by directing pull of straps toward body.
- Alternatively, 2" elasticized straps allow patient to control compression placed on arm.
- Line entire length of inside seam with Moleskin (Patterson Medical) or other thin liner. Overlap liner onto

itself by approximately 1" to minimize potential of pinching forearm skin between orthosis pieces.
- Consider lining proximal and distal borders with soft liner, such as Moleskin or Microfoam™ tape (Patterson Medical) to reduce migration.

Survey Completed Orthosis

- Stockinette or TubiGrip™ (Patterson Medical) under orthosis can provide comfort, aid with edema, and minimize orthosis irritation.
- Check for possible bony irritation and/or neurovascular compromise.
- Instruct patient to remove orthosis for hygiene only and to follow physician's protocol.

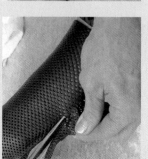
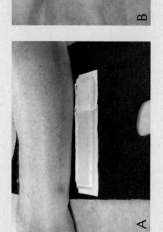
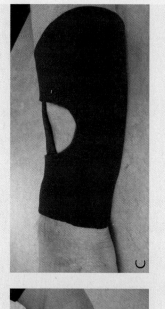

PP10-11

Circumferential design (elastic-coated material, Orfit® Colors™, Northcoast Medical) using pinch/cut technique to form seam.

PP10-12

A–C, Neoprene used to protect ulna osteotomy with silicone inserted over incision site.

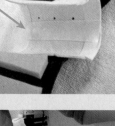
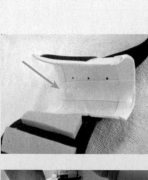

PP10-13

Used as base for mobilization orthosis.

PP10-14

Make certain to allow for full clearance of wrist motion.

PP10-15

Microfoam™ tape and foam on strapping to prevent migration (Patterson Medical).

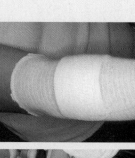

CLINICAL PEARL 10-7.
Use of Elasticized Sleeve to Help Molding Process

An elasticized sleeve can be used to secure circumferential orthosis such as a forearm guard or a proximal forearm orthosis. This technique allows for even pressure distribution while the material is setting. Do not use a size that is too tight, which may cause the orthosis' borders to dig in, possibly causing skin irritation. The patient can gently open and close the fist while the material is hardening, allowing the design to incorporate proximal forearm musculature.

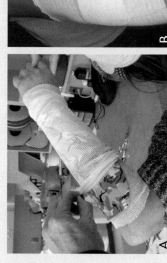

CLINICAL PEARL 10-8.
Protective Playing Orthosis

A, Foam padding can be added prior to fabrication and held in place with compressive stockinette. Thermoplastic material can then be applied. **B,** Shown here is a football player returning to sport with this protective orthosis status post fracture of the midshaft of the ulna. Note the use of small rivets to anchor one end of the neoprene straps for secure closure.

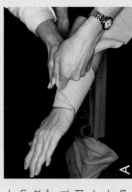
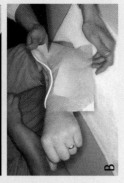

CLINICAL PEARL 10-9.
Circumferential Designs and Material Adherence

With circumferential designs, there are several techniques for preventing the thermoplastic material from adhering to itself. The best material of choice is one that has a coating; however, these materials will often "stick" together if they have been overstretched or overheated.

When there is no choice but to use uncoated material, try one of these techniques. (1) Do not overstretch the orthosis material. (2) Do not be too aggressive when pressing the pieces together. (3) Apply a wet Ace™ wrap or similar to the bottom piece (with an extra inch overlap directly onto the skin) and then wrap around gently over the entire orthosis **(A).** (4) Place a wet paper towel between the pieces just before overlapping **(B).** (5) Apply a thin layer of hand lotion on the warmed material's surface just before overlapping.

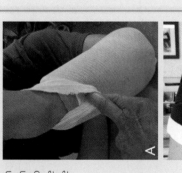
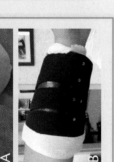

Proximal Forearm Orthosis (EO) (Fig. 10-11)

Common Names

- Tennis elbow strap
- Tennis elbow cuff
- Golfer's elbow strap
- Lateral epicondylitis strap
- Medial epicondylitis strap
- Counterforce brace

Alternative Orthosis Options

- Prefabricated orthosis
- Taping
- Neoprene orthosis

Primary Functions

- Decrease stress at proximal attachment of wrist extensors or flexors during functional use by providing counterforce and dispersing pressure about muscle bellies.

CLINICAL PEARL 10-10.
Proximal Forearm Orthosis to Address Combined Medial and Lateral Epicondylitis

Two pieces of silicone gel or ⅜" foam (2" by 2") can be added to a circumferential design to place pressure simultaneously over the proximal extensor and flexor muscle bellies. Occasionally, some patients present with lateral and medial epicondylitis simultaneously, likely because of overcompensating with the opposing muscle-tendon group.

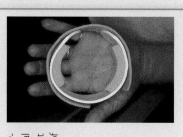

FIGURE 10-12

Common Diagnoses and General Optimal Positions

Lateral epicondylitis (tennis elbow)
Medial epicondylitis (golfer's elbow)

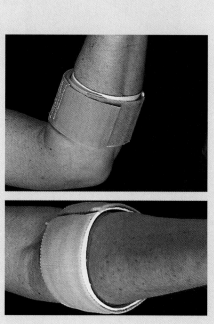

FIGURE 10-11

Fabrication Process

Pattern Creation (Fig. 10–12)

- Measure circumference of proximal forearm 1″ to 1½″ below epicondyles; subtract 1″ to obtain circumference of orthosis.
- Width of orthosis should be approximately 2½″.

Refine Pattern

- Check length and width.

Options for Materials

- Use ⅟₁₆″ or ³⁄₃₂″ material.
- Gel- or foam-lined thermoplastic materials eliminate added step of lining material over muscle bellies. When using traditional material, adhesive-backed foam or gel can be applied to molded thermoplastic in area over muscle bellies to disperse pressure.

Cut and Heat

- Position patient with elbow gently flexed, forearm neutral to slight pronation for lateral epicondylitis, or neutral with slight supination for medial epicondylitis.
- Heat thermoplastic material.
- Note that some gel- and foam-lined materials can be heated in sealed plastic bag to prevent water from saturating lining (refer to manufacturer's instructions for details).

Evaluate Fit while Molding

LATERAL EPICONDYLITIS

- Rest warm material over proximal extensor muscle bellies approximately two fingerbreadths distal to lateral epicondyle.
- Wrap material from ulnar aspect of arm to radial volar aspect, leaving slight opening along ulnar border.

- Stockinette can be used to allow material to set with even pressure distribution.
- Once material is secured on proximal forearm, have patient lightly open and close fist to get contouring about muscle bellies.

MEDIAL EPICONDYLITIS

- Rest warm material over proximal flexor muscle bellies approximately two fingerbreadths distal to medial epicondyle.
- Once material is secured on proximal forearm, have patient lightly open and close fist to get contouring about muscle bellies.

Strapping and Components

- After material has set, apply adhesive foam or gel on portion of orthosis that will be resting over flexor and/or extensor muscle bellies.
- Adhesive hook is applied to nearly full circumference of orthosis to provide even pressure distribution throughout orthosis.
- Consider that use of 2″ elasticized strap to allow orthosis to accommodate for forearm musculature is contracting and relaxing.
- Apply strap with even tension across entire circumference of orthosis.
- D-ring strap also works well for this type of orthosis.
- Direction of strap application should provide for easy donning and doffing.

Survey Completed Orthosis

- Smooth borders of orthosis's edges.
- Instruct patient in appropriate strap tightness and caution regarding signs of neurovascular compromise.
- Mark proximal and distal ends of orthosis and review proper orthosis placement.

🐾 PATTERN PEARL 10-16 TO 10-19

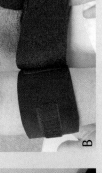

PP10-16

Foam-lined thermoplastic (approximately 2″ by 2″) over extensor or flexor muscle bellies with imbedded 2″ neoprene strap to secure.

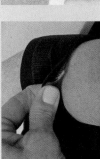

PP10-17

A and B, Custom neoprene strap uses adhesive hook/loop for closure. Sew corners of hook and loop for longevity.

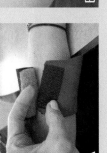

PP10-18

A and B, Custom neoprene strap combined with adhesive silicone gel.

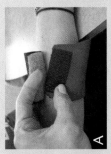

PP10-19

3pp® Tennis Elbow Strap (Photo courtesy of 3-Point Products).

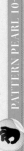

CHAPTER 10

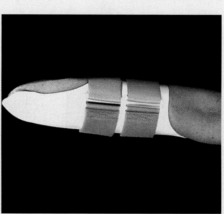

FIGURE 10-14

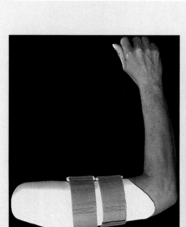

FIGURE 10-13

4 Arm-Based Orthoses

Humerus Orthosis (SO or EO) (Fig. 10–13)

Common Names

- Humeral fracture brace
- Sarmiento humerus brace

Alternative Orthosis Options

- Zipper-designed orthosis
- Cast
- Prefabricated orthosis
- Sling

Primary Functions

- Stabilize and protect humerus during fracture healing by applying gentle, circumferential compression to surrounding soft tissues.

Common Diagnoses and General Optimal Positions

Humeral shaft fracture

Fabrication Process

Pattern Creation (Fig. 10–14)

- Location of fracture along shaft dictates length of orthosis.
- For proximal shaft fractures, orthosis pattern should extend to proximal edge of acromion process, and distal edge can terminate just above elbow crease.
- For distal shaft fractures, orthosis pattern should extend just distal to acromion process, and distal edge can terminate over epicondyles medially and laterally.
- Both designs should support medial arm to axilla.

Refine Pattern

- Proximal border should allow nearly full shoulder motion.
- Distal border should allow unimpeded elbow motion.
- Check that there is enough material to encompass humerus circumferentially and add 1" to 1½" extra for overlap.
- Avoid irritation to epicondyles, olecranon, axilla, and ulnar nerve at cubital tunnel.

Options for Materials

- Use coated material so overlapped section can be popped open.
- For larger arms, ⅛" or ³⁄₃₂" materials provide needed support.
- For smaller arms, ³⁄₃₂" or ¹⁄₁₆" materials provide adequate support.
- Remember that elastic materials tend to shrink around the immobilized part; do not remove until orthosis is completely set.
- Use lightly perforated material that retains some degree of flexibility when set. Orthosis must bend slightly to be removed for hygiene; perforations help prevent skin maceration.

Cut and Heat

- Position patient seated with shoulder supported in slight abduction, it may help to have the assistant position extremity during fabrication process to minimize patient discomfort.
- While material is heating, prepad medial and lateral epicondyles using self-adhesive padding or silicone gel, if necessary.
- Carefully cut pattern from material. Pattern has many curves; try to be accurate in pattern design and transfer onto material.

Evaluate Fit while Molding

- Supporting entire piece of warm material, place along anterior humerus, aligning cut out for axilla and anterior elbow appropriately; open section is positioned along posterior humerus.
- If bracing for proximal shaft fracture, simultaneously extend warm material over humeral head to acromion process.
- If bracing for distal shaft fracture, extend material distally over epicondyles, making sure not to interfere with elbow mobility.
- Using both hands, carefully and gently stretch material anterior to posterior, under axilla, and over onto itself.
- Do not overstretch material, which may disrupt material's protective coating, causing inadvertent adherence.
- Gently flare material around proximal segment with careful attention to axilla (do not overlap material, which tends to irritate this sensitive region) and along distal borders.

Strapping and Components

- Use 2" self-adhesive D-ring straps, because they allow firm and easy closure; patient can make adjustments according to comfort.
- Attach D-rings so patient can tighten orthosis by directing pull of straps toward body.
- Line inside of orthosis with Moleskin or other thin liner. Overlap liner onto itself by approximately 1" to minimize potential of pinching forearm skin between orthosis pieces.
- Line proximal and distal borders with Microfoam™ tape or self-adhesive gel liners to decrease distal migration.

Survey Completed Orthosis

- Some patients may benefit from wearing stockinette or TubiGrip™ beneath orthosis to minimize orthosis irritation and aid with controlling perspiration.
- Check for migration and possible bony irritation or neurovascular compromise.
- Instruct patient to remove for hygiene only and to follow physician's protocol.

Discussion Points Questions

1. What is the purpose of a non-articular orthosis?

2. Describe the most common diagnosis and the purpose of a circumferential proximal phalanx orthosis.

3. Give an example of a common diagnosis for a hand fracture that would be treated with a non-articular orthosis?
   - Name two key fabrication points to consider during the fabrication process.
   - Describe the important fabrication modifications for a radial design and an ulnar design.

4. Give an example of a common diagnosis for an upper arm injury that would be managed with a non-articular orthosis.

5. Describe two or more fabrication considerations when constructing a circumferential humerus orthosis.

PATTERN PEARL 10-20 TO 10-24.

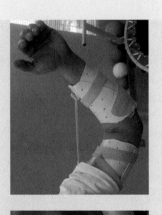

PP10-20

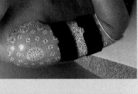

PP10-21

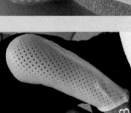
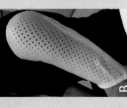

PP10-22

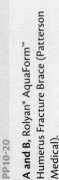
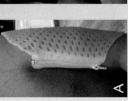

A and B, Rolyan® AquaForm™ Humerus Fracture Brace (Patterson Medical).

Elasticized circumferential strapping is an excellent choice for orthosis closure and additional fracture stabilization.

Two nonarticular orthoses can be joined together to form a mobilization orthosis.

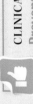

PP10-23

Lining proximal and distal ends of nonarticular orthosis may assist in reducing migration and minimizing tissue irritation.

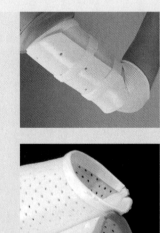

PP10-24

Rolyan® Preformed Humerus Brace (Photo courtesy of Patterson Medical).

CLINICAL PEARL 10-11.
Preventing Skin Irritation from Overlapped Segments

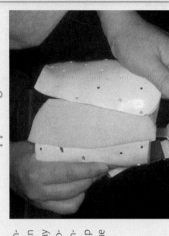

Lining the inside overlapped edge of circumferentially designed orthosis with Moleskin (Patterson Medical) (or a similar material) may reduce the potential for irritation at the orthosis/skin interface. The key is to overlap the lining onto itself to form an extra 1″ to 2″ soft flap on the inside of the orthosis. This technique can be used for most circumferential designs.

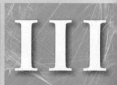

Optional Methods

11

Prefabricated Orthoses

Rebecca Harris, MS, OTR/L, CHT*

Chapter Objectives

After study of this chapter, the reader should be able to:

- Appreciate the various prefabricated devices that are available to address the multitude of upper extremity diagnoses.
- Understand what factors should be considered when choosing between a prefabricated and a custom orthosis.
- Describe how to properly fit a prefabricated orthosis.
- Give examples of modifications for customization of prefabricated orthoses to address specific patient needs.
- Recognize the various companies that offer prefabricated orthoses.

Key Terms

Continuous passive motion (CPM) machine

Dynamic and static progressive orthoses

Prefabricated orthoses

Introduction

Something that is designed to fit everyone fits no one well (Malick, 1982). One size fits none. As therapists, we are, by nature, skeptical of easy solutions to rehabilitation problems; and as hand therapists, we strive to design and create a comfortable and effective solution for the patient. The challenge of creating a well-fitting, purposeful orthosis for the patient provides many therapists with joy in their work. However, owing to time constraints, monetary issues, and/or perhaps the lack of product availability, it is not always practical or appropriate to make an orthosis from thermoplastic, plaster, fiberglass, or soft materials. Therefore, prefabricated orthoses offer an alternative treatment option and play an important role in the practice of upper extremity therapy.

This chapter outlines the considerations related to the use of **prefabricated orthoses** and includes information on how to become an educated consumer on the availability and application of these orthoses. Some of the commonly used and currently available orthoses are reviewed as well. Prefabricated orthoses can sometimes be used creatively for purposes other than what they were originally intended for; suggestions for these alternative uses are also provided.

---

*This chapter is based on the first edition chapter written by Janet Cope, MS, CAS, OTR/L.

Considerations for Fitting Orthoses

There are several issues to consider before choosing either a custom-made or a prefabricated orthosis. The skill of the therapist is sometimes a determining factor for using prefabricated devices. That is, some therapists custom fabricate orthoses only occasionally; therefore, they either do not have the skills to make the required custom orthosis or it would not be an efficient use of their time to do so. Adapting prefabricated orthoses may be helpful in these circumstances. Similarly, the setting in which a therapist works might dictate the choice of orthoses; those in home health-care settings without the necessary equipment for custom fabrication may find that prefabricated options are appropriate for some clients. In addition, one or any combination of the following factors may affect the selection of an appropriate orthosis for a particular patient:

- Specifics of the diagnosis
- Patient needs
- Time constraints
- Appropriateness and availability of the material
- Ease of application
- Cost effectiveness

Specifics of the Diagnosis

In assessing the patient's needs, one must consider what the best solution for the immediate situation will be. The therapist must clearly understand the patient's diagnosis and current status. Does the patient have a fracture with open wounds and a painful, edematous hand? Perhaps a preformed resting orthosis will save fabrication time and assist in immobilizing the upper extremity more quickly and with less molding and fitting requirements than a custom orthosis. Does the patient have an external fixator, pins, or other external hardware? Will the patient have specific needs for managing scar tissue? Patients with these particular requirements will most likely require customized orthotic fabrication. Does the patient require rigid immobilization or would a soft support suffice? For example, a patient with rheumatoid arthritis may use a prefabricated neoprene orthosis to minimize ulnar deviation of the digits during the day and a custom thermoplastic resting orthosis at night (Dell & Dell, 1996).

Patient Needs

The therapist and patient need to negotiate a safe and reasonable orthosis regimen for home use. "Poor compliance to splint wear is a common complaint of clinicians, a complaint that may stem, in part, from a flaw in prescription practices" (Pagnotta, Korner-Bitensky, Mazer, Baron, & Wood-Dauphinee, 2005). Patients are unlikely to wear an orthosis that interferes consistently with their daily activities, however much they require the device, unless time is taken to review rationale and potential outcomes. Patient education and involvement in the plan of care generally increase the likelihood of consistent implementation of the orthosis wearing schedule outside of the clinic. When selecting an orthosis designed to increase function, "fit, comfort, and effectiveness through a range of functional activities" (Melvin, 1995) should be evaluated before dispensing the device to the patient.

The therapist must carefully consider the needs of the patients. Can the patient wait for the prefabricated orthosis to be ordered? Does insurance allow the patient the additional visit that is required to properly fit the orthosis that has been ordered? The patient's requirements in both the home and work setting should be considered. For example, someone who is a heavy laborer may require a rigid orthosis that is easily washable for work but may be more comfortable in a soft prefabricated orthosis for home. Several other considerations are age, allergies (some materials contain latex), cognitive status, skin integrity, other current or previous injuries to the involved or uninvolved extremity, and a support system if assistance is required with donning and doffing the device.

Time Constraints

Time can be a major factor for all organizations and therapists. Today's demand for increased patient caseloads influences how much time the therapist has with each patient. The therapist must evaluate the need and weigh the benefits of a custom-made orthosis versus a prefabricated device. There are also precut options that can save the therapist time. Specific thermoplastic patterns can be ordered and come ready to heat and apply to the patient. This saves a great deal of time in pattern development and cutting. Is it more appropriate to use a prefabricated or precut elbow mobilization orthosis and to spend the patient's treatment time performing hands-on intervention, or to fabricate a custom orthosis? The therapist must decide what will be the best use of the available treatment time.

Appropriateness and Availability of the Material

The type of prefabricated orthosis selected or the material used to fabricate a custom-made orthosis can have an effect on patient comfort, tissue healing, and position options. Patients who are slender and have prominent bony structures may be more comfortable in an orthosis that is fabricated out of neoprene (see Chapter 14 on Neoprene Orthoses) or another soft, forgiving material. Thermoplastic is rigid and can be uncomfortable when constant use is required. Comfort is an important issue and is directly related to consistent wearing patterns (Rossi, 1988).

Thermoplastic material may be the most appropriate material to use if the patient is required to have his or her hands in water or soil for any reason during the day. Thermoplastic material is easy to clean and tolerates moisture better than most fabric-based orthoses. However, there are patients who perspire and are thus prone to tissue maceration when solid thermoplastic materials are used; a light fabric-based orthosis may be considered for these patients.

Adjustments can be simple to make on soft orthoses with flexible metal inserts. No equipment is necessary, and the orthoses can be modified at the patient's bedside or in the home. A thermoplastic wrist orthosis requires a heating source and patient compliance in upper extremity positioning while the material is molded; this may not always be possible. Thermoplastic material may be the wisest and most appropriate choice when, for example, treating a patient with a flexor tendon injury that requires exact joint positions.

Unfortunately, preferred materials may occasionally be unavailable from manufacturers or suppliers and, at times, discontinued. It is advisable to have several options on hand to ensure patient's needs are met within a reasonable time frame.

Ease of Application

Ease of application by the patient in the work or home setting is an important factor to consider when developing an orthotic intervention plan. The therapist must determine the simplest solution for the patient's requirements. A prefabricated digit extension mobilization orthosis may be easier for a patient to apply than a more complicated custom device. Using serial static casting might be the simplest solution for some patients.

If the patient has several issues (e.g., multiple joint contractures) that need to be addressed with multiple orthoses, they should be prioritized. The therapist must determine the feasibility of the orthosis plan for the patient in the home setting; an individual who lives alone must be able to don and doff the device independently. Immobilization of healing structures may be the most important problem to be addressed, but increasing function may be deemed most important by the patient. Making sure to balance these demands is essential to be sure that the best possible solutions are offered.

Cost-effectiveness

When evaluating the patient's needs, the therapist must consider all of the cost-related variables. Is the orthosis going to be worn for a short period of time or will it be required on a more permanent basis? Will the patient's insurance pay for a prefabricated or custom-molded orthosis? The insurance carrier may or may not cover either type of orthosis. In some situations, the prefabricated orthosis may be more affordable to the patient without compromising the quality of treatment. It is appropriate to educate the patient regarding the options and to include him or her in the decision-making process. In some cases, the patient may require several orthoses, worn alternately throughout the day and night. Some of these orthoses may be custom made and others prefabricated.

Educated Decision Making

An educated decision must be made each time an orthosis is selected for a patient. There is a wide variety of materials, components, and prefabricated orthoses available for almost every situation. It is challenging to keep abreast of all of the available prefabricated orthoses, but there are many ways to stay informed.

To keep up with new trends, therapists can attend upper extremity continuing education events, including lectures and hands-on labs on successful orthotic interventions. Larger conferences frequently feature vendor booths that allow therapists to investigate new materials and prefabricated orthoses. Therapists can try orthoses and equipment on and request further information. Vendors are eager to provide in-service training and information sessions at facilities, offer material samples, and help with specific patient problem solving. Company representatives are often therapists who have decided to enter the equipment provision aspect of the business; they are integral to the development of new product lines and improvements of existing ones. In working with therapists all over the country, they collect valuable information on trends and helpful hints and are willing to share the tips they have learned.

Catalogs and Web sites provide an expansive amount of information regarding orthotic fabrication, fitting, and therapy intervention. Updated frequently, they enable the therapist to stay abreast of therapy trends. See Appendix A for a list of vendors and rehabilitation companies along with contact information.

Therapists can also review articles in therapy and surgery publications to gain a better understanding of the theoretical basis behind decision making for the application of orthoses. There are many methods for solving every patient's situation. A custom orthosis might meet the biomechanical issues but may cause problems for the patient in the areas of maintaining skin integrity or comfort (Rossi, 1988). Solutions to many orthotic-related problems can be found by reviewing current literature.

Prefabricated Orthoses for the Upper Extremity

This section, which presents a review of prefabricated orthoses, is organized according to where on the upper extremity the orthosis is to be applied. For each region, various prefabricated orthoses are discussed and comparisons are made to highlight specific fitting issues. This discussion is not meant to be inclusive of all available prefabricated orthoses; each manufacturer has versions of the commonly used prefabricated orthoses, and available products are too numerous to mention all. It is recommended that a thorough review and update of billing rules, insurance coverage, and proper coding (if applicable) of these prefabricated orthoses be conducted in order to stay compliant and ethical with reimbursement (refer to Chapter 1, Concepts of Orthotic Fundamentals for additional information). Although **continuous passive motion (CPM) machines** can be considered a treatment modality, here, they are referred to as an additional prefabricated orthotic option.

Shoulder and Upper Arm Orthoses

The diagnoses commonly treated with prefabricated orthoses at the shoulder and upper arm are clavicle, scapula, and humerus fractures; humeral head dislocations or subluxations; and rotator cuff injuries and surgical repairs. The types of prefabricated orthoses used to treat these conditions include clavicle braces, slings, functional fracture braces, and shoulder immobilization orthoses.

Clavicle Brace

Clavicle braces are available in a limited variety from most of the major rehabilitation suppliers (Fig. 11–1). Some providers also stock pediatric sizes. When fitting a patient with a clavicle brace, a key point to evaluate is an appropriate fit through the axilla. The strap system should not be too tight through this area because it can create increased pressure on the brachial artery and plexus, which innervates the arm. A loose fit may encourage a flexed cervical posture and is also not appropriate for proper clavicular stabilization. The patient should be able to relax the shoulders while good cervical and thoracic posture is sustained. Slings may also

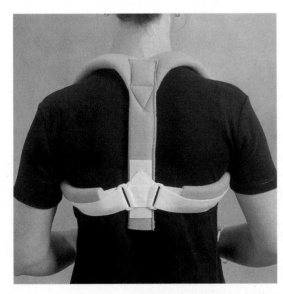

FIGURE 11–1 The Rolyan® Clavicle Posture Support. Observe the patient for 20 minutes after applying a clavicle brace to ensure proper fit. Check for any signs of neurovascular compression—numbness, tingling, coolness, or pain in the extremity—and readjust as needed. Photo courtesy of Patterson Medical (Warrenville, IL).

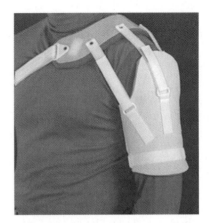

FIGURE 11–2 Hemiplegic slings—designed to support the head of the humerus in the glenoid fossa—are commonly recommended for patients who have had a stroke. Slings should be judiciously used to protect the extremity of patients with complex forearm and hand injuries, owing to the possibility of stiffness and edema. The AliMed® Hemi Shoulder Sling provides joint compression throughout the hemiplegic limb. Photo courtesy of AliMed (Dedham, MA).

be used for managing clavicle fractures and are often easier for patients to use. Discuss options and preferences with the referring physician.

Sling

There is a wide array of slings available that stabilize healing structures about the shoulder (e.g., rotator cuff, capsule, ligaments, bone, or neurovascular) and provide support and properly position the hemiplegic shoulder (Fig. 11–2). Hemiplegic arm slings are recommended for patients who have hemiplegia or a subluxating humeral head. There are several versions of the hemiplegic sling that have been used for many years; however, the newer GivMohr® Sling (Patterson Medical, Warrenville, IL) is an option that offers proprioceptive input in its design with the added benefit of reducing shoulder subluxation (Dieruf, Poole, Gregory, Rodriguez, & Spizman, 2005). The therapist must carefully monitor patients who are using slings to ensure that they are removing the sling and exercising the injured extremity, as recommended, to prevent complications of stiffness and distal edema.

There are a multitude of slings worn on the shoulder to provide support to an injured forearm, wrist, and/or hand (Fig. 11–3). Selection of an appropriate sling is contingent on the patient's diagnosis. Patients with a stable humeral fracture may wear a sling for support and comfort; it should be removed regularly throughout the day for appropriate exercise (Colditz, 1995). Patients who have undergone hand surgery also may be issued a simple version to be worn for comfort and protection of the upper extremity. Patient education with this population is key to minimize the dependent positioning of the hand that can encourage edema distally and appropriate exercises to prevent undue stiffness of the proximal joints.

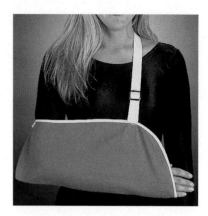

FIGURE 11–3 The Rolyan® Buckle Closure Arm Sling provides a way to rest the whole upper extremity following a surgery distal. Photo courtesy of Patterson Medical.

Humeral Fracture Brace

A prefabricated humeral fracture brace can be used for stabilizing a humerus fracture. A nonarticular design, which permits shoulder and elbow motion, may be chosen for midshaft fractures (Fig. 11–4) (Sarmiento & Latta, 2006). For more distal humeral fractures, custom components may be applied circumferentially to the humerus and the forearm with an elbow hinge connecting the two (Colditz, 1995).

Shoulder Immobilization Orthosis

A shoulder immobilization orthosis may be required for a fracture of the scapula, a rotator cuff injury and/or surgery, brachial plexus injury, and other shoulder surgeries. This orthosis immobilizes the humerus in the glenoid fossa and the scapula against the thoracic wall (Fig. 11–5).

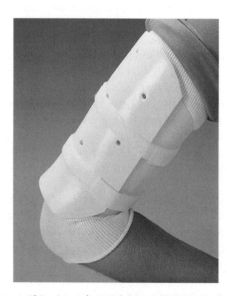

FIGURE 11–4 This circumferential brace (Rolyan® Preformed Humerus Brace) allows elbow and forearm motion while providing good immobilization and support to the healing fracture. Photo courtesy of Patterson Medical.

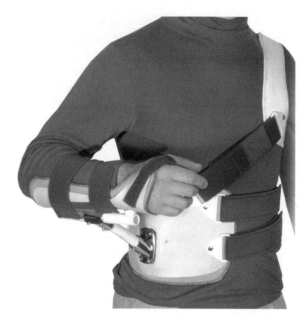

FIGURE 11–5 The FREEDOM® Gunslinger™ Shoulder Orthosis can be adjusted to place the humerus in any combination of abduction, flexion, and rotation. Photo courtesy of AliMed.

Continuous Passive Motion Machines

A shoulder CPM machine can be used for treating postoperative shoulders to prevent joint and soft tissue contractures. The Optiflex® S Shoulder CPM (Chattanooga, Vista, CA) is an example that is universal for left or right upper extremity use and has a memory chip card to store data for patients.

Elbow and Forearm Orthoses

The elbow is a complex and challenging joint to position properly and comfortably because it is composed of bony prominences and superficial nerves surrounded by forceful muscles. Some of the prefabricated orthoses that are used to treat the elbow are elbow protectors, neoprene compression sleeves, proximal forearm braces (counterforce braces), elbow mobilization orthoses, supination/pronation mobilization orthoses, and CPM machines.

Elbow Protector

Elbow protectors can be used before and after surgery for patients with cubital tunnel syndrome (ulnar neuropathy). The pad should be "worn over the posterior medial aspect of the elbow to protect the ulnar nerve from direct pressure or trauma" (Sailer, 1996). Available options incorporate a silicone gel pad insert to help reduce shock/vibration and apply light compression to a postoperative scar in the region of the ulnar nerve (Fig. 11–6).

Neoprene Compression Sleeve

Neoprene compression sleeves may be used to treat ulnar neuropathies, muscle strains, or provide comfort for arthritis of the elbow (Fig. 11–7). They offer gentle compression, warmth, and support to surrounding tissues as

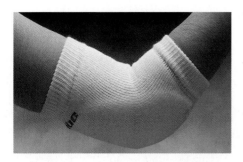

FIGURE 11-6 When fitting a patient with an elbow protector (Heelbo® shown), measure the distance circumferentially around the patient's elbow flexion crease, keeping in mind that the protector is intended to fit snugly. Photo courtesy of North Coast Medical (Morgan Hill, CA).

well as provide gentle feedback to the patient to restrict elbow flexion. The sleeve should fit snugly but not so tightly as to increase or induce any neurologic symptoms (tingling, pain, or numbness distally).

Proximal Forearm Brace (Counterforce Brace)

Lateral and medial epicondylitis straps and sleeves come in various options (Fig. 11–8A). Some have cushions that apply a gentle compressive force to the forearm muscles in an effort to change the fulcrum from the epicondyle to the muscle bellies; they also help reduce the intensity of the muscle contraction. When treating a patient with lateral epicondylitis, apply the pad over the forearm extensors just distal to the lateral epicondyle. With the elbow in extension, have the patient make a tight fist and then secure the strap firmly. Make sure to have the patient grasp, extend the wrist, and flex the elbow to check for comfort; pain at the lateral epicondyle should be diminished with the brace properly applied. Caution the patient not to secure the strap too tightly because the radial nerve is vulnerable to compression in this region (radial tunnel) with these particular braces (Aulicino, 1995; Kleinert & Mehta, 1996). A newer option—the Tendon Trak™—was designed to avoid direct pressure on irritated tissues allowing for circulation while continuing to provide support for the involved structures (Fig. 11–8B).

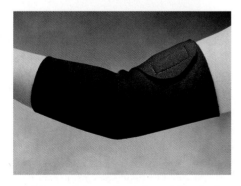

FIGURE 11-7 After applying a circumferential orthosis such as this Comfort Cool® Open Elbow Support, monitor the patient for a short time, watching for any signs of neurologic symptoms. Photo courtesy of North Coast Medical.

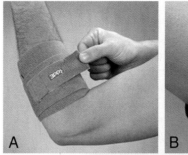
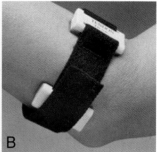
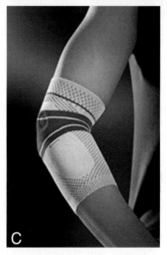

FIGURE 11-8 **A,** The 3pp® Tennis Elbow Strap should reduce the patient's pain; adjust the amount of compression applied as needed to increase patient comfort. Photo courtesy of 3-Point Products (Stevensville, MD). **B,** The Tendon Trak™ is therapist designed and features adjustable pads that should "bracket" the involved tissues and can be used for lateral or medial epicondylitis. Photo courtesy of North Coast Medical. **C,** The user-friendly Bauerfeind EpiTrain® Elbow Support combines the benefits of a compressive elbow sleeve with a tennis elbow brace. Photo courtesy of Bauerfeind USA, Inc. (Marietta, GA).

Many of the straps and sleeves designed for the treatment of lateral epicondylitis can also be used in the treatment of medial epicondylitis by rotating the pad to apply pressure on the medial forearm muscles. A multipurpose sleeves and straps can be used to treat patients who are diagnosed simultaneously with medial and lateral epicondylitis. These devices are designed to apply compression to both the extensor and the flexor muscle groups simultaneously (Fig. 11–8C).

Elbow Mobilization Orthoses: Dynamic and Static Progressive

Stiffness secondary to fractures and dislocations at the elbow can be treated with various prefabricated **dynamic and static progressive** elbow orthoses that provide a corrective force to the tissue. Devices such as the Elbow Extension or Flexion Dynasplint® System (Dynasplint® Systems, Inc., Severna Park, MD) and Progress™ Elbow Hinge Orthosis (North Coast Medical, Morgan Hill, CA) have neoprene or foam cuffs with malleable metal attachments both proximal and distal to the elbow. These orthoses are flexible and comfortable for the patient and can be easily adjusted when there is a decrease in bandages or edema. Patients can wear this type of orthosis with the load adjusted to provide a gentle stretch for sleep or intermittent daytime use. To maintain the gains in range of motion (ROM), the orthosis can be locked at a specific degree if desired, providing a means of static progressive positioning. Dynasplint® Systems offers these orthoses in pediatric and infant sizes as well as adult sizes; separate units for extension and flexion required.

A static progressive stretch orthosis developed by Joint Active Systems (JAS®, Effingham, IL) can be used to treat elbow flexion and extension contractures in one unit (Fig. 11–9). The application of a gentle stretch over a long period of time improves tissue extensibility and yields permanent tissue lengthening (Bonutti, Windau, Ables, & Miller, 1994). The device has proximal and distal cuffs, which can be adjusted to fit various limb lengths, and a load-adjustable hinge centered at the olecranon. Patients with spinal cord injuries at C5–C6 frequently develop elbow flexion contractures and may benefit from this type of orthosis. Mackie Elbow Brace (Ortho Innovations, Rochester, MN) offers a static progressive stretch in either flexion or extension in the same unit. The recently introduced elbow supination pronation (ESP) device from Lantz Medical (Indianapolis, IN) allows for addressing elbow flexion/extension and supination/pronation limitations either with a dynamic or static progressive approach all in one device.

Prefabricated hinged orthoses can also be used for restricting ROM in one direction while allowing unrestricted motion in the other direction (Fig. 11–10). For example, when treating patients with a biceps tendon repair, the brace

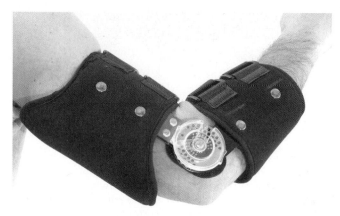

FIGURE 11–10 The hinge on this brace (Freedom® Comfort ROM Elbow Brace) can be adjusted to allow a specific restricted ROM. Photo courtesy of AliMed (Dedham, MA).

can be locked out to restrict full elbow extension, thereby preventing tension on the repaired tendon while allowing passive flexion and active extension exercises. As healing progresses, the extension restriction can be modified to increase ROM appropriately.

Supination/Pronation Orthoses

A tone and positioning (TAP) orthosis is a simple and comfortable alternative to a custom-molded supination/pronation orthosis. The Comfort Cool® Spiral Arm Splint (North Coast Medical) provides a gentle, low-load supination or pronation stretch to aid in increasing functional hand position (Fig. 11–11). This device, although originally developed for patients with neurologic conditions, can be beneficial in facilitating supination or pronation ROM if the tissue at the forearm and wrist is not too dense (soft end feel). This orthosis is not capable of delivering the torque required for patients with hard end feel or long-standing limitations in ROM. Other options for applying a stretch include dynamic and static

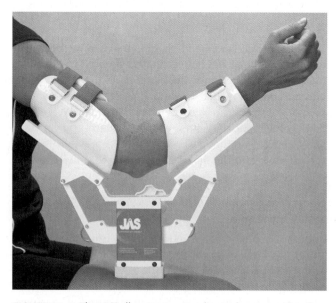

FIGURE 11–9 The JAS® elbow system can be used to treat either flexion or extension contractures at the elbow. The patient can easily don this orthosis and adjust the tension until a mild stretch is felt. Photo courtesy of Joint Active Systems (Effingham, IL).

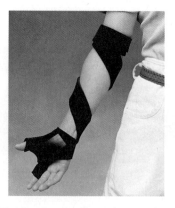

FIGURE 11–11 The Comfort Cool® Spiral Arm Splint is made of neoprene and is easily fitted, in either supination or pronation, to patients of all age groups. The neoprene strap can be used with the included glove component or can be used with a custom-made thermoplastic volar wrist support. Photo courtesy of North Coast Medical.

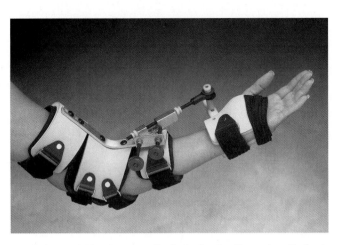

FIGURE 11–12 The Progress-Plus™ Supination/Pronation Orthosis from North Coast Medical allows for addressing both limitations in one device. Photo courtesy of North Coast Medical.

progressive devices such as the Progress-Plus™ Supination Pronation Orthosis (North Coast Medical) (Fig. 11–12).

Continuous Passive Motion Machines

An elbow CPM machine may be used to increase ROM. These are typically tabletop devices that can be set up to address limitations in flexion and extension at the elbow and supination and pronation of the forearm.

Wrist Orthoses/Wrist and Hand Orthoses

The wrist is made up of several joints that allow multidirectional movement, which can be complicated to support properly. When immobilization is the goal of an orthosis,

it is essential to provide adequate support to the wrist in all planes of motion. When mobilization is the goal, it is essential to facilitate intended movement patterns. Some prefabricated orthoses used for treating diagnoses at the wrist are wrist orthoses, wrist and hand orthoses, CPM machines, and wrist mobilization orthoses. Other diagnoses involving the digits also require the wrist to be included for adequate support and will also be included in this section.

Wrist Orthoses

"Commercially available wrist supports do not fit most distal radius fracture patients comfortably and can block full finger and thumb ROM" (Laseter & Carter, 1996). There are several issues to consider when fitting a patient with a prefabricated wrist and hand orthosis, including clearance of the distal palmar crease, thenar eminence, and first web space as well as proximal fit at the forearm to reduce migration, allow digit movement, and ensure appropriate wrist position.

Adequate distal clearance is necessary for unrestricted grasp and pinch activities. The patient should be able to flex all fingers fully and comfortably with little or no interference from the distal portion of the wrist support, especially the radial portion. The opposite problem may also be encountered when some designs may actually not extend distal enough, preventing the wrist from being immobilized adequately. Patients with large forearms and narrow wrists have inherent problems with distal migration of wrist orthoses and improper fit. The Liberty™ Flare (North Coast Medical) is a prefabricated orthosis that is designed specifically to accommodate this population (Fig. 11–13A). If a prefabricated orthosis is unable to provide the patient with adequate use of the digits or a comfortable fit proximally, a custom-fabricated orthosis may be indicated.

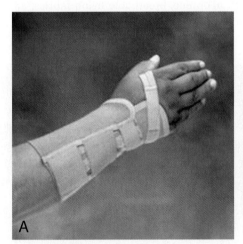
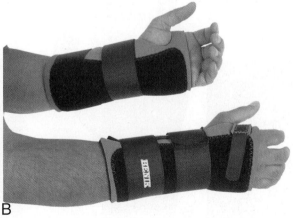

FIGURE 11–13 **A,** This wrist orthosis (Liberty™ Flare Splint) is a valuable option for patients with large forearms compared to wrist size. Photo courtesy of North Coast Medical. **B,** The Benik Corporation (Silverdale, WA) offers the W310 Wrist Splint that combines neoprene with a thermoplastic panel that can be heated and shaped to conform to the patient. Please note that customized designs are available directly through Benik to meet specific patient requirements. Photo courtesy of Benik Corp (Silverdale, WA).

The actual position of the wrist should be visualized while the prefabricated orthosis is on the patient and adjusted appropriately as per the specific diagnosis. For example, a patient with a wrist sprain is usually positioned for comfort, whereas an individual with a distal radius fracture is ideally positioned in 20 to 30° wrist extension after cast removal. If the patient is unable to obtain the desired range of extension, a prefabricated orthosis with a flexible metal or thermoplastic insert can be molded to the current wrist extension and later modified (Fig. 11–13B).

CARPAL TUNNEL SYNDROME

Prefabricated volar wrist supports are commonly prescribed to patients with carpal tunnel syndrome as a conservative method of treatment (Keith et al., 2009). It is recommended that patients with carpal tunnel syndrome be immobilized in a neutral position to provide maximum space at the carpal tunnel and reduce compression on the median nerve (Brininger et al., 2007) (Fig. 11–14A).

The Med Spec GelFlex® Wrist Brace (Medical Specialties, Inc., Charlotte, NC) has a gel cushion along the volar surface to provide gentle, conforming compression to the incision site after carpal tunnel surgery (Fig. 11–14B). This elastic canvas wrist wrap provides protection to the incision site and gives gentle feedback to the patient to avoid extreme positions of wrist flexion and extension postsurgery. A neoprene wrist wrap is a nice transitional option for a patient who is weaning off long-term use of a volar wrist support.

The Dynasplint® Carpal Tunnel System (Dynasplint® Systems, Inc.) was recently introduced and promotes stretching

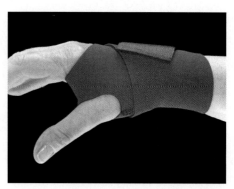

FIGURE 11–15 The thumbhole of this AliMed® Neoprene Wrist/Hand Wrap can easily be modified by simply trimming with scissors. Photo courtesy of AliMed.

the transverse carpal ligament over time to eliminate symptoms; it is still in preliminary stages of research.

ARTHRITIS

Volar wrist supports afford mobility at the hand and digits and are frequently prescribed for people with arthritis as a means to rest the affected wrist joint. Although wrist supports can be beneficial, patient compliance for wearing them is relatively low (Pagnotta et al., 2005). Patient concerns regarding wrist supports (whether prefabricated or custom) include comfort, interference with activities, appearance, cost, and reduced freedom of movement.

There are various wrist supports designed specifically to meet the needs of patients with arthritis. Neoprene wrist wraps are comfortable and warm but may provide less support than their foam and fabric-based counterparts (Fig. 11–15). Most suppliers have wrist supports that also provide metacarpophalangeal (MP) and/or thumb positioning (Fig. 11–16). Wrist and wrist/finger supports are available in neoprene, breathable nylon fabrics, and preformed thermoplastic options.

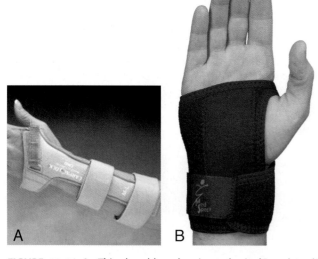

FIGURE 11–14 A, This dorsal-based wrist orthosis (Carpal Lock® Wrist Splint) positions the wrist in neutral, allowing unrestricted digital motion. Photo courtesy of North Coast Medical. **B,** The GelFlex® Wrist orthosis provides scar management within the design ideal for postoperative patients. Photo courtesy of Medical Specialties, Inc. (Charlotte, NC).

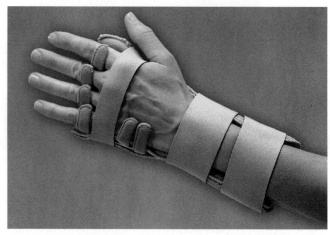

FIGURE 11–16 3-Point Products offers a forearm-based orthosis called the Comforter™ Splint which has extra padding and is intended for night use. Photo courtesy of 3-Point Products.

When treating patients with arthritis, the therapist needs to clearly define all relevant issues and goals to help determine which regime best suits the needs of the patient (see Chapter 17, Arthritis for more details). Some patients have problems with hyperhidrosis and prefer a light, breathable fabric orthosis, whereas others find orthoses that help keep the area warm to be helpful. Patients who are working or who are physically active tend to prefer the least restrictive orthosis. Patients may not tolerate MCP support during the day but will use a wrist-hand-finger orthosis (WHFO) to comfortably position the hand while sleeping.

Wrist-Hand-Finger Orthoses

Individuals with various diagnoses may require a WHFO for day and/or night use. There are several designs available for the treatment of patients with such diagnoses as arthritis, burns, nerve palsies, crush injuries, and spasticity. These orthoses come in various designs including volar, dorsal, and circumferential. There are soft versions that provide a gentle continuous stretch to spastic muscles and more rigid plastic orthoses that provide immobilization to healing structures (Wallen & O'Flaherty, 1990). The SaeboStretch® (Saebo Inc., Charlotte, NC) orthosis is an example of a flexible prefabricated WHFO that provides support used for patients with mild-to-moderate increased tone (Fig. 11–17A). Dynapro™ WHFOs (Ongoing Care Solutions, Inc. [OCSI], Pinellas Park, FL) offer support for those with moderate-to-severe spasticity. To address issues such as decreased functional use, increased tone, and contractures in the pediatric population, Comfy™ Hand Orthoses (Lenjoy Medical Engineering, Inc., Gardena, CA) offer various options that are terry cloth lined in multiple colors (Fig. 11–17B). The Benik Corporation W-700 series (Benik, Silverdale, WA) offers patients with radial nerve palsy several options for wrist and/or digit support in a low-profile design (Fig. 11–17C,D). See Chapter 21 for more details about the neurologically involved patient and Chapter 19 for peripheral nerve injuries.

Wrist Mobilization Orthoses: Dynamic and Static Progressive

Prefabricated dynamic and static progressive wrist orthoses are commonly prescribed to increase wrist ROM. The JAS® Progressive Splint (Joint Active Systems) is designed to increase wrist flexion and extension. The Static-Pro® Wrist Orthosis (DeRoyal Industries, Powell, TN) provides an alternative for wrist flexion and extension mobilization (Fig. 11–18A). Dynasplint® Systems also offers dynamic wrist extension and flexion orthoses in both adult and pediatric sizes (Fig. 11–18B).

Continuous Passive Motion Machines

Wrist CPM machines are frequently used to aid in increasing ROM at the radiocarpal joint. The Kinetec Maestra Hand and Wrist Machine (Patterson Medical) is a tabletop wrist CPM unit that can produce flexion and extension and radial and ulnar deviation at the wrist joint. Portable wrist machines

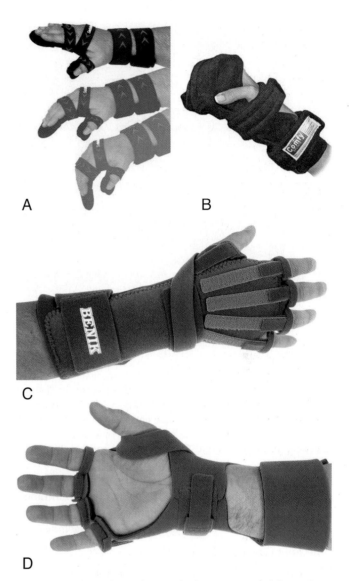

FIGURE 11–17 A, The SaeboStretch® is recommended for patients with neurologic conditions such as mild-to-moderate spasticity. Photo courtesy of Saebo, Inc. (Charlotte, NC). **B,** This Comfy™ Hand/Thumb Orthosis is washable and easily modified to obtain a custom fit. Many options are available including the thumb and dorsal-based designs. Photo courtesy of Lenjoy Medical Engineering, Inc. (Gardena, CA). **C and D,** This Benik W711 Forearm-Based Radial Nerve Splint is a low-profile option for long-term orthotic management. Note that this device is also offered in a hand-based design for patients without wrist involvement. Photo courtesy of Benik Corp.

include the Kinetec 8091 (Patterson Medical) and the JACE Wrist W550 (JACE Systems, Cherry Hill, NJ) (Fig. 11–19). These CPM machines provide adequate force throughout the ROM for patients with a soft end range.

Hand and Finger Orthoses

Because the hand is unique, the therapist is faced with many challenges in balancing the medically necessary restrictions with the patient's need for functional use. Some of the

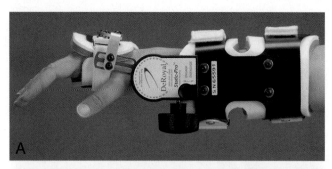

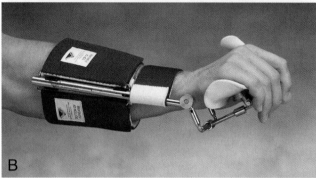

FIGURE 11–18 **A,** The Static-Pro® Wrist Orthosis offers a static progressive stretch at the joint's end range. Photo courtesy of DeRoyal (Powell, TN). **B,** This Wrist Extension Dynasplint® System provides a stretch in one direction only; multiple units are required to address multiple areas of stiffness. These units can be rented or purchased. Photo courtesy of Dynasplint® Systems, Inc. (Severna Park, MD).

prefabricated orthoses used for treating the hand are immobilization orthoses, dynamic and static progressive digit orthoses, ulnar deviation orthoses, gloves, and CPM machines.

MCP Joint Deviation Orthoses

The therapist should closely follow patients who have rheumatoid arthritis and are using supportive devices to slow the progression of carpal collapse and the resulting ulnar deviation

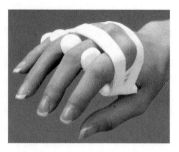

FIGURE 11–20 An LMB Soft Core Ulnar Deviation Splint is worn to support the MCP joints in extension and prevent radial deviation, which enables the patient to better perform functional grasp activities. Photo courtesy of DeRoyal.

at the MCP joints (Dell & Dell, 1996). Patients with ulnar drift may benefit from being supported with an ulnar deviation orthoses (Fig. 11–20). Short and long versions of this orthosis and other suggested prefabricated orthoses for this population are reviewed in Chapter 17, Arthritis. Another deviation orthosis is available to address proximal interphalangeal (PIP) joint deformity. The company 3-Point Products (Stevensville, MD) offers the 3pp® Side Step™ Splint with adjustable tension to correct/prevent joint deformity (Fig. 11–21).

PIP Joint Immobilization Orthoses: Boutonniere Deformity

Boutonniere deformity, or the disruption of the central slip of the extensor tendon mechanism as it inserts onto the base of the middle phalanx, is acutely treated with immobilization (Palchik et al., 1990). Aronowitz and Leddy (1998) treat all patients with acute boutonniere deformities with a device that positions the PIP in extension, leaving the distal interphalangeal (DIP) free to move actively or to be moved passively (Fig. 11–22A). Oval-8® (3-Point Products) and SIRIS™ Boutonniere Splint (Silver Ring Splint Company, Charlottesville, VA) may be used for the correction of a

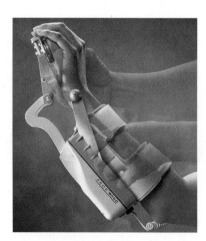

FIGURE 11–19 The JACE W550 Wrist CPM Machine allows for control of end-range stretching including programmable tension and time parameters. Photo courtesy of JACE Systems (Cherry Hill, NJ).

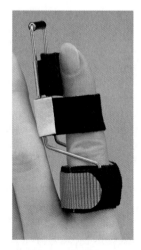

FIGURE 11–21 This 3pp® Side Step™ Splint can be used to address deviation issues at the DIP or PIP joint. Photo courtesy of 3-Point Products.

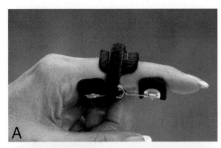

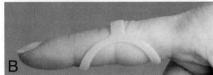

FIGURE 11–22 **A,** Note how the DIP joint is left unrestricted to allow for lateral band gliding exercises with this Bunnell™ Mini Modified Safety Pin Splint. Photo courtesy of North Coast Medical. **B,** Oval-8® Finger Splints may be used for management of a more chronic deformity. Photo courtesy of 3-Point Products.

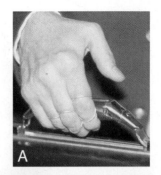

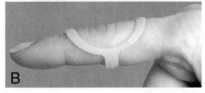

FIGURE 11–23 **A,** Silver Ring Splints are both functional and attractive. Photo courtesy of Silver Ring Splint Company (Charlottesville, VA). **B,** Oval-8® Finger Splints are offered in multiple sizes and can be modified with a heat gun. Photo courtesy of 3-Point Products.

boutonniere deformity and offer a more cosmetic solution for long-term deformity (Fig. 11–22B). Active and passive ROM at the DIP joint, while extension is passively maintained at the PIP joint, facilitates optimal anatomic positioning of the lateral bands.

PIP Joint Extension Restriction Orthoses: Swan-Neck Deformity

Swan-neck deformity, hyperextension of the PIP joint, and flexion of the DIP joint is commonly seen in patients who have rheumatoid arthritis or chronic volar plate injuries at the PIP joint. SIRIS™ Swan Neck Splint from Silver Ring Company (Fig. 11–23A) and orthoses such as the Oval-8® from 3-Point Products (Fig. 11–23B) offer a low-profile, attractive, and extremely effective option to maximize function of the digit in this chronic deformity. These devices restrict PIP extension allowing for functional flexion; they prevent the often painful "snapping" of the lateral bands as they slide dorsally when the PIP joint goes into hyperextension.

DIP Joint Immobilization Orthoses: Mallet Finger

DIP extension orthoses, including aluminum-padded orthoses and Stax Splints (North Coast Medical), are commonly used in the treatment of a mallet finger injury, which is the disruption of the terminal tendon at its attachment on the distal phalanx (Fig. 11–24A). The goal of treatment is to immobilize the terminal tendon so that it may scar down during an uninterrupted period of 6 to 8 weeks (Alexy & De Carlo, 1988). One concern for the treating therapist and physician is maintaining tissue integrity on the dorsum of the DIP joint during the immobilization period. A benefit of the clear plastic Stax Splint is that it affords visualization of the tissue; one downside is that you are not able to alter the joint position.

Aluminum orthoses are easily fitted to any digit and can be bent to modify extension at the DIP joint. To increase the stability of the orthosis (beneficial for maintaining dorsal tissue integrity), trim the foam to a thickness of ⅛″ and then cover the device with silk tape. Aluminum orthoses can be held in place with ½″ tape (Fig. 11–24B). Garberman, Diao, and Peimer (1994) report that as long as the injured digit is continuously kept immobilized in extension for 6 to 10 weeks, the type of orthosis used is insignificant in the successful outcome of mallet finger deformity. Customized casts and digit orthoses may be more appropriate for some populations (see Chapter 7, Immobilization Orthoses for details).

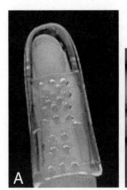

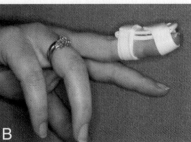

FIGURE 11–24 **A,** The Open-Air™ Stax Finger Splint is perforated, allowing air circulation and decreasing the likelihood of tissue maceration. Photo courtesy of North Coast Medical. **B,** An aluminum orthosis secured with Microfoam tape. Applying the tape obliquely to the volar fingertip and then crossing it over the dorsum of the device provides maximum distribution of pressure and secures the distal phalanx in good extension while the terminal tendon is healing (E. Rosenthal, personal communication, 1997).

CHAPTER 11

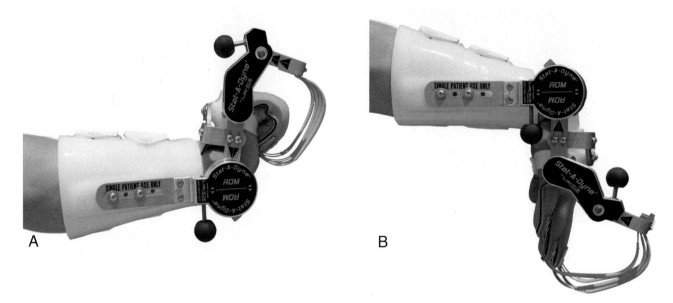

FIGURE 11–25 **A and B,** The Stat-A-Dyne® WHFO provides the therapist with the ability to isolate the tissue stretched by positioning the wrist and digits accordingly. This device also allows for a synergistic stretch into a functional grasp and release pattern as shown. Photos courtesy of Lantz Medical (Indianapolis, IN).

Finger Mobilization Orthoses: Dynamic and Static Progressive

Various prefabricated dynamic and static progressive finger orthoses are available to address stiffness (see Chapter 15, Stiffness). Full ROM at the PIP joints is imperative for hand function; therefore, both dynamic and static progressive PIP orthoses are commonly used in the clinic. A loss of extension at this joint can limit a person's ability to grasp large objects or collect change with an open palm. A loss of flexion at this joint can severely limit the ability to grasp objects or even shake hands (Prosser, 1996). The Stat-A-Dyne® WHFO uniquely provides for full ROM in both wrist and digit extension and flexion (Lantz Medical) (Fig. 11–25A,B). The SaeboFlex (Saebo, Inc.) is an orthosis for the neurologically involved patient that positions the fingers and wrist in a functional extension position via springs but allows active grasping. The dynamic nature of this device provides the release or extension (Fig. 11–26).

PIP JOINT EXTENSION

There are various digit-based spring-loaded PIP extension mobilization orthoses for the treatment of PIP joint flexion contractures. The amount of padding, length, and ability to alter force depend on the design. The LMB Spring Finger Extension Assist Splint (DeRoyal) is one example of this common orthosis (Fig. 11–27A). These come in various lengths; be sure to properly fit the device to the digit watching for any undue stress on adjacent joints.

Digit extension neoprene sleeves, such as the AliMed® Dynamic Digit Extensor Tube Splint (AliMed, Dedham, MA), can also be used to treat patients with PIP joint flexion contractures that have a soft end feel (Fig. 11–27B). Patients may tolerate wearing this orthosis longer because the heat generated by wearing a neoprene material can increase tissue extensibility

and blood flow while decreasing joint stiffness, pain, and muscle spasms (Michlovitz, 1990). Patients should be instructed in tissue monitoring because maceration of the skin can occur owing to excessive perspiration (Clark, 1997).

Other PIP joint mobilization orthoses include the PIP Extension Dynasplint® System, the JAS® EZ Finger orthosis (which offers extension and flexion with a single device), and variations of the Bunnell™ Safety Pin Splint (Patterson Medical) that provide a dynamic force via a spring coil (Fig. 11–27C). A Rolyan® Sof-Stretch Coil Extension Splint (Capener) (Patterson Medical) is commonly used in the treatment of boutonniere injuries postoperatively and PIP joint flexion contractures (Fig. 11–27D) (Capener, 1967;

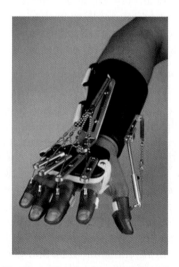

FIGURE 11–26 The SaeboFlex is custom fabricated to provide a custom fit to the patient with neurologic condition. Photo courtesy of Saebo, Inc.

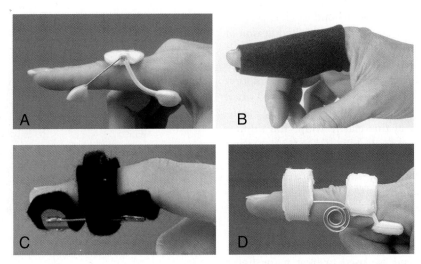

FIGURE 11–27 **A,** The LMB Spring Finger Extension Assist Splint can be adjusted to provide more (straightening the orthosis) or less (squeezing the proximal and distal pads together) force to the patient's PIP joint. The lateral wires can also be pulled out a little to accommodate edema. Photo courtesy of DeRoyal. **B,** The AliMed® Dynamic Digit Extensor Tube is made of neoprene and applies a low-tension load. This banana-shaped device is comfortable to wear and comes in various sizes. Photo courtesy of AliMed. **C,** The Bunnell™ Mini Spring Wire Safety Pin Splint to address DIP joint flexion contracture. A variation of this design is available to stretch the PIP joint as well. Photo courtesy of AliMed. **D,** Rolyan® Sof-Stretch Coil Extension Splint (Capener) used to position the PIP in extension. Photo courtesy of Patterson Medical.

Colditz, 1990; Iselin, 1997; Prosser, 1996). In an investigation by Prosser (1996), patients reported that the low-profile (streamlined) Capener Splint was easy to wear during the workday. Patients are more likely to use a comfortable, low-profile orthosis, thus spending more time in the device. Time spent at total end range is a significant factor; the greater the wearing time, the greater gains made in treating a PIP flexion contracture (Flowers & LaStayo, 1994; Prosser, 1996).

PIP JOINT FLEXION
The flexion glove is a staple found in most hand therapy clinics (Fig. 11–28A). It can be used alone or in conjunction with a volar wrist support to apply a passive flexion stretch to the MCP and interphalangeal (IP) joints as well as the extrinsic extensors. The wrist may need to be immobilized because it tends to collapse into flexion when a flexion force is applied to stiff digits. The patient can easily apply the glove and adjust it to a comfortable level of stretch. Customization of the glove includes converting the force applied from dynamic to static progressive by replacing the rubber bands with static line for those patients not responding to the dynamic stretch.

PIP/DIP flexion straps are fabricated and sold by many companies to provide a flexion stretch to the PIP and DIP joints simultaneously (Fig. 11–28B). However, the therapist can easily fabricate this simple strap with ¾" pajama elastic forming an adjustable loop. Patients can readily increase the tension by sewing, stapling, or securing a safety pin to make the loop tighter. Orthoses are available that can be used for multiple fingers that require increased flexion at the PIP and MCP joints (Fig. 11–28C).

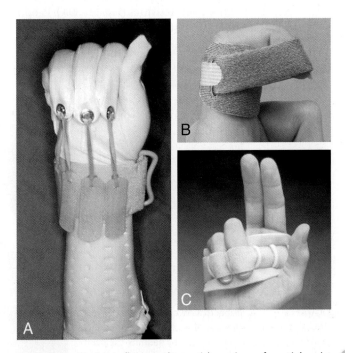

FIGURE 11–28 **A,** A flexion glove with a circumferential wrist orthosis. The wrist orthosis is worn to prevent compensatory wrist flexion when force is applied to the digits. **B,** The 3-Point Products Final Flexion Wrap is simple to use, adjustable, offers a flexible and comfortable material, and can be used for other purposes in addition to PIP/DIP flexion (see Table 11–1). Photo courtesy of 3-Point Products. **C,** The Norco™ Cinch Strap provides a stretch for combined MCP and PIP limitations. Photo courtesy of North Coast.

Elasticized wraps, such as Coban™ and CoFlex® (Patterson Medical), can also be used to address limited flexion of the fingers. This reusable wrap is self-adherent, making it easy to apply, hold in place, and reuse. The 2″ to 4″ rolls are useful for wrapping all fingers into flexion if limited motion is consistent across the digits. The 1″ rolls are best used when the fingers require individual levels of stretch. Many manufacturers have a version of this elastic wrap. The thinner wraps are useful for applying a stretch wrap to the digits and then dipping in paraffin because the wax can seep into contact with the fingers fairly readily. The thicker wraps are best for gentle edema wrapping because they provide support to a swollen, painful finger.

BUDDY STRAPS

Buddy straps are readily available in different forms from most major medical supplier and are used to treat many finger injuries including amputation, fractures, dislocations, sprains, and extensor tendon injuries (Fig. 11–29) (Alexy & De Carlo, 1988). These straps can be prefabricated or custom made and are easily adjusted to fit to swollen or slender fingers (see Buddy Strap fabrication in Chapter 10, Mobilization Orthoses).

Gloves

Various types of gloves are available, including short-fingered work gloves, bicycle gloves, and weight-training gloves, which are used to protect the hand from vibration, cold, contact stress, or repetitive work activities (Fig. 11–30A). People who use wheelchairs frequently wear palmar-padded gloves to increase their ability to grasp and decrease the wear and tear on their hands.

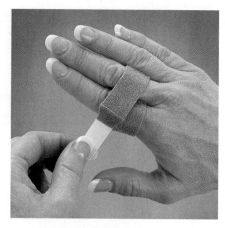

FIGURE 11–29 The 3pp® Buddy Loops® are one example of prefabricated buddy straps and are commonly used to ease the transition out of an immobilization orthosis. Photo courtesy of 3-Point Products.

For patients with peripheral nerve injury, the Robinson InRigger Gloves (AliMed) provide dynamic digit extension dorsally while allowing full finger flexion for function. Various "in-rigger" systems are available to meet the needs of different patients (Fig. 11–30B,C). Patients are fitted with a glove and components are added to accommodate for losses secondary to the specific nerve injury.

For patients with significant scarring to either the dorsal or the volar surface of the hand, the Bio-Form® Pressure Glove (North Coast Medical) can help control edema and hypertrophic scarring (Fig. 11–30D). This glove is available

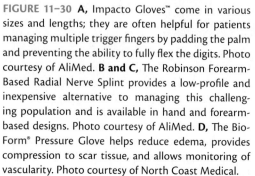
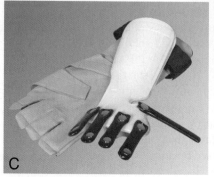
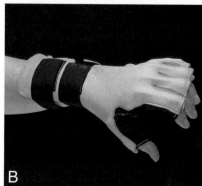
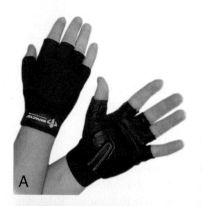
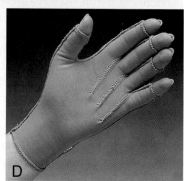

FIGURE 11–30 A, Impacto Gloves™ come in various sizes and lengths; they are often helpful for patients managing multiple trigger fingers by padding the palm and preventing the ability to fully flex the digits. Photo courtesy of AliMed. **B and C,** The Robinson Forearm-Based Radial Nerve Splint provides a low-profile and inexpensive alternative to managing this challenging population and is available in hand and forearm-based designs. Photo courtesy of AliMed. **D,** The Bio-Form® Pressure Glove helps reduce edema, provides compression to scar tissue, and allows monitoring of vascularity. Photo courtesy of North Coast Medical.

with or without open fingertips, which can provide opportunity for vascular monitoring and sensory input. For scar management alone, fully lined silicone gloves are available. For edema alone, various compression gloves, such as Iso-toner® gloves, are available from most medical suppliers.

Continuous Passive Motion Machines

Hand CPM machines can be used to treat patients with severe burns (Fig. 11–31A,B). Early goals for rehabilitation of patients with burn injuries to their hands include restored soft tissue coverage and "rapid advancement of active range of motion" at the MCP joints (Barillo et al., 1997). Patients with burns who are unable to flex the MCP joints to at least 70° and those who are unable to flex the digits actively secondary to the side effects of medication may use a CPM for 4 to 8 hours during the day and possibly while they sleep.

CPM machines are more commonly used to treat patients with stiff edematous fingers, a common complication of many injuries of the upper extremity. The CPM can be used to facilitate gentle ROM throughout the fingers or can be used to achieve increased motion at a specific joint. Note that obtaining full DIP flexion is a challenge when applying these devices. Furthermore, the unaffected joints often compensate by maximally flexing, thus decreasing the force aimed at the target joints. For example, when addressing tight PIP joints, the MCP joints may hyperflex, thus prohibiting optimal stretch at the PIP joints. The therapist should carefully monitor the patient's use of a CPM machine and the settings should be checked frequently.

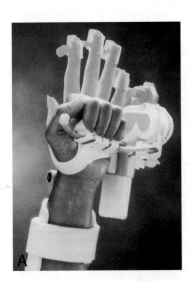
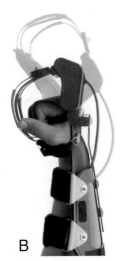

FIGURE 11–31 A, Hand CPM machines (JACE H4440 Hand CPM shown) may be used in the early treatment of patients with severe burn injuries. This system can also be used to assist patients in obtaining a composite fist. Note that the force applied promotes maximal DIP flexion. Units are available that provide the option for dynamic tension as well as continuous motion. Photo courtesy of JACE Systems. **B,** The Vector1 has an easy-to-apply glove design that allows for individualization of each digit. Photo courtesy of Lantz Medical.

Thumb Orthoses

The thumb is responsible for approximately 40% of hand function (Swanson & de Groot Swanson, 1990). When supporting a patient's thumb, the therapist must consider that the thumb is involved in all tasks requiring grasping, pinching, or stabilizing an object or requiring sensory information to operate (King, 1992). The therapist can be extremely challenged to find an orthosis, prefabricated or custom made, which is comfortable and functional while providing the proper support and positioning for the thumb joints. A painful carpometacarpal (CMC) joint can limit pinch or grip and severely impair hand function. An ideal orthosis for osteoarthritis at the CMC joint is one that stabilizes the joint in midpalmar/radial abduction, restricts adduction, and allows for full flexion at the IP joint (Melvin, 1995). A recently introduced functional orthosis is the MetaGrip® (HandLab, Raleigh, NC) that supports the CMC joint (MP and IP joints free). This device is adjustable, extremely durable, available in multiple sizes, can be cleaned in a washing machine, and will not lose shape in the heat (Colditz & Koekebakker, 2010) (Fig. 11–32A,B).

Restriction Orthoses

Neoprene wrist and thumb orthoses (either prefabricated or custom) can provide warmth and support to the thumb and wrist (see Chapter 14, Neoprene Orthoses for details). Custom-made thermoplastic orthoses for CMC arthritis are quite effective in immobilizing the thumb joint in a position of rest. Unfortunately, this immobilization orthosis can significantly hinder normal hand function and is often bothersome to the patient's skin and bony prominences. Patients often complain that the orthoses are uncomfortable and interfere with their daily routines. The 3pp® ThumSling® NP (3-Point Products) is designed to stabilize the CMC joint while allowing some mobility (Fig. 11–33A). The Comfort Cool® Thumb CMC Restriction Splint (North Coast Medical) is another functional orthosis commonly used for CMC

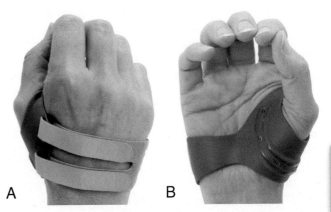

FIGURE 11–32 A and B, The MetaGrip® allows for maximum thumb and hand function while still offering optimal CMC joint positioning. An aluminum insert is adjustable to fit the individual patient. Photo courtesy of HandLab (Raleigh, NC).

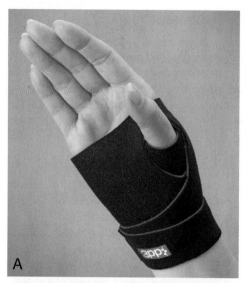

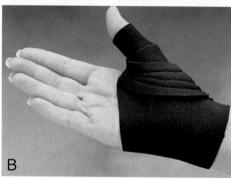

FIGURE 11–33 **A,** The 3pp® ThumSling® NP provides adjustable compression and support about the thumb. Note that a longer version including the wrist is also available. Photo courtesy of 3-Point Products. **B,** The unique strap design of this Comfort Cool® Thumb CMC Restriction Splint provides support to the CMC joint. Photo courtesy of North Coast Medical.

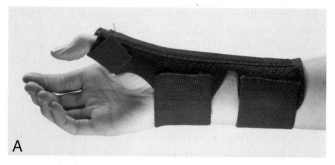

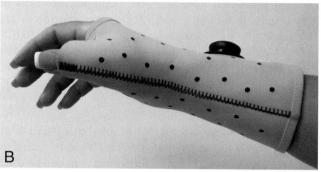

FIGURE 11–34 **A,** The Target Hitchhiker Thumb Orthosis allows IP joint motion while immobilizing the wrist and thumb MP/CMC joints. Photo courtesy of Corflex (Manchester, NH). **B,** The Long Thumb Spica Fracture Brace from Exos Corporation (distributed by DJO Global, Vista, CA) provides an alternative to casting or a circumferential orthosis. This unique prefabricated device allows for a customizable fit by dry heating the precut form and molding it directly to the patient. This orthosis includes a BOA® closure system to provide adjustable compression to accommodate for edema changes and patient comfort. This orthosis can be washed, or worn while bathing or swimming without risk of skin maceration due to perforations and unique material characteristics. Photo courtesy of Exos Corporation (Arden Hills, MN).

dysfunction including instability and arthritis (Fig. 11–33B). The neoprene material provides the joint warmth, gentle support, and protection. A version of this design is available that includes a moldable thermoplastic piece to provide a rigid stay at the CMC joint (Comfort Cool® CMC Abduction Orthosis, North Coast Medical). A longer version of this restrictive orthosis, the Comfort Cool® Wrist and Thumb CMC Restriction Splint (North Coast Medical), includes the wrist and is commonly used to treat deQuervain's tenosynovitis, inflammation of the thumb tendons at the radial wrist.

Immobilization Orthoses

At times, it is necessary to rigidly immobilize the patient's thumb, and there are various prefabricated and preformed thumb immobilization orthoses available from almost every manufacturer (Fig. 11–34A,B). The greatest challenge with these prefabricated devices is finding a version that places the thumb in an optimal functional position (midway between palmar and radial abduction); commonly in the prefabricated options, the thumb is placed in a greater

degree of palmar abduction or the distal edge prevents full IP joint motion making functional use difficult.

The therapist must pay close attention to proper biomechanical fit and comfort when applying an orthosis to a patient's thumb. The requirements for positioning of the thumb depend on the specific diagnosis. Deciding to use a radial versus circumferential design may depend on the rigidity needed and the functional demands of the patient. When less rigidity and more mobility is required, a radial-based design may be more comfortable and functional for the patient.

Prefabricated Orthoses Adaptations

Keeping abreast of all of the information on available orthotic materials, components, and prefabricated options is both challenging and interesting. Therapists must be able to use all available resources to best meet the needs of their patients. Sometimes, this means adapting prefabricated

TABLE 11–1

Creative Uses of Prefabricated Orthoses

Prefabricated Orthosis	Intended Use	Expanded Use	Adaptations
Reverse knuckle bender	PIP extension	FDP or FPL exercise tool	Move orthosis to distal phalanx
LMB	PIP extension	Increase tissue extensibility	Use in combination with paraffin and hot packs
Digit extension tube	PIP extension	Increase PIP extension	Add ³⁄₃₂″ thermoplastic insert volarly
Padded palmar work gloves	Reduce shock and vibration in palm and digits	Reduce MCP flexion in treating trigger finger	Patient wears glove to sleep or for functional use during day as needed
Isotoner® glove	Edema reduction	As flexion glove in combination with volar wrist support	Punch holes at tips and run rubber bands to apply flexion force
Silipos Digicap	Scar management	Edema management	Wear for edema management
Figure-8 (Oval-8® or Silver Ring)	PIP extension	Isolated DIP flexion	Clear DIP proximally, use as exercise blocking orthosis
Coban™	Edema control	Flexion wrap	Apply to individual digit or all digits in full fist position
Wrist Hand Orthosis	Wrist support	Digit and wrist support for radial nerve palsy or other nerve-related issues or for stiffness	Add finger loops around proximal phalanx of involved digits (i.e., 3pp® Final Flexion Wrap or cut custom neoprene finger loops) and attach with Velcro to dorsum of orthosis for digit MCP support

FDP, flexor digitorum profundus; *FPL*, flexor pollicis longus.

orthoses for purposes other than what they were originally intended to do. Table 11–1 provides a few creative ways to use prefabricated orthoses.

*C*onclusion

Prefabricated orthoses play an integral part in the practice of upper extremity therapy. The therapist should carefully evaluate each patient and then determine which type of orthosis is most appropriate. When determining what orthosis to use, the therapist must consider the biomechanical goals, requirements for the treatment of a specific diagnosis, and, most important, the patient's goals. Sometimes, a custom-made orthosis is more appropriate; and at other times, a prefabricated orthosis is the better choice.

Chapter Review Questions

1. What factors should be considered when choosing between a prefabricated and a custom orthosis?

2. Give an example of a modification that can be made to a prefabricated orthosis in order to address a specific patient need.

3. What diagnoses would be most appropriate for a prefabricated orthosis? Which would not?

4. How can a therapist keep abreast on the wide variety of prefabricated orthoses available?

5. Give two examples of prefabricated mobilization orthoses and their function, advantages, and disadvantages.

12 | Casting

Karen Schultz, MS, OTR/L, FAOTA, CHT; updated for 2nd edition by MaryLynn Jacobs, MS, OTR/L, CHT

Chapter Objectives

After study of this chapter, the reader should be able to:

- Define and discuss key concepts and terms related to casting.
- Identify key factors to consider when selecting the most appropriate cast technique.
- Appreciate the variety of material choices available for casting the joints of the upper extremity.
- Describe the most common diagnoses or conditions that would be appropriate for the casting techniques presented.
- Explain the general precautions relative to the use of the various casting materials.

Key Terms

Bivalved
Casting motion to mobilize stiffness (CMMS)
Drop-out cast

Fiberglass casting materials
Functional cast therapy (FCT)
Orficast™
Plaster of paris (POP)

QuickCast 2
Serial static
Soft casting materials
Univalved

Introduction

Casting is the circumferential application of rigid or semirigid material to a part of the body. The materials used include **plaster of paris (POP)**, rigid or soft casting tape, and digit casting tapes. Often, the cast has no opening for removal, but it can be **univalved** or **bivalved** to allow the cast wearer to remove and reapply it. Serial stretchers, often made of POP, incorporate half the extremity circumference (Tribuzi, 1990). A **drop-out cast** is circumferential on one side of a joint and incorporates half the extremity circumference on the other side. This design blocks joint motion in one direction but allows motion in another; thus, the patient may use active motion to help resolve a passive limitation but cannot regress to a prior posture (Hill &Yasukawa, 1999). Although the cast, drop-out cast, and serial stretcher have no moving parts and are often considered immobilization orthoses, they can provide or augment the functions of a mobilization orthosis (Bell-Krotoski, 1987, 2011). Colditz (2011) describes the use of casting materials for the mobilization of chronically stiff joint(s). This concept is reviewed briefly in this chapter but in greater detail in Chapter 15 on stiffness (Box 12–1).

BOX 12–1

Types of Casts

Univalved cast: opened only on one side normally to increase space secondary to edema or discomfort; can be secured with hook and loop or a circumferential wrap (Fig. 12–12A)

Bivalved cast: cut on both sides for easy removal; can be secured with hook and loop or a circumferential wrap (Fig. 12–12B)

Drop-out cast: part of the extremity can be moved within the cast; restricts motion in one or more directions (Fig. 12–12C)

Cylindrical cast: typical circumferential fracture cast needs to be removed using a saw (Fig. 12–12D)

Plaster slab/stretcher cast: these incorporate half the surface/circumference of the body part; most often used to give rigid support to a joint and used with a circumferential wrap or to apply a stretch to extrinsic tendons and tight tissues (Fig. 12–12E)

Indications for Use

Clinicians find casting to be a powerful weapon in their treatment arsenals. The casting technique helps solve several challenging problems that the therapist frequently identifies during the patient evaluation. Because casting provides optimal pressure distribution and a cast usually remains on 24 hours per day, the patient population for casting often includes those with sensory, motivation, and cognitive problems (Bell-Krotoski, 1987, 2011). Casting maintains the maximum tolerable end range position and thus maximizes end range time. As described by Flowers and LaStayo (1994, 2012), the greater the end range time, the faster the contracted tissue lengthens and passive range of motion (PROM) increases.

Indications for casting include the following:

- **Swollen, painful proximal interphalangeal (PIP) joints**—common after joint dislocation and joint reconstruction (Bell-Krotoski, 1995, 2011; Colditz, 2002)
- **Acute, closed central slip avulsion without fracture** (Colditz, 2002; Coons & Green, 1995; Evans, 2011; Rosenthal & Elhassan, 2011; Schneider & Smith, 1987)
- **Acute, closed terminal extensor tendon rupture or avulsion** (Brzezienski & Schneider, 1995; Rosenthal & Elhassan, 2011)
- **Extrinsic muscle–tendon unit tightness**—a sequelae to protective positioning and common after many types of injuries, including extensive soft tissue injury to the hand or wrist, crush injury, tendon and nerve laceration, replantation, and fracture (Colditz, 2002; Tribuzi, 1990)
- **Hard end feel contractures of any joint**—may be secondary to fracture; amputation; dislocation; tendon rupture, laceration, or repair; nerve repair; volar

plate avulsion; and burn (Bell-Krotoski, 1995; Colditz, 2002; Schultz-Johnson, 1992, 1999; Tribuzi, 1990)
- **Muscle–tendon unit imbalance at a joint**—may be the result of ulnar nerve palsy, arthritis, tendon avulsion, or tendon laceration and repair (Bell-Krotoski, 1987)
- **Proximal joint loss of PROM**—improvement requires long lever arms via a mobilizing orthosis (Bell-Krotoski, 1987; Colditz, 2002)
- **Chronically stiff hand**—casting motion to mobilize stiffness (CMMS) (Colditz, 2000a, 2000b, 2002, 2011)
- **Compliance problems** (Bell-Krotoski, 2011; Colditz, 2011; Sailer & Salibury-Milan, 2000)
- **Loss of PROM owing to spasticity** (Goga-Eppenstein, Hill, Seifert, & Yasukawa, 1999)

Casts can be used for various purposes, including the following:

- To rest and/or protect a joint, especially when edema needs to be controlled (Bell-Krotoski, 1995, 2011)
- To coapt acutely ruptured tendons or bony avulsion and to immobilize the part to allow anatomical healing (Brzezienski & Schneider, 1995; Coons & Green, 1995; Schneider & Smith, 1987)
- To increase PROM by holding articular and periarticular structures at the maximum tolerable length for long periods of time, remodeling tissue (Flowers & LaStayo, 1994, 2012; Glasgow, Tooth, Fleming, & Hockey, 2012)
- To transfer a muscle–tendon unit force to adjacent joints (Bell-Krotoski, 1987; Colditz, 2011)
- To rebalance flexor and extensor mechanisms at the PIP joint (Bell-Krotoski, 1987)
- To increase the effective lever arm, and thus the force at a proximal joint when distal joints are casted (Bell-Krotoski, 1987)
- To act as a base for mobilizing orthoses when distributing pressure and minimizing migration are essential
- To mobilize multiple joints by casting specific joints in positions of function and allowing self-mobilization of noncasted joints via active range of motion (AROM) (Colditz, 2000a, 2000b, 2011)
- To mobilize a joint by blocking motion in one direction and allowing motion in another (Goga-Eppenstein et al., 1999)
- To decrease tone and increase soft tissue length in spastic extremities (Colditz, 2002, 2011)

Swollen, Painful PIP Joints

After joint dislocation or reconstruction, the PIP joint may require rest in the maximum available extension (Fig. 12–1A,B). This position reduces the incidence of PIP flexion contractures and places the joint structures in the optimal position to regain function. Dorsal dislocations or fracture dislocations are exceptions and require an orthosis to block extension in order to protect the healing volar structures (Baltera, Hastings, Sachar, & Jitprapaikulsarn, 2010; Lubahn, 1988). A cast reduces edema and provides excellent pressure distribution. The hard

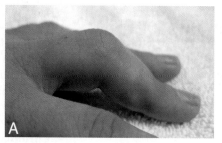
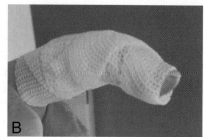

FIGURE 12–1 **A,** Central slip disruption following a blunt trauma to the dorsal PIP joint, resulting in an inability to actively extend the PIP joint. Note the posturing of the DIP joint into hyperextension. **B,** Initial cast includes the PIP in extension with the DIP flexed to overcome the strong tendency to revert back into the deformity.

shell offers protection from external forces. However, the cast may stress the PIP joint during removal, even if it is soaked first to soften it. Thus, for highly acute joint involvement that results in extreme tenderness, the therapist may need to choose another form of orthotic intervention other than casting.

Acute, Closed Central Slip Avulsion and Zone III Extensor Tendon Repair

Casting is one treatment method for acute, closed central slip avulsion and zone III extensor tendon repair (Fig. 12–2A–C) (Evans, 1995, 2011; Rosenthal & Elhassan, 2011). The sooner this injury is identified and treated, the better. However, even weeks and months after injury, if the finger still appears to be inflamed, the tendon may still benefit from a period of undisturbed extension in a cast. When the tendon is allowed to rest in the stress-free, shortened position, it may heal without surgical intervention. Positioning the finger with the PIP in neutral and the distal interphalangeal (DIP) left free coapts the ends of the torn central slip and allows the rebalancing of the extensor mechanism at the DIP joint. It also helps elongate the oblique retinacular ligament (ORL) and improve DIP flexion. Evans (1995, 2011) adds a nail hook and rubber band to the cast with a proximal rubber band attachment on the

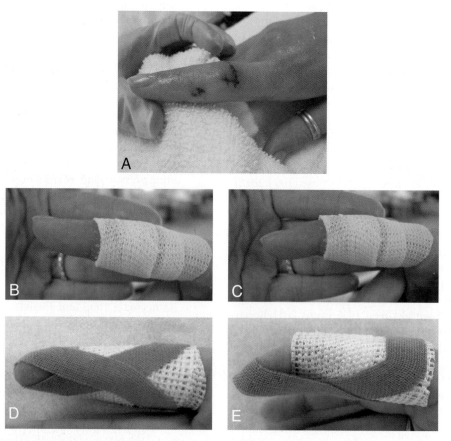

FIGURE 12–2 **A,** A lacerated and repaired zone III extensor tendon injury is managed in much the same way as a closed central slip avulsion. **B,** The PIP is positioned in full extension, and the DIP is free to move. **C,** Note the tight ORL with attempts at flexing the DIP joint with the PIP extended. **D and E,** Elastic therapeutic tape is applied to impart a gentle dynamic flexion stretch to ORL. The amount of tension applied can be easily adjusted by the patient.

volar side of the cast to increase DIP flexion in the finger with a tight ORL. Another option to consider when the digit presents with a tight ORL (instead of a nail hook) may be to use a strip of elastic therapeutic tape (such as Kinesio® Tex Tape or similar elastic therapeutic tape) or a soft Microfoam™ tape to apply gentle flexion force. To use this approach, start on the dorsal proximal surface of the cast and direct the tape over the DIP joint with gentle pressure ending on the volar proximal surface of the cast (Fig. 12–2D,E).

Ideally, if the finger demonstrates full PIP extension, the cast is left in place for approximately 6 weeks. If the finger has developed a flexion contracture, then the PIP needs to be serially casted until full extension is reached. Once the PIP flexion contracture is resolved, the 6-week period of immobilization commences. Some clinicians recommend starting small arc guarded active motion at 3 weeks; however, this must be done with great care and with a responsible patient (Evans, 1995, 2011). If the patient flexes the PIP abruptly during this time, the therapist can assume that the continuity of the central slip has been compromised, and the 6 weeks of extension must begin again. Making this information clear to the patient facilitates compliance. At the 6-week point, the patient is gradually weaned from the cast and can begin wearing a removable orthosis. Discontinuing extension positioning abruptly can compromise the end result.

Extrinsic Muscle–Tendon Unit Tightness

Extrinsic muscle–tendon unit tightness occurs after many types of injuries, including extensive soft tissue injury to the hand or wrist, crush injury, tendon and nerve laceration, replantation, and fracture. It can also be a sequela to protective positioning. The therapist has many treatment options for minimizing the muscle–tendon unit shortening, one being the POP stretcher, which can be very effective if constructed well (Fig. 12–3).

The advantage of plaster lies primarily in its extreme rigidity. The initial plaster costs little. However, if the patient requires many serial stretchers, the price of the material added to the cost of setup and cleanup may equal or even exceed the cost of thermoplastic material. The **serial static** treatment process necessarily involves progression of the orthosis' shape to position the tissue at ever-greater lengths. Although plaster cannot be remolded the way thermoplastic material (elastic based) can, it often gives superior results. The type of thermoplastic material that can withstand frequent remolding is often not rigid enough to maintain the joint at end range. Highly rigid thermoplastics cannot tolerate frequent remolding and must be discarded for new material. Reinforcing the thermoplastic requires effort each time the orthosis is revised. With a minimum of practice, therapists can fabricate POP stretchers efficiently and cost effectively.

Another essential advantage is POP's superior drape and ability to distribute pressure. When pressure is distributed well along the skin surface, the patient can withstand higher forces (Brand, 1988). The limitations in the amount of force that can be generated in an orthosis are related to skin tolerance because this is usually the weak link in force delivery. However, if the force is well distributed, the target tissue can often withstand higher loads (Brand, Hollister, Giurintano, & Thompson, 1999a). It is theorized that higher loads may have the potential to increase tissue length faster. Thus, plaster provides the opportunity to increase PROM faster than materials that are less conforming and less efficient at distributing the load.

Hard End Feel Joint Contractures

Brand (1988) was the first clinician to use serial casting on hard end feel contractures of the PIP joints (see Chapter 15 on Stiffness for details). Since then, therapists all over the world have used this technique on PIP joints and other joints of the upper extremity with great success (Fig. 12–4). Serial

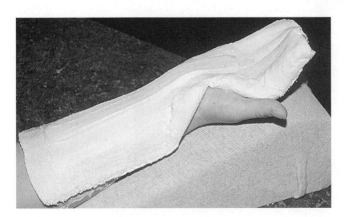

FIGURE 12–3 A POP stretcher is used to lengthen the muscle-tendon unit itself as well as any muscle–tendon unit adhesions.

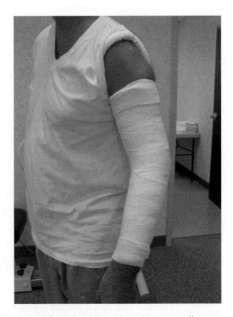

FIGURE 12–4 Serial static approach to improve elbow extension using POP. Note the generous length proximally and distally to maximize pressure distribution and patient comfort.

casting positions shortened tissue at maximum length but not beyond it, the way mobilizing orthoses with elastic traction tend to do. This positioning applies a mechanical stress to tissue, causing it to remodel in a longer form. Clinical experience has shown that almost any contracture involving live tissue, even one that is years old, will benefit from serial casting. Notable exceptions are Dupuytren's disease and contractures caused by fibrotic tissue (see Chapter 15, Stiffness for details). Heterotopic ossification and exostosis do not respond to casting.

Tissue that has been overstretched will shorten when placed on slack for a significant duration in a cast. Clinical experience suggests that tissue remodeling to increase length occurs more rapidly than remodeling to shorten overstretched tissue. In the case of a PIP flexion contracture, the cast may reestablish enough length in the palmar tissues to allow full passive PIP extension. However, the overstretched dorsal hood extensor mechanism often will not be able to accomplish full active extension; thus, surgery may be necessary. The surgical procedure creates an inflammatory response in the extensor hood. If immobilized long enough (usually 3 to 4 weeks) to allow collagen cross-linking to form and then mobilized at just the right speed, extension and flexion may be restored at 8 to 10 weeks postsurgery without reproducing the previous extensor lag. The patient will not be a candidate for the extensor procedure until the flexion contracture resolves.

Muscle–Tendon Unit Imbalance

Addressing the AROM and PROM limitations induced by nerve injury, Bell-Krotoski (1987) noted that casting can help "rebalance externally what has become imbalanced internally by a selective muscle loss." After paralysis of the hand's intrinsic muscles, an imbalance of the extensor mechanism—overpull of the proximal phalanx by the extensor digitorum communis (EDC) into extension and absent translational forces of the intrinsics on the dorsal hood—prevents the fingers from being fully extended at the interphalangeal (IP) joints (Fig. 12–5A). In addition, the metacarpophalangeal (MCP) joints lose their primary flexor, and these joints flex only after flexion of the IP joints by the flexor digitorum superficialis (FDS) and flexor digitorum profundus (FDP).

Bell-Krotoski (1987) explained that casting of the IP joints into extension allows the fingers to be brought into full extension by the EDC and into flexion at the MCP joints by the FDS and FDP (Fig. 12–5B,C). Thus, casting allows external rebalancing of the fingers and can be used temporarily before and after intrinsic replacement surgery in lieu of dynamic mobilization. The hyperextension in the intrinsic minus hand commonly present at the MCP joint does not usually continue after the casts are applied because the primary flexion of the MCP joint has been restored.

Another example is with weakened muscles from a nerve injury or compression such as carpal tunnel syndrome (Fig. 12–6A). The abductor pollicis brevis (APB) is a very powerful and important muscle about the thumb innervated by the median nerve. Strengthening this muscle is a challenge secondary to the strong compensatory pull of the thumb extrinsic muscles. To assist in blocking these extrinsic muscle–tendon units, simply cast the thumb IP joint in extension. This will help isolate the action of thumb palmar abduction by isolating the APB muscle (Fig. 12–6B,C).

Casts can also be used as an exercise tool. To improve tendon glide and joint motion, provide the patient with DIP and PIP casts to apply during exercise sessions (Fig. 12–7A,B). These are a helpful addition to a home program to maximize glide and joint motion.

Lengthening Lever Arms

Occasionally, the therapist identifies a situation in which a contracture requires the use of higher force levels. In such cases, the physics of levers may help deliver the force. Casting is an excellent method for stabilizing a joint to increase mechanical advantage. As described in Chapter 4, Mechanical Principles, the farther away the sling or loop is placed

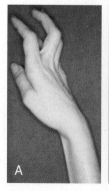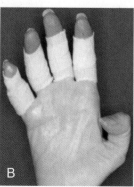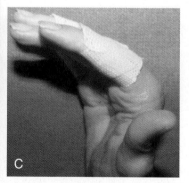

FIGURE 12–5 A, Combined ulnar and medium nerve injury leading to intrinsic paralysis and an imbalance of the extensor mechanism prevents the fingers from being fully extended at the PIP joints. Casting of the PIP joints into extension allows the MCP joints to be brought into full extension by the EDC **(B)** and full flexion by the FDS and FDP **(C)**.

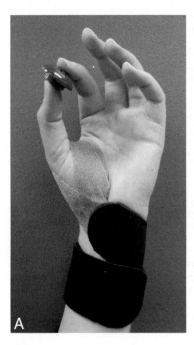
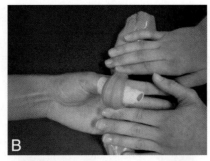
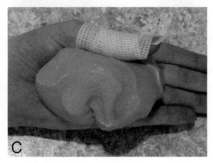

FIGURE 12–6 A, Orficast™ tape used to position thumb out of the palm with patient, demonstrating loss of thenar muscle function after median nerve injury; tape adheres directly to neoprene strap, securing orthosis around the wrist. Exercise orthoses: **(B)** Thumb IP extension immobilization cast assists in redirecting the power of thumb palmar abduction to the APB muscle and MP flexion to the flexor pollicis brevis (FPB) muscle **(C)**.

from the affected joint, the higher the force that the orthosis can generate. For example, when an orthosis is fabricated to increase MCP joint flexion, the sling can be placed distal to the stabilized PIP to increase the force at the MCP. Without PIP stabilization, the distally placed sling will instead act on both the PIP and the MCP. This stabilizing technique is especially desirable for small fingers—the short proximal phalanxes result in a decreased mechanical advantage (Fig. 12–8A,B). The therapist who uses long lever arms must first take note of joint stability and then closely listen to the patient for complaints of joint pain (Fig. 12–8C–E) (Brand, Hollister, Giurintano, & Thompson, 1999b).

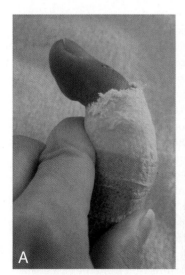
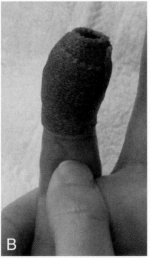

FIGURE 12–7 Blocking casts can assist with home program; PIP cast for encouraging DIP/FDP glide **(A)** and DIP cast for PIP/FDS glide **(B)**.

Chronically Stiff Hand

Effectively treating chronic stiffness of multiple joints of the hand and upper extremity can seem overwhelming. Strategically casting specific "looser" joints of the hand while leaving stiffer joints free for mobilization via AROM has proven effective when other approaches have failed (Colditz, 2000a, 2000b, 2002, 2011).

Hand therapists have been taught to fabricate mobilization devices that increase joint motion in one direction but cautioned that gains in one direction should never be at the expense of losing motion in the opposite direction. An additional principle taught is that immobilization of *any* joint that is not absolutely necessary to be within the orthosis should be avoided. Colditz (2000b, 2002, 2011) makes the exception with her approach: **casting motion to mobilize stiffness (CMMS)**. She describes a process of using circumferential casting to recover motion in the hand with multiple chronically stiff joints (Fig. 12–9). This technique requires careful molding of a *POP* cast to immobilize proximal joints so as to focus and redirect all the power of active movement to the targeted "stiff" distal joints (Bell-Krotoski, 2011; Colditz, 2011). Active movement of the distal joints is possible in both directions of flexion and extension, reestablishing differential glide of the soft tissue layers necessary for normal joint motion.

The advantages of CMMS are the following:

- The consistent light pressure of the cast and the active motion within the circumferential cast facilitates lymphatic flow, thus mobilizing chronic edema.
- The patients are able to focus active motion on the stiffest joints, which they have previously been unable to effectively move to gain joint range.

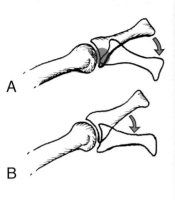
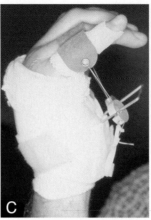
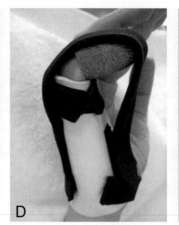
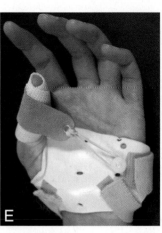

FIGURE 12–8 Applying stress to a joint can result in undesirable tilting **(A)** or desirable gliding **(B)**. **C,** This PIP casting technique can be used when an MCP extension contracture and a PIP flexion contracture coexist. **D,** The small finger (SF) DIP joint is casted in order to increase the lever arm for better mechanical advantage when applying dynamic stretch to the PIP joint via the strip of neoprene. **E,** Adding this thumb IP joint cast allows for isolated stretch at MP joint.

- The targeted, repetitive active movement of the stiff joint(s) enables cortical reintegration and recreates functional movement patterns.
- POP is inexpensive, therapy visits are fewer and less frequent (decrease in co-payments), and cast changes are infrequent because the cast is left in place for prolonged periods to allow retention of joint movement gained (Colditz, 2000a, 2000b, 2011).

Compliance Problems

Motivation, cognition, family demands, and maturity can each affect compliance. Therapists and physicians need to recognize that a fairly high percentage of patients are not fully compliant when issued a removable orthosis (Sanford,

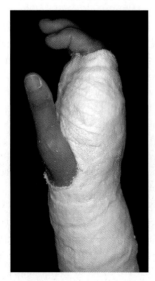

FIGURE 12–9 Wrist and MCP extension cast fabricated from POP used to encourage motion at the IP joints.

Barlow, & Lewis, 2008). When compliance becomes a major concern in patient treatment, the therapist/physician should consider a circumferential, nonremovable cast (Colditz, 2011). This will offer the best opportunity for achieving treatment goals because it requires no judgment or cooperation. The patient need only keep the cast on and in good condition. If a caregiver is involved, then the clinician must instruct the caregiver to watch for signs of cast intolerance, vascular compromise, and how to remove the cast. The cast eliminates difficulties that result from donning and doffing the orthosis improperly and inconsistently.

Casting for Central Nervous System Disorders

Traumatic brain injury, stroke, and cerebral palsy commonly result in muscle tone and muscle synergy disorders that create joint contractures (see Chapter 21, Adult Neurologic Dysfunction for more information). Because patients with these disorders often lack the cognitive and sensory awareness to monitor their own status, their orthoses must distribute pressure optimally or harm to skin and joints can result (Schultz-Johnson, 1999). A frequently used technique to increase PROM for central nervous system (CNS) disorders is serial casting (Colditz, 2011; Goga-Eppenstein et al., 1999). The circumferential design provides even pressure distribution, edema control, and scar remodeling via pressure. Because the ROM problems confronting these patients are mostly owing to hypertonicity of muscle in consistent patterns, the clinician usually does not need to worry about losing motion in the opposite direction from the cast goal.

The therapist must carefully consider the number of joints incorporated into the cast, since hypertonicity controlled at one joint may increase tone at adjacent joints. For example, if an elbow cast does not control the wrist, flexor tone (now controlled at the elbow) may increase at the wrist, causing dramatic wrist flexion posture and potential median nerve compression against the distal volar end of the cast.

CNS Casting Materials

Many therapists use synthetic casting tape lined with cast padding to treat spasticity because it is strong yet lightweight. Some therapists still favor plaster, especially for use around the fingers, thumb, and palm, because it conforms well and allows air exchange (Fig. 12–10).

Fabrication

Casting an adult, especially one in an agitated state, most often requires additional positioning assistance. The patient's joint is placed in a tolerable position—usually a submaximal position for the joint—while the clinician applies the casting material. All plaster casting materials heat the extremity during fabrication, which in turn can warm soft tissue structures, making the extremity more flexible. If the cast fabricator takes advantage of the increased PROM, the joint position obtained during casting may be too extreme for the patient to tolerate. Therefore, caution should be taken during fabrication not to overstress the tissue. As the joint/tissue position progresses, some swelling may occur; should this happen, reassess cast position, cast tightness, and any other conditions that may have caused this. If the edema is due to dependent positioning, then simple elevation may suffice.

Precautions

Casting for patients with CNS injuries has its own set of precautions and concerns. The clinician must frequently check for signs of cast intolerance by looking for color and temperature changes, swelling, and subtle signs of discomfort. To avoid the possibility of cast-caused trunk abrasions, the therapist may choose to cover the cast with a soft material or wrap, such as Moleskin, stockinette, or an Ace™ wrap. The clinician must instruct the family and/or nursing staff to be sure that the patient does not put things into the cast. Taping the cast's edges prevents this possibility. All caregivers must remember to keep the cast dry.

CNS Cast Regimen

Particularly important with this patient population is to not initiate casting on a Friday if the patient cannot be checked over the weekend. If the setting permits, the therapist should check the first cast a patient receives several times a day. In an outpatient facility, the therapist must make sure that the patient and/or caregiver understand all precautions. If the patient does well, the cast can be left in place 3 to 6 days, after which it is removed. If it is clear that the patient has tolerated casting well, then the clinician may immediately replace the cast and leave it on for up to 2 weeks or as the medical doctor (MD) recommends. Careful monitoring must continue.

Casting over a prolonged period can lead to muscle atrophy. Although considered a contraindication or negative side effect in the primarily orthopedic patient, in the patient with CNS dysfunction, this loss of muscle strength is considered a goal. The atrophy helps reduce flexion posture and subsequent joint contracture (see Chapter 21, Adult Neurologic Dysfunction for detailed information).

Casting Materials and Equipment

Plaster of Paris

Therapists have used gauze impregnated with POP to cast finger contractures, especially PIP flexion contractures (Fig. 12–11) based on the work of Paul Brand, MD. Plaster is the material first used by Dr. Paul Brand for patients with Hansen's disease in India and then in the United States (Wilson, 1965). Brand developed a technique of applying

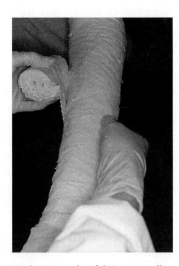

FIGURE 12–10 POP being used to fabricate an elbow cast to combat spasticity in a patient with a neurologically involved upper limb.

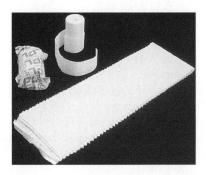

FIGURE 12–11 POP comes in rolls and sheets of various widths.

POP casts that imparted a gentle stretch to the tissue as it was being applied. He slowly and serially corrected the clubfoot deformity that many patients with Hansen's disease presented with. Through his work and documentation, hand therapists have fruitfully used this technique for smaller joints of the hand and upper extremity. Every clinician is encouraged to read his book, *Clinical Mechanics of the Hand* (Brand & Hollister, 1985, 1993), and a letter he wrote shortly before his death to the *Journal of Hand Therapy*, "Lessons from Hot Feet" (Brand, 2002). Plaster has been one of the preferred materials of choice because it is readily available, inexpensive, breathable, friendly to skin and wounds, and accurately conforming. Patients can be instructed in how to remove and apply plaster for use in a home program.

POP's primary disadvantage is that it is vulnerable to moisture. POP softens and loses its strength when exposed to water. Plaster is heavier and often thicker than thermoplastic. Although POP is messy to apply, the practiced therapist can develop a system to minimize cleanup. When POP and water mix, an exothermic chemical reaction takes place. Cases of burns caused by the application of POP have been reported; thus, the therapist must observe the patient carefully for this possible complication (discussed in detail later in this chapter) (Becker, 1978; Grazer, 1979; Haasch, 1964; Kaplan, 1981; Lovell & Staniforth, 1981; Schultze, 1967; Staniforth, 1980) (Box 12–2).

Fiberglass (Rigid)

With the advent of **fiberglass casting materials** (gauze impregnated with a water-activated resin), therapists have been able to take advantage of its lightweight quality to make larger casts (Fig. 12–12A–E). Fiberglass is rigid, durable, and lightweight, making it a good alternative for casting large joints. It is available in bright colors and all sorts of patterns. A few available products for rigid immobilization include Scotchcast™ Plus Casting Tape (3M™, St. Paul, MN), Cellacast® Xtra Cast Tapes (Patterson Medical, Warrenville, IL), and Delta-Lite® (BSN medical Inc., Charlotte, NC).

BOX 12–2

Why Consider Plaster over Thermoplastics?

- Excellent conformability, thus decreases the possibility of pressure sores
- Absorbs perspiration due to its porous nature
- Generates neutral warmth, which allows for gentle stretching as it sets
- Cutaneous stretch receptors rapidly adapt to the change in length with serial casting
- Provides more even skin pressure (cylindrical)
- Aids in edema reduction because of the circumferential "snug" application
- Can be made as nonremovable; changed only by therapist

BOX 12–3

Plaster versus Fiberglass

Plaster
- Longer drying time
- More prone to indentations that can lead to breakdown
- Stronger
- Heavier
- Less costly

Fiberglass
- Shorter drying time
- Higher risk of splintering
- Harder
- Lighter
- More resistant to dirt
- More durable
- More costly

These materials can be used for serial casting of wrists and elbows; however, they are not an option for casting fingers. Unfortunately, the skin does not tolerate the chemicals in the fiberglass and such casts require padding; thus, finger casts are too bulky and nonconforming. Fiberglass casts must be removed with a cast saw, and it also has a shorter shelf life than plaster (Box 12–3).

Soft Casting (Semirigid)

Application of a soft cast offers an alternative to traditional rigid casting when some degree of mobility is indicated. Commonly available products include Scotchcast™ Soft Cast (3M™, St. Paul, MN), Cellacast® Soft Cast tape (Lohmann & Rauscher, Topeka, KS), and Delta-Cast® Soft (BSN medical Inc.). This category of soft materials is unique in the world of casting materials. They remain somewhat flexible and never set rigidly, as does their fiberglass and POP counterparts. These characteristics offer two major advantages. First, because they never become rigid, soft casting tapes can be used for patients who will benefit from slightly flexible immobilization. Second, they do not require a cast saw for removal, so they can be used for patients who cannot tolerate a cast saw or who may need to remove the cast when away from the facility. This material cannot be made into a bivalved cast. This is applied directly on the skin or over light stockinette; no padding is necessary underneath the material. The soft cast material has no shelf life once the package is opened; any cast material not used must be discarded. Other materials such as thermoplastics or a plaster slab can be creatively incorporated into the cast orthosis to increase overall rigidity or block a direction of motion.

Soft casting is a great transition modality from a hard cast to semirigid one. Soft casting is often used with athletes for return to sport with the appropriate padding on the outside of the orthosis (see Chapter 20, The Athlete, for greater

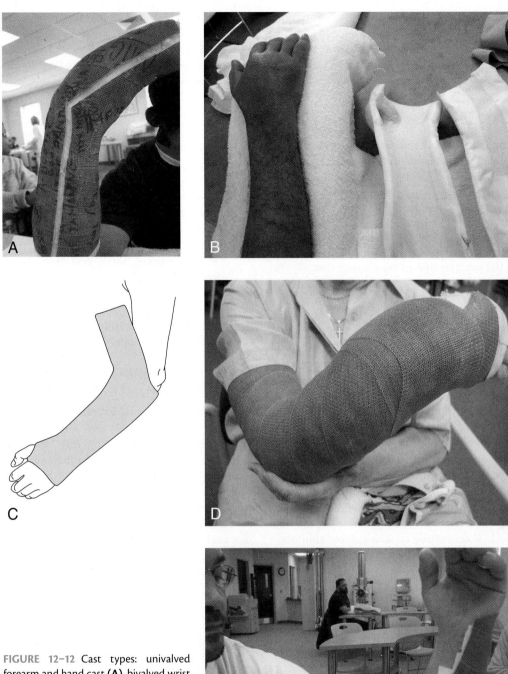

FIGURE 12–12 Cast types: univalved forearm and hand cast **(A)**, bivalved wrist cast **(B)**, drop-out cast **(C)** (Photo borrowed from Deshaies, L. D. [2008]. Upper extremity orthoses. In M. V. Radomski & C. A. Trombly Latham [Eds.], *Occupational therapy for physical dysfunction* [p. 440]. Philadelphia, PA: Lippincott Williams & Wilkins), cylindrical long arm cast **(D)**, and posterior elbow slab/cast **(E)**.

detail). Increasing the layers increases the durability and rigidity; however, this makes the cast heavier and bulkier. The overall setting time for this material is approximately 5 to 6 minutes. If univalved or upon permanent removal, a cast spreader is used to open the cast. Once open, the borders are lined with a Moleskin or Moleskin-like material to decrease irritation from possible rough edges. Securing the cast on the extremity can be done with any type of circumferential wrap. During contact sports, the athlete will need to have additional padding to protect opposing players.

Delta-Cast® Conformable: Functional Cast Therapy

Gaining popularity is the concept of **functional cast therapy (FCT)**, formerly referred to as focused rigidity casting (FRC), based on the premise that using a device that allows functional use while providing protection and stabilization to the injured structure(s) prevents many of the harmful consequences of prolonged immobilization. The theory is that an early return to function helps minimize muscle atrophy and joint stiffness and improves circulation to the healing area. These orthoses are made from Delta-Cast® Conformable Casting Tape (BSN medical Inc.)—a knitted, elastic, polyester fabric, imbedded with a clear resin. This product can be used as an alternative to traditional thermoplastic orthoses; it may allow for increased function and more comfort than a traditional fiberglass cast. Due to a three-way stretch, Delta-Cast® Conformable provides for a smooth, contoured application resisting wrinkling around the wrist and digits (Fig. 12–13A). The cast is applied over a terry cloth stockinette, removed with simple bandage scissors, and edged with felt. The number of layers determines whether the final cast will be flexible or rigid. A zip-cutting stick, a flexible thin barrier that is slid under the cast exactly where it is to be cut off with bandage scissors, is used to avoid harming the patient

because there is minimal padding between skin and cast. These washable casts are ultimately secured to the area with hook-and-loop closure (Fig. 12–13B). Indications for use are similar to all other casting materials, commonly used as an alternative to an immobilization orthosis or circumferential cast.

Some benefits of Delta-Cast® are as follows:

- Latex- and fiberglass-free formulation
- Durable—same device can be used throughout all phases of healing
- Fit may be adjusted by trimming if edema changes
- Easy to trim and remove with cast scissors (Patterson Medical)—no cast saw required
- Washable (device can be hand washed and then dried with hair dryer or air dried)
- Multidirectional (three-way) stretch providing wrinkle-free application
- Excellent conformability and good rigidity
- Smooth finish, which helps to increase patient comfort
- Working time: 0 to 3 minutes; setting time: 3 to 20 minutes
- Available in various widths from 1″ to 4″

Digit Casting Tapes (QuickCast 2, Orficast™ Tapes)

QuickCast 2 (Patterson Medical) and **Orficast™** (North Coast Medical, Morgan Hill, CA) are two nonplaster options currently available for digit casting. They have become very popular in hand therapy, offering the therapist a means to make a low-profile, circumferential digit orthosis quickly and with excellent conformability. The slight tackiness of these materials helps to obtain maximal contouring. QuickCast is an elastic fiberglass mesh, impregnated with heat-softened thermoplastic. The material shrinks when it is heated with a hair dryer (Fig. 12–14A). Orficast™ tape is composed of threads of thermoplastic that are knitted together, making it breathable,

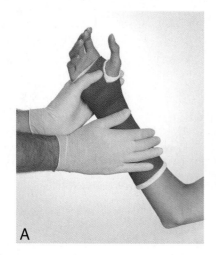
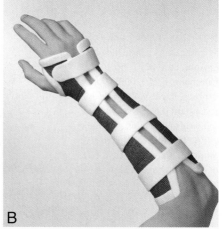

FIGURE 12–13 Delta-Cast® Conformable Casting Tape used for FCT technique: application requires gloves to protect hands **(A)** and final cast shown with hook-and-loop closure **(B)**. Photos courtesy of BSN medical Inc. (Charlotte, NC).

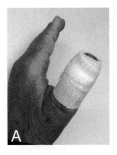
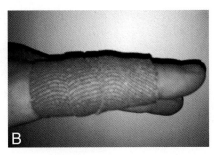

FIGURE 12–14 **A,** QuickCast 2 used to fabricate this thumb IP immobilization orthosis following a terminal tendon injury. **B,** Orficast™ conforms well to create a smooth PIP immobilization orthosis after a central tendon injury.

and is most commonly activated (softened) in hot water (Fig. 12–14B). Orficast™ is available in 3 cm and 6 cm rolls; once molded to the digit, this material can be dry heated to bond together and to adhere strapping if needed. With both of these materials, once heated, the individual strips can be applied either directly onto the skin or over some type of light cotton stockinette. For a firm cast, only one or two layers of tape are required; the more layers that are applied, the more rigid the final cast will be (and the more bulky). Not only do these casts create a comfortable orthosis, but, because the material is so thin as compared to POP, they also allow the therapist to cast adjacent fingers without forcing them into extreme abduction. These casting tapes set up quickly, several minutes faster than plaster or fiberglass, making it a time-efficient material. The setup and cleanup for a QuickCast or Orficast™ orthosis is minimal compared to plaster. The therapist does not need to wear any gloves during application. A finger cast made from these tapes can sometimes be removed (discussed later in this chapter), reheated, and reused as long as there has not been excessive wear and it does not have to be cut off the finger. This is in sharp contrast to plaster, where the therapist must discard these casting materials after removal. The therapist can create univalve finger casts to make them removable with Serial Cast Scissors. The short blades, with blunt ends, are contoured for safety when cutting close to the skin, and the proportionally long handles provide excellent mechanical advantage.

Clinical Example: Serial Static PIP Joint Extension Orthosis

Activation of QuickCast 2

The most common method to activate QuickCast 2 tape is to use a hair dryer that is long nosed, 1,600 W with high airflow. This type of dryer heats the tape effectively and quickly. It is important that it is long nosed because the dryer will not shut off when hot air is funneled back into the end. Short-nosed dryers shut down when hot air returns into the nose, which often occurs when heating QuickCast 2. The tape is

placed on a towel or silicone surface so that when the airflow is applied, it will not "fly" off the surface. The activation time is approximately 60 seconds. The working time is approximately 30 seconds, which may be challenging for a clinician that is not familiar with this material. However, with handling experience, this working time should be sufficient. **Caution:** Do not use a heat gun with QuickCast 2.

Activation of Orficast™

Orficast™ thermoplastic tape is activated by heating at a minimum temperature of 149°F. Possible activation sources include hot water bath, heat gun, heating plate, or microwave oven. The activation time depends on the heat source and varies from 30 seconds to 2 minutes. When activated on a heating plate or in a microwave oven, Orficast™ thermoplastic tape should be placed on silicone paper to prevent adherence to the surface. When using a heat gun, the tape should be placed on a towel to avoid migration; the heat gun should be set at minimum airflow and held at least 6″ from tape. Orficast™ has more stretch and elastic properties than its counterpart, QuickCast 2. Although this property can be used to the clinician's advantage, caution should be taken to avoid excessive stretch, which could lead to excess compression of tissues.

Casts fabricated from both of these tapes, if in good condition, can be gently unwrapped, reheated, and reapplied. The reader is referred to the manufacturers' instructions for more detailed information on the specific properties, advantages, and areas for caution for each material. Overheating of either of these materials will cause breakdown of the material itself. Patients can expose their fingers to water with these materials; however, they must dry the cast thoroughly to prevent skin maceration or softening of the cast. The patient can dry the cast with a towel or hair dryer on a low setting. Patients should use caution with getting these casts wet whenever possible due to the potential loss of cast rigidity and joint position.

Materials and Method

Making a tape cast requires the following materials:

- QuickCast 2 or Orficast™ tape
- Activation source (as mentioned previously):
  - QuickCast 2: hair dryer
  - Orficast™: hot water, heat gun, microwave oven
- Serial Cast Scissors (Patterson Medical)
- Towel
- Spray bottle with water (optional)
- Petroleum jelly (optional)
- Cast padding (optional)
- Tincture of benzoin (or similar; optional) (Patterson Medical)

To begin the cast fabrication process, cut the length of the preferred tape needed for the finger. The length depends on the length and circumference of the finger and the number of joints involved (Fig. 12–15A). The finger cast requires only a single layer of material with about $^1/_8$″ overlap.

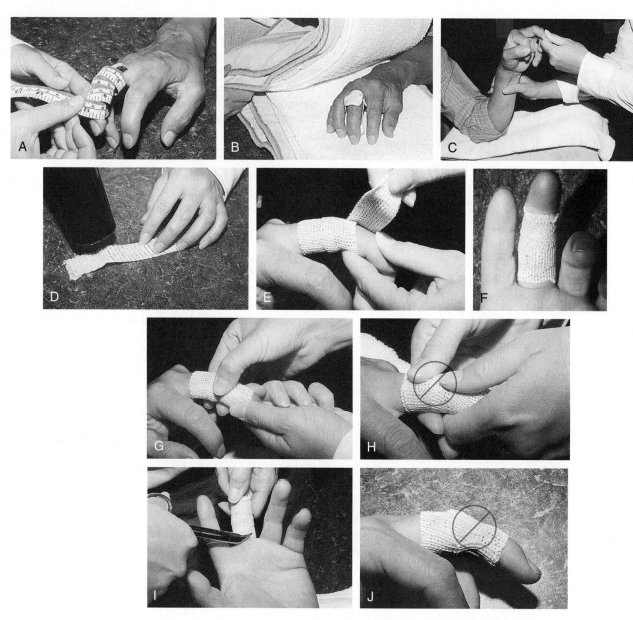

FIGURE 12–15 **Steps for fabricating a QuickCast 2/Orficast™ finger cast. A,** Estimate the amount of tape needed by spiraling a cloth dressmaker's tape around the finger in the same configuration as the planned cast. **B,** Heat in combination with a digit extension mobilization orthosis to precondition the finger to gain maximum PROM just before casting. **C,** Extend the patient's PIP joint using axial traction. **D,** Hold the dryer above the QuickCast tape, which will shrink as it becomes soft and hot. Keep the dryer steady; avoid moving it back and forth. If using Orficast™, activate in hot water for about a minute. **E,** Keeping the tape stretched cautiously (QuickCast 2 can tolerate more stretch than Orficast™, where too much stretch can lead to vascular compromise), wrap all the way around the proximal phalanx once and then begin to spiral distally, wrapping once for each layer and overlapping the previous layer. **F,** Wrap the finger so the DIP joint is free to move. **G,** Use a continuous rotary motion to conform the material closely to the finger and obtain an optimal fit. **H,** To avoid point pressure, do not poke at the cast with your fingertips; instead, use the length of your fingers for maximal pressure distribution. **I,** Use the Serial Cast Scissors to contour and smooth the edges. **J,** If there are any indentations, the cast must be removed and remade.

Preconditioning the Finger

The cast results are more rapidly achieved and of greater magnitude when the joint is preconditioned or stretched out just before casting (Flowers & LaStayo, 2012; Glasgow et al., 2012). The therapist should use one of the following techniques to gain maximum PROM just before casting: compression and/or massage for edema reduction, heat and stretch, joint mobilization, active and passive exercise, and therapeutic activities (Fig. 12–15B).

Position and Technique

Before making the cast, decide on patient and finger positions. Practice with the patient. Be sure the patient understands the materials, technique, and rationale for cast application. Position the finger as follows:

1. Remove any rings from the finger to be casted.
2. Seat the patient, placing the elbow of the affected extremity on a firm but padded surface.
3. Have the patient (or an assistant) hold the finger to be casted at the distal phalanx, leaving the DIP crease free, and then pull the finger using axial traction while the patient (or an assistant) pulls the hand away from the traction force by extending the wrist or bending the elbow (Fig. 12–15C). The force must take the PIP joint to maximum available extension without causing pain.
4. Activate the cut tape (Fig. 12–15D), and when softened, pick it up and stretch it back to maximum length.
5. Sustain the traction force until the cast is set.

Take note that with QuickCast 2, after the tape is applied on stretch to the finger, it will not significantly shrink back down and overcompress the finger. However, with Orficast™, only apply a light stretch to avoid vascular compromise. Because the tape will be tacky, the therapist should moisten his or her hands with water to prevent the tape from sticking and to make the material easier to work with. Taking care to avoid the fragile skin of the finger web space, place the tape as far proximally as possible on the proximal phalanx. Keeping the tape cautiously stretched, wrap it all the way around the proximal phalanx and then begin to spiral distally, overlapping each wrap by about $1/8''$ over the previous wrap (Fig. 12–15E). If the DIP joint is to be left free to move, end approximately $1/16''$ proximal to the DIP joint flexion crease, but extend the cast fully to the DIP joint dorsally (Fig. 12–15F). Once the tape has been applied to the entire finger, use a continuous rotary motion of the fingers to "screw" the material down onto the digit (Fig. 12–15G). **Caution:** Avoid point pressure against the tape at all times (Fig. 12–15H). Keep fingers moving on the cast tape.

Check and Revision

Inspect the palmar joint crease at the MCP joint and be sure the patient can flex the MCP without the proximal-palmar end of the cast pressing into the joint crease. If this occurs, use the Serial Cast Scissors to carve out some of the material and allow unimpeded movement (Fig. 12–15I). Next, check the DIP crease to be sure that the DIP joint can fully flex. Again, either push the material away from the crease or use the Serial Cast Scissors to trim the cast if needed. Finally, check the web spaces and contour or trim as needed. The Serial Cast Scissors present minimal risk to the patient's skin. All of the edges must be smooth to prevent skin irritation. Observe the cast closely for any signs of indentation along the substance of the cast. If any indentation is evident, remove the cast and start over (Fig. 12–15J).

If the cast appears unsatisfactory, simply unwind the material—this is an option even a few minutes after the cast is completed. After the tape is off the finger, simply repeat the heating process and reapply the same material. Unwinding the material becomes more challenging once the tape is fully hardened. The cast will set up in 1 minute or less. **Caution:** Do not use the hair dryer (or heat gun) to reheat the tape when it is on the finger. The heat can cause great discomfort and may burn the tissue.

Occasionally, the cylindrical cast will become loose enough that it may slide off the finger, especially after the first few applications. This may be due to a decrease in edema and/or a loosening of the tape due to body heat and extended wear. If the cast comes off at a time where the patient cannot come back to the clinic for remolding, the patient should always be instructed on how to keep the cast on in these situations. Microfoam™ tape, Coban™, and similar self-adherent type wraps can be applied to both the proximal portion/border of the cast and exposed skin in order to anchor the cast on the finger (Patterson Medical). This should be sufficient enough to hold the cast in place until the patient can return to the clinic.

Using Plaster of Paris

Materials and Preparation

Making a PIP extension cast from POP requires the following materials (Fig. 12–16):

- POP rolls cut into $2\,1/2''$ strips, folded in half
- Hot water
- Small clean bowl
- Serial Cast Scissors
- Tissue
- Petroleum jelly
- Cast padding (optional)
- Drapes to protect work surfaces and patient's clothes

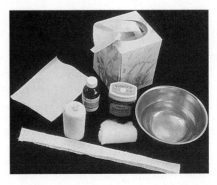

FIGURE 12–16 Materials and equipment needed to fabricate a POP finger cast.

For best results, use 3″ wide POP folded in half and then trimmed to a 1 ¹/₄″ width. Choose the fastest setting plaster obtainable and one that has a fine texture and, in the end, creates a smooth, strong cast that sets quickly. There are numerous products on the market that have these qualities; one example is Gypsona® (BSN medical Inc.).

Prepare the clinic for POP application and gather the required materials and equipment needed. To protect surfaces from plaster drippings, cover them with disposable waterproof covers. Place drapes over the patient's clothing. The therapist may wish to wear an apron. The therapist and patient should remove watches and rings.

Fill a small clean bowl with hot water. The hotter the water, the faster the plaster will set. Cut the length of POP needed for the finger; the length depends on the length and circumference of the finger and the number of joints involved. Estimate the amount of POP needed by spiraling a cloth dressmaker's tape around the finger in the same configuration as planned to make the cast and then double the length (Fig. 12–17A). Remember that each layer of the cast requires two wraps of POP, and each layer overlaps the preceding one by 50% or ³/₄″.

Method

Precondition the finger as described for making a finger cast earlier in the previous section (Fig. 12–15B). Positioning for POP casting is virtually the same as that for the casting tapes (Fig. 12–15C), with a few exceptions.

To begin the cast fabrication process, coat the finger with petroleum jelly (Fig. 12–17A), which protects against the drying effects of the plaster. Dip the length of plaster into the water, and then run the POP between two fingers to remove excess water (Fig. 12–17B). Taking care to avoid the fragile skin of the finger web space, place the tape as far proximally as possible on the proximal phalanx. Wrap all the way around the proximal phalanx twice and then begin to spiral distally, wrapping twice for each layer and overlapping

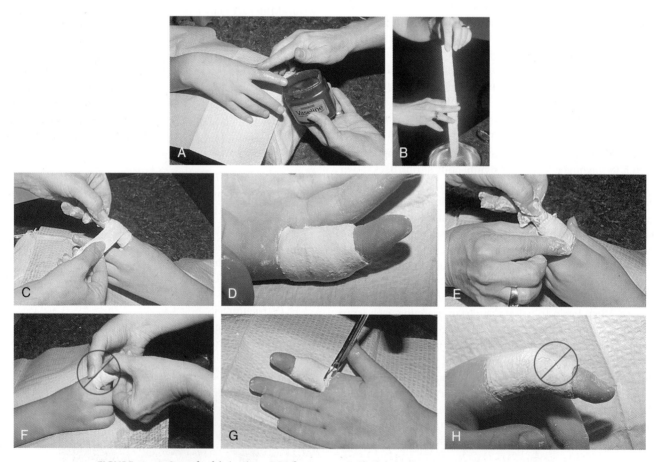

FIGURE 12–17 Steps for fabricating a POP finger cast. A, The lubricating process helps protect the finger from the drying effects of the POP. **B,** Squeeze to remove excess water. **C,** Wrap all the way around the proximal phalanx twice and then spiral distally, wrapping twice for each layer and overlapping the previous layer. **D,** To allow the DIP joint to move freely, end just short of the DIP flexion crease. **E,** Use a continuous rotary motion to closely form the material to the finger and obtain optimal fit. **F,** To avoid point pressure, do not poke at the cast with your fingertips; instead, use the length of your fingers for maximal pressure distribution. **G,** Use the Serial Cast Scissors to contour and smooth the edges. **H,** If there are any indentations, the cast must be removed and remade.

the previous layer halfway or by about $^3/_4''$ (Fig. 12–17C). To allow the DIP joint to move freely, end approximately $^1/_{16}''$ proximal to the DIP joint flexion crease but extend the cast fully to the DIP joint dorsally (Fig. 12–17D). Once the material is applied to the entire finger, use a continuous rotary motion of the fingers to coax the material down onto the finger (Fig. 12–17E). **Caution:** Avoid point pressure against the material at all times (Fig. 12–17F).

Check and Revision

Once the POP has been applied and with traction sustained on the finger, check the cast. Inspect the palmar joint crease at the MCP joint and be sure the patient can flex the MCP without the proximal-palmar end of the cast pressing into the joint crease. If this occurs, push or roll the damp plaster back away from the crease or use the Serial Cast Scissors to carve out some of the material to allow unimpeded movement. Next, check the DIP crease to be sure that the DIP joint can fully flex. Again, either push or roll the damp plaster back away from the crease or trim the cast if needed. Finally, check the web spaces and contour or trim as needed (Fig. 12–17G). The Serial Cast Scissors pose a minimal risk to the patient's skin. Of course, under optimal conditions, the cast will not need trimming. Observe the cast closely for any signs of indentation along the substance of the cast. If indentation is evident, remove the cast and start over (Fig. 12–17H).

If the cast appears unsatisfactory after making it, the therapist can remove the plaster and begin again with a clean bowl; clean water; and new plaster, petroleum jelly, and tissue. It may be possible to raise the end of the POP cast and unwind it. The patient may soak the POP cast off in very warm water. Alternatively, Serial Cast Scissors can be used to cut into the plaster either at the proximal or distal end to help remove it.

Helpful Techniques for Finger Casting

Cast Removal

Both the patient and the therapist must be familiar with techniques for cast removal. The patient should leave the clinic only after indicating a clear understanding of how to remove the cast. The patient must be instructed that the cast cannot be removed with a cast saw because there is no padding.

If the patient's contracture is approximately 30° or less, then the patient will most likely be able to pull the cast off. For patients with unstable MCP joints (such as with rheumatic disease), the proximal phalanx will need to be stabilized before pulling off the cast. If the joint is too tender for this removal technique, if the joint is quite swollen, or if the contracture is more severe, then the cast removal is more involved.

UNWINDING

For the first few casts, mark the distal end of the tape with a pen; this will help with cast removal in an emergency and help assure the patient that he or she can unwind the cast (Fig. 12–18A). The patient can immerse the casted finger in the warmest tolerable water to soften the material and unwind the cast (Fig. 12–18B). The patient should soak the cast in the warmest water tolerable for 5 minutes or longer. Once the distal flap of the casting material is raised, it is possible to unwrap the cast. This "unwinding" can be challenging; however, it is frequently done with QuickCast 2 or Orficast™ tape in order for the piece to be reused. It may need to be resoaked several times before the cast can be removed. If the tape has served its purpose, it can simply be cut off with the Serial Cast Scissors. The therapist or patient can soak the cast to soften it partially and then use Serial Cast Scissors to cut it off.

PARAFFIN

Another technique that may be used when the purpose of the cast is to be used intermittently (such as for just night wear or exercise sessions) is to apply one layer of paraffin to the finger prior to cast application. This technique can be used with all digit circumferential materials detailed in this chapter. The paraffin seeps through the porous holes in the tape/plaster, making for a smooth nonabrasive surface

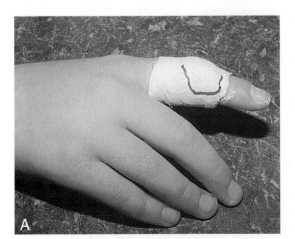
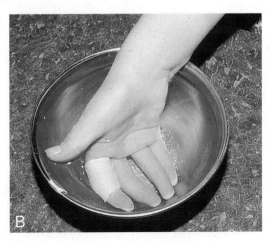

FIGURE 12–18   **A,** Mark the end of the cast to ease removal. **B,** Remove a cast by soaking it in warm water.

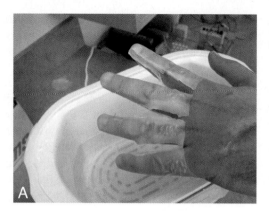
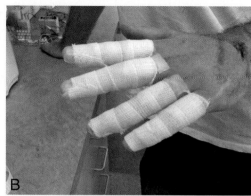
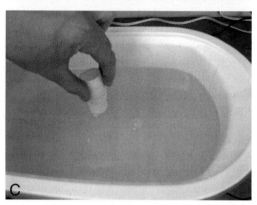

FIGURE 12–19 **A and B,** One layer of paraffin wax can be applied to the fingers prior to casting tape application (works with QuickCast 2, Orficast™, and POP). The paraffin will, in turn, make the casts easy to remove and provide a smooth gliding surface for repeated donning/doffing. Caution should be taken as to not apply the warmed tape material until wax is fully dry. These casts are being used as exercise orthoses in order to isolate and encourage MCP extension/flexion. **C,** The proximal and distal borders of the cast are being lightly dipped in paraffin to smooth out irregular/sharp and potentially irritating edges.

for the digit to slide within. This technique may also be used for those with fragile or sensitive skin (Fig. 12–19A,B). The distal and proximal borders of a circumferential cast can also be dipped in order to provide a smooth surface, maximizing comfort during wear and donning/doffing (Fig. 12–19C).

CUTTING

The therapist may choose one of two approaches to cut the cast for removal. Bell-Krotoski (1987, 2011) described a window technique by which the dorsal aspect of the cast is cut out along the proximal phalanx. With this section of the cast removed, the patient can usually slip the cast off (Fig. 12–20A).

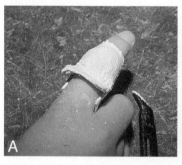
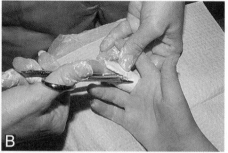
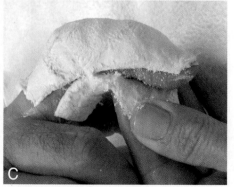

FIGURE 12–20 Window **(A)** and univalve **(B)** cutting techniques for cast removal. **C,** Gently pull apart material to remove the cast.

The other option is to create a univalve in the cast with a longitudinal cut along either the radial/palmar or the ulnar/palmar border (Fig. 12–20B,C). The location for these cuts has two advantages. The palmar skin has more subcutaneous padding than the dorsal skin, and the volar approach avoids the PIP condyles. Cutting over a bony prominence usually creates discomfort for the patient. Either the window or the univalve approach can be used to make the cast removable for intermittent wear.

Securing the Cast in Place

Occasionally, the patient will have trouble keeping the cast on. This occurs rarely but is most frequently seen with very small fingers that are approaching full extension and fingers that were edematous when the cast was applied and have since lost volume. When presented with this problem, the cast maker must be certain that the cast was applied properly. Three techniques are helpful for maintaining cast position on the finger when the proper casting technique does not result in a secure cast:

1. **Circumferential wraps.** The patient can wrap the cast and adjacent skin with self-adherent wraps, such as Coban™, or with various adhesive tapes such as Microfoam™ tape, elastic therapeutic tape, or athletic tape. The wrap can be applied around the cast and proximal (Fig. 12–21A–C). The type of wrap chosen will depend on how the patient intends to use the digit with the cast on.
2. **Additional tape material.** The therapist can cut an additional piece of material, laminate it to the proximal end of the cast, and continue wrapping through the first web space and around the palm (Fig. 12–22). DIP casts can be secured proximally to the digit with circumferential wraps as described previously or creatively positioned with a thin rolled piece of additional material (Fig. 12–23).
3. **Preparing skin.** Tincture of Benzoin, Tuf Skin Taping Base (Patterson Medical), and Skincote™ Protective Prep Pads (Patterson Medical) are products that create a tacky surface on the skin. A tiny amount of these can be dabbed on the skin before applying the cast. The products can be removed with rubbing alcohol when desired. Applying these products will assist in keeping the cast in place.

Protecting Adjacent Fingers

Sometimes, the finger adjacent to the casted finger becomes irritated from rubbing against the cast. To prevent this or to relieve it once it occurs, the patient may cover the cast with Moleskin, a bandage (such as a Band-Aid®), finger stockinette, or light Coban™ wrap (Patterson Medical).

Reinforcing the Cast

After the casting process is complete and it is apparent that the rigidity is not enough to hold the joint position, the cast can be reinforced with additional material. Heating and applying an additional strip of the casting material circumferentially can work, but this increases the overall bulk of the cast. If this is a concern, instead a scrap piece of thermoplastic can be added to the cast for reinforcement (Fig. 12–24).

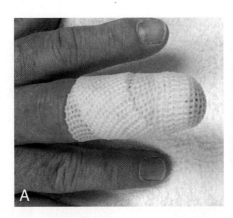
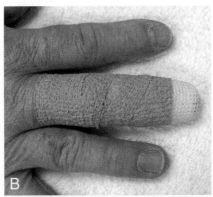
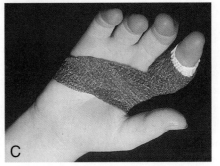

FIGURE 12–21 A and B, QuickCast 2 DIP extension orthosis with Coban™ applied on the cast and then onto the proximal phalanx to prevent slippage. **C,** For securing a PIP cast, Coban™ (or similar material) can be wrapped around the cast and anchored through the palm.

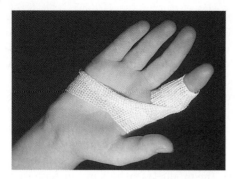

FIGURE 12–22 Another technique for securing a finger cast includes using additional casting material attached to the cast and wrapped through the web space and palm.

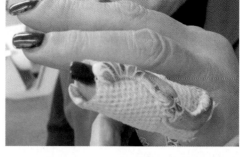

FIGURE 12–24 Thermoplastic material can be adhered directly to the casting tape to improve rigidity in an area without increasing the bulk of the orthosis.

Precautions for Finger Casting

Material Tolerance

If the patient does not tolerate the cast tape directly against the skin or if additional padding is desired, one or more layers of tubular finger bandage may be applied to the finger before making the cast. In the case of wounds or the use of padding, the patient must avoid getting the finger wet. Techniques for keeping the finger dry in a cast range from putting a plastic bag around the whole hand, using a "finger cot" to cover the digit (available at local drugstores), or cutting a finger from a surgical glove and placing it over the cast (Fig. 12–25A,B).

Hand therapists' reports of POP intolerance are minimal; however, the therapist should be aware that by increasing the dipping water temperature for the POP material and increasing the number of layers of POP applied can significantly increase the temperature within the setting cast (Conroy, Ward, & Fraser, 2007). Covering the POP with a towel or pillow while the material is setting can significantly increase the internal temperature (Gannaway & Hunter, 1983; Lavalette, Pope, & Dickerson, 1982) (Box 12–4 and Box 12–5).

Casting over Wounds

Each clinician must use personal judgment when the finger still has open wounds. POP casts can be applied over open wounds and over dressings and are generally tolerated well. The nature of the POP material assists in absorbing wound drainage (Colditz, 2002, 2011). QuickCast 2 can be applied over open wounds that are dressed (Brand & Yancey, 1997). The thinnest possible dressing, the better, in order to gain the most benefits from the conforming properties of the material and even pressure distribution. A layer or two of petroleum gauze such as Xeroform™ (Patterson Medical, 3M™, St. Paul, MN) may be all that is needed. The person applying the cast must take care to keep the dressing in place during cast application. Casts can be used to secure scar management products to an area of the hand. Elastomer™ (Patterson Medical) products adhere into the fabric of the casting tapes (Fig. 12–26).

Indications for Cast Removal

The therapist must thoroughly instruct the patient in symptoms that signal an ill-fitting cast. A poorly made cast can compromise nerve, vascular structures, and/or skin. The

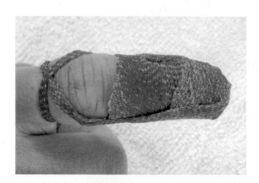

FIGURE 12–23 To secure this DIP cast, a proximal "strap" made from thinly rolled Orficast™ tape was used.

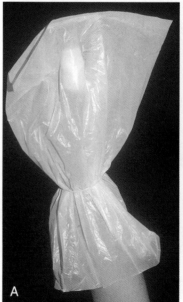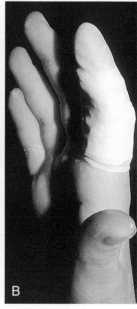

FIGURE 12–25 To keep a finger cast dry, use a plastic bag **(A)** or a surgical glove **(B)**.

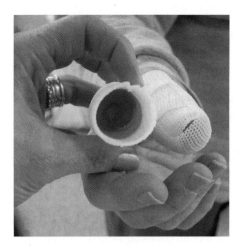

FIGURE 12–26 The cast provides the means of holding the scar mold in place.

symptoms that signal pressure on a nerve are tingling, numbness, and unusual pain. Point pressure directly against a digital nerve can cause a neuropraxia. The symptoms that signal vascular compromise are tingling, numbness, unusual pain, color change, unusual coolness, and persistent throbbing. The symptoms that signal skin compromise from sharp edges are unusual pain and red skin just proximal or distal to the cast. Excess pressure can produce significant redness over the affected area, commonly seen at the PIP joint dorsally.

SENSORY COMPROMISE
Casting the patient with sensory compromise places an even greater responsibility on the therapist to make a well-fitting cast. The patient with numbness will not have the primary signal (pain) to warn that the cast is causing problems. However, it is helpful to know that Brand's (1988) initial casting population suffered extreme sensory compromise from Hansen's disease but did extremely well with POP casting. It is precisely the pressure-distributing nature of the circumferential cast that makes it appropriate for this at-risk population.

Placing a three-point pressure orthosis on a numb part is often not an option that can be considered. Still, the therapist must strongly emphasize the potential risks to the patient and teach him or her to inspect the skin regularly to check for problems that the nervous system may miss.

VASCULAR COMPROMISE
When the cast is completed, the therapist must inspect the color of the fingertip. It may appear slightly darker red than the adjacent fingers or can change color so much as to appear purplish, which indicates difficulty with venous outflow (Fig. 12–27). The finger may also become white or dusky, indicating difficulty with arterial inflow. The patient must remain in the clinic until the color of the finger normalizes. This usually happens within 5 to 10 minutes; however, it may take more than 20 minutes before vascular tone normalizes for vascular outflow difficulty. Usually, the

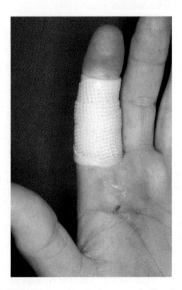

FIGURE 12–27 Vascular compromise noted distally worsens with attempts at DIP flexion.

discoloration occurs in a patient who is receiving a first cast, and the problem does not recur. The person applying the cast must use judgment to determine whether the color of the finger means that the cast should be left on or removed and redone. A sustained color change can signal that focused pressure against major arteries or veins exists and must be relieved.

SKIN TOLERANCE

If the patient presents initially with erythema of the dorsal aspect of the PIP joint or develops this over a period of time in the cast, casting does not have to be discarded or discontinued (Fig. 12–28A). Vascular compromise dorsally, if not dealt with, can cause skin breakdown. Bell-Krotoski (1987, 2011) described a technique using clouds, or wisps, of cast padding to protect vulnerable tissue (Fig. 12–28B). To make the cloud, pull a small fluff of cast padding from the roll. Apply petroleum jelly over the area where the padding will go to keep the cloud in place during cast fabrication. With the padding over the dorsum of the PIP, the normal casting procedure can begin. The therapist must be sure that the padding stays in place during cast fabrication. Bulkier approaches

to padding the cast usually do not have a satisfactory result (Bell-Krotoski, 1987, 2011). Sharp cast edges—proximally or distally—can also compromise skin integrity (Fig. 12–28C). Another issue regarding tissue integrity is when maceration occurs beneath the cast if the patient gets the finger wet. This persistent moisture can eventually cause skin breakdown if not addressed with a period of "drying out" and a prompt cast change (Fig. 12–28D).

Skin Lubrication

Popular is the application of petroleum jelly (or like lubricants) to the skin before POP cast application. As mentioned, petroleum jelly helps lubricate the skin under the moisture-robbing plaster. It also helps secure small amounts of padding. As described earlier, a single layer of paraffin can also be considered before casting with POP, QuickCast 2, or Orficast™. A layer of paraffin fully cooled can be used under the application of these casts. The paraffin allows for easy removal and a very light coating against the skin to soften the harshness the materials may have on sensitive skin. However, if the paraffin is not allowed to cool and POP (with its heating qualities) is applied, the skin under this material

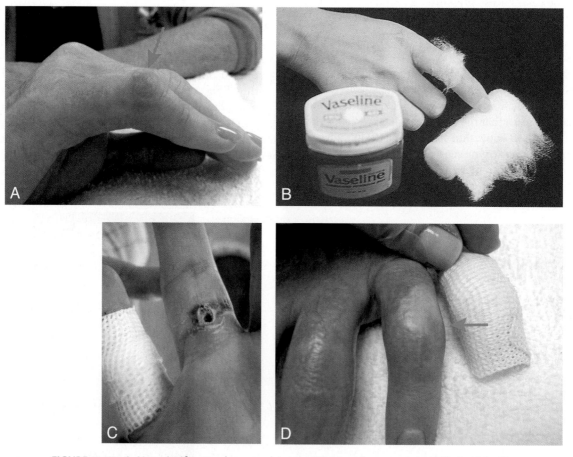

FIGURE 12–28 **A,** Note significant redness overlying the PIP joint after cast removal. **B,** A minimalist approach to padding relieves pressure over the PIP in the cast. Petroleum jelly helps stabilize the wisp of padding. **C,** Tissue breakdown from the proximal edge of a finger cast. **D,** Area of maceration on the dorsum of the digit after cast got wet a few days prior.

may become reddened and severely irritated. Caution and sound clinical judgment should be used (Fig. 12–19A,B). Paraffin can also be used to coat irregular edges on a cast that is intended to be removable (Fig. 12–19C).

Casting Regimen

Frequencies of cast changes vary with the characteristics of the patient. Diagnosis, severity and duration of contracture, and wound and sensory status all help determine the number of times a week or month a patient will be seen for a cast change (Flower & LaStayo, 2012). The issues of geography, financial status, patient schedule, and motivation usually have more impact on the regimen than the medical factors.

Some patients seem to benefit from less frequent cast changes, whereas others have the best results with frequent cast changes. Theoretically, the more frequent cast changes will have better results because a new end range is captured with each cast change, enhancing the mechanical signal to the tissue to remodel.[1]

Clinical Example: Serial Static POP Stretcher for Modifying Scar Tissue

Materials and Preparation

The materials needed to make a POP stretcher are as follows (Fig. 12–29):

- Approximately 10 plies of POP cut from rolls or strips
- Stockinette
- Additional POP strips for finishing
- Hot water
- Clean bowl
- Bandage scissors
- Tissues
- Drapes to protect work surfaces and patient's clothes
- Finger loops of vinyl with line attached or flexible surgical drain tubing
- Cast padding (optional)
- Draped arm wedge (optional)
- Banding metal, thermoplastic strips, or additional POP strips for reinforcement (optional)

The number of initial POP strips depends on the size of the arm to be managed. The hotter the water, the faster the plaster will set; but be careful not to burn the patient. Finger loops are especially necessary if flexor tightness differs significantly among the digits. The optional arm wedge may be foam or solid.

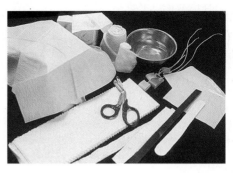

FIGURE 12–29 Materials and equipment needed to fabricate a POP stretcher.

Prepare the clinic for POP application. Gather the required materials and equipment. To protect surfaces from plaster drippings, cover them with disposable, waterproof covers. Both the therapist and patient will want to protect their clothing with drapes or aprons and should remove watches and rings.

Determine the amount of POP required for the stretcher (Fig. 12–30A,B) by measuring the greatest width of the extremity, generally the palm or proximal forearm. Be sure to include the drape of the material halfway down the forearm or palm in the measurement. Measure length from longest fingertip to two-thirds of the way up the forearm to determine POP strip length. Round the corners of the plaster. Lay the plaster down on the hand to determine the location of the thenar eminence (Fig. 12–30C). Cut a slit in the plaster at the midway point of the thenar eminence. This will be turned back to leave the thumb free, and the overlap will reinforce this thinner part of the orthosis (Fig. 12–30D). Finally, fill a large clean bowl with hot water.

Method

Tissue Preconditioning

As for finger casting, gains in PROM of the forearm are more rapid and of a greater magnitude if the tissue is preconditioned or stretched out just before orthosis application (Schultz-Johnson, 2003). Methods of preconditioning were discussed earlier in this chapter. Note that patients with sensory compromise may not be candidates for tissue preconditioning.

Position and Technique

Before making the POP orthosis, decide on patient and joint positions. Practice with the patient. Be sure the patient understands the materials, technique, and rationale for cast application. Position the patient and prepare the tissue as follows:

1. Clean and dry the area of the arm to be covered.
2. Seat the patient and place the affected extremity on a firm but padded surface (a foam wedge is excellent) with the forearm supinated and position the joints as desired.
3. Start with the wrist in neutral and place the MCP and IP joints in maximum available extension; once the fingers demonstrate full passive extension, begin progressing the wrist into extension while maintaining digit extension until full composite extension is achieved.

---

[1]This section has been adapted and reprinted with permission from Schultz-Johnson, K. S. (1999). *PIP serial casting with QuickCast 2*. Edwards, CO: UE Tech.

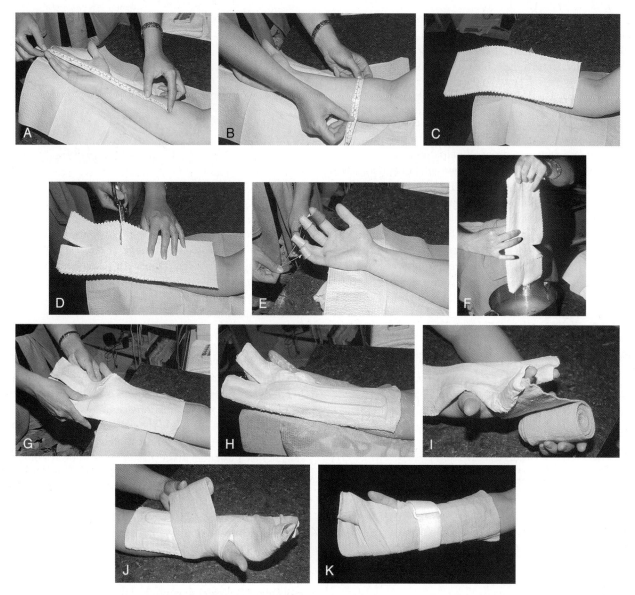

FIGURE 12–30 Steps of applying a forearm POP stretcher. A and B, Determine the appropriate plaster dimensions by measuring the length and greatest width of the extremity. **C,** Check that the plaster is of the proper dimensions. **D,** Cut a slit in the plaster at the midway point of the thenar eminence. If the range of motion of the fingers differs significantly, cut the plaster longitudinally between the fingers to position the fingers at different angles. **E,** This traction maneuver maximizes the stretch on the affected tissue. The fingers may be stretched individually as well. **F,** Immerse the plaster in water for 5 to 10 seconds and remove any excess water. **G,** Gently mold the POP to the arm, avoiding point pressure. **H,** If reinforcement is desired, contour the plastic or metal to the stretcher and cover it with two or three layers of POP to secure it in place. **I and J,** Tuck the end of the wrap in between the index finger and POP stretcher and wrap proximally. The tips of the digits are left uncovered so a patient with diminished sensation can check color and temperature. **K,** D-ring hook-and-loop straps help secure the stretcher in position and distribute the pressure.

4. To position the fingers, especially if the flexor tightness varies significantly between digits, place vinyl finger slings or loops with line attached or place flexible surgical drain tubing over the fingertips and have the patient or an assistant place the fingers under traction into maximum tolerable extension (Fig. 12–30E). **Caution:** Avoid point pressure at all times.

Applying the Plaster of Paris Stretcher

As the process begins, keep in mind that even with extra–fast-setting plaster, the therapist will have adequate time to contour the POP to the arm. The POP will set in 3 to 5 minutes. Tribuzi (1990) described the application of padding or stockinette before applying the POP. However, this author has never used an interface between the POP and the skin in the fabricating process and has never encountered a complication.

Using care to fully saturate all of the POP, all the strips are immersed as a group into the water. Remove the POP as a unit and gently squeeze along the length of the strips to remove excess water (Fig. 12–30F). The wet plaster is then placed on the patient's arm and over the fingers (or fingers in the slings, if used). Using all of the POP layers as a single unit, mold the POP to the arm, carefully contouring the forearm, palm, fingers, and spaces between the fingers (Fig. 12–30G). No pressure need be applied to the POP. The person positioning the fingers controls the finger and wrist joint angles, and the person forming the stretcher simply follows the shape and position of the hand and arm.

When the POP is set, remove it from the arm. Although the plaster is dry on the surface, it is still wet in the deeper layers and will still be soft enough to smooth edges by hand or with plaster scissors. At this point, the therapist may add any reinforcement desired to increase the rigidity of the orthosis. Thermoplastic and banding metal are both effective reinforcement materials. The reinforcement bar should extend over most of the length of the stretcher (Fig. 12–30H). Additional strips of POP secure the reinforcements to the POP base.

Securing the Plaster of Paris Stretcher

Once the final POP stretcher revisions are made, the patient puts it on and wraps it into place with an elasticized bandage. The therapist must carefully instruct the patient in proper wrapping technique to avoid vascular compromise. To start the wrap, the patient tucks the end of the wrap in between the index finger and POP stretcher and then starts wrapping proximally in a Figure-8 or spiral fashion (Fig. 12–30I,J). D-ring hook-and-loop straps may be added to reinforce the wrist or finger position (Fig. 12–30K).

If the arm underwent preconditioning before stretcher fabrication, the therapist must instruct the patient in cast application when the lengthened tissue returns to its shorter length. When first applied, the arm will not fit perfectly into the stretcher. The wrap will have to be readjusted over time as the patient wears the stretcher and tissue once again lengthens. Some patients do not tolerate this readjustment process well. For them, avoid tissue preconditioning. Patients with sensory compromise are not candidates for the readjustment period because pressure distribution is poor, and the risk of skin injury is high.

Check and Revision

Check the stretcher for sharp edges, cracks, and pressure areas. Sharp edges can be rounded with the application of hot water. A pair of sharp plaster scissors is also effective. Should cracks appear in the plaster, apply warm water to the cracked area and add two or more strips of plaster. These strips do not need to be the length of the whole orthosis but must be long enough to adhere well and give adequate reinforcement.

Precautions for POP Stretcher

Material Properties

Care must be taken to avoid stressing the POP before it has fully set. It takes several hours before the POP will have its full strength. After the initial exothermic heat reaction, the plaster will be quite cold for the next few hours until it fully dries. Some patients may find this uncomfortable. However, providing the patient with a stockinette (preferably polypropylene) may resolve this problem. Tolerance to the material was discussed in detail earlier in this chapter (Box 12–4).

As always, the patient must have a thorough understanding of the signs and symptoms that indicate orthosis removal. Vascular, dermal, and neurologic symptoms were discussed earlier in this chapter (Box 12–5).

Skin Lubrication

POP wicks moisture from the skin and can be very drying. Having the patient wear a stockinette as an interface between the arm and the POP can improve skin lubrication. Patients who wear a POP stretcher may need to apply a skin lubricant more frequently.

Pressure Areas

The patient must be instructed to check for the deep red marks in the skin that indicate pressure areas and to report these to the therapist. Teach the patient to attempt to resolve pressure areas with repositioning the stretcher, adjusting the wraps and straps, or inserting small temporary bits of tissue or cotton. Pressure problems that do not respond to these interventions indicate that the stretcher cannot be worn until the therapist can make the appropriate revisions.

Casting over Wounds

Casting over wounds was discussed in detail earlier in this chapter. Plastic wrap placed over a dressing protects the dressing during stretcher formation and will keep it free from POP and moisture. Clinical experience suggests that POP aids wound healing. Experts have noted that POP wicks away exudate when it is applied either directly to the wound or over a light dressing. Although some clinicians may fear that the wound will stick to the plaster, the adherence aids in wound healing because it prevents shear stress (the greatest enemy to wound healing) (Bell-Krotoski, 2011; Colditz, 2002).

Thermal Effects of POP

When POP and water mix, an exothermic chemical reaction takes place. The literature does report cases of thermal burns with the application of POP bandages (Becker, 1978; Grazer, 1979; Haasch, 1964; Kaplan, 1981; Schultze, 1967; Mahler, Pedowitz, Byrne & Gershuni, 1996). When working with plaster, therapists should keep this thermal effect in mind. Tribuzi (1990) noted that casts reach maximum temperature in 5 to 15 minutes after application. Tribuzi listed several variables that may increase the temperature of the exothermic reaction, including the following:

- High room temperature
- High humidity
- Cast thickness of more than eight plies
- Undersaturation or oversaturation with water
- Use of fast-setting plaster
- Dipping temperature
- Inadequate ventilation during the drying period

Inadequate ventilation can occur from overwrapping the freshly applied plaster with cotton or elastic bandages, covering the plaster with blankets, or placing the cast or orthosis near a pillow or mattress (Johnson and Johnson Orthopaedic Division, 1985; Kaplan, 1981; Lavalette et al., 1982).

Bell-Krotoski (1995, 2011) postulates that these injuries may actually be caused by pressure from an improperly applied POP rather than from heat. When working with plaster, the clinician must always use clean water because the plaster residue left in the dipping container from previous casts is thought to act as an accelerator and increase the exothermic reaction. In addition, shards of set plaster can accidentally be incorporated into the orthosis and cause irritation and discomfort.

Although Tribuzi (1990) noted that POP should never be applied directly to the skin, Bell-Krotoski (2011) and others state that there is no contraindication to this practice (Bell-Krotoski, 2011; Brand & Yancey, 1997; Colditz, 2002; Tribuzi, 1990). Certainly, any time a clinician would like to include cast padding to a circumferential plaster cast, the padding must be placed first. A cast saw cannot be used if there is no padding under the cast.

Stretcher Regimen

Deciding when to fabricate a new stretcher is easier than deciding how frequently to change a serial cast because the extremity demonstrates what it needs. When a patient is consistently able to lift out of the stretcher by 5° at the target joint(s), the time has come for a new stretcher.

It is the responsibility of the therapist to assess the characteristics of each patient to determine a safe and effective wearing schedule. As with any removable orthosis, the patient should initially wear the orthosis for a trial period of 20 to 30 minutes to determine skin tolerance. Once tolerance is established, the patient can gradually increase time in the orthosis. Nighttime tolerance is a goal. This achieves 6 to 8 hours of end range positioning and then leaves the extremity free during the day for exercise. When the goal is stretcher wear during sleep, the therapist may want to decrease the amount of stretch placed on the tissue during stretcher fabrication or may avoid preconditioning before fabrication.

For the patient who cannot sleep while wearing the stretcher, the therapist must achieve a balance between stretcher wear, activities of daily living, and exercise. Remember that the more the patient wears the stretcher, the faster the patient will reach the therapeutic goals. A minimum amount of time in the stretcher (which depends on the individual patient) must occur for the stretcher to affect tissue change (see Chapter 15, Stiffness for details) (Flowers & LaStayo, 2012; Flowers & Michlovitz, 1988; Glasgow et al., 2012). The therapist may consider combining other orthoses or POP finger casts with stretchers. Applying the finger orthosis or casts before stretcher fabrication may help achieve optimal IP joint position.

Conclusion

Casting is a powerful treatment technique that has the ability to provide outcomes that no other orthotic intervention can offer. The circumferential approach has many benefits, including improved pressure distribution and minimized shear and migration. Casting offers an efficient and effective means to decrease contractures, including those with a hard end feel. Even patients with cognitive and sensory impairment can benefit from casting.

As with any treatment approach, the therapist must carefully consider the nature of the problem before applying the cast. Patients with PROM limitations owing to soft tissue abnormalities that will not respond to low-load, prolonged stress should not receive a cast. Joint limitation caused by heterotopic ossification, exostosis, or loose body will also not benefit from casting. The circumferential design of the cast allows mobilization of a joint that might not be a candidate for conventional orthotic management, for example, in the case of some forms of joint instability and acute inflammation. However, avascular necrosis, infection, unstable fracture, marked demineralization, myositis ossificans, and stress across healing structures without adequate blood supply or tensile strength to withstand tensile stress remain contraindications to cast application.

The family of casting products continues to increase, offering patients and clinicians even more options. Keeping current and familiar with the characteristics of each new product helps the therapist choose the material that best meets the patient's needs. This chapter reviewed only a few of these materials, and the reader is encouraged to research and stay abreast of all casting options that are made available. Circumferential and noncircumferential casting techniques to serially increase PROM require skills that are unique to this modality. This chapter describes several of these. Continued innovation in the use of casting will benefit patients in new and effective ways.

ACKNOWLEDGMENT FROM SECOND EDITION

Sincere thanks to Judy Colditz, OTR/L, CHT, FAOTA, for her guidance with integrating information on casting motion to mobilize stiffness (CMMS) and Debby Schwartz, OTD, OTR/L, CHT for her insight regarding the use of Orficast™ from Orfit Industries.

ACKNOWLEDGMENTS FROM THE FIRST EDITION

Many thanks to Trudy Hackencamp, OTR/L, CHT, for the information she provided regarding casting spasticity. Thanks also to Judy Bell-Krotoski for our many discussions over the years regarding the use of POP and serial casting of fingers. Finally, thanks to Jessica Hawkins, my patient of many years, who has worn more casts than anyone can count and has given me invaluable feedback.

Chapter Review Questions

1. Name three of the most common indications for casting.

2. Explain the material choice and rationale for use of a cast for zone III extensor tendon injuries.

3. Give a clinical example of a serial static mobilization orthosis using two types of cast material. What is the injury and why did you choose this material?

4. What are the general precautions of plaster of paris (POP) casting and how is the plaster removed?

5. What are the advantages of soft casting materials? Name two types.

13 | Taping Techniques

Ruth Coopee, OTR/L, CHT, CLT, LMT

Chapter Objectives

After study of this chapter, the reader should be able to:

- Appreciate three popular taping methods: athletic taping, McConnell taping, and elastic therapeutic taping (Kinesio taping method).
- List the commonly encountered injuries for each taping application.

- Describe the differences between each type of taping application and the specific goals for each type of tape.
- Understand the precautions for each taping technique.

Key Terms

Anchor
Athletic taping
Correction technique

Elastic therapeutic taping (Kinesio taping method)
Figure-8 or locking strip
"I," "Y," "X," FAN, and Buttonhole cuts

McConnell taping
Spray adherent
Prewraps
Undertapes

Introduction

Research supports the theory of encouraging early motion to improve healing time and the quality of tissue repair (Cyr & Ross, 1998). Casting and immobilization in rigid orthoses, although beneficial at certain stages of healing, do not allow motion (Fess & McCollum, 1998). Hinged braces and orthoses are often cumbersome and not practical for performing activities of daily living (ADLs). Silicone and soft orthoses that offer semirigid support have been introduced to provide protected motion during return to activity and to prevent injury or reinjury of soft tissue (Birrer, 1994; Canelon, 1995; Henshaw, Satren, & Wrightsman, 1989). These types of orthoses are helpful but time consuming and are not always cost-effective.

From sports medicine and athletic training to professional athletes and the Olympic arena, strapping and/or taping techniques have been used successfully for pain reduction associated with edema, early protected return to activity (Ewalt, 2010; Hilfrank, 1991; Ozer, Senbursa, Baltaci, & Hayran, 2009), and scar modification (Atkinson, McKenna, Barnett, McGrath, & Rudd, 2005; Niessen, Spauwen, Robinson, Fidler, & Kon, 1998; Reiffel, 1995). Taping the upper extremity is a cost-effective treatment alternative for many common injuries and overuse syndromes seen in the clinic and does not interfere with overall gross function and grip strength (Chang, Chou, Lin, & Wang, 2010; Rettig, Stube, &

Shelbourne, 1997) (Fig. 13–1). Taping is not applicable for conditions requiring the protection of rigid devices, but it may be incorporated along the recovery continuum to allow for protected mobilization or to assist in neuromuscular retraining (Bennell, Duncan, & Cowan, 2006; Hsu, Chen, Lin, Wang, & Shih, 2009; Jaraczewska & Long, 2006; McConnell, Donnelly, Hamner, Dunne, & Besier, 2011; McConnell & McIntosh, 2009; Ozer et al., 2009; Salsich, Brechter, Farwell, & Powers, 2002; Yasukawa, Patel, & Sisung, 2006). A skilled and extensive evaluation to determine the appropriateness and the timing for proper implementation is necessary before incorporating taping. As with many such modalities, effective taping is employed as a complement to a comprehensive rehabilitation program (Fig. 13–2).

This chapter provides a brief overview of three popular taping methods and application techniques: traditional **athletic taping**, **McConnell taping**, and **elastic therapeutic taping (Kinesio taping method)**. The use and application of any of these three methods is only limited by the creative skills of those trained to apply these tapes. The applications are endless and can be used far beyond what is described in this chapter. This chapter will provide an overview of each taping method and its various applications as well as highlight the commonly encountered upper extremity injuries a therapist may be asked to tape. Table 13–1 compares these distinctly different taping methods and provides a summary of their features. Note that this table highlights the most commonly used tapes as the date of this publication. The reader is encouraged to stay abreast of new products as they become available.

Specialized training is recommended for each technique to provide proficiency and improve comprehension of the underlying mechanisms and associated therapeutic programs. Instruction is offered through various venues; refer to a listing of helpful Web sites at the end of this chapter. Accessibility to some training programs may be limited based on clinical training or expertise (e.g., training in spinal manipulation) and on the scope of practice laws in individual states. The clinician must have an extensive clinical knowledge of anatomy, kinesiology, and the physiology of healing to determine if taping is indicated and, if so, to determine the best choice of technique and material. Note that each patient and injury is unique and requires a comprehensive evaluation by the physician and therapist before therapy intervention (Austin, Gwynn-Brett, & Marshall, 1994). The evaluation should include knowledge of the physical demands and requirements of the patient, the structure(s) involved, the degree of injury, and the stage of healing. Table 13–2 is a general guide to the application of taping based on the specific degree of injury.

Patients using taping techniques should be closely monitored. Frequent reevaluation of the injured body part, healing process, tension, and tape placement as well as the taping materials themselves is essential to maximize the success of taping as a method of treatment. Inspection of the completed taping should be conducted to ensure proper support and proper taping application. Patients are at risk for significant harm if they return to activity with inadequate support or limitation of movement. Therefore, sound professional clinical judgment and proper diagnosis are imperative to ensure a positive outcome. Treatment may also include instruction of proper tape application and removal by the patient, family member, or other caregiver. It is important to educate the patient about the precautions and to stress the necessity of frequent monitoring of the body part for changes in skin integrity and neurovascular and lymphatic function.

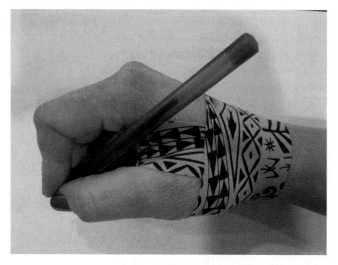

FIGURE 13–1 Dynamic Tape™ (Patterson Medical) used to address CMC joint instability by providing gentle support to the joint with activities such as writing.

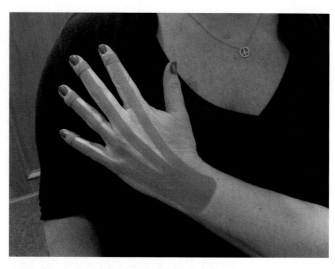

FIGURE 13–2 Kinesio® Tex Tape applied to the dorsum of hand to decrease edema.

TABLE 13–1

Comparison Chart

Method	Athletic	McConnell	Elastic
Materials	Adhesive spray Prewrap (i.e., M-Wrap by Mueller) Padding adhesive tape	Undertape (i.e., Cover-Roll®) Brown adhesive tape (i.e., Leukotape®)	Kinesio® Tex Tape Balance Tex Tape Dynamic Tape SpiderTech™ Tape PerformTex Tape Rock Tape
Evaluation	Muscle Joint Soft tissue	Analysis of structural alignment and dysfunctional biomechanics	Analysis of muscle, soft tissue, and fascial dysfunction and its relationship to pathology
Indications	Joint injury Ligament injuries grades 1–3 Muscle injury Rigid yet flexible protection	Postural reeducation Muscle retraining Joint alignment	Scar and soft tissue modification Relieves myofascial pain Edema reduction Muscle support and reeducation Joint support (correction) Postural reeducation Increase circulation
Technique/ Methodology	Provides a progressive amount of support and immobilization to healing tissues and prevents reinjury while allowing continued participation in activity	Passively repositions soft tissue and "holds" bony structures into proper alignment to retrain and restore normal static and dynamic functional biomechanics	A specially developed elastic tape is used to facilitate the neurosensory and physiologic mechanisms of skin and muscle, affecting soft tissue, fascia, and muscle tension while modifying functional biomechanics and reducing pain.
Advantages	Maximum support to healing structures	Provides support to very weak structures and allows full range of motion	Gentle approach to treatment of myofascial pain and soft tissue injuries allows full range of motion.
Disadvantages	Tape trauma and irritation Needs to be replaced and checked often for maximum support Patient false dependency	Tape trauma and irritation Pulling of the tape may be "pain" restrictive in exercise Not appropriate for grade 3 injuries	Complexity Tape allergy Not appropriate for grade 2–3 injuries, although may be used in combination with athletic tape

TABLE 13–2

Injury Classification List and Recommendations

	Degree of Injury	Stability	Suggested Taping Application
First-degree injury	Damage with little or no elongation of ligaments or soft tissue	No instability	Tape 3–10 days
Second-degree injury	Overstretch with partial tear and moderate ligament involvement	Some laxity to joint	Tape 4–6 weeks
Third-degree injury	Complete rupture with abnormal movement on stress testing	Major loss of joint ligament integrity and structural function Medical evaluation	Tape for a minimum of 4 months with close monitoring

Taping Materials

There are many types of athletic or sports tapes and products on the market, each with its own indications. The increased popularity of elastic "therapeutic" taping in the sports arena has led to an ever growing variety of products with variations in the tape adhesive and the amount of elastic recoil. The practitioner should exercise increased caution in application of these tapes intended for the young healthy athlete. The reader is referred to the listed Web sites to gain further information on the exact properties of the tape he or she is working with. Tape should not be confused with bandages or cohesive circumferential wraps that do not adhere directly to the skin such as Coban™ tape. All tapes should be stored flat to maintain the roll shape and in a cool dry location to maintain its adhesive quality. Table 13–3 lists commonly

used taping materials along with their functions (Arnheim & Prentice, 2000; Austin et al., 1994).

Athletic Taping

General Principles

The main function of athletic taping is to restrict or immobilize specific joint structures while allowing for some degree of active movement (Arnheim & Prentice, 2000; Austin et al., 1994; J. Wallis, personal communication, 2000, 2001). This can be done with nonelastic or elastic type adhesive athletic tapes. Multiple layers of *nonelastic* adhesive tape are applied across a joint to provide rigid stability for ligament injuries, outside support, and restrict forces that would apply stress to

TABLE 13–3

Commonly Used Materials and Function

Skin tougheners Adhesive sprays	These are applied to the skin in either a pad or spray method before taping to improve adhesion of tape to the skin and decrease chemical tape irritations. Tougheners have an additional astringent to prepare the skin. Note that these products can also cause irritation if used for prolonged periods.
Undertapes	An adhesive backed, nonelastic material used as a base to which a sports tape is applied. It also serves as a light padding to protect skin or bony areas and prevent skin blisters and cuts.
Prewraps	Similar to undertape, except that it does not have an adhesive backing; it is composed of a fine, porous polyester foam material that has a slight stretch to help conform to contours. It provides increased padding to skin and bony areas but requires a spray adherent to increase skin contact.
Adhesive tapes	Rated by number of vertical fibers per inch; this relates to tensile strength and weight; available in ½", 1", 1½", and 2" widths; often referred to as "white tape," zinc oxide, or linen tape. They are inelastic and provide a high degree of joint support and immobilization.
Elastic tapes	Dependent on the percentage of elastic stretch to allow for controlled movement in a joint and functional muscle support; rated by percentage of elastic stretch or recoil. Increasing popularity of this method with athletes has led to development of a larger choice of products, some with higher elastic recoil. Caution should be exercised with these products because they are intended for the young healthy athlete. Higher recoil will increase shearing forces on the skin and may lead to blister formation or tissue injury.

an injured part. *Elastic* tapes are used for contractile tissue injuries (muscle and tendon) and to provide localized pressure. Tape can also support and protect a weakened muscle by limiting tendon excursion. Depending on the technique of application, athletic taping can provide minimal-to-moderate constraint of healing tissues while allowing joint motion for controlled, protected healing. Encapsulating acutely injured joint structures assists in edema control via compression and active muscle pumping. To reduce edema associated with muscle contusion, an elastic tape can be used to provide localized compression and allow supported contraction and relaxation.

Goals of Athletic Taping

- Support and protect weakened joint structures.
- Limit harmful movement and assist in planes of movement.
- Provide a progressive method to achieve pain-free functional movement.
- Allow for movement of an injured part to improve circulation and healing.
- Assist in controlling edema.

- Prevent worsening of injury and muscle atrophy.
- Improve kinesthetic awareness in an acutely injured joint.
- Allow early return to function.

Indications for Use

Athletic taping is most often used in the treatment of sprains, strains, subluxations, and dislocations with ligament tears or ruptures resulting in unidirectional or multidirectional instability (Ewalt, 2010; Kaneko & Takasaki, 1996; Ozer et al., 2009). When a thorough medical evaluation determines it appropriate and if applied properly, taping creates a rigid support and provides for maximal soft tissue control. This technique is particularly effective in the conservative management of subacute second- and third-degree injuries. For grade 3 injuries or after repetitive injury, taping is combined with activity restriction to allow tissue healing.

Technique

The manner in which the tape is applied determines the degree of mobility or immobility across a joint. Table 13–4

TABLE 13–4

Techniques and Methods Used in Athletic Taping

Anchor	Circumferential pieces of tape placed proximal and distal to the injury form a base to attach tape strip ends; may use elastic tape if room for muscle expansion is needed.
Stirrup	A U-shaped loop of nonelastic tape used to create lateral stability (ankle)
Vertical strips	Tension is applied as the tape is attached moving from the distal to the proximal anchor. Increase stability of the affected joint is achieved through joint compression and fascial restriction.
"Butterfly" or check reins	Multiple strips of tape are applied at angles to each other with the apex at the joint to limit movement in unidirectional or multidirectional planes (X or star). A variation of this technique to inhibit abduction in the fingers is applied with anchors to adjacent digits. The tape between the anchors is twisted onto itself to create a "rein"-limiting movement.
Locks	A smooth roll application with increased tension at key points of support and reinforce joint stability yet allow protected functional movement (Figure-8 with cross-point at the support point)
Figure-8 or locking strip	Used to complete a taping, covers open areas and tape strip ends while adding stability
Compression	An elastic adhesive tape is stretched from the center and applied directly down with pressure over a muscle injury. No tension is applied at the ends to avoid vascular constriction. This provides support to the muscle and fascia while assisting in edema reduction.
Closing up (in) Cover-up	Strips of tape are applied to cover all open areas and finish taping job. This increases durability and provides consistent coverage to prevent blisters and constriction with focal edema.
Strip method	One strip of tape is laid down in a specific direction with highly controlled tension from one anchor to the other.
Smooth roll method	Refers to the use of one single continuous uninterrupted piece of tape; it may begin and end at the same anchor as with joint locks.

lists common techniques and methods used in athletic taping (Arnheim & Prentice, 2000; Austin et al., 1994). The skin overlying the area to be taped needs to be cleansed of all oils, perspiration, hair, and old adhesive before application of a skin toughener or **spray adherent**. This creates a microscopic layer to protect the skin from tape irritants and increases the adhesive quality of the tape. **Prewraps** are types of protective tapes that can be used before tape application in order to protect the skin from the tape itself. They also eliminate or minimize the need to shave hair prior to taping. Prewrap (i.e., M-Wrap by Mueller, Prairie du Sac, WI) can also be applied to protect bony prominences, soft skin creases, or superficial nerves and arteries. See summary in Table 13–3 for further clarification of the specific variations and uses for these wraps.

In addition, prewrap may be used to hold additional padding in place. Tape anchors are applied proximal and distal to the joint being taped (Fig. 13–3). The joint is placed in a well-supported unstressed position. Depending on the degree of injury, the target joint is taped in either an anatomical neutral position or placed in a slack position to restrict movement stress on healing structures. The person applying the tape should be in an efficient and comfortable position to help proper application technique. The amount of support and joint restriction is dictated by the degree of injury and is achieved by the technique and tension applied during taping. The joint should be evaluated on completion to determine if there is adequate restriction of motion to protect from reinjury. There should be no pain. Inspection must include evaluation for distal patency and surrounding tissue assessment to ensure there is no occlusion or impairment of circulatory or lymphatic function.

Taping may be used for a particular event or may stay in place for several days. The taping becomes progressively looser with activity and should be checked regularly so the joint does not become vulnerable. Tape removal should always be performed carefully so as not to damage or accidentally tear the skin. Blunt-ended bandage scissors are used on the opposite side of the injury to tunnel under the tape and slowly ease the tape off of the skin. Slowly cut and gently peel the tape away by pressing down on the exposed skin while drawing the tape parallel to the surface of the skin. Do not pull up on the tape because this may tear the skin and cause subcutaneous hemorrhaging. Close inspection and evaluation of the skin are imperative for preventing breakdown from adhesives, chronic shearing forces, or tape irritation.

Precautions

The patient should be counseled against developing a false sense of security and/or dependency on taping. Examination of circulation and tape performance should be completed after application and throughout the day. Inspection of the skin between tapings is necessary to check for possible skin breakdown in the form of maceration, blister formation, or rash; taping should be suspended or discontinued if these signs are noticed. Do not tape over abrasions, blisters, lacerations, or cuts. Decreased sensibility from ice or edema may mask tissue response and sensation of pain during taping, resulting in injury. Do not use ice or heat before taping, particularly in the subacute phase. Reduction in interstitial tissue volume from the ice application may create a progressive tightening of the taping as the tissue warms up. Conversely, tissue volumes may decrease after heat application, resulting in reduction of support. It is important to note that improper application can aggravate an existing injury or create a new one.

Helpful Hints

- Place joint in position to be stabilized or protected.
- Overlap at least half the width of the underlying tape strip to prevent separation.
- Avoid using continuous smooth roll method. Apply only one turn around a joint then tear. Continuous wrapping increases tension and becomes constrictive.
- Smooth and mold each strip as it is laid on the skin, allowing it to flow around the natural contours of body. This is more difficult with heavier, stiffer tapes.
- Maximum control is achieved by (1) the amount of tension applied to the tape (if elasticized tape) and (2) the position the joint is in if using a traditional non-elasticized tape.
- Do not tape immediately after application of heat or cold; wait until the tissue returns to normal temperature.

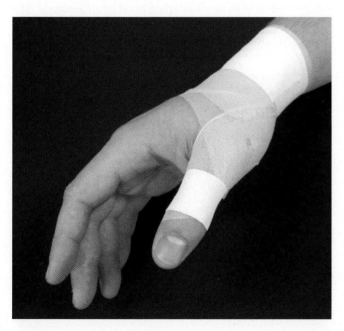

FIGURE 13–3 Proximal and distal anchors applied over underwrap in preparation for the MP joint taping.

McConnell Taping

General Principles

This taping method developed in 1984 by Jenny McConnell, an Australian physical therapist, was initially used for the conservative management of patellofemoral pain (J. McConnell, personal communication, 2001; Bennell et al., 2006; Derasari, Brindle, Alter, & Sheehan, 2010; Pfeiffer et al., 2004; Salsich et al., 2002; Tremain, 1996). Later, she successfully expanded her philosophy and treatment techniques to the spine and upper extremity (McConnell et al., 2011; McConnell & McIntosh, 2009). The McConnell technique involves an extensive muscle evaluation, analysis of individual biomechanics, and posture. Treatment of structural misalignment in conjunction with poor movement patterns is addressed through a comprehensive rehabilitation program with taping serving to assist in the physical reeducation of the body. McConnell taping is applied not to restrict normal movement but to facilitate proper joint alignment, muscular function, and biomechanics.

Goals of McConnell Taping

- Position a joint into more appropriate alignment.
- Increase stability of a joint (ligament support).
- Correct articular orientation by inhibiting short, tight muscles.
- Facilitate firing capacity of weak, lengthened, overstretched muscles.
- Enhance muscle retraining by balancing tissue length/tension relationship.
- Assist in both static and dynamic neuromuscular reeducation.

The McConnell Program includes the following:

- Mobilization of the spine
- Stretching exercise
- Therapeutic exercise to improve motor control and coordination
- Biofeedback

Indications for Use

Taping is used as a vehicle to directly control fascia and establish proper structural alignment for improved muscular recruitment and neuromuscular retraining. These techniques help reduce pain, which encourages compliance in an exercise program, usually designed to strengthen and lengthen the muscular structures involved in pathology. Proper analysis of the underlying pathology is essential to maximize the effectiveness of the method, which focuses on reestablishing a proper length/tension relationship and motor control. The following issues respond well to McConnell taping: subluxation, unidirectional or multidirectional instability, impingement, postinjury or postoperative retraining, overuse, and poor alignment (Bennell et al., 2006; Derasari et al.,

2010; McConnell et al., 2011; McConnell & McIntosh, 2009; Pfeiffer et al., 2004; Salsich et al., 2002; Tremain, 1996).

Technique

A thorough evaluation is completed to determine the pathologic mechanisms involved and how best to correct them. Specific taping materials are used in this technique owing to their tensile strength and durability. First, a white adhesive undertape (such as Cover-Roll®) is applied to the skin without tension. This provides a protective bed for application of a heavyweight working brown adhesive tape (which is sold by many different names and brands such as Leukotape®). The undertape is extremely important because it protects the skin from shearing forces and the strong holding adhesive of the brown tape (Fig. 13–4). Taping with a vertical strip technique gains control of muscle tissue and fascia. If applied correctly, there should be an immediate reduction in pain and no restriction of normal movement. Taping should be completed before exercise to allow proper pain-free exercise performance. To support joint alignment and ligaments, the working tape uses the surrounding fascia to hold the joint in a corrected, tension-free position. To treat shortened tissues or inhibit overactive muscles, the goal is to create a multidirectional stretching force to the muscle belly or shortened tissue. The working tape is applied with tension, perpendicular to the alignment of muscle fibers and with downward force to create both a lateral and compressive stretch to the muscle fibers and fascia. To treat lengthened or weak muscles, the working tape is used to draw the fascia or muscle proximally to passively shorten the fibers. This provides support through somatosensory feedback and prevents overstretch. To ensure proper joint and bone alignment during application of the working tape, the desired position is maintained manually by the nontaping hand or an assistant. The tape will then maintain the body in the proper position to assist in neuromuscular and postural reeducation. Return to

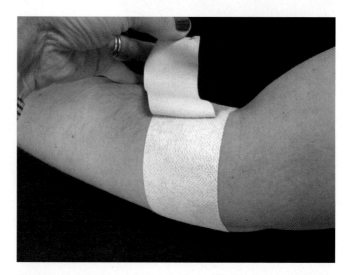

FIGURE 13–4 White undertape protects skin from strong adhesive of brown tape.

previous poor postural movement patterns are discouraged through sensory feedback. The tape may remain in place for 1 to 3 days before replacement is necessary. Remove the tape as described earlier for athletic tape. The skin should be evaluated and cleansed thoroughly before reapplication.

Precautions

Avoid taping patients with known allergies to tape. Do not apply to fragile, thin, or healing skin or tissue that is susceptible to stress injury. Skin integrity and examination for irritation or sensitivity should be continuously evaluated, and taping should be discontinued as necessary. During application, care should be taken not to apply strong tension because this can create shearing forces to adjacent as well as target tissues. When taping the shoulder, be careful not to compress the brachial plexus as it crosses the humerus. Remember that the patient should experience immediate improvement and reduction in pain; if the patient experiences an increase in pain, the tape should be removed immediately. This continued pain may be the result of improper evaluation of causal factors or improper taping procedure. It is important to have received training by a certified instructor, which will improve effectiveness and proficiency in the technique. Taping is just one part of the McConnell multifaceted treatment approach to correcting structural dysfunction. Instruction in evaluation techniques to determine individual taping needs and a comprehensive exercise program to retrain full-body maladaptive movement patterns is important to the successful implementation of this technique.

Helpful Hints

- A skin toughener may be helpful in reducing skin irritation.
- There should be at least a 50% reduction in symptoms.
- The tape should improve symptoms immediately.
- If there is no change in symptoms, discontinue use.

Elastic Therapeutic Taping (Kinesio Taping Method)

General Principles

In this section of this chapter, the author has chosen to focus on the Kinesio taping method because this is the basis for the original Kinesio® Tex Tape application. The emerging popularity of elastic therapeutic tape has led to the development of similar products and a multitude of creative uses for this type of tape. It has gained rapid popularity over the past decade, evolving as a mainstay in therapy clinics, sports arenas, and chiropractic offices and as a treatment intervention for professional and Olympic athletes. Kinesio taping method has been used extensively in Japan and was introduced to

the United States in 1994 (Kase, 1994; Kase, Hashimotom, & Okane, 1996). The concept for the development of a special highly elastic therapeutic tape and later the taping method were initiated by Dr. Kenzo, a Japanese chiropractor. After chiropractic training in the United States in 1973, he specialized in rehabilitation and therapeutic medicine. Intrigued with conservative ways of treating traumatized soft tissue, he used sports tape to assist in soft tissue control. Not satisfied with the stiff restriction of athletic tapes, he searched for an elastic material that would work with the flexibility of muscle, fascia, and skin to facilitate healing. His futile search for a manufacturer in the United States to work with him in the development of an elastic therapeutic tape brought him to the Nitto Denko Corporation in his native Japan. Kase worked with the tape using his knowledge of kinesiology and anatomy to develop the Kinesio taping method. Proper application of the tape does not restrict soft tissue movement, as do conventional adhesive tapes, but rather relies on the movement of skin for multilevel effects. The elastic recoil of the tape is used to provide support to weak muscles and encourages full joint movement (Fig. 13–5). The movement of taped skin and soft tissue creates a massaging effect that promotes lymph and blood flow (Shim, Lee, & Lee, 2003), decreasing pressure on mechanoreceptors, thus reducing pain and edema. Sensory receptors located in the skin also act on ascending and descending neurologic pathways to reduce pain and assist in control of muscle tension via Golgi tendon organ input (Leonard, 1998). The application technique may specifically address sensory receptors in the skin, lymphatic movement for edema and circulation, muscle tension control, or joint support. An advanced application skill, the **correction technique**, can be used to offer support to a target ligament. In this taping application, the center portion of the tape is fully stretched (100%) and then placed straight onto the involved joint/ligament structure. This allows the elastic properties of the tape to recoil, pulling the fascia to the center of the tape (Fig. 13–6).

Goals of Elastic Therapeutic Taping

- Decrease pain and abnormal sensation in skin and muscle.
- Reduce edema and inflammation.
- Normalize muscle tone and abnormality of fascia involved in pathology.
- Support a weakened muscle in movement (expanding effects) by preventing overstretch and reducing fatigue.
- Reduce spasm or overcontraction of a shortened muscle.
- Improve range of motion (ROM).
- Provide muscle and proprioceptive reeducation.
- Reestablish muscular balance to correct misalignment of a joint.
- Support normal joint alignment for rehabilitation.
- Prevent injuries in exercise or ADLs.
- Improve kinesthetic awareness of proper posture and structural alignment.
- Increase circulation.

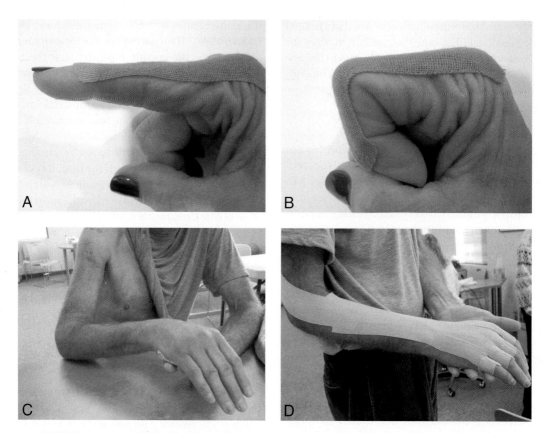

FIGURE 13–5 **A and B,** Application of elastic tape dorsally with tension can assist the weak intrinsic muscles in their efforts to extend the proximal interphalangeal (PIP) joint. **C and D,** This patient presented with a humerus fracture along with radial nerve involvement affecting the wrist and digit extensor strength. Elastic tape was applied under the orthosis, to further assist these weakened muscles to allow for a more functional grasp and release pattern as the nerve healed.

Indications for Use

Elastic therapeutic taping (Kinesio taping method) is used to address soft tissue pathology created by muscle imbalance and assists in removing chemical substances and edema while retraining the body in improved structural alignment. An indirect approach, it works on the neurologic,

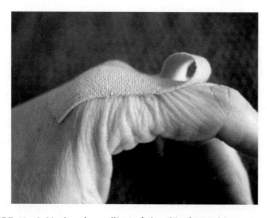

FIGURE 13–6 Notice the pulling of the skin from this tape applied with tension dorsally.

somatosensory, and physiologic processes of the body (Liu, Chen, Lin, Huang, & Sun, 2007; Murray & Husk, 2001). The tape, in combination with the method, has multisystemic effects on vascular, lymphatic, soft tissue, joint, and muscular dysfunctions (Kaya, Zinnuroglu, & Tugcu, 2011; Shim et al., 2003). A thorough and comprehensive understanding of pathology and its relationship to muscle physiology and kinesiology is essential to the success of this form of taping. An evaluation of muscle, fascia, soft tissue continuity, and structure is completed to determine the causal factors of the pathology.

Elastic therapeutic taping is used to complement a rehabilitation program and can be easily taught to patients, family members, or other caregivers for continued application in chronic conditions/situations for self-management (Jaraczewska & Long, 2006; Yasukawa et al., 2006). This technique is effective in treating many acute and chronic orthopedic and complex conditions such as subluxations, sprains, impingement syndromes, complex regional pain syndromes, fibromyalgia, overuse, edema, adhesions and scars, and muscle dysfunctions; it also facilitates postural reeducation (Fig. 13–7) (González-Iglesias, Fernández-de-Las-Peñas, Cleland, Huijbregts, & Del Rosario Gutiérrez-Vega, 2009; Hsu

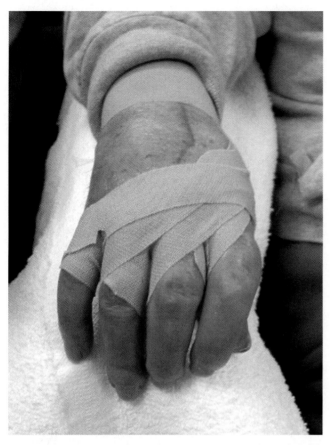

FIGURE 13–7 Kinesio taping was used to position the MCP joints into an extended and radially deviated position 1 month post-MCP arthroplasty after the orthosis was discontinued.

et al., 2009; Jaraczewska & Long, 2006; Kalichman, Vered, & Volchek, 2010; Kase, Wallis, & Kase, 2003; Kase, 1994; Kaya et al., 2011; Liu et al., 2007; Murray & Husk, 2001; Paoloni et al., 2011; Schneider, Rhea, & Bay, 2010; Slupik, Dwornick, Bialoszewski, & Zych, 2007; Thelen, Dauber, & Stoneman, 2008; Yasukawa et al., 2006).

Product Variations

Kinesio® Tex Tape was specifically developed to be used with this technique. The Nitto Denko company obtained a patent for the original elastic therapeutic tape in 1987, and it was sold exclusively under the name of Kinesio® Tex Tape until 2007 (Towatek Co. Ltd., personal communication). Since that time, the Kinesio® Tex Tape product has gone through multiple changes in design and manufacturer and the Nitto Denko company continues to produce the original product but under different names in the international marketplace. Many of the elastic tapes use the same formula as the Nitto Denko company but with some variation. The increasing popularity in the use of "elastic taping" techniques with athletes has yielded an ever-expanding market of products with higher elastic recoils and stronger adhesives/patterns to enhance performance and endurance in sports activities.

An Internet search under "**elastic adhesive tape**," "**elastic therapeutic tape**," or "**elastic sports tape**" will provide information, and several Web sites are included at the end of this chapter that offer products as well as guidelines for taping techniques. Web sites will include information regarding manufacturer and differences in elasticity of the tape in percentage relative to stretch. Tape elasticity is noted in percentage and can be a bit confusing. A tape is said to be 100% at rest, and the additional amount of stretch added would make the difference. Therefore, a tape of 140% would lengthen 40%. Caution must be employed with the use of all elastic tapes to avoid shearing forces on the skin that could result in tissue injury.

Properties of Tape and Technique of Application

The high elastic recoil of the tape combined with proper application affects the superficial fascial structures in the skin and creates a lifting or "ripple effect" in resting tissue. These changes cause a reduction in subcutaneous interstitial pressure, improving lymphatic drainage of toxic chemicals and edema reduction. During normal movement, there is a constant tactile stimuli to low-threshold cutaneous mechanoreceptors of the skin. This stimulates muscle, decreases pain, and enhances proprioception for neuromuscular reeducation. The high elastic recoil of the tape also provides support to weak muscles, reducing fatigue. The thickness and weight of the tape is approximately the same as skin so it does not perceive the tape. It stretches in the longitudinal axis only up to 40% of its resting length. The tape is made of a 100% woven cotton fabric and there is no latex or medicinal properties in the tape. An acrylic, heat-activated adhesive forms a "fingerprint" glue pattern with holes between to allow for passage of perspiration and air. The tape is applied to a paper substrate with a 25% stretch and is available in 2″ and 3″ widths. Multiple colors are also available. Most tapes are "water resistant" using a light paraffin spray coating to increase wearing time when exposed to perspiration or water. The tape may be worn for up to 4 days (or longer depending on the patient's skin qualities and area of body part application), and the patient is able to shower with the tape in place. The digits, thumb, and volar palm of the hand can be challenging in terms of prolonged adherence partially due to exposure to water and other liquids. Care should be taken when drying as not to roll up the edges of the tape. The tape is dried using a dry terry cloth (or absorbent) towel or paper towel because they both will wick the moisture from the tape. A thorough evaluation is critical in obtaining positive results because taping needs to address both the pain and the cause of the pain to provide correction of the pathology. The specific taping technique is determined by the target fascia and tissue to be treated, which also affects how the tape is cut. The most commonly used cuts are the "Y"- and "I"-shaped cuts from 2″ wide tape. Table 13–5 lists techniques and methods

Techniques and Methods Used in Kinesio Taping

"I" or single strip cut	May be used on all muscles across a joint in a correction technique or to encourage rotation; it is applied moving along the center of the muscle. A 1″ width is used for a small muscle.	
"Y" cut	Used to surround multiple or a large muscle belly; the base of the letter is used as the anchor. The separation of the ends or tails assists in changing the tension of the tissue between, lifting it to increase lymphatic flow.	
"X" cut	Used to stabilize at a joint for treatment of rhomboidal-shaped muscle or in a correction technique	
"FAN" cut	Used primarily for edema reduction; the anchor serving as the drawing point to which you want the lymph to drain toward	
"Buttonhole" cut	Used as an anchor in forearm tapings to prevent rolling; athletic or bandage tape may be used to secure the short end if using partial hand coverage as illustrated in lateral epicondylitis taping.	

used in Kinesio taping, and Table 13–6 defines appropriate tape tension.

To treat a tight, shortened muscle and decrease spasm, the tape is anchored on the insertion or movable segment. Move the body so the muscle and skin are on stretch and apply the tape around the lateral and medial margins of the target muscle, ending at the origin or fixed aspect of the muscle (insertion to origin) (Fig. 13–8).

To provide support to a weak muscle, anchor the tape at the origin or fixed part of the muscle. Move the body so the muscle and skin are on stretch and apply the tape around the lateral and medial margins of the target muscle, ending at the insertion or movable aspect of the muscle (origin to insertion) (Fig. 13–9). When providing treatment to the cause of the disability, it is important to reestablish balance at the joint by addressing both the agonist and the antagonist (e.g., to effectively treat an overstretched upper

Proper Tape Tension

No tension	There should be no "pull" at the anchor or end of the tape.
25%	"Pull-off" paper stretch is the most effective tension (i.e., edema, lymphedema, pain).
50%	Tape may be slightly stretched if applied to nonstretched skin (i.e., joint contracture or contraindications to joint movement).
75%–100%	Tape is applied with all elastic stretch taken out only when using a "correction" technique (i.e., adhesive scars).

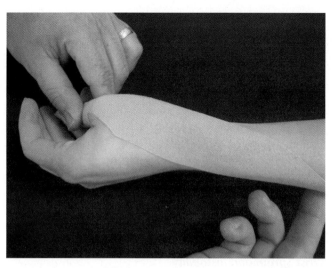

FIGURE 13–8 Tension applied from insertion to origin when addressing deQuervain's tenosynovitis.

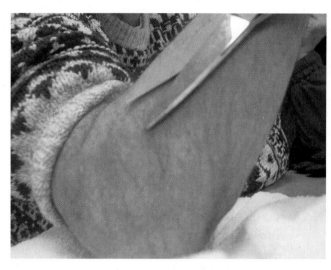

FIGURE 13–10 Trimming hair prior to tape application can ease the discomfort of tape removal.

trapezius, the shortened, tight pectoralis minor must also be addressed).

After application, lightly rub the tape to activate the heat-sensitive glue. The tape may be applied over fine hair, but more coarse hair should be clipped short with scissors or shaved (Fig. 13–10). Once rubbed to activate the glue, the tape may not be reapplied. For best adherence, it should be applied 20 to 30 minutes before activity so it can better tolerate perspiration. It is not necessary to use an adhesive spray before application, except when applying the tape to moist tissue areas or when the patient's skin is sensitive to the adhesive. Athletes who will be training and sweating profusely and water athletes may benefit from the use of an adhesive spray applied prior to tape application. To remove the tape, it is best to start at the proximal end and work distally, moving with the direction of hair growth. Brushing the tape briskly while rolling it onto itself is most effective for overstimulating sensory receptors and decreasing discomfort. To reduce

trauma to the skin, a thin, viscous oil (such as olive oil) may be rubbed and absorbed into the tape to loosen the adhesive prior to removal.

Precautions

Do not stretch the tape unless using one of the correction techniques. The elasticity of the tape provides the therapeutic effect and, if improperly applied, will increase pain. If applied correctly, there should be immediate pain relief. Some patients have experienced sensitivity to the adhesive and, often, to test a strip in an unaffected area for 24 hours prior to prolonged taping is prudent (Fig. 13–11). Application of a skin barrier or spray adherent may prevent irritation. Application of dry heat (such as a hair dryer) to the adhesive *prior* to application will activate the adhesive and increase bonding to difficult areas such as the palm. This technique does not work to reattach the tape because small cellular debris will limit adhesion. The multiple effects of Kinesio taping often create an evolutionary process in

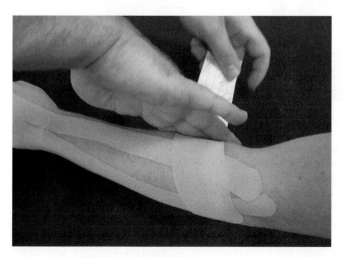

FIGURE 13–9 Tension applied from origin to insertion when addressing the supinator in this lateral epicondylitis taping.

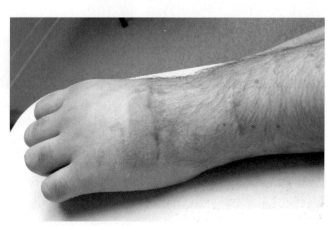

FIGURE 13–11 Redness present after tape removal indicating tape sensitivity.

symptom presentation. A tissue and muscle reevaluation prior to each application is therefore critical to the successful correction of underlying pathology. It is not uncommon to alter tapings from one treatment to another in response to the changes and individual needs of the patient. Due to the complex nature of this taping method, formal training from an experienced and certified instructor is highly recommended to obtain optimal results.

Helpful Hints

- Complete a thorough evaluation for both the pain and cause of pain.
- Move through an ROM before applying the tape to maximize tissue movement.
- Clean the skin of any oils or lotions and dry thoroughly.
- Use a spray adherent, if necessary.
- Cut the tape into the appropriate shape to address the target tissue or function (edema).
- Apply the anchor of the tape securely without tension while the body is in neutral position.
- The target muscle and fascia are moved into maximal elongation (end ROM) when treating a shortened, tight or spastic muscle-tendon unit.
- Apply the tape with "pull-off" paper tension (25%) unless used in a correction technique.

- Place the tape so it surrounds the muscle or as appropriate to the cut shape of the tape.
- Apply tape without tension at the end attachment points.
- Be sure of proper placement prior to smoothing down the tape; work from the center outward to prevent lifting of the ends.
- Use white tape substrate as a pattern for home use.
- Consider taking photos with phone to ensure proper home application.

Clinical Examples

Clinical Examples of Athletic Taping

Wrist Sprain and Instability

APPLICATION

When using athletic taping for the wrist, consider shaving the skin, if necessary, and apply a spray adherent to the areas to be taped (Fig. 13–12) (Arnheim & Prentice, 2000; Austin et al., 1994). The materials required are 1½″ to 2″ wide white adhesive or linen tape and prewrap. If additional support is needed, a dorsal X taping may be used before closing in. After taping, check for appropriate application and motion restriction.

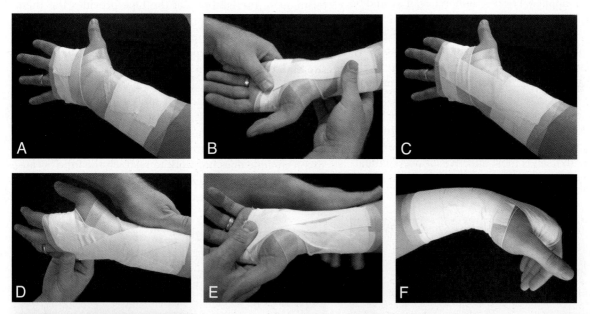

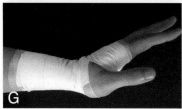

FIGURE 13–12 Athletic taping for a wrist sprain or instability. A, Apply undertape or prewrap circumferentially to protect the forearm; place white tape anchors around the proximal forearm and at the metacarpals. The skin may be further protected with an adhesive spray or prep pad. **B and C,** Place the wrist in neutral position (unless otherwise indicated) and apply a strip of white tape, with tension, from the distal anchor to the proximal anchor both dorsal and volar. To provide more support or restriction to extension, another strip may be placed, overlapping and parallel to the longitudinal piece along the ulnar aspect. **D,** Apply two strips, with tension, from the distal anchor (dorsal and volar), forming an X to support the radial aspect of the wrist. **E,** Repeat this process on volar and ulnar aspects of the wrist. Note the positions of the X supports. (Additional X supports may be added to further limit motion, if necessary.) Complete the taping by applying a top anchor strip to secure the distal ends. Close in the forearm by applying overlapping circumferential strips, moving distal to proximal. **F and G,** Final taping with restriction in flexion and extension noted.

GENERAL CONSIDERATIONS

The therapist must understand which structures require the most support to allow proper positioning of the wrist; if necessary, apply an additional tape strip for maximum protection. Tape strips are placed on tension to provide support but should not be so constrictive as to impinge on the skin or vascular structures. The patient instructions should include periodic evaluations to ensure proper support and appropriate timing for replacement. If possible, teach the patient how to apply the tape. The wrist taping may stay in place for 2 to 4 days depending on the degree of restriction and the activity level of the patient. Instruct the patient to remove tape immediately if there is an increase in pain or adverse vascular signs. A backup orthosis may be necessary to protect the wrist between tapings or as needed. Athletic taping achieves support and restriction through the quality of the material, the specific technique used, the tension applied by the tape, and the number of layers used to restrict movement. Keeping this in mind will assist in customization for individual needs and diagnosis.

Thumb Ulnar Collateral Ligament Injury

APPLICATION

Before using athletic taping for a thumb ulnar collateral ligament (UCL) injury, shave the area, if necessary, and apply adhesive spray (Fig. 13–13) (Arnheim & Prentice, 2000; Aus-

tin et al., 1994). The material required is 1″, 1½″, or 2″ wide white adhesive tape. Because there is increased tension on the UCL, parallel ½″ strips of tape may be placed from the interphalangeal (IP) anchor to the wrist for added support. After taping, check for appropriate application and motion restriction.

Thumb MP Joint Hyperextension Injury

Before using athletic taping for a thumb volar plate sprain or hyperextension injury, apply adhesive spray (Fig. 13–14) (Arnheim & Prentice, 2000; Austin et al., 1994). The material required is 1″ wide white adhesive tape strips. After taping, check for appropriate restriction of thumb MP extension with unrestricted flexion.

GENERAL CONSIDERATIONS

For both the volar plate and ligaments surrounding the thumb MP, consideration should be given to avoid undue stress to injured structures during the taping procedure. Instruct the patient in self-evaluation of the taping. The patient should replace the tape if gapping or loosening is noted and should remove the tape immediately with pain, numbness, or vascular changes. The tape should be replaced in 2 to 3 days depending on the activity level of the patient. When placing the strips, be sure to overlap tape strips slightly to prevent gapping.

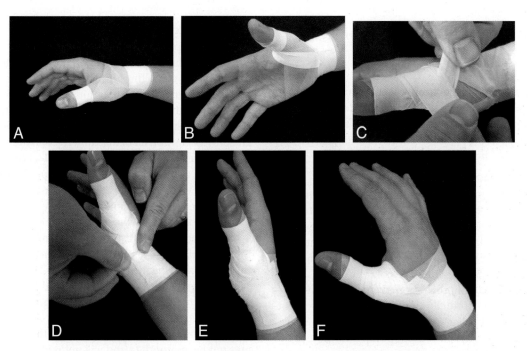

FIGURE 13–13 Athletic taping for a thumb UCL injury. A, Apply undertape or prewrap circumferentially to protect the hand and thumb. Apply circumferential anchors with light tension at the wrist and distal proximal phalanx. **B,** Form a diagonal anchor by attaching a strip to the distal anchor and directing it through the web space to the volar aspect of the proximal anchor. **C,** Using a Figure-8 design with a downward equal pull, form the crosspiece and repeat several times until the thumb is encapsulated. **D,** Anchor the dorsal attachment on the diagonal strip with pressure to adduct the thumb and restrict abduction. **E and F,** To complete the taping, repeat the diagonal and circumferential wrist anchor strips to secure the Figure-8 strip ends. Note position of MP joint in slight ulnar deviation to protect the UCL.

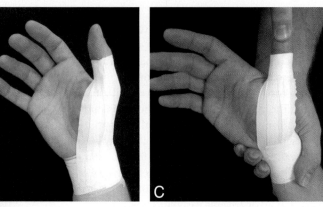

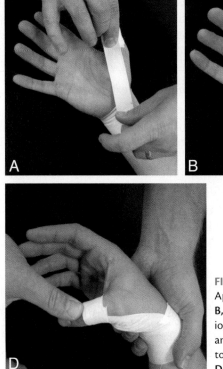

FIGURE 13–14 **Athletic taping for a thumb hyperextension injury.** Apply prewrap and anchor strips as shown in Figure 13–13A. **A and B,** Position and maintain the MP joint in desired degree of MP flexion and begin to apply multiple strips of tape volarly from proximal anchor to distal anchor in direction per photo. **C,** Add anchor strips to proximal and distal borders and check for restriction of extension. **D,** Notice unrestricted MP flexion in final taping.

Clinical Examples of McConnell Taping

Postural Correction

APPLICATION

McConnell taping can be used for postural correction (Fig. 13–15) (C. Bailey, personal communication, 2001). The materials required are brown heavyweight adhesive tape and an undertape. A spray adherent or skin toughener may be used to protect the skin from irritation.

GENERAL CONSIDERATIONS

Taping for postural correction serves as a gentle reminder to the patient. Exercise caution when applying the longitudinal tape; do not upwardly compress the joint capsule, which can lead to shoulder impingement or bursitis. If the patient experiences paresthesias, increased pain, or discomfort, the tape should be removed. Taping should be combined with a comprehensive program to improve strength and proper muscular recruitment and coordination during active movement. The therapist should place the extremity in the proper position. Do not overcorrect, which may be uncomfortable to the patient and inhibit normal use of the extremity.

Shoulder Subluxation

APPLICATION

When taping for a shoulder subluxation, use a spray adherent or skin toughener to protect the skin from irritation, if necessary (Fig. 13–16) (J. McConnell, personal communication, 2001). The materials required are brown heavyweight adhesive tape and an undertape.

GENERAL CONSIDERATIONS

McConnell taping for the shoulder may cause increased irritation depending on the condition of the muscle carrying the weight of the arm. This taping does not address multidirectional instability, only the anterior subluxation commonly seen in patients who have undergone cerebrovascular accidents (CVAs). The vertical strip serves to support the weight of the arm and provide upward lift of the humerus, and the transverse strip supports the humeral head in the glenoid serving as a reinforcement of the anterior ligaments. When taping a patient who has suffered a CVA or who has weakened deltoids, the use of two vertical, parallel, and overlapping strips may assist in reducing the load on the skin. Also when applying the vertical working tape, avoid pulling straight up, which may create additional stress to the skin. Rather, move parallel to the skin and gently taking up the slack, observing the skin on the edges for signs of excess tension. If the patient experiences increased pain or paresthesias, remove the tape immediately. This taping may stay in place for 3 to 4 days depending on the patient's age, overall medical condition, diagnosis, and skin condition. The technique shown here may not be appropriate and will not replace a sling or outside supportive device for heavy extremities or large subluxations of 2 cm or greater. Use caution with all shoulder tapings employing nonelastic tape. Excess force and pressure can have adverse effects on joint and soft tissue structures. This technique should be combined with a comprehensive strengthening program for the muscles affecting the joint to provide extrinsic stability and prevent further damage or stretching of supporting ligaments and joint structures. McConnell taping for shoulder subluxation

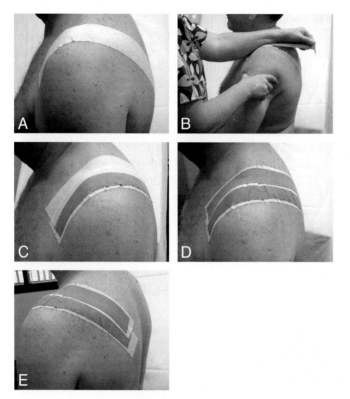

FIGURE 13–15 McConnell taping for postural correction. A, Place the undertape from the anterior aspect of the glenohumeral joint across the acromion process, ending at the medial inferior border of the scapula. **B,** Use the nonworking hand to position the extremity in the proper desired posture of external rotation while using the taping hand to apply downward pressure on the trapezius and secure the tape diagonally across the scapula. **C,** To increase scapular retraction, repeat step A, positioning the second tape just medial to the first tape. **D,** Completed taping. **E,** Placement of posterior tape after completion.

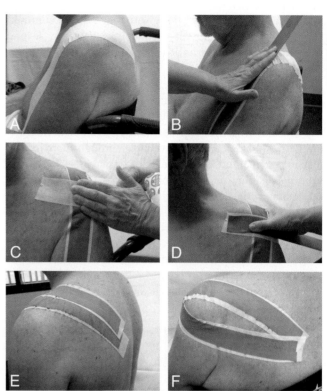

FIGURE 13–16 McConnell taping for shoulder subluxation. A, Apply the vertical undertape over the anterior surface of the upper arm beginning at the elbow and ending just medial to the scapula. **B,** When applying the brown adhesive tape on top of the undertape, use the nonworking hand to approximate the head of the humerus up and back while applying the working tape, ending at the medial scapula. **C,** Place the next undertape perpendicular to the first starting medial to the coracoid process. **D,** Use the nonworking hand to approximate the humerus while applying the working tape for anterior capsular support and external rotation of the humerus. **E,** Position of anterior tapes at completion. **F,** Position of tapes across scapula when complete.

also works well for anterior instability because the tape strips create a perpendicular capsular support. In this case, a shorter vertical strip may be used to avoid upward compressive forces that may result in subacromial impingement.

Lateral Epicondylitis

APPLICATION
Lateral epicondylitis can be treated with McConnell taping. Use a spray adherent or skin toughener, if necessary, to protect the skin from irritation (Fig. 13–17) (C. Bailey, personal communication, 2001). The materials required are brown heavyweight adhesive tape and an undertape cut into 1″ strips. The taping technique shown uses a diamond unloading pattern to shift the fascia and soft tissue restrictions away from the lateral epicondyle.

GENERAL CONSIDERATIONS
The patient should experience immediate decrease or relief of symptoms after taping. The taping can remain in place for 2 to 3 days before needing to be replaced. Be careful to maintain the adhesive tape on the undertape to prevent skin contact and irritation on removal. The taping for lateral epicondylitis should be combined with a comprehensive stretching and strengthen-

ing program for the upper extremity, focusing on the forearm extensors. Do not pull up on the tape, rather glide the fascia parallel to the skin. When the taping has been completed, there will be a puckering and lifting of the skin over the lateral epicondyle.

Clinical Examples of Kinesio Taping

Lateral Epicondylitis

APPLICATION
Kinesio taping for lateral epicondylitis addresses the tight forearm extensor muscles by applying the tape from insertion to origin and providing assistance to the overused supinator muscle (Fig. 13–18). The technique requires 2″ wide combination "buttonhole" and Y-cut tape for the extensors. The buttonhole technique is used to secure the tape on the hand and prevent removal during functional activities. Use a short, or half, version for this application because the tape is applied to the dorsum of the arm only. A 1½″ to 2″ end is needed to provide a secure anchor in the palm. The long end is then cut down the middle to approximately 4″ (or two boxes, if using the demarcations on the back of the

substrate) from the buttonhole. Note that this is a common taping method for lateral epicondylitis; however, several other application patterns do exist.

GENERAL CONSIDERATIONS

If the patient has long or coarse forearm hair, it may need to be shaved or trimmed to ensure adhesive contact. Shave the hair only where the tape is to be applied. Cosmetic shavers with 1″ blades are now available through many of the elastic tape manufactures. These shavers create a "track" for tape application, allowing only hair loss where necessary (Web sites at the end of this chapter will have further information). Apply tape with pull-off paper tension. The patient should experience rapid relief of symptoms, unless he or she has a chronic condition. For chronic lateral epicondylitis, a few days are required to reduce the edema in the tissues and for the patient to experience relief. There should be no irritation from the tape, unless it was applied with too much

tension or the patient is allergic. Allergic responses to the adhesive are seen as a blister-type rash or hives. To ensure that the patient is not allergic to the acrylic adhesive, apply a small piece of tape without tension on an area of skin that does not pass across a joint. This will remove human error during application as the cause of any reaction. Round the corners of the tape to prevent lifting of the anchor or ends. Anchors should be a minimum of 1″ and secured by rubbing before moving the fascia into the taping position. The anchors and ends of the tape are secured while the patient is in a neutral position. The paper substrate may be torn through the cotton tape; but if torn on the edge and pulled, it will tear across and will not affect the elastic tape. To improve tension control, tear the paper substrate just after the anchor and fold back the edge of the paper to create a handle. Keeping the tape parallel and close to the skin, pull on this handle with one hand and follow behind with the index finger of the opposite hand, smoothing the tape onto

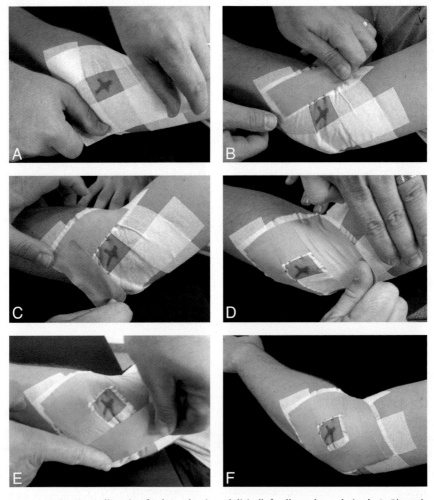

FIGURE 13–17 McConnell taping for lateral epicondylitis (left elbow, lateral view). A, Place the undertape in a diamond configuration to surround the area of pain (noted with marker). **B,** Attach the brown tape at the inferior anterior section of the diamond starting at the inferior apex. Stretch the fascia superior and anterior along the course of the undertape and attach it at the anterior apex of the diamond. **C,** Repeat the process, placing the tape in the direction of the inferior posterior aspect of the diamond. **D,** Repeat, placing the tape at the posterior superior aspect of the diamond. **E,** Place the last tape at the anterior superior aspect to complete the diamond. **F,** Completed diamond deloading.

the skin while moving toward the end attachment site. Rub to create friction heat to secure.

The demarcations on the back of the substrate indicate the stretch direction (longitudinal marks) and 2″ boxes. These can be used to help measure and cut the tape and when providing directions to the patient for self-application. There may be some redness after removal, but it should resolve in about 30 minutes. To remove the residual glue from the skin, rub skin adhesive remover, oil, or skin lotion (or cream) into the tape or use soap during bathing to decrease the removal trauma.

Carpal Tunnel Syndrome

APPLICATION

Kinesio taping for carpal tunnel syndrome uses a space correction technique to lift the skin, creating a space in the area of inflammation or pain to improve lymph and vascular

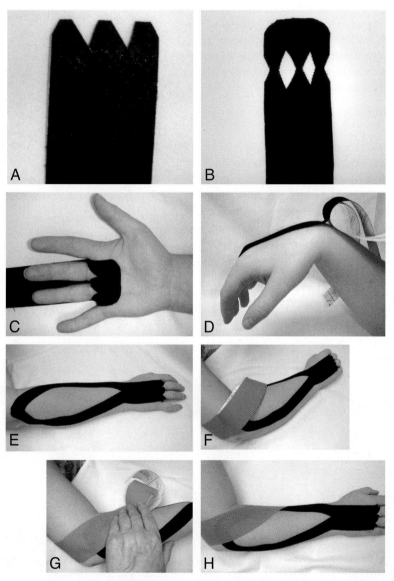

FIGURE 13–18 Kinesio taping for lateral epicondylitis. A, Fold the tape, cut two triangles (finger holes), and snip the corners at an angle (to accommodate digit web spaces). Proximal end of tape should be split into a "Y" cut. **B,** Completed "buttonhole" cut. **C,** Place the middle and ring fingers through openings and secure with a 1″ to 2″ volar anchor. **D,** Position the wrist in maximum flexion and apply the tape over the dorsum of the hand to the wrist. The split should be located at the dorsum of the proximal wrist (over the muscle belly). **E,** Maintaining the wrist position, extend the elbow and apply the tape around the medial and lateral margins of the extensor muscle wad, ending at the lateral epicondyle. **F,** Apply an additional "I"-cut tape to help the supinator muscle relax, because a contracted muscle may put pressure on the radial nerve, creating similar symptoms. Apply the tape anchor just proximal to elbow, on an angle at the midline of the humerus. **G,** Position the forearm in pronation with the elbow in slight flexion to prevent compensatory movement of the humerus. Apply the tape over the lateral epicondyle and supinator, terminating on the medial ulnar side of the forearm. **H,** Completed taping.

movement (Fig. 13–19). The target tissue is the retinacular ligament. The material required is a 2″ wide I-cut tape.

GENERAL CONSIDERATIONS

The tape may be applied to either the volar or the dorsal aspect of the wrist depending on the response of patient. The patient may experience changes over a 24-hour period and may benefit from the edema taping in combination with this correction technique. Do not apply tension to the ends of the tape from the midline of the wrist to the final attachment to the skin. To best handle the tape for this technique, tear the edge of the substrate and pull—this will run the tear centrally across the paper. Fold back the substrate to form two handles. Hold these in a lateral pinch fashion and draw them apart directly over the area to be taped. Apply direct downward pressure then smooth for good contact.

DeQuervain's Tenosynovitis

APPLICATION

The target tissues for Kinesio taping for deQuervain's tenosynovitis are the inflamed extensor pollicis brevis and abductor pollicis longus; therefore, the tape is applied from insertion to origin (Fig. 13–20). Retinacular ligament taping uses a correction technique to lift the skin and fascia over the first dorsal compartment and carpometacarpal (CMC) joint, reducing edema and improving vascular flow. The materials required are a 2″ wide I-cut tape measured from the IP of the thumb to the origin of the abductor pollicis longus, a 2″ wide I-cut tape (as described earlier for carpal tunnel syndrome),

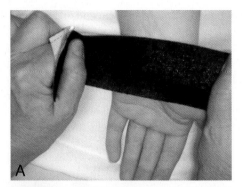

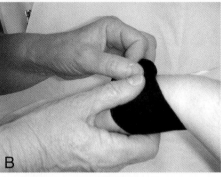

FIGURE 13–19 Kinesio taping for carpal tunnel syndrome. A, Position the hand in tolerable active wrist extension. Apply correction tape ("I"-cut tape with all the stretch taken out of the center and applied directly down onto the area) over the transverse carpal ligament. **B,** Move the wrist into relaxed flexion and apply the ends without tension.

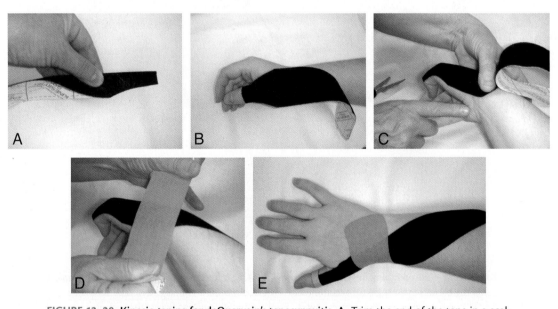

FIGURE 13–20 Kinesio taping for deQuervain's tenosynovitis. A, Trim the end of the tape in a scallop or curved form to prevent circumferential restriction of the proximal phalanx. **B,** Place the anchor just proximal to thumb IP joint. **C,** With the elbow flexed, position the thumb into flexion and ulnarly deviate and flex the wrist as tolerated. Apply the tape along the radial aspect of the wrist and up onto the extensor surface, ending at the mid forearm (origin of the abductor pollicis longus). **D,** Maintain the wrist position. A correction tape (all the stretch taken out) is placed over the retinacular ligament at the radial aspect of the wrist. Then apply the ends with no tension and the wrist relaxed in a neutral position. **E,** Circumferentially secure the distal thumb anchor with crosscut pieces of ½″ wide Kinesio® Tex Tape (no tension).

and two ½″ crosscut pieces of tape or white tape to secure at the IP and prevent rolling.

GENERAL CONSIDERATIONS

The ½″ securing tapes for the anchor should be applied loosely so as not to constrict. They may be applied after the muscle taping. This taping is also effective for relieving associated sensory radial nerve signs and provides support to the CMC joint, reducing pain and associated edema with use of the "lifting strip" at the retinacular ligament. To increase the I-tape conformity on the thumb and web space, fold the tape and scallop it slightly to create a 1″ area of tape contact on the dorsal thumb, gradually increase to cover the thenar area of the thumb.

Edema Management

APPLICATION FOR EDEMA

The target tissue for Kinesio taping for edema management is tight flexor and extensor muscles that inhibit lymphatic flow (Fig. 13–21). The movement of the fascia during normal activity also assists in lymph drainage, causing decompression and space correction. In theory, the elastic recoil demonstrated by the tape once applied to the overextended skin lifts the connective tissue fibers. This contributes to improved lymphatic mobility and secondarily decreases pressure on the underlying structures, which in turn may aid in lessening pain. When worn, the stretch properties of the tape during dynamic movement functions much like a soft tissue massage by increasing blood flow and decreasing edema. The material required is a length of 2″ tape, buttonhole cut (as described for lateral epicondylitis).

GENERAL CONSIDERATIONS

This technique is effective for treating postoperative pain and edema, but caution should be taken when addressing acutely healing tissues. Taping may be placed on the dorsum, avoiding contact with surgical areas when apparent and still be effective in reducing edema. The taping should be combined with active motion because this creates movement and massaging of the skin to improve lymphatic return. To assist in proper adherence in finger web spaces, gently pull the tape and then relax to allow it to settle and improve skin contact.

Scar Management

APPLICATION FOR SCAR

The target tissue for Kinesio taping in scar management is adherent scars or those incision areas that may be at risk for adherence such as the dorsum of the MP joints or the radial styloid area as shown in Figure 13–22. The creative application of the tape over an adherent scar can gently "lift" or lightly "pull" the skin and underlying soft tissue away from the structure to which it is fixed or adhered. By keeping the tape on,

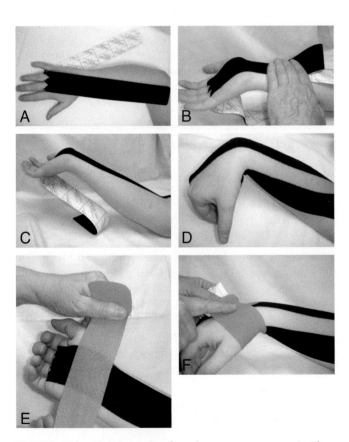

FIGURE 13–21 Kinesio taping for edema management. A, Place "buttonhole"-cut tape through the middle and ring fingers. **B,** With the wrist in maximum extension, apply the tape to the volar surface of the hand to the wrist. **C,** Apply the tape over the flexor muscle mass, ending at the medial epicondyle. **D,** Move the wrist into maximum flexion. Apply the tape over the dorsum of the hand, wrist, and extensor muscles, ending at lateral epicondyle. **E,** Place the scar (volar) on stretch and apply a correction tape (all the stretch out) perpendicular to the first taping. **F,** Then move the wrist into flexion and apply the tape without tension to the edge of the dorsal strip to prevent circumferential restriction.

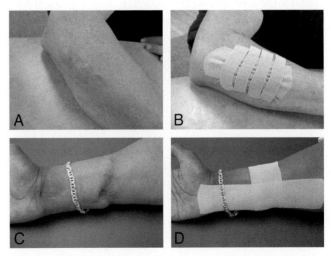

FIGURE 13–22 Kinesio taping for scar management. A and B, Kinesio taping used over an adherent surgical scar. Strip placement was changed at each therapy visit to provide the tissue with various tension to improve soft tissue mobility. **C and D,** Kinesio taping applied over this traumatic scar to decrease adherence of skin to underlying tissue. Tape was worn throughout the day to allow for active motion to promote tissue mobility.

the movement of the fascia under the tape during normal activity creates a gentle shear stress, which in turn may aide in facilitating gentle independent gliding of the tissue. This would be considered a correction technique because the tape is stretched beyond the pull-off paper tension. The materials required are dependent on the size of the scar or incision.

GENERAL CONSIDERATIONS

This technique is effective for treating potential scar formation or managing adherent scars. Caution should be taken with application over acutely healing tissues; however, if placed lightly and correctly, the tape can gently lift the skin, allowing an increase in nutrition and blood flow, thus promoting active healing. When appropriate, taping should be combined with active motion because this creates movement between the superficial adherent tissue and those that lie beneath.

Conclusion

Taping is not for every patient or therapist and should be employed with caution and sound clinical judgment. In addition, taping should not be viewed as a replacement for traditional forms of orthotic management because it holds a special place in upper extremity rehabilitation. The advantages of soft tissue support and increased joint mobility that taping provides place it in a class of its own. Athletic taping has had a longer history and is supported by more clinical research studies than the other taping methods. The effectiveness of McConnell taping and elastic therapeutic taping to date has been primarily the result of years of anecdotal reports, clinical experience, and individual case reports. These, along with growing research studies, support the effects of these taping techniques.

Web sites provide information on educational opportunities and links or resources for obtaining taping supplies. Some sites offer instructional vignettes to assist the novice. The limitations found with the application of orthoses may also be found with taping. For example, patients may not want to wear the tape in public or may object to wearing the tape for a prolonged period of time. Patients may become frustrated when learning to handle and manage the tape. A strong patient–therapist educational base is important; but as with all new skills, it takes time and practice to develop proficiency. The growing use of taping to treat injuries is rapidly evolving. Clinicians should master these taping techniques and add them as an additional tool to further enhance a patient's treatment possibilities. Taping is an expanding area of practice and, as with all modalities, should be performed by a skilled clinician and only a part of a comprehensive rehabilitation program. Clinicians should stay abreast of new tapes and products as they enter the market because this will allow opportunities for further study in developing unique taping applications to address specific populations.

Many Thanks to Kevin Auffrey, ATC for his input, guidance and many photographs of the 3 taping techniques reviewed in this chapter.

Chapter Review Questions

1. What are three popular taping methods discussed in this chapter and how do they differ?

2. For what injuries is athletic taping most often used? Give three specific examples.

3. Before the application of athletic tape and McConnell taping, are there any additional procedures that must be done?

4. Name a minimum of three indications of use for elastic therapeutic taping.

5. What are the precautions for each taping technique?

14 Neoprene Orthoses

Sabrina Cassella, MEd, OTR/L, CHT
Jessica Griffin Scheff, MS, OTR/L

Chapter Objectives

After study of this chapter, the reader should be able to:

- Appreciate the history and evolution of neoprene materials and its unique application within the field of upper extremity rehabilitation.
- Report the properties and characteristics of various types of neoprene materials.

- Develop the clinical reasoning skills and techniques required to reproduce the orthoses described.
- Appreciate the innovative characteristics and boundless possibilities that neoprene offers the clinician when faced with alternative orthotic management.

Key Terms

Breathoprene
Comfortprene
Contact dermatitis
Direction of stretch

Hook receptive
Latex allergies
Neoplush
Neoprene

Polychloropene
Prickly heat (maliaria rubra)
Seam tape
Unbroken loop

Introduction

This chapter is written to inspire and stimulate the creative use of **neoprene** material in daily practice. Threaded throughout this chapter, the reader will find highlights from the first edition blended with new and innovative uses of neoprene. Within this chapter, it is unrealistic to include all of the possibilities that can be made with this versatile material. It is the authors' intent to provide a frame of reference and, in doing so, inspire the reader's imagination. This chapter is predominately based on experience because there is little research available on custom neoprene orthotic fabrication. Throughout this chapter, the reader will find case studies and clinical pearls that portray the creative process of using this unique and adaptable material. The content encompasses the results after trial and error, patient feedback, physician support, and collegial contributions.

The goal is to keep it simple by using materials commonly found in the average hand therapy clinic. There is no cookbook approach to making a neoprene orthosis especially because there is little need for pattern usage. The historical use of neoprene, quick and easy alternative fabrication techniques, and a host of strapping methods will be discussed. The scope of orthotic management with neoprene is vast, owing only to one's creative imagination and the complete understanding of the underlying diagnoses to which these devices are applied.

---

*This chapter is based on the first edition chapter written by Nicole Jacobs, OTR/L, CHT and Christy Halpin Wright, OTR/L, CHT.

History of Neoprene

Neoprene was invented by DuPont scientists in 1930 to provide an alternative to natural rubber as the demand and price for this resource increased. It was the first synthetic rubber product ever created and also goes by the name **polychloroprene**. Neoprene is a synthetic, latex-free polymer, making it an excellent option for the growing number of people with **latex allergies**. During World War II, all the available neoprene went toward war efforts to make products like tires, hoses, and fan belts. Neoprene is still used today for products such as wet suits, automobile tires, and the soft coating around exercise weights (American Chemistry Council, 2012; Colditz, 1999).

Neoprene conforms and drapes, making it easy to work with. This unique orthotic fabrication alternative can offer support to the incorporated joint(s) while still allowing for some mobility (Colditz, 1999). There are many neoprene products available on the market. Besides traditional neoprene, there are also neoprene-like products such as **Breathoprene™**, **Neoplush™**, and **Comfortprene™**. The reader is referred to the resource section for a current list of neoprene suppliers and products.

Characteristics of Neoprene

There are many characteristics of neoprene that make it an excellent choice for orthotic fabrication.

- Neoprene is available in various thicknesses ranging from 1.5 to 6.0 mm (or $\frac{1}{16}''$ to $\frac{1}{8}''$). These measurements pertain to the rubber core and do not take into account thickness of the material added by backings, such as nylon knit or loop (Colditz, 1999).
- Neoprene is more resistant to water, oils, and heat than natural rubber (American Chemistry Council, 2012).
- Traditional neoprene is nonperforated, which makes it an excellent insulator. Perforated options may help patients who tend to sweat readily or for athletes to use during competition.
- Neoprene is elastic in nature. Neoprene's rubber core has equal stretch in all directions. The laminated top layers, commonly nylon knit, terry cloth, or loop material can affect the direction of stretch (Colditz, 1999).
- Neoprene can be directly adhered to thermoplastic materials and tapes.
- Custom neoprene orthoses can be fabricated to immobilize, mobilize, or restrict motion.
- The "wetsuit" properties of neoprene also allow patients to wear the strapping or orthosis during "wet" activities. This characteristic may increase wear compliance and patient satisfaction.
- Neoprene can be easily cut/trimmed without risk of fraying edges and material breakdown.

Direction of Stretch

The **direction of stretch** should be kept in mind depending on the goal of the orthosis. If the goal is to restrict motion, then the degree of *least* stretch would be applied *lengthwise* to the joint. If support during motion is the goal, then the direction of *most* stretch is applied *around* the joint (Colditz, 1999).

Mobilization Force

With the rising cost and decreasing reimbursement in rehabilitation, fabrication of mobilization orthoses can be an expensive treatment option. Based on the elastic properties of neoprene, the material can be used as a "dynamic" force in the fabrication of mobilization orthoses instead of using traditional rubber bands. "Orthoses made of neoprene material have the advantage of being pliable and at the same time can be constructed as dynamic orthoses" (Punsola-Izard, Rouzaud, Thomas, Lluch, & Garcia-Elias, 2001).

Types of Layers

The following are types and characteristics of the laminated top layers commonly found on neoprene.

Unbroken Loop *(defined in this chapter as "***hook receptive***")*

- Feels similar to loop strapping material; readily attaches to hook material
- Adds bulk to the neoprene (is thick)
- Reduces the amount of stretch and drape
- Offers maximum durability for exterior or interior linings
- Feels cushiony, fuzzy, and warm against the skin
- Takes no time to add fasteners (use hook strap directly anywhere)
- Bonds well with iron-on seam tape
- Allows quick application of supportive straps for any orthosis

Nylon

- Adds no bulk to the neoprene (is thin)
- Allows full stretch and drape
- Provides moderate durability of exterior or interior linings
- Does not have ability to attach to hook or loop material directly
- Takes time to add fasteners (needs iron-on hook and loop)
- Feels slick and cool against the skin
- Bonds best with iron-on seam tape

Terry Cloth

- Adds no bulk to the neoprene (is thin)
- Allows full stretch and drape
- Provides maximum durability for interior linings (rarely used on exterior)

- Takes minimal time to add fasteners (use hook strap for short term, iron-on fasteners for permanent use)
- Feels soft and cool against the skin
- Bonds well with iron-on seam tape

Precautions and Care of Neoprene

Although it is rare, there are reported cases of allergic **contact dermatitis** (ACD) and **prickly heat (miliaria rubra)** caused by neoprene use (Colditz, 1999; Stern, Callinan, Mark, Schousboe, & Yutterberg, 1998). When dispensing a prefabricated or custom neoprene orthosis, it is important to instruct patients to monitor skin integrity frequently. The warm compressive qualities of neoprene may be very inviting to some patients; but for others, it may be intolerable. Caution should be used when dispensing these orthoses for use during strenuous exercise, heavy manual labor, or for use in very warm climates. Skin breakdown and maceration may become problematic (Colditz, 1999).

To reduce the risk of skin irritation, the orthosis should be frequently hand washed with mild soapy water or machine washed in a gentle cycle with all hook and loop fastened (Colditz, 1999). Neoprene orthoses should be thoroughly air dried before reapplication to prevent skin breakdown and irritation. Patients wearing neoprene straps during wet activities such as swimming will require a second set of straps to allow complete drying of wet straps prior to reapplication. Wearing stockinette sleeves under a neoprene orthosis may help to absorb sweat, but will not act as a barrier to ACD (Stern et al., 1998). Perforated neoprene may be useful in minimizing these issues by increasing airflow.

Why Choose a Custom versus Prefabricated Neoprene Orthosis?

Custom options allow flexibility to make adjustments and alterations based on specific patient needs and evaluation findings. Patterns or designs can be adjusted and easily modified to accommodate the special requirements of each patient. Using the alternative fastening techniques described in this chapter, fabrication time for these custom neoprene orthoses is significantly reduced.

The traditional fabrication of custom-made neoprene orthoses required sewing or the use of iron-on seam tape and glue. This process was lengthy and not all clinics were equipped with a sewing machine or special dowels to accommodate for using seam tape. In a fast-paced rehabilitation setting, this option may be impractical for some therapists due to time constraints, thus making a prefabricated neoprene orthosis the desired alternative. Proper fit of prefabricated devices can be challenging as well as costly in that a clinic must stock all the necessary inventory of types and sizes available (Colditz, 1999). The fabrication techniques described in this chapter offer another alternative and cost-effective way to customize these soft orthoses without the use of a sewing machine, seam tape, or glue.

Traditional Fabrication and Fastening Techniques

Traditional custom neoprene orthoses fabrication techniques required an iron and seam tape or sewing and glue. Fastening methods described in this chapter have eliminated the need to use these methods. The following are directions to fabricate a neoprene thumb orthosis, which is one of the more complex custom neoprene patterns adapted from the previous edition of this book (Fig. 14–1). The materials needed for fabricating a traditional neoprene orthosis (Fig. 14–2) are as follows:

- Neoprene material
- Scissors
- Iron-on seam tape
- Iron-on hook-and-loop tape or strips
- Seal cement (glue)
- Disappearing-ink marking pen or chalk
- Thenar web space thermoplastic form (Fig. 14–3) (Simin, 2000)
- Small dowel

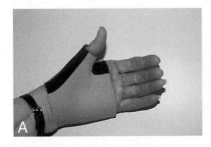
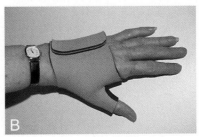

FIGURE 14–1 **A and B,** Custom neoprene thumb orthosis for CMC arthritis.

TRADITIONAL NEOPRENE THUMB ORTHOSIS

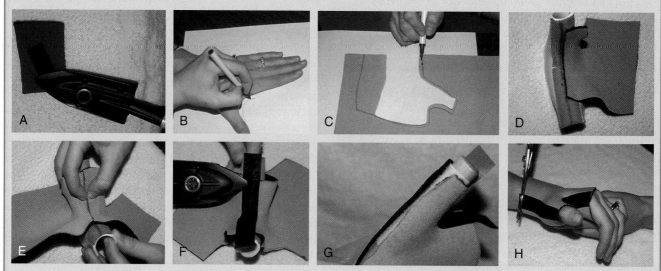

FIGURE 14–2 Steps for fabricating a traditional neoprene thumb orthosis.

A

- Set the iron to the midrange on the dial and let it heat. Test a small area of the neoprene and heat-sensitive seam tape. If the neoprene and tape do not adhere within 15 seconds, increase the temperature and test again.

B

- Trace the patient's hand on paper from the MCP joints to the wrist, making sure the wrist is in neutral and not excessively radial or ulnarly deviated. Trace the thumb in full radial abduction, paying special attention to tracing the web space as precisely as possible.

C

- Place two pieces of neoprene material, wrong sides facing, and use folded-over adhesive-backed hook between the layers to help keep the two pieces together and stabilized while continuing to make the pattern. The piece of neoprene that will be the dorsal piece should be 2″ to 3″ wider than the other.
- Trace the pattern onto the top (dorsal) piece of neoprene material. Trace 1/4″ wider than the pattern along the radial side to allow for the seam.
- Add 2″ to 3″ of width to the top piece along the ulnar side.

D

- Cut out the pattern. Remember that the top (dorsal) piece is wider than the bottom (volar) piece. It is important for the two pieces to be attached with hook so they are cut exactly the same. Keep the scissors perpendicular to the neoprene to maintain a flat edge, which is necessary for bonding of the radial-side seam.
- Take the volar piece of neoprene and place the web space area from the neoprene pattern onto the thermoplastic web space form. Match up the neoprene with the line drawn down the middle of the piece of hook on the web space form.
- Lightly apply the seal cement (glue) to the black core material of neoprene in the web space area of the dorsal piece.

- Heat the seal cement with a heat gun until small bubbles are seen indicating cement is ready.

E

- Now attach the web spaces from both pieces together onto the web space form, using the line drawn onto the hook for alignment.
- Pinch the edges together, moving from distal to proximal. Allow a few moments for the seam to set up before moving on to the next area.

F

- Press the seam tape over the seam while it is still on the web space form. Apply the iron directly to the tape for 15 seconds at a time. Look for melted glue to show along the edges of the tape. Be careful; if the iron is held in one spot too long, the seam glue can heat and come apart.
- The edges can be finished by either folding or heating the seam tape around edges of the neoprene or by trimming any excess.

G

- Remove the orthosis from the web space form.
- Apply glue to the next seam and use a dowel to align edges to form the thumbhole. Follow the same steps, substituting the dowel for the web space form.
- Remove the orthosis from the dowel.
- Attach the iron-on hook strip to the neoprene by placing a piece of paper towel between the iron and the hook material to prevent burning of material. Apply the iron for 15 seconds at a time, and look for the melted glue on the edges of the hook strip.
- Let the hook cool for at least 30 minutes before applying stress.

H

- Check the fit, and trim as necessary.
- Trim any excess seam tape.

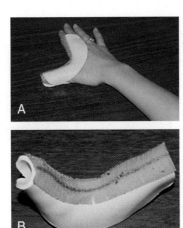

FIGURE 14-3 Thumb web space form on (**A**) and off (**B**) the patient. Note that a marker was used as a guide to line up the two pieces of material during the gluing process.

Creative Fabrication and Fastening Techniques

The following are the fabrication and fastening techniques used by the authors. Many of the tools and supplies used are common items found in the hand therapy clinic.

Fabrication Supplies

- Neoprene material (preferably hook receptive)
- Scissors
- Rivets (various sizes from small to large)
- Blunt-nosed pliers
- Heat gun
- Foam or Moleskin

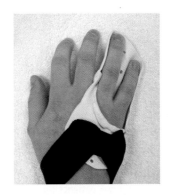

FIGURE 14-4 Neoprene is a nice option for functional orthoses, allowing muscle movement beneath the strapping as seen in this digit immobilization orthosis.

- Adhesive hook
- Solvent

There are several options to consider for fastening and creating a custom neoprene orthosis. The techniques described attempt to keep the fabrication process simple with no sewing, gluing, or seam tape required. Strong hook receptive backing on neoprene has decreased the need to sew or iron-on strap attachments (Beasley, 2011).

Attaching Neoprene to Thermoplastic
Adhesive Hook (Fig. 14-4)

- Apply adhesive tab to desired location on thermoplastic orthosis.
- Place trimmed and previously fitted neoprene strap.

Rivet (Fig. 14-5A-E)

- To prevent removal of strap, a speedy rivet can be used in combination with the adhesive hook.

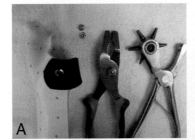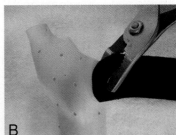
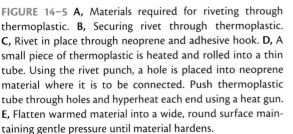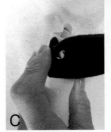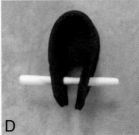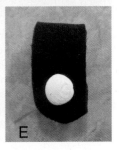

FIGURE 14-5 A, Materials required for riveting through thermoplastic. **B,** Securing rivet through thermoplastic. **C,** Rivet in place through neoprene and adhesive hook. **D,** A small piece of thermoplastic is heated and rolled into a thin tube. Using the rivet punch, a hole is placed into neoprene material where it is to be connected. Push thermoplastic tube through holes and hyperheat each end using a heat gun. **E,** Flatten warmed material into a wide, round surface maintaining gentle pressure until material hardens.

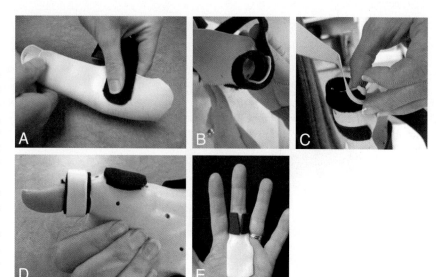

FIGURE 14–6 **A,** Direct adherence of neoprene to thermoplastic material. **B,** A piece of neoprene can be used as a volar support to the thumb proximal phalanx within an immobilization orthosis. **C,** A rivet or thermoplastic strip can be added for extra reinforcement. **D,** A ring of thermoplastic can be adhered over neoprene if increased stabilization of the thumb is necessary. This is an excellent alternative for those patients who do not tolerate thermoplastic against skin. **E,** This concept can be applied to other digits as shown in this MCP immobilization orthosis for trigger finger. The neoprene provides a flexible "strap" to secure the orthosis allowing donning/doffing over an enlarged PIP joint.

- Using a hole punch, make a small hole through all three layers of material (thermoplastic, adhesive hook, and neoprene).
- A rivet can then be placed through this hole and set with blunt-nosed pliers.
- Homemade rivets can be easily made using small scrap pieces of thermoplastic.

Direct Adherence (Fig. 14–6A–E)

- When using a coated thermoplastic material, apply solvent to desired area.
- Using a heat gun, warm thermoplastic material for 5 to 10 seconds until area is tacky but does not lose shape.
- Place and hold neoprene to this area for 15 to 20 seconds with good compression.

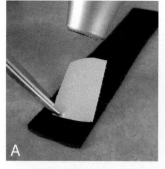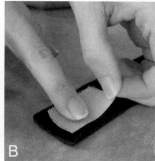

FIGURE 14–7 **A,** Hyperheat adhesive hook to apply to neoprene. Scissors or pliers can be used to hold a piece of adhesive-backed hook while using a heat gun to activate the adhesive. Hold the tab approximately 2″ from heat gun for 5 to 10 seconds. This method is intended to hyperheat the adhesive backing. The warm "tacky" glue should then penetrate and seep into and between the fabric fibers of the neoprene, further securing the hook onto the neoprene. **B,** Applying pressure to secure adhesive hook.

- If necessary for added security, an additional piece of thermoplastic material can be added over the top of adhered strap, spilling over the strap borders onto the thermoplastic base.

Attaching Neoprene to Neoprene

Heated Hook Material (Fig. 14–7A,B)

- Using a heat gun, hyperheat the precut length of adhesive-backed hook for 5 to 10 seconds until edges begin to curl.
- Place hook on desired location of neoprene and apply moderate pressure, paying special attention to the edges to ensure a good bond.
- This technique can work alone or can be used in conjunction with rivets for a more secure application (see instructions in the following text).

Rivets (for use as a closure) (Fig. 14–8)

- Using a heat gun, hyperheat the precut length of adhesive-backed hook for 5 to 10 seconds.
- Place hook on desired location of neoprene and apply moderate pressure, paying special attention to the edges to ensure a good bond.

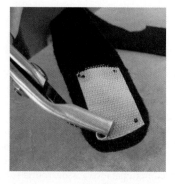

FIGURE 14–8 Securing rivet through adhesive hook and neoprene.

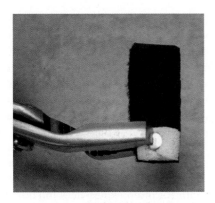

FIGURE 14–9 Securing rivet using a foam "washer."

- Using a hole punch, create small holes for rivets on all four corners of hook. The rivets should be of adequate size; a rivet that is "too large" may lead to irritation of the skin against the rivet.
- Place a rivet through each hole and secure with blunt-nosed pliers.

Rivets with Hook, Foam, or Moleskin (to act as a washer) (Fig. 14–9)

- In cases where rivets are attached to neoprene without adhesive hook, it is recommended to apply foam, a small piece of adhesive hook, or Moleskin type material to the neoprene at the area where the rivet will be applied.
- This will in turn function as a "washer," preventing the material from pulling through the riveted area after repeated use.
- The authors have found that using this technique disperses the pressure of the rivet head, therefore increasing the life span of the custom orthosis.

Seam Tape (Fig. 14–2F)

- Place the heat-sensitive seam tape (adhesive glue side down) over the two pieces of neoprene that will be joined.
- Using medium pressure, hold the heated iron in place over seam tape for 10 to 20 seconds until melted glue begins to show around edges of the tape. The time to set/bond the two pieces will depend on individual heat iron settings.
- Hook material or seam glue can be used to help stabilize the two pieces while attempting to attach the seam tape, thus helping to prevent gapping.
- If the iron is too hot, searing of seam tape and neoprene may occur; this can be prevented by using a small piece of paper towel between the iron and the material.

Creative Uses of Neoprene

A wide variety of conditions exist that may benefit from soft neoprene orthoses. Many patients prefer soft orthoses, which may improve orthosis wear compliance, and often these soft devices are more easily tolerated versus thermoplastic ones (Beasley, 2011). Custom orthoses can promote independence with daily activities, help decrease pain and stress on joints, and facilitate patients returning to self-care/work following injury or surgery. Custom neoprene orthoses can be flexible or semiflexible, depending on the fabrication techniques chosen and the addition of thermoplastic stays or supports (Beasley, 2011). Therapists are only limited by their own imagination! The following are examples of how the authors have used neoprene for patients with a wide variety of diagnoses.

Thumb and Digits

Interphalangeal Joints

Using small or scrap pieces of ⅟₁₆″ or ³⁄₃₂″ neoprene material, custom orthoses can be fabricated for the digits. Patients following digital nerve repairs or amputations may benefit from custom neoprene digit sleeves. These patients often present with hypersensitivity to touch and/or vibration and temperature intolerance. Digit sleeves can offer protection while still allowing flexibility to incorporate the affected digit in activities (Fig. 14–10A,B). Buddy strapping can be helpful following collateral ligament repairs, complex fractures, tendon repairs, or arthroplasty to encourage or maintain proper digital alignment (Beasley, 2011) (Fig. 14–11A,B). To mobilize the proximal interphalangeal (PIP) joints, distal interphalangeal (DIP) joints, and intrinsics, dynamic PIP/DIP straps can be made using a safety pin or staple for closure. This allows for a gentle progression of stretch as a patient's range of motion (ROM) improves. The extrinsic extensors can be stretched by immobilizing the metacarpophalangeal (MCP) joints in a custom thermoplastic orthosis in flexion and applying a dynamic stretch via neoprene distally to the PIP and DIP joints (Fig. 14–12A–C). Immobilizing the MCP joints in extension, in combination with PIP/DIP

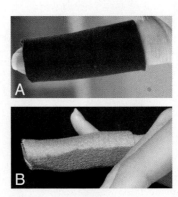

FIGURE 14–10 A, Protective digit sleeve for patient following a digital nerve repair using seam tape for closure. **B,** Digit sleeve using Orficast™ Tape for closure and to provide gentle digit extension mobilization. This same orthosis can be made using a thin strip of thermoplastic for closure as well.

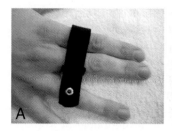
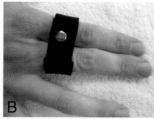

FIGURE 14–11 A, A proximal phalanx orthosis (Buddy strap) showing adhesive hook riveted to neoprene. Strap was fabricated with hook receptive backing facing away from skin. **B,** Orthosis/Buddy strap shown applied to patient.

mobilization straps, will provide an isolated stretch to the intrinsic muscles. This simple approach allows for an easy, quick, and inexpensive alternative to traditional mobilization orthoses (Fig. 14–12D,E).

First Carpometacarpal Joint

Patients with first carpometacarpal (CMC) joint osteoarthritis (OA) can benefit from pain relief with the use of a properly constructed neoprene orthosis (Beasley, 2011). Traditionally, patients with thumb OA are prescribed hard thermoplastic thumb orthoses. Many patients are intolerant of this option and/or have difficulty using these for daily activities including work-related tasks. Orthoses are commonly used to decrease pain and joint stress, minimize deformities, and provide support (Beasley, 2012). Studies have shown that patients with CMC and MCP joint OA prefer soft neoprene orthoses when compared with the traditional hard plastic option (Weiss, LaStayo, Mills, & Bramlet, 2004). Patients with MCP and/or CMC joint OA may benefit from a soft, flexible support to complete the simplest activities of

daily living (ADLs) (Leonard, 1995). The authors of this chapter have had great success using custom neoprene orthoses for this patient population as an alternative to, or in conjunction with, traditional thermoplastic devices. Patient feedback supports the use of orthoses during all activities with improved comfort and pain relief. Patients that need to wear gloves at work report that a glove can be easily applied over this low-profile orthosis (Fig. 14–13A–I).

For patients with rheumatoid arthritis (RA), neoprene orthoses can ease stress on joints when manipulating objects and prevent further advancement of joint deformity. The patient with RA often experiences inflammation, pain, and sensitivity about the affected joints (Beasley, 2011). Studies have shown that the use of a stabilizing orthosis to reduce joint mobility during times of acute inflammation can decrease joint friction and prevent excessive joint loading (Beasley, 2012). In a study by Callinan and Mathiowetz (1996), it was found that 57% of patients with RA preferred soft orthosis options as compared to those fabricated from traditional rigid thermoplastic materials. Compliance with the use of soft orthoses was 82% compared to 67% with hard orthoses (Fig. 14–14A–D).

Nerve Injury

Following nerve repair, patients require an orthosis to help maintain proper joint positioning and facilitate functional use of the involved extremity while awaiting nerve return. This is often referred to as antideformity orthotic management. The authors have used neoprene to create some alternative options to traditional orthotic fabrication techniques for this patient population.

ULNAR NERVE
Some patients have difficulty tolerating thermoplastic MCP extension restriction orthoses (traditionally termed *anticlaw*

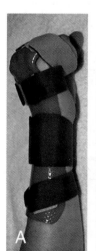
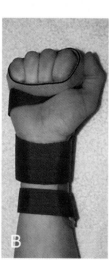
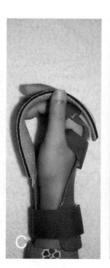
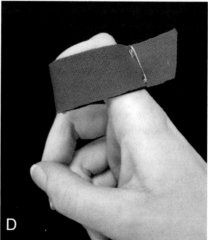
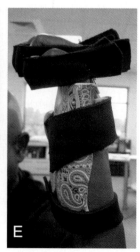

FIGURE 14–12 A–C, Multiple views of composite digit flexion orthosis using neoprene and thermoplastic materials. **D,** Traditional PIP/DIP orthosis utilizing nylon-backed neoprene and a safety pin. **E,** MP extension immobilization orthosis combined with PIP/DIP mobilization straps for isolated intrinsic stretching.

CUSTOM NEOPRENE FIRST CMC ORTHOSIS

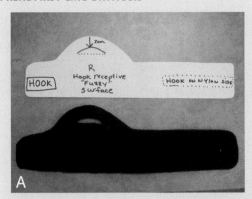

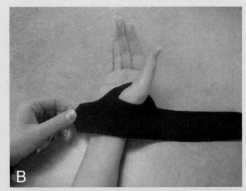

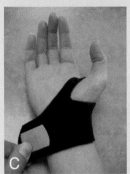

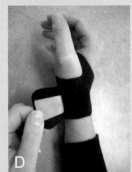

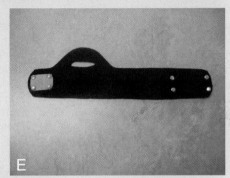

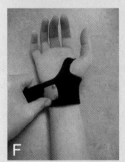

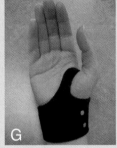

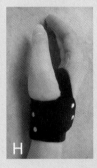

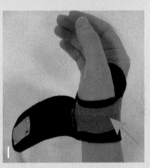

FIGURE 14–13

A

- Create pattern as shown, being attentive to which hand, right or left, the orthosis is being fabricated for. One generic template can be used, making adjustments for wrist and hand size; orthosis pattern demonstrated here is for a right hand. Note that for clarity of this pattern fabrication, the soft hook receptive side will be termed the *fuzzy* side. This becomes important when attaching the closures.
- Trace pattern using school chalk onto the fuzzy side of neoprene.
- Cut out pattern from neoprene.
- Mark and center the thumb placement by measuring approximately 2 cm from the apex of the pattern. The shape of the thumb opening should follow the general curve of the neoprene pattern.
- Fold material in half to line up traced thumb marking and cut along this line. This cut should resemble a thin crescent moon shape rather than an oval or circle.

B

- Place neoprene on patient to assess size (nylon surface should be against skin).
- Check for fit of thumb opening, adjusting as needed. Ideally, the orthosis should rest on the midshaft of the first metacarpal.

C

- Trim the volar ulnar arm (ulnar tab–like piece) of the neoprene material to end at the midulnar border of the hand.
- Cut a piece of adhesive hook approximately 4 cm in length (make sure to round corners to reduce lifting of borders).
- Apply the adhesive hook on the ulnar tab of the neoprene (fuzzy side). The placement of this adhesive hook acts as a catch to maintain proper position of the "wrap around" nature of the orthosis.

D

- Next, address the dorsal radial arm of the material by gently pulling it around the dorsum of the hand to meet the "ulnar tab."

(continued)

CUSTOM NEOPRENE FIRST CMC ORTHOSIS (Continued)

- Once the dorsal strap has met this "tab," continue to wrap in a radial dorsal direction as shown.
- This is the time to measure for the length of this segment. Trim any excess that may go beyond the head of the second metacarpal.
- Cut a piece of adhesive hook approximately 7 cm in length. This piece of adhesive hook should begin approximately at the flexor carpi radialis (FCR) insertion and end at the midshaft of second metacarpal.
- Attach this piece of adhesive hook to the nylon side of the radial segment as shown.

E

- Ensure orthosis fits patient comfortably and the adhesive hook pieces are correctly placed.
- Using a rivet punch, make holes on all four corners of each piece of adhesive hook. This helps to prevent lifting of the corners of the adhesive hook for longevity of the orthosis. If irritation occurs with rivets placed at ulnar tab, consider applying two rivets at each end instead of the four described here.
- Placement of rivets:
  - Radial arm: Ensure that the cap segment (not stem) of the rivet is on the **opposite** side of the material that the adhesive hook lies on.

- Ulnar arm: The stem segment should be placed against the skin with the cap segment on the **same** side of the material that the adhesive hook lies on (as the cap segment may irritate the skin).

F

- With the forearm supinated as shown, apply neoprene material through thumb opening.
- The description that follows is for patient instruction on proper application of the orthosis: Pull the ulnar arm of neoprene toward pisiform, simultaneously grab the radial arm, and pull in a volar ulnar direction, aiming to meet the adhesive hook on the ulnar tab. Once connected, continue to wrap across the volar wrist, capturing the radial thumb column and terminating about the midshaft of the second metacarpal.

G

- Volar view of completed orthosis.

H

- Radial view of complete orthosis.

I

- In this neoprene thumb orthosis, the Orficast™ Tape provides additional stabilization to the first CMC joint. Other materials such as uncoated thermoplastic material (sticky) or QuickCast tape can be added to an area where extra support is desired.

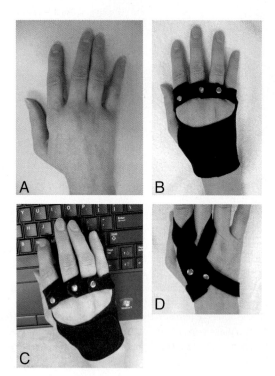

orthoses)—a well-accepted protocol following ulnar nerve repair. This soft alternative is best for people with more subtle clawing of ulnar digits as seen with high ulnar nerve lesions (refer to Chapter 19 for more detail). Thermoplastic reinforcement can be added to the neoprene, over the dorsal digits, to improve pressure distribution and offer increased stability if necessary (Fig. 14–15A,B).

MEDIAN NERVE

Following median nerve repair, opposition straps are commonly fabricated to assist in maintaining a wide first web space and thumb opposition/palmar abduction. This orientation places the thumb in a functional position for pinching and fine motor activities (refer to Chapter 19 for more detail). The authors have used a combination of Orficast™ adhered to neoprene to increase and maintain the pull into opposition, creating proper purchase about the first CMC joint (Fig. 14–16A,B). These designs can be modified to meet the needs of other neurologic diagnoses including post cerebrovascular accident (CVA) and spinal cord injuries.

RADIAL NERVE

Fabricating custom orthoses for patients with radial nerve or posterior interosseous nerve palsies can be challenging. Traditional functional custom orthoses may be bulky and often time consuming to fabricate, also requiring frequent adjustments and repairs. Orthoses can be fabricated using neoprene alone or in conjunction with a thermoplastic

FIGURE 14–14 A, Patient presents with ulnar drift deformity at MCP joints from RA. **B,** Custom-fabricated neoprene orthosis demonstrating improved digit alignment. **C,** Patient using orthosis during functional activity. **D,** A similar design for a patient requiring only index and middle finger realignment.

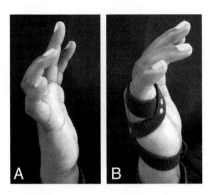

FIGURE 14–15 **A,** Patient with claw deformity following a high ulnar nerve injury waiting return after motor nerve grafting. **B,** Custom neoprene MCP extension restriction orthosis.

material to provide a low-profile option for these often frustrated patients. Because of neoprene's elastic properties, the dynamic force it imparts can be used to support the weakened digit and/or wrist extensors. In the radial nerve injured hand, this can translate to a low-profile design, assisting the weakened or absent extensors while allowing unimpeded wrist and/or digital flexion (Fig. 14–17A–F).

Wrist and Hand

Wrist Instability

From simple wrist irritation to complex instability issues, many patients can benefit from custom wrist neoprene orthoses. Simple circumferential wrist wraps can be fabricated with ¹⁄₁₆″ neoprene to provide light support and compression for patients, including athletes or workers with mild wrist pain or discomfort (Beasley, 2011) (Fig. 14–18A,B).

Patients experiencing wrist instabilities may require more support to decrease pain during active ROM, especially with forearm rotation. This can be accomplished with a thicker ³⁄₃₂″ neoprene or neoprene combined/adhered to thermoplastic material. As noted by Beasley (2011), foam

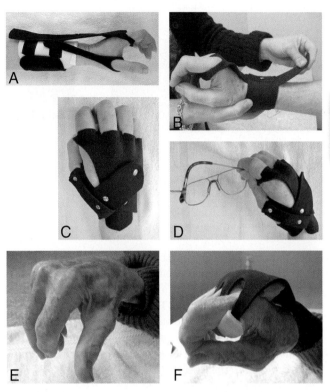

FIGURE 14–17 **A,** Using a thermoplastic forearm cuff, neoprene is attached to provide both dynamic wrist, thumb and digit extension. **B,** Dynamic distal forearm-based composite light wrist and digit extension orthosis for patient with returning radial nerve palsy. **C,** Dynamic hand-based digit and thumb extension orthosis for a patient with posterior interosseous nerve (PIN) palsy. **D,** Patient demonstrating functional pinch using custom orthosis. **E,** Patient presenting with loss of extensor digitorum communis (EDC). **F,** Custom orthosis fabricated with foam applied over the dorsum of the MCPs to promote functional pinch and gentle digit extension.

padding can be strategically added to help increase compression provided by these soft orthoses (Fig. 14–19A–D).

Wrist and Thumb

For patients with a combination of thumb and wrist pain, a custom neoprene orthosis can be designed to provide dynamic support and compression allowing earlier return to previously painful activities. DeQuervain's tenosynovitis is a common diagnosis resulting in thumb and radial wrist pain. A neoprene orthosis can be created to assist in dynamic thumb extension. These soft devices can be especially welcoming to those who are sensitive over the first dorsal compartment. Thermoplastic material or casting tape "struts" can be simply adhered to the neoprene material giving it additional reinforcement to decrease the load on the inflamed tendons. Due to neoprene's elastic nature, it can provide compression and support for repetitive motions for populations like musicians or new mothers (Beasley, 2011) (Fig. 14–20).

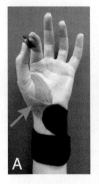 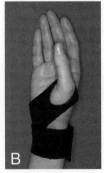

FIGURE 14–16 **A,** Opposition strap using Orficast™ Tape adhered to neoprene. **B,** This thumb abduction/opposition strap is being used 6 weeks after median nerve repair to improve functional position of the thumb column for prehension.

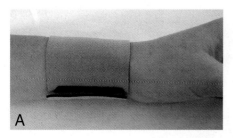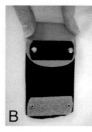

FIGURE 14–18 **A,** Simple circumferential wrist orthosis fabricated from nylon-backed neoprene. **B,** Adhesive hook and adhesive loop riveted to material for closure.

Forearm

Many patients following wrist or elbow fractures have difficulty regaining forearm rotation. Straps made from neoprene can be used to provide a dynamic passive stretch into supination and/or pronation. These straps can be used alone or in combination with a distal thermoplastic component (such as a forearm-based wrist and thumb immobilization orthosis) to better isolate forearm rotation and distribute forces directed to the forearm (Fig. 14–21A–D).

Elbow

Proximal Forearm Straps

A common condition seen among manual laborers and athletes is medial and/or lateral epicondylitis involving the proximal insertions of the wrist muscles. Counterforce braces/orthoses have been used to help disperse force and strain on the involved tendons for many years. In application of these devices, caution has been promoted to avoid compression of radial nerve over the supinator muscle (Carin, Borkholder, Hill, & Fess, 2004). Custom neoprene orthoses allow for these proximal devices to be fabricated with optimal fit, taking into consideration the size of the arm, location of pain, and where the patient feels the greatest amount of

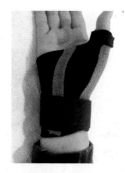

FIGURE 14–20 Custom wrist and thumb orthosis fabricated for an active patient with a history of mild CMC OA and deQuervain's tenosynovitis who requires support to engage in recreational activities such as kayaking and golf. Notice the Orficast™ Tape adhered to provide rigidity and extra support to the design.

relief when compression is applied. Foam or silicone inserts can be used under the orthosis to increase the specificity of the force being applied (Fig. 14–22A–D). Similar straps can be fabricated to treat bicep or triceps tendonitis as well.

Elbow Sleeves/Straps

Custom elbow sleeves can be used to protect sensitive structures about the forearm and elbow. Padding can be added to provide cushioning over bony prominences, soft tissues, or nerves that are irritated. Patients with cubital tunnel often complain of pain during activities; protective padding of the medial elbow may offer some relief (Beasley, 2011) (Fig. 14–23A–E).

Many patients who undergo an ulnar shortening osteotomy experience extreme sensitivity over hardware. The

CUSTOM NEOPRENE WRIST WRAP

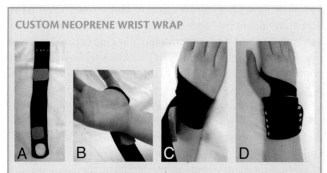

FIGURE 14–19 **A,** Pattern for custom wrist wrap. **B,** Application of wrist wrap with dorsal to volar pull aligning foam pad over ulnar head. **C,** Second foam pad placed over same location for increased pressure volarly to stabilize ulnar wrist. **D,** Completed wrist wrap with riveted adhesive hook for closure.

CUSTOM NEOPRENE FOREARM SUPINATION/ PRONATION ORTHOSIS

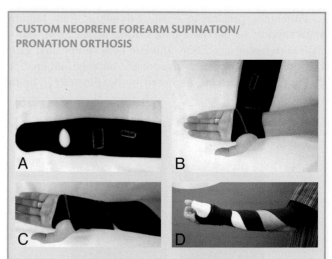

FIGURE 14–21 **A,** Pattern for forearm supination mobilization orthosis. **B,** Orthosis application with chalk outline for the angle of pull across palm and hook to prevent neoprene from separating. **C,** Showing proximal application of orthosis on patient. **D,** Patient status after open reduction internal fixation (ORIF) for a distal radius fracture using a supination mobilization orthosis combined with a wrist/thumb immobilization orthosis.

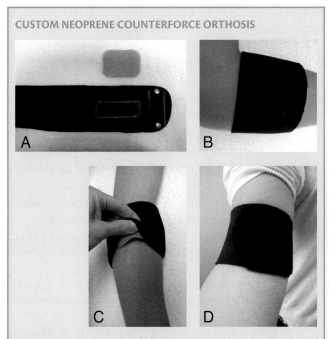

FIGURE 14–22 **A,** Pattern for custom neoprene counterforce orthosis. **B,** Custom neoprene counterforce orthosis on patient. **C,** Foam applied over proximal extensor carpi radialis brevis (ECRB) muscle belly to provide counterforce. **D,** Similar pattern used for patient with distal bicep tendonitis, using hook-backed silicone as counterforce to prevent distal migration of orthosis.

plate often needs to remain in place until there is evidence of complete bony healing. Patients may find relief and protection from a custom elbow/forearm sleeve combined with silicone or foam padding placed over the sensitive region to relieve pressure and function as a barrier to external forces (Fig. 14–24A,B). This may help patients to resume daily activities or return to work sooner. A clinician may encounter a patient who has a sensitive scar after carpal tunnel release, trigger finger release, or a nerve repair. These patients often have pain with grasping and weight bearing through the affected wrist and hand. Silicone gel sheeting or elastomer molds can be held in place using neoprene over the affected area providing protection and improved tolerance to temperature and vibration (Beasley, 2011).

Creative Neoprene Strapping with Custom Thermoplastic Orthoses

Neoprene's soft elastic nature makes it a comfortable and conforming strapping option. Elastic materials are helpful in maintaining more constant and consistent pressure as patients move and function during ADLs and work tasks; allowing muscles to contract and relax beneath the straps (Beasley, 2011). The authors have experienced that the life

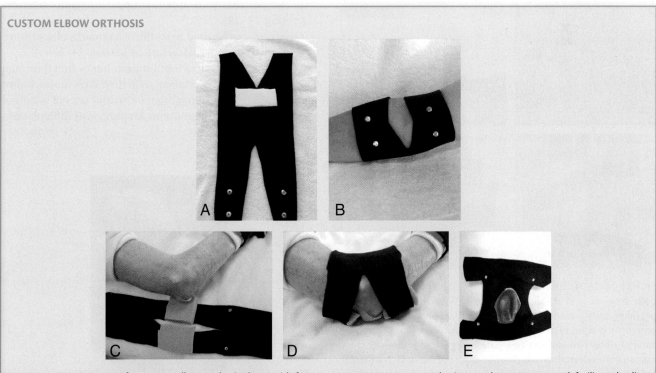

FIGURE 14–23 **A,** Pattern for custom elbow orthosis/sleeve with foam padding placed over the cubital tunnel. **B,** Elbow orthosis shown on patient. **C,** A patient with scleroderma with chronic olecranon ulcer using custom neoprene orthosis to reduce pressure and facilitate healing. **D,** Custom orthosis shown on patient. **E,** Gelbodies™ silicone insert used in custom neoprene elbow sleeve to pad olecranon.

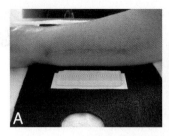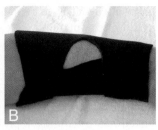

FIGURE 14–24 A, Sensitive ulnar forearm scar following ulnar shortening osteotomy with custom orthosis and silicone insert for protection and scar management. **B,** Orthosis shown on patient.

span and durability of neoprene straps is far greater than the traditional loop or hook receptive strapping products available. Neoprene allows for creative and custom strapping options with minimal to no fraying and material breakdown. For example, straps can be cut extra wide to more evenly distribute pressure over an edematous hand or wrist. Custom neoprene straps can be split to increase orthosis stability or increase conformity about joints and/or bony prominences (Fig. 14–25A–E). These characteristics make it a great strapping option and may help to

maintain stability of a custom thermoplastic orthosis while patients engage in their daily activities. Colditz (1999) noted that neoprene straps are an excellent option for people with pain, hypersensitivity, edema, or sensitive bony prominences.

Alternative Uses

Neoprene allows for many other creative uses in a therapy clinic.

- Traditional finger loops can be replaced with custom neoprene loops. Neoprene provides the ability to custom fit each finger loop to meet specific patient needs with the fabrication of mobilization orthoses (Fig. 14–26).
- Neoprene can be used to apply a gentle dynamic stretch to a targeted joint with mobilization orthoses (Fig. 14–27A–C).
- A piece of neoprene can be used as a dynamic "low-profile" mobilization force when attached to a base with a homemade thermoplastic outrigger. The strip of neoprene is cut with several small slits throughout the length and is caught by the hook. This allows for the patient to control the progression of the dynamic stretch being applied to the tissue (Fig. 14–28).
- Neoprene can also be used to fabricate custom slings for patients with proximal upper extremity fractures (Fig. 14–29).
- Straps can be used to stabilize a nonarticular orthosis such as a humeral fracture brace (Fig. 14–30).
- Patients experiencing limited hand function may encounter other challenges in their daily life, including donning and doffing braces. Creative uses of neoprene can help provide solutions for previously difficult tasks (Fig. 14–31).

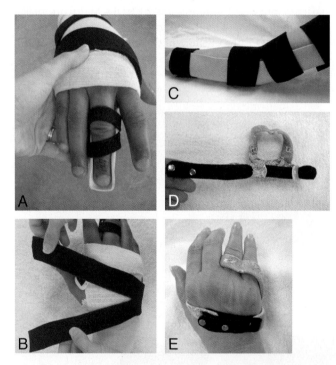

FIGURE 14–25 A, Split strap maintaining PIP extension stabilizing both proximal and middle phalanges. **B,** Bivalved neoprene strap providing stabilization through first web space and around wrist to prevent migration of orthosis. **C,** Large neoprene strap placed over anterior elbow to maintain elbow positioning within orthosis. Strap is split on both sides to increase contour about the elbow. **D,** Traditional MCP extension restriction (anticlaw) orthosis with single neoprene strap pulled through holes in thermoplastic; strap is weaved through neoprene similar to buddy strap design described earlier. **E,** Shown on patient with strap closed.

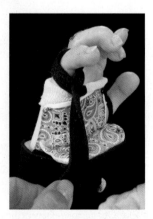

FIGURE 14–26 Soft and dynamic finger loop option created by weaving one end of strap through small slit placed in opposite end for gentle MCP flexion mobilization.

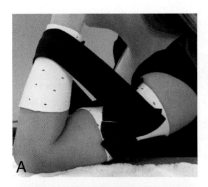

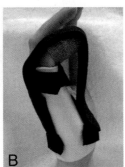

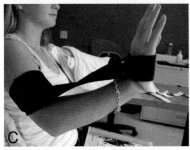

FIGURE 14–27 A, Elbow flexion mobilization orthosis using forearm and humeral cuff with neoprene strap for a patient following open reduction internal fixation (ORIF) of an olecranon fracture. **B,** Dynamic PIP flexion mobilization orthosis with a DIP extension immobilization cast in order for the flexion forces to be solely directed to the PIP joint. **C,** Dynamic wrist extension and elbow flexion mobilization orthosis following an elbow joint debridement in this college gymnast.

- Prefabricated orthoses can be customized to meet individual patient needs. For example, a prefabricated neoprene thumb and hand orthosis can be quickly converted with a custom neoprene strap to incorporate the wrist for a patient with deQuervain's tenosynovitis who requires a flexible wrist support to return to work (Fig. 14–32A–C).

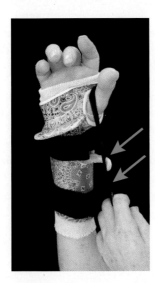

FIGURE 14–28 Strap used within an immobilization orthosis for progressive thumb web space mobilization.

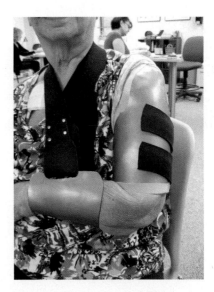

FIGURE 14–29 Custom "cuff and collar" sling for patient following humeral fracture.

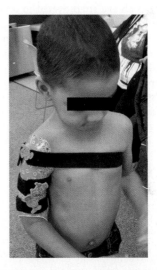

FIGURE 14–30 Strap shown on a Sarmiento-type orthosis to stabilize proximal border of orthosis and prevent migration. The brace is adorned with stickers for increased compliance and acceptance of orthosis.

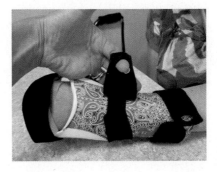

FIGURE 14–31 Neoprene loops added to this custom made dorsal-volar wrist/hand immobilization orthosis for a patient with increased flexor tone. The loops within the straps provide for ease of donning and doffing when bilateral dexterity and outside assistance is limited.

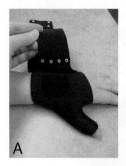 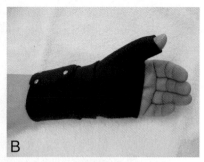

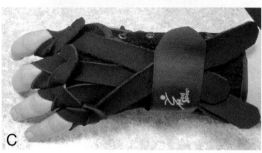

FIGURE 14–32 A, Neoprene strap riveted to a prefabricated neoprene hand and thumb orthosis. **B,** Illustrates completed design with additional custom wrist support. **C,** Neoprene 'dynamic' MCP extension loops added to a prefabricated wrist immobilization orthosis for a patient with a radial nerve injury. Note how a 'slit' in the distal end of the neoprene straps allows for the proximal end to feed through and form a 'sling' to assist in MCP extension yet allow functional flexion. The straps attach to the hook on the proximal border of the orthosis. Dynamic finger extension loops added to prefabricated wrist immobilization orthosis for patient with radial nerve palsy.

Conclusion

Neoprene is a versatile soft orthosis option based on its characteristics as described in this chapter. The use of neoprene as an orthotic material is appropriate for a wide variety of patients including those with arthritis, neurologic conditions, and orthopedic diagnoses to name a few. The authors have only touched the surface of orthotic fabrication possibilities with neoprene; it is up to therapists to use these tips, practice their skills, and tap into their creativity to fabricate a truly custom device to meet the needs of their unique patient.

CASE STUDY SECTION

The case studies presented here are meant as a teaching guideline only. Treatment and orthosis protocols vary greatly from surgeon to surgeon and from therapist to therapist. The therapist should check with the referring physicians and colleagues to define the preferred treatment and appropriate orthotic intervention.

CASE STUDY 1: Rheumatoid Arthritis

A 47-year-old female patient presents with RA affecting bilateral hand and wrists, with pronounced symptoms in the right hand (Fig. 14–14A). All digits present with ulnar drift at the MCP joints, with radial side of index MCP joint being acutely tender to palpation. Her wrist and hands are most painful at work as an administrative assistant with activities such as typing, sorting papers, and opening binder clips. She reports increased pain with home tasks such as gardening and cleaning. Bilateral custom immobilization orthoses were fabricated for night use (resting orthoses). A trial of Kinesio® Tape was applied to her right hand to aid in passively realigning her second and third digit MCP joints into radial deviation. This helped determine if a custom neoprene orthosis would be of benefit. Patient reported increased lateral stability (during lateral prehension activities) and decreased pain with the use of this tape. It was therefore concluded that a custom, more permanent strapping system should be devised to replicate the positioning offered by the Kinesio® Tape.

A custom neoprene ulnar drift orthosis was created (Fig. 14–14B). The orthosis was fabricated for all digits and was helpful in realigning the digits (specifically the proximal phalanges) during active use. The patient reports that the neoprene orthosis reduces her pain and increases her function with work and home tasks that were previously bothersome (Fig. 14–14C).

Prior to fabrication of such an orthosis, consider factors such as the following:

- Number of digits requiring support within the orthosis
- Amount of force required to realign the digit and whether force can be generated with neoprene alone or with an added piece of rigid thermoplastic
- Type of closure best suited for the patient for easy donning and doffing of orthosis (i.e., permanent closure vs. adjustable tabs with adhesive hook)

Additional case studies can be found on the companion web site on thePoint.

Chapter Review Questions

1. Describe the various types of neoprene materials that a clinician can choose from.

2. Why is the unbroken loop side of the neoprene important?

3. What are the advantages of a custom neoprene orthosis versus a prefabricated neoprene orthosis?

4. Give two examples of a diagnosis and neoprene orthosis management. Describe the advantages of the neoprene versus a thermoplastic orthosis in these two cases.

5. Give an example of two ways to apply adhesive-backed hook to a piece of neoprene material?

Orthotic Intervention for Specific Diagnoses and Populations

15 Stiffness

Karen Schultz, MS, OTR/L, FAOTA, CHT; updated for 2nd edition by MaryLynn Jacobs, MS, OTR/L, CHT

Chapter Objectives

After study of this chapter, the reader should be able to:

- Understand the causes and contributing factors to why an upper extremity becomes stiff.
- Explain the common contractures that occur in the upper extremity after injury.
- Describe the mobilizing orthoses that can be used with managing the stiff extremity.
- Appreciate the role of casting motion to mobilize stiffness.
- Give an example of each type of mobilizing orthosis and the rationale for their use.

Key Terms

Adaptive shortening
Adhesion
Casting motion to mobilize stiffness (CMMS)
Dynamic orthoses
Hard end feel

Low-load, prolonged stress (LLPS)
Mobilization orthosis
Plaster of paris
Scar formation
Serial static orthoses
Static progressive orthoses

Soft end feel
Springy end feel
Stiffness
Stress
Torque-angle range of motion

We should regard the hand as a mobile organ and never let it stiffen. It must move to survive.

—STERLING BUNNELL, 1947

Introduction

In the 1999 keynote address at the American Association of Hand Surgeons Seminar on Joint Stiffness, Hardy noted that, although the profession has made great strides in hand surgery and rehabilitation, joint stiffness continues to remain a challenge. **Stiffness**, the loss of normal passive range of motion (PROM) and active range of motion (AROM), remains one of the most common reasons for visiting an upper extremity therapy specialist (Copeland, 1997; Means, Saunders, & Graham, 2011). Although the clinician has many weapons in the therapy armamentarium for improving PROM, orthotic intervention is one of the most powerful.

But how do clinicians know when to apply an orthosis and what type will offer the best outcome for the patient? To find the answer, therapists combine a thorough understanding of the diagnosis with a comprehensive evaluation. The clinician also needs the well-honed ability to see into the future. This does not suggest the ability to be clairvoyant but rather states the importance of knowing according to the tissues affected, the predictable effects of position, edema, the progression of wound healing (see Chapter 3 Tissue Healing for more information), cortical reintegration, and the potential contractures.

The reader should keep in mind that although this chapter reviews several orthotic approaches in the mobilization of stiff tissues—dynamic, serial static, static progressive, and casting motion to mobilize stiffness (CMMS)—there is yet no agreed-on optimal approach (Michlovitz, Harris, & Watkins, 2004).

This chapter describes how the therapist applies knowledge of wound healing and of the unique anatomy and mechanics of each joint to predict and avoid or to evaluate and treat joint stiffness. After reviewing the nature and cause of joint stiffness, the effect of an orthosis on tissue length is presented. The contribution of various clinical entities to the loss of PROM is discussed along with a joint-by-joint review of the structures that, when wounded, adversely positioned, or affected by scar, leading to limited PROM. Table 15–1 summarizes the common contractures seen in the upper extremity.

Passive Range of Motion Loss

Trauma, especially in conjunction with necessary prolonged immobilization, often results in decreased tissue elasticity and PROM (Akeson, Ameil, Avel, Garfin, & Woo, 1987; Akeson, Ameil, Mechanic, Woo, Harwood, & Hamer, 1977; Akeson, Ameil, & Woo, 1980; Ameil, Woo, Harwood, & Akeson, 1982; Colditz, 2011; Enneking & Horowitz, 1972). This loss of joint flexibility has two major sources: **scar formation** and **adaptive shortening** (Flowers & Michlovitz, 1988). Both create formidable barriers to motion.

Scar Formation

Formed to repair tissue defects, scar is deposited not only between discontinuous structures but also in noninjured tissues surrounding the wound. All wounded and some non-wounded structures become attached, resulting in the one wound/one scar phenomenon (Peacock, 1984) (Fig. 15–1). An **adhesion**, the pathologic attachment of one structure to another via scar, limits the excursion of articular and periarticular structures, restricting useful joint motion. As the scar matures over time, it contracts and becomes denser (Akeson et al., 1980; Frank, Ameil, Woo, & Akeson, 1985).

Adaptive Shortening

Inflamed tissue undergoes remodeling in a shortened form when it is immobilized in a slack position and deprived of constant stress in the form of motion (Brand, 1985). Brand (1985) theorized that this adaptive shortening occurs when lack of stress signals the body to reduce tissue constituents, creating

TABLE 15–1	
Common Contractures of the Upper Extremity	
Joint	**Contracture(s)**
DIP	Flexion or extension (decreased extension or flexion)
PIP	Flexion (decreased extension)
MCP	Extension (decreased flexion)
Thumb MP	Flexion (decreased extension)
Thumb CMC	Adduction (decreased abduction)
Wrist	Flexion and ulnar deviation (decreased extension and radial deviation)
Forearm	Pronation (decreased supination)
Elbow	Flexion (decreased extension)
Shoulder	Decreased flexion, abduction, and external rotation

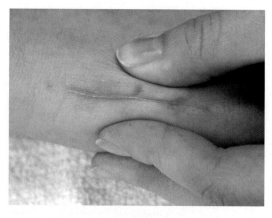

FIGURE 15–1 Adherent incision along the ulnar aspect of the hand interferes with tissue mobility and tendon excursion.

structures with less length. Research has proven this true for the biceps muscle (Williams & Goldspink, 1978). Inadequate tissue length limits joint motion. Both scar and normal tissue may become adaptively shortened and contribute to loss of motion.

Stress and Restoration of Passive Range of Motion

To reverse the motion-robbing effects of scar and adaptive shortening, the clinician faces the challenge of changing the length and density of the adhesions and shortened tissue. To achieve the desired length change, the clinician controls the environmental demands on the tissue and applies the mechanical stimulus of **stress**. Living tissue, including scar, will reorganize and change in response to stress. The stress stimulus of tension triggers an increase in the length of the tissue (Arem & Madden, 1976).

The scientific community has not yet quantified the exact amount of stress required to stimulate change in tissue length. Clinically, it is apparent that the amount of stress required increases as the maturation of the scar progresses. Research supports the hypothesis that the longer tissue remains at maximum tolerable length, the more it will increase in length (Cyr & Ross, 1998; Flowers & LaStayo, 1994, 2012; Glasgow, Tooth, Fleming, & Hockey, 2012; Glasgow, Tooth, Fleming, & Peters, 2011). Typically, the clinician employs experience and data from repeated evaluation to determine optimal stress loads. In addition to intensity, the clinician must also consider the effect of the variables' duration and frequency because they mediate total stress delivery (Flowers & LaStayo, 2012; Flowers & Michlovitz, 1988; Glasgow et al., 2012; Glasgow et al., 2011).

Optimal Stress Application: Delivery Approach

Clinical experience, observation of some cultures' success at altering the body's configuration, and the orthodontic and orthopedic literature support the use of **low-load, prolonged stress (LLPS)** over any other combination of load and stress for achieving permanent increase in tissue length and, therefore, in PROM (Arem & Madden, 1976; Flowers & LaStayo, 1994, 2012; Glasgow et al., 2012; Glasgow et al., 2011; R. M. Hotchkiss, 1995, n.d.; Light, Nuzik, Personius, & Barstrom, 1984) (Fig. 15–2). Clinically, low-load, brief stress (LLBS); high-load, brief stress (HLBS); and high-load, prolonged stress (HLPS) have failed to demonstrate effectiveness in producing permanent length change. Although the mechanism of action is unknown, LLPS appears to work by providing a mechanical stimulus that causes scar to remodel biologically into a permanently lengthened form. Clinically, the most effective way to apply LLPS is initially to stress the tissue to maximum length with LLBS. Then the tissue is maintained in its lengthened state with light to moderate force for a prolonged period

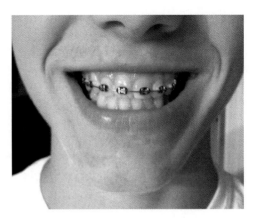

FIGURE 15–2 The theory of LLPS is also applied in the practice of orthodontia.

of time. Thus, the key to reducing a PROM limitation is an extended time of low-load stress to position the shortened tissue at or near the end of its currently available length.

Low-Load, Prolonged Stress

The clinician has several options for applying LLPS to tissue. However, the most powerful LLPS technique of the longest duration is orthotic intervention. An orthosis maintains the tissue elongation gained during therapy, a home program, and functional use of the hand. Using low tension, it maintains the newly gained length over long periods of time. Brand (1985) theorizes that the application of mechanical stress via an orthosis signals contracted tissue to grow or add cells while the body absorbs redundant tissue. In the clinic, therapists note that an orthosis applied at end range brings about increases in PROM much more quickly than LLBS and exercise (Fig. 15–3).

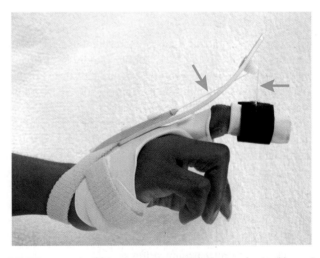

FIGURE 15–3 A PIP extension mobilization orthosis (dynamic approach) using the Digitec system is applied with tension generated through a rubber band. Note the exact 90° angle of pull between the monofilament and the middle phalanx. Also note that if tension generated through the rubber band is too much, this patient may develop a pressure area at the dorsum of the PIP joint.

Sometimes an orthosis creates increases in PROM that were previously unavailable by any approach short of surgery. McKee, Hannah, and Priganc (2012) caution the clinician that the duration of immobilization at end ranges may impair the nutrition of tissues and undesirably compresses articular cartilage. This is something the clinician should consider when using any orthotic intervention.

Characteristics of Approaches in Orthotic Intervention

When increasing PROM is the goal of the orthosis, the clinician may choose one of three passive mobilization approaches: **dynamic**, **serial static**, or **static progressive**. The American Society of Hand Therapists' nomenclature classifies each of these three types of orthoses as a **mobilization orthosis** when it is used to passively mobilize a joint. Colditz (2011) has described **casting motion to mobilize stiffness (CMMS)** or active redirection for management of the *chronically* stiff hand that is not responding to a more standard therapy approach. To address a severely stiff hand, Colditz (2011) recommends application of a nonremovable cast to mobilize stiffness. This concept has become increasingly more popular among therapists in order to manage this difficult population. This technique is described later in this chapter.

When describing the three passive mobilization (dynamic, serial static, and static progressive) approaches, clinicians often incorrectly describe orthoses designed to mobilize joints as dynamic (Cassanova, 1992). The following discussion shows that the term *dynamic* has a different and specific meaning.

Dynamic Orthoses

Dynamic orthoses have self-adjusting resilient or elastic components—such as spring wire, rubber bands, or springs—that create "a mobilizing force on a segment, resulting in passive or passive-assisted motion of a joint or successive joints" (Fess, 2011; Fess & Phillips, 1987; Glasgow et al., 2011). In addition, dynamic orthoses allow active-resisted motion in the direction opposite of their line of pull. The dynamic tension generated continues as long as the elastic component can contract, even when the shortened tissue reaches the end of its elastic limit (Fig. 15–4A–C). Glasgow et al. (2012) and Glasgow et al. (2011) found that with dynamic intervention, the most important predictors of outcome were the following:

- Degree of pretreatment stiffness
- Type of deficit (flexion improves faster than extension)
- Length of time since injury (<12 weeks) the dynamic orthosis was applied
- Amount of time throughout the day the device was worn

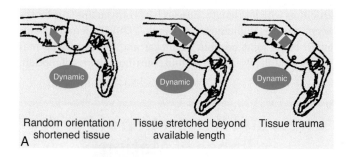

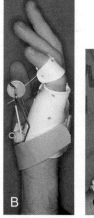
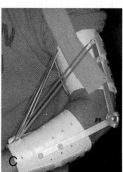

A   Random orientation / shortened tissue   Tissue stretched beyond available length   Tissue trauma

FIGURE 15–4 A, A dynamic orthosis generates tension as long as the elastic component can contract, even when the shortened tissue reaches the end of its elastic limit; thus, tissue trauma can result. **B,** A dynamic PIP flexion mobilization orthosis using a Phoenix outrigger. **C,** A dynamic elbow flexion mobilization orthosis using a Phoenix elbow hinge.

Static Progressive Orthoses

Static progressive orthotic intervention involves the use of inelastic components, such as hook-and-loop tapes, static lines, progressive hinges, turnbuckles, and screws. These components allow progressive changes in joint position as PROM changes without needing to change the structure of the orthosis. Only the line of pull must be changed as PROM progresses. A static progressive orthosis holds shortened tissue at its maximum length. Because the components lack the elasticity of those used in a dynamic approach, the appropriately set tension of the orthosis does not continue to stress tissue beyond its current maximum length limit (Fig. 15–5A–C) (Schultz-Johnson, 1992). Custom static progressive orthoses have also been described to facilitate stretch into both flexion and extension within one device. When applied to the wrist, these orthoses are most effective with joint limitations of 15° of flexion and 25° of extension (Sueoka & DeTemple, 2011).

Serial Static Orthoses

Serial static orthotic intervention differs from a static progressive approach in that the clinician must remold the orthosis to accommodate increases in mobility.

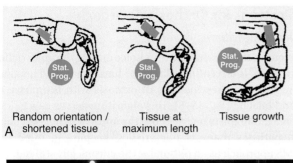

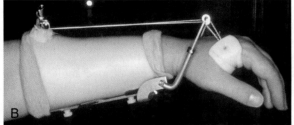

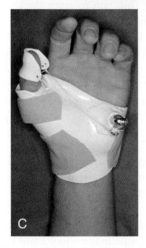

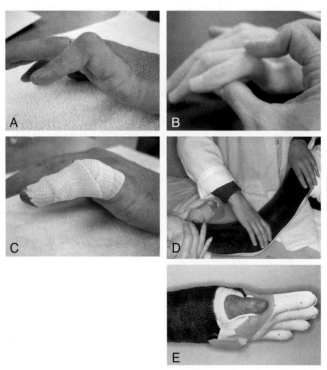

FIGURE 15–6 PIP flexion contracture (**A**), note the limitation in passive extension (**B**), serial static extension mobilization orthosis applied using QuickCast 2 casting tape (**C**), example of serial static approach to gain elbow extension (**D**), and a serial static digit extension orthosis to increase length of shortened extrinsic flexor tendons secondary to cast immobilization (**E**).

FIGURE 15–5 **A,** Because static progressive components lack the elasticity of those used for dynamic orthotic intervention, the appropriately set tension of the orthosis does not stress tissue beyond its current maximum length limit. Tissue lengthening occurs without tissue trauma. **B,** A wrist extension mobilization orthosis using a Phoenix wrist hinge and MERiT™ component. **C,** A thumb IP flexion mobilization orthosis using a MERiT™ component.

Proximal interphalangeal (PIP) serial casts and serial wrist extension orthoses exemplify this approach. The clinician establishes the tension of the orthosis to maximum tolerable end range. Therefore, the orthosis does not continue to stress tissue beyond its current maximum length limit (Schultz-Johnson, 1992). No change in joint position occurs until the clinician modifies the orthosis (Fig. 15–6A–E). Flowers and LaStayo (1994, 2012) have gathered data to substantiate Dr. Paul Brand's suggestion that a joint held in a lengthened position for a significant period of time will adapt to that length, causing growth of connective tissue about the joint. They have shown that the most effective form of stress delivery is to maximize the length of time that stress is delivered. Although their

research was on the PIP joint, they propose that this principle could be applied to other synovial joints of the body (Flowers & LaStayo, 2012).

Casting Motion to Mobilize Stiffness

Orthotic courses and the literature have stressed the importance of never increasing joint motion in one direction at the cost of losing motion in another direction as well as never immobilizing any joint that is not absolutely necessary to include within the orthosis. Colditz (2000, 2002, 2011) describes use of a nonremovable cast to direct *active* motion only toward the stiffest joints. The cast is used for the chronically stiff hand; but occasionally, a removable orthosis may be used for very early management of stiffness (Fig. 15–7). (*Chronic* is defined as hard end feel joint motion regardless of time since injury.) This technique is referred to as CMMS. Colditz (2011) purports this technique "simultaneously mobilizes stiff joints, reduces edema, and generates a new pattern of motion to revive the cortical representation of normal motion." The reader is encouraged to further study CMMS (Colditz, 2011) and make this approach an option for management of the chronically stiff hand. In this technique, a carefully molded cast from **Plaster of paris** (POP) is applied. It is important to use a "highly compliant material" (Colditz,

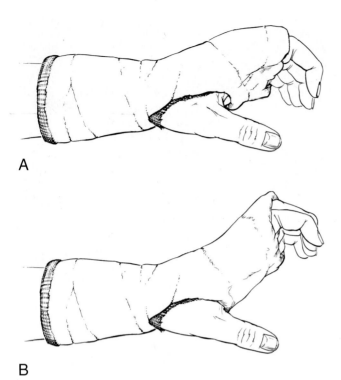

FIGURE 15–7 A, A circumferential wrist and MCP extension orthosis (without hood) isolates the PIP joints for active flexion and extension. **B,** This intrinsic stretching cast positions the MCP joints in full extension to encourage lengthening of the tight intrinsic muscles. (Photos courtesy of Judy C. Colditz ©.)

2000), such as POP, to obtain an intimate fit and allow for prolonged wear with minimal risk of soft tissue irritation. Immobilizing the proximal joints, including the wrist when the goal is mobilizing the digits, is necessary in order to focus and redirect all the power of movement to the targeted distal joints (Bell-Krotoski, 2011; Colditz, 2011). Chapter 12 Casting reviews the application of POP in detail.

The advantages of CMMS (Colditz, 2011) are the following:

- Circumferential nature and light pressure applied by the cast aids in mobilization of edema
- Joint motion is possible in both flexion and extension.
- Targeted repeated movement facilitates cortical integration.
- Cost of POP material is low.
- Therapy visits and cast changes are less frequent than with traditional therapy methods.

Challenges of CMMS (Colditz, 2011) are the following:

- Determined optimal cast design (decided by deficits in tightness and altered patterns of movement)
- Precise application of the cast (refer to Chapter 12 on Casting)
- Adequate amount of time in the cast
- How to wean from the cast and not lose gains made

Indications for Orthosis Approach

Orthosis Algorithm

As a foundation for making the choice among the approaches for orthotic intervention, clinicians have developed an algorithm that matches the type of orthosis with the phase of wound healing (Fig. 15–8). This algorithm serves as a guideline only; therapists must choose the approach that best suits each patient's many characteristics, keeping in mind the CMMS approach as an option for the chronically stiff hand.

Based on this algorithm, many clinicians have delayed using the static progressive approach until the later phases of wound healing because they consider it a high-load generator. This is a misconception. A static progressive force generator has a wide range of load application from extremely low to extremely high. Because the static progressive force generators are infinitely adjustable, the range of force is more diverse than that achievable from a rubber band or spring. Thus, any tissue that can tolerate dynamic traction can tolerate static progressive traction. In addition, tissues that cannot tolerate dynamic orthotic intervention may tolerate static progressive traction. It is up to the clinician to establish the correct amount of tension or load for the given tissue and to set up the orthosis appropriately (Schultz-Johnson, 2000). Table 15–2 compares the approaches (Schultz-Johnson, 2000).

Torque-Angle Range of Motion

Assessment of **torque-angle range of motion (TAROM)**, the quantification of the amount of torque force required to gain a certain amount of PROM at a joint, helps the therapist decide what type of orthosis will resolve the patient's PROM limitations (Roberson & Giurintano, 1995). If a joint requires a significant amount of torque to gain maximum PROM and the torque-angle curve has a rapidly rising slope, then the joint will have a **hard end feel** (Fig. 15–9A). Serial static or static progressive intervention is probably the only means to increase PROM. However, if a joint requires only a low amount of torque to gain

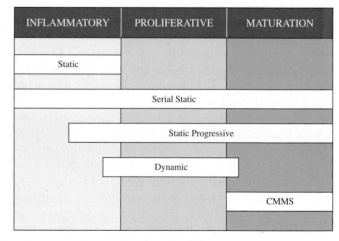

FIGURE 15–8 Algorithm for matching the type of orthosis with the phase of wound healing.

TABLE 15–2

Comparison of Orthotic Passive Mobilization Approaches

Characteristic	Dynamic	Serial Static	Static Progressive
Force and ROM adjustment	• Elastic tension is not readily or precisely adjustable; when applied to a joint, it exerts a given force and places the joint at a given point in its PROM. • Extremely difficult to establish a tolerable elastic tension that places tissue at maximum length but not beyond • Patient can pull against the dynamic force, shortening the tissue on an intermittent basis, which thwarts the purpose of the orthosis (to hold the tissue at its maximum length for long periods of time).[a]	• Creates constant tension and joint positioning • End range position with tolerable tension is easily achieved. • Patient cannot move from the end range established by the clinician; orthosis holds tissue at its current maximum length.	• Static progressive tension and joint positioning are infinitely adjustable. • Always possible to establish a static tension that places tissue at maximum length but not beyond it • As tissue remodels into a longer form, orthosis can immediately be adjusted to capture increased length and PROM. • Patient remains at end range until orthosis is readjusted to optimize the combination of ROM and tension.
Tension	• Dynamic component continues to shorten even when tissue has reached the end of its available length, which causes microtears and increased scar. • Microtears, in turn, undergo the normal phases of wound healing. • As the scar matures, it contracts and further limits PROM.	• Holds the tissue at maximum length and does not stress beyond it	• Holds the tissue at maximum length and does not stress beyond it
Force control	• Springs and elastics deform over time. • Neither clinician nor patient has control of forces.	• Clinician has control over forces.	• Clinician can maintain control over forces or instruct patient in proper use, so the patient has control.
Orthosis tolerance and time dose	• Because dynamic component continues to shorten, it frequently stresses tissue beyond its available length, leading to poor orthosis tolerance and the inability to wear the orthosis for as many hours as required to achieve permanent length change.[a]	• Appropriate stress fosters consistent orthosis wear, resulting in tissue growth and reorganization in a longer form and creating a permanent length change.	• Appropriate stress fosters consistent orthosis wear, resulting in tissue growth and reorganization in a longer form and creating a permanent length change.
Orthosis tolerance and sleep	• Because patient often cannot tolerate the orthosis during sleep, the orthosis must be worn during the day, which interferes with functional use of the hand. • If the dynamic force is light enough to allow sleep, it probably is not taking the joint to end range.	• Patient can tolerate the orthosis during sleep, minimizing need for daytime wear.	• Patient can tolerate the orthosis during sleep, minimizing need for daytime wear

(continued)

TABLE 15–2			
Comparison of Orthotic Passive Mobilization Approaches (Continued)			
Characteristic	**Dynamic**	**Serial Static**	**Static Progressive**
Joint end feel	• Improves PROM in joints with soft end feel but is ineffective for hard end feel joints	• Improves ROM of soft end feel joints faster than do dynamic orthoses • Improves PROM in joints with soft or hard end feel[a,b]	• Improves ROM of soft end feel joints faster than do dynamic orthoses • Improves PROM in joints with soft or hard end feel[a,b]
Efficiency	• Requires many more weeks or months in orthosis and in therapy than do static approaches	• Highly effective in increasing PROM, especially for patients with compliance and sensory problems	• Increases PROM faster than any other approach and, sometimes, when no other treatment approach is successful[c]

[a]Bell-Krotoski, J. A. (1987). Plaster casting for the remodeling of soft tissue. In E. E. Fess & C. Phillips (Eds.), *Hand splinting: Principles and methods* (2nd ed., pp. 453–454). St. Louis, MO: Mosby; Bell-Krotoski, J. A. (2011). Tissue remodeling and contracture correction using serial plaster casting and orthotic positioning. In J. M. Hunter, E. J. Mackin, & A. D. Callahan (Eds.), *Rehabilitation of the hand: Surgery and therapy* (6th ed., pp. 1599–1609). St. Louis, MO: Mosby; Fess, E. E. (2011). *Orthosis for mobilization of joints: Principles and methods* (6th ed., pp. 1588–1598). St Louis, MO: Mosby.

[b]Fess, E. E., & Phillips, C. (Eds.). (1987). *Hand splinting: Principles and methods* (2nd ed.). St. Louis, MO: Mosby.

[c]Bonutti, P. M., Windau, J. E., Ables, B. A., & Miller, B. G. (1994). Static progressive stretch to re-establish elbow range of motion. *Clinical Orthopaedics and Related Research, 303,* 128–134.

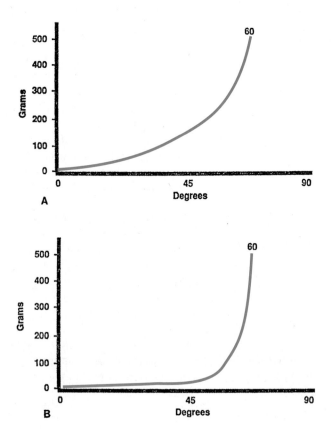

FIGURE 15–9 **A,** A hard end feel joint requires a significant amount of torque to gain maximum PROM and has a torque-angle curve with a rapidly rising slope. **B,** A soft end feel joint requires only a low amount of torque to gain maximum PROM and has a torque-angle curve with a slowly rising slope.

maximum PROM and the torque-angle curve has a slowly rising slope, then the joint will have a **soft** or **springy end feel** (Fig. 15–9B). A soft end feel joint can benefit from serial static, static progressive, or dynamic orthotic intervention. However, clinical experience has shown that the dynamic approach requires more time than the static approaches to produce the desired result (Schultz-Johnson, 1992).

A soft end feel joint indicates either a) relatively young scar tissue that has not yet formed significant cross-linking or b) transient physiologic changes that have occurred, such as swelling or malnourished cartilage. A joint contracture has been produced which has a soft and spongy end range of motion. At this point the body still has to work to absorb the abnormal cells in the area in order for that joint to regain normal motion (Bell-Krotoski, 1987, 2011). A hard end feel joint indicates mature scar tissue with advanced cross-linking, the presence of a check rein, or the absorption of tissue required for normal passive motion (e.g., a PIP flexion contracture when the body absorbs volar skin and joint capsule, see Fig. 15–6A) (Bell-Krotoski, 1987, 2011).

Clinical experience has shown that using static approaches to PROM limitations offers fast results. However, when optimal results require tissue excursion and the joint limitation feels soft, a dynamic orthosis provides the best solution. The clinician can design an orthosis that incorporates both static progressive and dynamic approaches, so the wearer can alternate between the two (Fig. 15–10A,B). The analysis of the duration and nature of the contracture, coupled with the information gained from TAROM measurements, helps the therapist select the appropriate orthosis. McKee et al. (2012) have suggested that although static approaches to

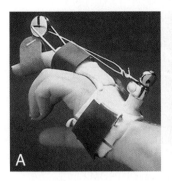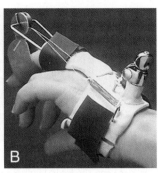

FIGURE 15–10 This PIP extension mobilization orthosis incorporates both static progressive **(A)** and dynamic **(B)** approaches. The patient is able to alternate between the two approaches. Shown using Phoenix outrigger and MERiT™ component.

managing joint stiffness achieve positive outcomes in tissue lengthening, one should appreciate that continued joint immobilization may impair nutrition to tissues and adversely compress articular cartilage.

TAROM can also help the therapist discover the quality of the stiffness. Sometimes, the pure AROM or PROM measurement does not change over time; however, the patient will note that the joint feels better. This description does not generally indicate a decrease in pain. Further assessment may reveal that the arc of motion is more easily available, which means that either the clinician does not have to push as hard during the PROM evaluation and/or the patient does not have to contract the muscle as hard to achieve the arc of motion. If the clinician had been performing TAROM evaluations all along, it would be obvious that the plotted slope of the torque-angle curve was becoming less steep. Thus, the quantification of the degree of stiffness relative to both noninvolved joints and to previous evaluations of the joint in question is a valuable piece of information in the battle against stiffness. Such data can help the clinician in treatment planning and orthosis assessment.

Contraindications to Orthotic Intervention

Just as it is important to know the indications for mobilizing orthoses and for approaches that match a given problem, it is important to know the contraindications for orthoses that seek to mobilize joints.

Common contraindications include the following:

- Joint instability
- Avascular necrosis
- Neurovascular deficiencies
- Acute inflammation
- Infection
- Unstable fractures
- Marked demineralization
- Myositis ossificans
- Heterotopic ossification
- Exostosis formation
- Loose body in joint
- Stress across healing structures without adequate blood supply or tensile strength to withstand tensile stress
- Patients with claustrophobia
- Patients with altered mental status

In addition, three special diagnostic categories that are most always contraindications to mobilizing orthoses require special comment: Dupuytren's contracture, motion loss due to irradiation, and Ashworth's disease.

Dupuytren's contracture does not respond to LLPS (Abbott, Denney, Burke, & MGrouther, 1987; Sampson et al., 1992). Owing to its nature, Dupuytren's tissue, made up of myofibroblasts, does not remodel in the same way as normal tissue or scar. Only in the postmedical intervention period (surgery or injection/manipulation) will Dupuytren's contracture respond to orthotic intervention because the intervention removes the unresponsive tissue and replaces some of it with scar.

Irradiated tissue does not usually respond to LLPS. The tissue is mostly fibrotic and does not possess the same viscoelastic properties as normal connective tissue. It lacks the live cells required to respond to the mechanical stimulus and to reorganize.

The last category, which this the author of the first edition of this book calls Ashworth's disease, has no formal name in the literature. Late hand surgeon Charles R. Ashworth (personal communication) described the condition as nameless and extremely rare. Dr. Charles Ashworth believed he had seen more of this than any other physician in the United States. Ashworth's disease is a congenital anomaly that causes its bearer to have supernumerary muscles. The condition may present in a limited manner in a part of the upper extremity or may involve the entire extremity, including the shoulder and neck. Before puberty, it causes no limitation and, in fact, can provide some cause for pride in patients who value extra muscle bulk and strength. However, at puberty, the disease becomes active and causes the supernumerary muscles to fibrose and contract, often creating severe deformity. The contracting tissue is powerful enough to sublux joints. Clinical experience shows that this fibrotic tissue does not respond to orthosis management.

Whenever the clinician applies an orthosis—and especially when any doubt about orthosis appropriateness or tolerance exists—he or she must rigorously check for the following signs that indicate a problem with this device:

- Pain (dolor)
- Heat (calor)
- Redness (rubor)
- Edema
- Decreased ROM
- Decreased strength
- Decreased sensation

If any of these symptoms and signs is seen, the therapist must thoroughly check the orthosis for fit and pressure distribution. It is important for the clinician to rethink the rationale for orthosis application to be certain of its appropriateness.

Causes of Joint Stiffness

When discussing joint stiffness, the nature of the limitation in joint PROM must be addressed. Changes in the soft tissue structures surrounding a joint, the periarticular structures (e.g., ligament, joint capsule, volar plate, and sagittal bands), can cause such motion limitation. Changes in the structure of the articular surfaces of the bones forming the joint can also lead to loss of PROM. The relationship of adjacent bones to one another also affects arc and ease of motion (Fig. 15–11).

Spasticity and congenital anomalies may cause joint stiffness (see Chapters 21 Adult Neurologic Dysfunction and 22 The Pediatric Patient for further information). Although metastatic and primary bone tumors and Paget's disease can lead to stiffness, they will not be specifically addressed here (Copeland, 1997).

As noted, periarticular structures may adaptively shorten when positioned on slack for a significant period of time; inflammation hastens this process. Arem & Madden (1976) described how periarticular structures may fold upon themselves, like an accordion, and become stuck in that position when scar forms between these folds (Fig. 15–12). Spotwelding of periarticular structures may also occur during scar formation when the scar attaches the normally mobile tissue to less mobile tissue (Fig. 15–1). This leads to a decrease in extensibility and glide (Flowers & Michlovitz, 1988).

The aforementioned changes in periarticular tissue and the joint surface have long been part of the literature pertaining to joint stiffness. Mulligan (1999), a physiotherapist from New Zealand, described a theory in the search for understanding the cause of decreased motion. When he combined joint mobilization techniques with passive physiologic motion, Mulligan found he was able to restore

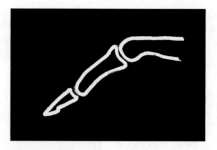

FIGURE 15–12 The accordion phenomenon is caused by scar formation between the folds, leading to decreased PROM.

normal, pain-free motion in many patients. This success was achieved even in many cases in which the loss of motion and pain had existed for years. Although Mulligan has spent years honing his techniques for restoring motion, he has not used the scientific method to examine why his techniques are so often effective. Mulligan postulates that the reason for many PROM limitations is a "positional fault" that "mobilization with movement" corrects. Once the correct joint relationship is restored, the joint moves normally and pain diminishes. Mulligan advocates the use of taping techniques to enhance his mobilization approach (Fig. 15–13).

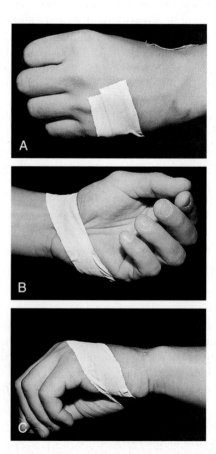

FIGURE 15–13 Dorsal (**A**), volar (**B**), and ulnar (**C**) views of Mulligan taping, which mimics orthosis intervention. Orthosis/tape combinations can be used to augment this often effective technique.

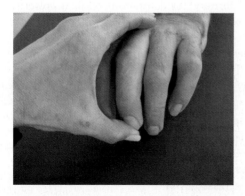

FIGURE 15–11 Limited passive motion noted at IP joints secondary to stiffness from immobilization after fracture dislocation of MF PIP joint.

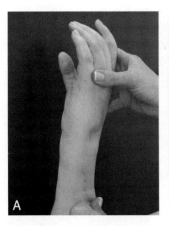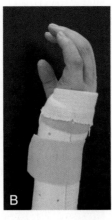

FIGURE 15–14 **A,** Note the pitting and brawny edema on the dorsum of the hand. **B,** This wrist immobilization orthosis with elastic stockinette and wide straps aids in reducing edema along with active hourly digital ROM and other edema management techniques.

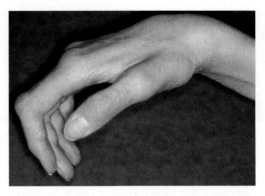

FIGURE 15–15 The position of ease with wrist flexed, MCPs extended, and IPs flexed.

Each joint possesses a unique anatomy that when subjected to trauma or autoimmune processes and to inflammation produces predictable patterns in the limitation of flexibility. When presented with the diagnosis and duration postinjury or since onset, the clinician uses knowledge of these patterns to plan treatment. Often, the treatment consists of orthotic intervention to prevent or decrease the effect of the pathology.

Precipitating Conditions for Stiffness

Edema

Chronic edema is the clinician's worst nightmare. When not managed, edema will progress to the infiltration of tissue spaces, become brawny and pitting, and eventually lead to fibrosis (Villeco, 2011) (Fig. 15–14A,B). In the worst scenario, edema will disrupt blood and nutrition to vital tissues. Therefore, intervention of the edematous hand is paramount.

In the presence of diffuse edema, the hand assumes the position of ease: wrist flexed, metacarpophalangeal (MCP) joints extended, and interphalangeal (IP) joints flexed (Grigsby deLinde & Miles, 1995). This position minimizes tension on the dorsal skin of the hand, on the ligaments, and on the periarticular structures. When the edema remains and the hand is left untreated, the wrist loses extension, the MCPs develop extension contractures, and the IPs develop flexion contractures (Fig. 15–15). The clinician must immediately seek to control edema and position the hand appropriately. Orthotic intervention provides the desired extremity posture. Traditional strapping applied to the edematous hand may obstruct lymphatic flow and cause "window" edema or pooling of edema proximal and distal to the strap placement (Villeco, 2011). This warns the clinician that the placement of the strap is causing harm (Colditz, 2011). Strategic fabrication of the orthosis, such as a circumferential design, may better assist in even pressure distribution. Gentle circumferential compression wrapping or wide neoprene-like straps are another alternative for light distribution of pressure. Both of these techniques can effectively hold an orthosis in place while assisting in edema control (Fig. 15–16A,B). Once

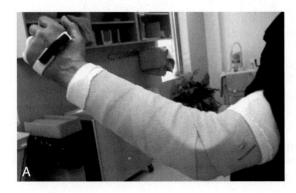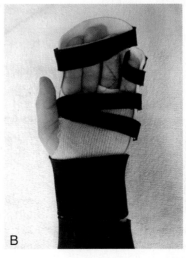

FIGURE 15–16 **A,** An elasticized wrap is used to hold this elbow flexion mobilization orthosis (serial static approach) in place to evenly distribute pressure and manage edema. **B,** Wide neoprene straps are used in this wrist/hand extension restriction orthosis post–flexor tendon repair.

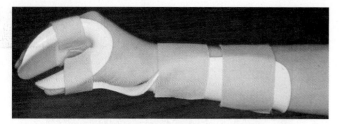

FIGURE 15–17 The antideformity position is the position of choice for minimizing or preventing hand stiffness and deformity.

edema subsides, the wide straps or wraps can be replaced with traditional strapping methods.

The position of choice for minimizing or preventing hand stiffness and deformity is called the antideformity position (Fig. 15–17): wrist in 20 to 25° extension, if available; maximum tolerated MCP flexion; and maximum tolerated IP extension. Even if the PROM limitations do not permit the initial orthosis to secure the desired position, serial adjustments to the orthosis should generally accomplish the goal.

Paralysis

Paralysis of the primary IP extensor and MCP flexor occurs with loss of ulnar or combined ulnar and median nerve motor function. This leads to sustained flexion of the IP joints and hyperextension of the MCP joint as the patient attempts to straighten the fingers with only the extrinsic extensor digitorum communis (EDC) (Fig. 15–18A,B) (Brand & Hollister, 1999). Over time, this unopposed flexion alone can produce IP flexion contractures owing to adaptive shortening (Fig. 15–19A,B). The hyperextension at the MCP joint further facilitates the loss of IP flexion and subsequent contracture as noted in Figure 15–18A. Left to the whims of the extrinsic flexor, the MCP joint flexes only after both IP joints have done so. The combination of MCP hyperextension (when the patient attempts to open the palm for function) and lack of functional MCP flexion facilitate the loss of MCP flexion.

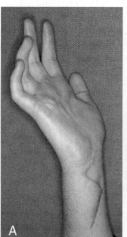
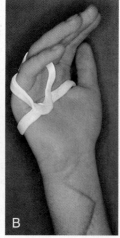

FIGURE 15–18 A, Claw deformity is commonly seen with ulnar nerve injury. **B,** An MCP extension restriction orthosis.

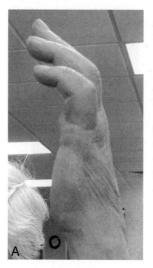
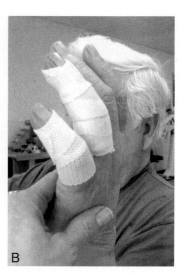

FIGURE 15–19 A, IP flexion contractures developed subsequent to a long-standing ulnar nerve injury. **B,** Serial static IP extension mobilization orthoses applied to achieve full IP extension.

The presence of edema and/or of inflammation often hastens the contracture. When the therapist notes loss of ulnar or combined ulnar and median nerve function, the treatment plan must immediately include MCP flexion orthotic intervention (Fig. 15–18). With the MCP joint flexed, the power of the EDC transfers to the IP joint and reestablishes active IP joint extension (Brandsma, 1993). Edema or inflammation indicates the need for an IP extension immobilization orthosis to prevent contracture. Established IP flexion or MCP extension contractures require a mobilizing orthosis to increase PROM (see Chapter 19 Peripheral Nerve Injuries for details).

Loss of the ulnar nerve innervated intrinsic muscles produces the loss of ulnar finger metacarpal rotation and results in the loss of the cupping function of the palm (Fig. 15–20A,B). When the metacarpals remain immobile and the intrinsic muscles become fibrotic, the transverse metacarpal arch is lost. The palm assumes a narrow and flattened appearance, a sign of intermetacarpal contractures. Orthoses that incorporate the palm must be carefully contoured to preserve the metacarpal arch (Malick, 1972).

Intrinsic Tightness

Injury or disease can create spasm or scarring of the intrinsic hand muscles. Intrinsic tightness causes loss of simultaneous MCP extension and IP flexion. When these movements are impaired, the clinician should perform a test of intrinsic length (Fig. 15–21A–D) (Aulicino, 1995). If intrinsic tightness is noted, the therapist begins the appropriate orthosis and exercise regimen to increase composite MCP extension and IP flexion. Intrinsic tightness can create an imbalance that results in swan-neck deformity at the PIP and distal interphalangeal (DIP) joints (Melvin, 1989). Loss of intrinsic function can result in loss of the intermetacarpal movement,

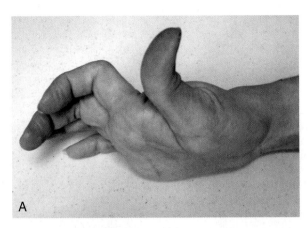
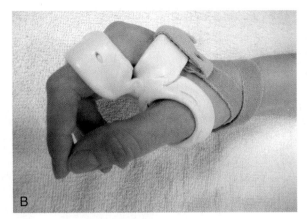

FIGURE 15–20 A, With paralysis of the intrinsics postmedian and ulnar nerve injury, there is a loss of the arches in the hand. **B,** An MCP extension restriction (with thumb opposition) orthosis applied to this hand to better balance and harness the functioning muscle–tendon units.

as described earlier. When intrinsic muscles become fibrotic, they seem to be resistant to orthotic intervention and exercises geared to increase their length. It is possible that fibrotic tissue lacks an adequate number of living cells to respond to tension stimuli and to reorganize in a manner conducive to length increase.

Extrinsic Tightness

Injury and overuse are the primary culprits of extrinsic tightness (Lowe, 1992). Extrinsic tightness can occur in either the flexor/pronator or extensor forearm muscles. Extrinsic extensor tightness condition leads to the loss of composite finger flexion (MCPs and IPs simultaneously) or the loss of composite finger flexion combined with wrist flexion (Fig. 15–22A–E). Just the reverse is true for extrinsic flexor

tightness; it creates the loss of composite finger extension (MCPs and IPs simultaneously) or the loss of composite finger extension combined with wrist extension (Fig. 15–23A–C). When the problem is the result of overuse, it usually disappears with proper stretching exercises. However, when scarring is the cause, composite extension or flexion orthotic intervention is often necessary to lengthen adhesions and increase motion.

Extensor Tendon Injury

Extensor tendon injury creates motion loss at different joints, depending on the level of injury. Zones I and II tendon disruptions cause loss of active DIP extension (Brzezienski & Schneider, 1995; Rosenthal & Elhassan, 2011), which if left untreated leads to a DIP flexion contracture. Lack of

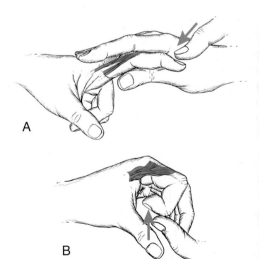
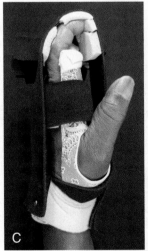
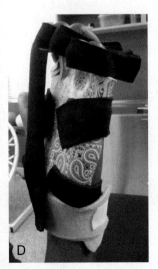

FIGURE 15–21 A and B, The intrinsic tightness test. Note the loss of simultaneous MCP extension and IP flexion. **C and D,** The MCP extension position in this orthosis allows for maximum available flexion stress to tight intrinsic muscles. In **C,** the IF demonstrates a greater flexion loss and therefore is managed with a gentle composite flexion strap. In **D,** a neoprene PIP/DIP strap is used to gain IP flexion.

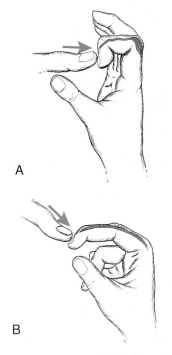

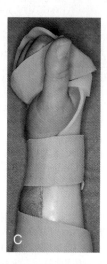

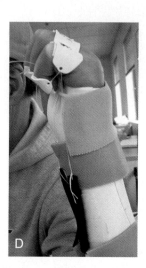

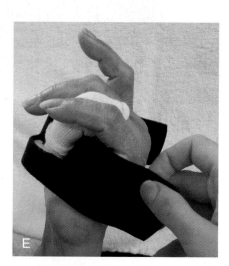

FIGURE 15–22 A and B, The extrinsic tightness test. Note the loss of composite finger flexion. Two variations of a composite digit flexion mobilization orthoses: dorsal "dynamic" approach using a neoprene strap **(C)** and volar "static progressive" approach with monofilament lines and hook/loop adjustments **(D). E,** Hand-based split strap with foam to apply composite flexion stretch.

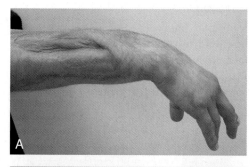

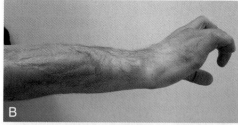

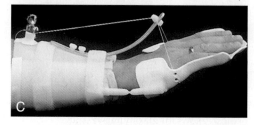

FIGURE 15–23 A and B, Extrinsic flexor tightness presenting with loss of combined wrist and digit extension. **C,** A wrist and digit extension mobilization orthosis (static progressive approach).

treatment over many months creates an imbalance at the IP joints, resulting in overpull at the lateral bands, shifting them dorsally. Eventually, a swan-neck deformity, with PIP hyperextension and its concomitant loss of flexion at the PIP, occurs (Fig. 15–24A–D). The adhesions caused from nonoperative or operative treatment can limit DIP flexion, leading to a DIP extension contracture (Fig. 15–25).

A zone III or IV tendon disruption results in loss of active PIP extension (Coons & Green, 1995; Rosenthal & Elhassan, 2011), causing loss of passive PIP extension. If left untreated, a PIP flexion contracture results. Lack of treatment over many months creates an imbalance at the IP joints, shifting the lateral bands volarly. This leads to a boutonniere deformity, with PIP flexion and its concomitant loss of flexion at the DIP (Fig. 15–26A–C). When the oblique retinacular ligament (ORL) adaptively shortens, it creates a DIP hyperextension deformity and loss of flexion at the DIP (Fig. 15–27A–E). The adhesions that result from nonoperative or operative treatment can limit wrist, thumb MP, MCP, and IP flexion, leading to a one or more joint extension contractures (see Chapter 18 Tendon Injuries for further information).

Flexor Tendon Injury

To repair a zone II flexor tendon laceration, the surgeon must invade the flexor tendon sheath. The finger is then positioned in flexion for many hours a day owing to inflammation, edema, and scar synthesis (Fig. 15–28). As described earlier, this combination creates the perfect situation for the

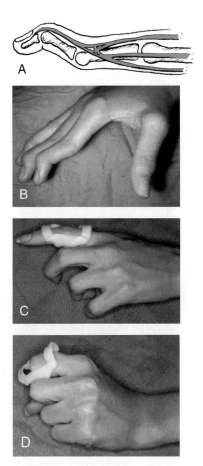

FIGURE 15–24 **A and B,** Swan-neck deformity; note the PIP hyperextension and DIP flexion. A PIP extension restriction orthosis with extension **(C)** and flexion **(D)**.

formation of IP flexion contractures (Stewart & van Strien, 1995). Flexor tendon injury in other zones may also cause IP flexion contractures, owing to the flexion posture of the digit coupled with the generalized edema and inflammation that often involves much of the hand.

When the flexor digitorum superficialis (FDS) ruptures or is transferred to another location, an imbalance

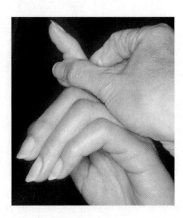

FIGURE 15–25 Adhesions following zone I extensor tendon injury limit active DIP flexion.

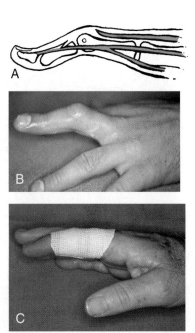

FIGURE 15–26 **A and B,** Boutonniere deformity; note the PIP flexion and DIP hyperextension. **C,** A PIP extension immobilization orthosis using QuickCast 2.

is set up that can lead to swan-neck deformity as shown in Figure 15–25A,B (Brand & Hollister, 1999). As noted, when left untreated, the faulty mechanics can lead to loss of motion at the IP joints (see Chapter 18 Tendon Injuries).

Burn Injury

Partial-thickness burns cause joint stiffness primarily via adaptive shortening of periarticular structures. Tight skin positions these structures on slack in the presence of inflammation, edema, and scar formation. Healing scar contracts, pulling the joints along with it (Fig. 15–29A,B). Skin damage across motion creases is the most likely to create joint stiffness (Chapter 23 Burns, provides more details). Full-thickness burns can also damage tendon. The loss of active motion, coupled with the adaptive shortening, creates a powerful mechanism for joint stiffness. The clinician must be aware of the tendon's vulnerability to thermal injury. The orthosis should not only prevent primary joint contracture but also protect vulnerable tendon structures such as the central slip of the extensor hood mechanism (dorsum of the PIP) (Grigsby de Linde & Miles, 1995).

Fracture

Fracture causes joint stiffness via several mechanisms. For example, edema and inflammation accompany most fractures. Cartilage defects also produce loss of PROM, which occurs in a predictable cascade of increased friction, leading to inflammation that in turn creates pain and edema. The normal reflex arc and the patient's normal response to pain limit active motion at the joint. When the joint fails to

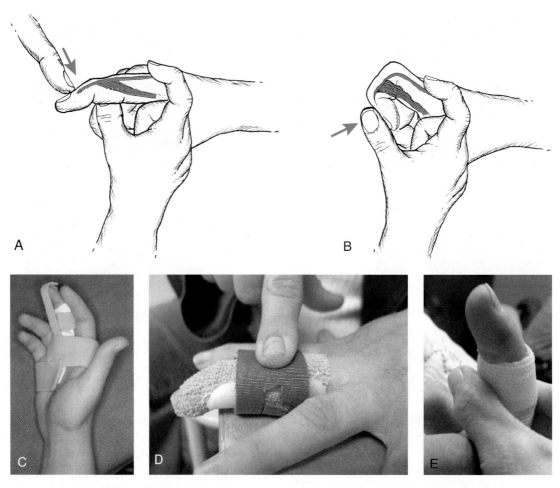

FIGURE 15-27 A and B, The ORL tightness test. Note the lack of isolated DIP flexion. **C,** A DIP flexion mobilization orthosis using loop strapping for a static progressive approach. **D and E,** PIP immobilization orthosis applied to allow isolated AROM at the DIP joint.

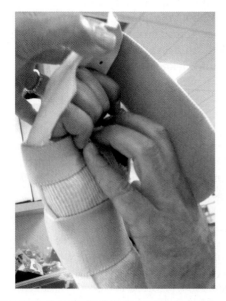

FIGURE 15-28 During the initial phase of flexor tendon repair, IP flexion contractures are not uncommon due to the extended period of time the digits must be protected in flexion.

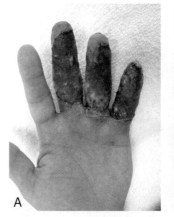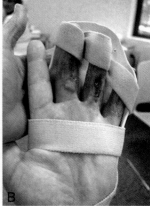

FIGURE 15-29 Third-degree burns of the volar surface of the hands **(A),** healing wound is being kept in extension to prevent contracture. The patient takes this off for gentle exercises in flexion and extension **(B).**

go through its full arc of motion, periarticular structures shorten; and eventually, the joint will lose motion.

A fracture may produce loose bodies in an adjacent joint (Raney, Brashear, & Shands, 1971). A loose body limits joint motion mechanically. If the loose body persists and the joint limitation is sustained, the periarticular structures may adaptively shorten, causing joint stiffness.

Structures that glide over bone may become trapped in the scar callus that heals the bone. This may lead to extrinsic tightness or may involve a prime joint mover, such as a wrist extensor. When this occurs, the muscle–tendon unit does not have adequate excursion, and the ability to restore and maintain joint motion is severely compromised (Fig. 15–30) (see Chapter 16 Fractures, for details).

Ligament Injury or Dislocation

A sprain directly compromises structures supporting the joint. Ligament injuries tend to heal slowly owing to poor vascularity (Levine, 1992). They also tend to be painful for months and even years after they are healed. Clinical experience shows that edema after ligament injury of the small IP and MCP joints tends to linger much longer than for other types of injuries (Mannarino, 1992). The edema and pain severely limit motion. The therapist must fabricate an orthosis carefully to prevent joint contracture and balance this with carefully guided exercise. Once a joint contracture establishes itself, the therapist must carefully note sprain classification, swelling, color, and temperature to avoid aggravating the joint while attempting to restore motion.

Infection

As part of the initial evaluation of a trauma patient with wounds or percutaneous pins, the therapist should obtain information about the patient's risk for infection. When risk factors are present, the therapist must be on constant alert for signs of infection. Infection causes an acute and severe inflammatory reaction. Edema always accompanies infection and is the primary reason that infection frequently

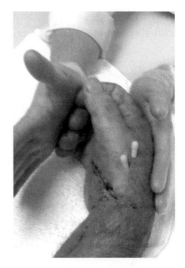

FIGURE 15–30 Note the tight extrinsic extensors as the therapist assists with ROM.

results in stiffness. Some organisms not only trigger inflammatory reactions but also produce toxins that destroy tissue. Frequently, infection management involves immobilization of the involved part, which contributes to joint stiffness. Sepsis has the capacity to turn a good surgical result into a poor one because of its motion-robbing effects (Nathan & Taras, 1995).

Diabetes

The patient with diabetes has a greater risk for hand stiffness as commonly seen with chronic stenosing tenosynovitis, also known as trigger finger (Means et al., 2011) (Fig. 15–31A,B). The patient may present with the involved digit locked in either flexion or extension due to long-standing tenosynovitis. Over time, a PIP joint flexion or extension contracture may develop interfering with simple activities of daily living (ADLs) and life tasks. Conservative treatment is aimed at edema reduction and serially casting the digit in the desired direction of correction. Surgical intervention is a last resort

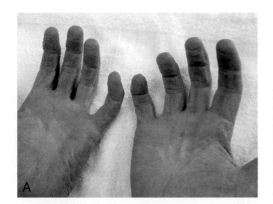
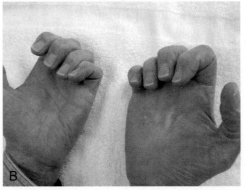

FIGURE 15–31 Severe stenosing tenosynovitis bilaterally. A, Note limitation in digit extension **(B)** and composite flexion. This patient has already developed contractures in which only surgical intervention will restore functional use.

because these patients may have a greater risk for postoperative complications secondary to the complexity of the disease process.

Psychopathology

No discussion of stiffness is complete without addressing the contribution that psychopathology can make to PROM loss. The problems take many forms, including but not limited to the following:

- Contribution to causing an accident (Hirschfeld & Behan, 1963)
- Self-inflicted wound (Wallace & Fitzmorris, 1978)
- Noncompliance with postinjury care
- Clenched fist syndrome (Vranceanu, 2011)
- Refusal to move a joint via nonfunctional cocontraction (Simmons & Vasile, 1980)
- Refusal to move a joint for a significant period of time (Brand, 1988)
- Secondary gain issues (Vranceanu, 2011)

Improving PROM in a patient with these tendencies usually involves some form of psychotherapy. The patient perceives attempts to increase motion as undesirable and will resist. Empathy and skilled communication is paramount along with a supportive and consistent multidisciplinary team approach (Vranceanu, 2011).

Stiffness at Specific Joints

Distal Interphalangeal Joint

The DIP joint is vulnerable to stiffness in both flexion and extension. The DIP presents a unique challenge in that once the joint becomes stiff, the short length of the distal phalanx offers little in terms of a lever arm to torque the joint into the desired ROM. The joint is unique in that the motor sensors surrounding the joint are singular and do not have the redundancy that is available at the other joints of the hand.

Thus, if one of the motors becomes injured or ineffective, stiffness is likely to result.

The DIP has a dense volar plate that can become folded and adherent in scar in the presence of inflammation. The resultant flexion contracture often occurs with zone I or distal zone II flexor tendon injury, especially in the case of flexor digitorum profundus (FDP) advancement (Evans, 1990). With advancement, the flexed position of the DIP is encouraged with the introduction of a pull-out wire and button that introduce even more scar and inflammation (Fig. 15–32A). Although some loss of DIP extension might be considered desirable in the face of lost flexor excursion, the resulting extreme flexion contractures can be disfiguring and disabling. The therapist must respect the time for tendon healing but should begin to extend the DIP as soon as the type of repair and the health and cooperation of the patient permit. Progressive isolated DIP extension orthotic intervention improves PROM and minimizes stress on the flexor tendon (Fig. 15–32B). However, even though such an orthosis attempts to extend only one joint in the series that the FDP affects, intervention so close to the repair can lead to attenuation or rupture.

When the extensor of the joint is avulsed from its insertion in the case of a mallet injury, the joint cannot actively extend. If left untreated, the volar structures undergo adaptive shortening, and a flexion contracture results. An untreated mallet injury can also lead to imbalance of the entire extensor mechanism of the finger and affect the PIP joint. The mallet injury must be immediately placed in extension to coapt the tendon ends and allow restoration of extension (Fig. 15–33A–C). Clinical experience has shown that after days or even weeks have elapsed since the time of injury, if the dorsal aspect of the DIP remains reactive, it is possible that instituting an extension orthosis will restore tendon continuity.

With a diagnosis of a PIP central slip injury, the therapist must include a program of DIP flexion to prevent ORL tightness as shown in Figure 15–27D. If the injury is old, the DIP has already lost flexion, and the PIP is beginning

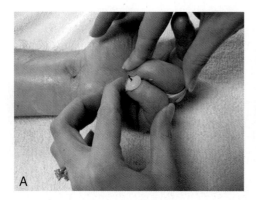
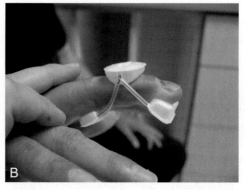

FIGURE 15–32 **A,** Pull out suture (button) on the dorsum of the small digit in the management of a zone I flexor tendon injury. **B,** Prefabricated digit extension mobilization orthosis; note the use of small size to isolate the DIP joint.

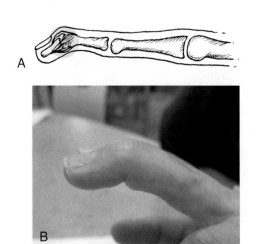

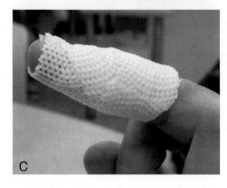

FIGURE 15–33 **A and B,** Rupture of the terminal extensor tendon, "mallet finger." **C,** DIP extension immobilization cast fabricated from QuickCast 2 material. Note the clearance of the PIP joint crease and the opening distally to check for signs of impaired vascularity. These small casts are worn uninterrupted for 6 to 8 weeks.

to contract (see Fig. 15–6A,B), the clinician must progress the patient through a combination of PIP extension/DIP flexion orthoses and exercise to restore normal PROM as shown in Figure 15–27C (R. B. Evans, 1995). As mentioned, scarring of zone I or II extensors can lead to loss of extensor tendon glide/DIP extension. This inability to extend the DIP joint, left untreated, may lead to DIP flexion contractures. There are many options available to manage

combined PIP and DIP flexion deficiencies (Fig. 15–34A,B). A circumferential PIP joint immobilization orthosis can be used for exercise to promote FDP gliding and DIP AROM; this is a device that can be dispensed to be used on an independent basis as part of a home exercise program (Fig. 15–27D).

Proximal Interphalangeal Joint

The PIP joint can become stiff in either flexion or extension (Figs. 15–6, 15–19, 15–26, and 15–35A–E). However, it is the PIP flexion contracture that is the most challenging to resolve for the following reasons (Glasgow et al., 2012; Lluch, 1997; Sokolow, 1997):

- Tendency for the volar plate to shorten or fold on itself after trauma
- Prevalence of a flexed finger posture in the position of ease and during function
- Vulnerability of the extensor mechanism (it is thin, superficial, and intimate with the underlying bone)
- Length loss caused by proximal phalanx fractures, leading to redundancy in extensor mechanism length and causing lack of full active extension
- Extensor hood attenuation from prolonged positioning in flexion, rendering the mechanism too long to provide full extension even when the contracture has resolved (Brandsma, 1993)
- Density of the PIP volar plate, making it prone to adaptive shortening, and the thickness of the structure, making its lengthening difficult

PIP joints are usually held in flexion, and hands are used in flexion. When a patient uses his or her hands for normal function during the day, the PIP joints are frequently in some degree of flexion (Fig. 15–36). The position of comfort and rest is flexion. In the face of pain and edema, the PIPs are held in flexion to place the periarticular structures on slack. During sleep, the PIP joints assume a flexed position.

Many types of trauma to the finger cause the extensor mechanism to become adherent to the bone and skin. This

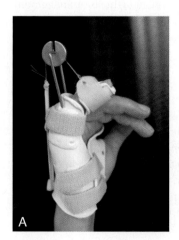

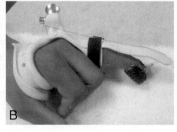

FIGURE 15–34 DIP flexion contractures can be difficult to manage secondary to the short lever arm of the distal phalanx. Both of these are providing simultaneous extension forces to the PIP and DIP joints. **A,** A dynamic approach using a Phoenix outrigger. **B,** A static progressive approach.

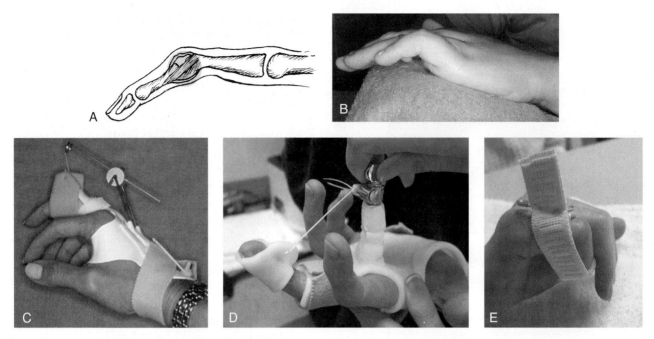

FIGURE 15–35 **A and B,** Small finger (SF) PIP joint flexion contracture. **C,** A PIP extension mobilization orthosis using a dynamic approach via a Rolyan® outrigger. **D,** A static progressive orthosis being used to manage a PIP extension contracture. Note the built-up platform that the MERiT™ component sits on in order to provide the proper line of pull. **E,** Combined PIP–DIP flexion mobilization strap using pajama elastic and a safety pin; this allows for adjusting tension.

adhesion of the dorsal hood creates loss of excursion. Without full excursion, the PIP joint cannot actively assume full extension (Mannarino, 1992; Rosenthal & Elhassan, 2011). If the patient fails to perform PROM consistently, the volar structures adaptively shorten, causing a flexion contracture.

Proximal phalanx fractures can result in shortening of the bone. However, the extensor hood length remains the same. This length redundancy makes complete active extension mechanically impossible. As for dorsal hood adhesions, with active extension lost, the volar structures adaptively shorten.

If the PIP flexion contracture remains for any significant period of time, the extensor hood becomes attenuated. The discrepancy in length between bone and tendon creates a

mechanical deficit. The extensor mechanism cannot generate adequate tension to extend the joint fully. For this reason, even though many therapists argue for prioritizing PIP flexion to regain functional use of the hand, others prioritize PIP extension, especially in the face of an FDP with good excursion, evidenced by good DIP flexion. Hand surgeon Robert Ashworth (personal communication, 1987) offered the following clinical gem: When the IP joints lack flexion, if the FDP has the ability to take the DIP through full available PROM, then the outcome for IP flexion is good. Over the years, Ashworth's indicator has proven itself to be consistently correct. Once the extensor hood length increases, the likelihood of its shrinking to normal proportions again is nil. Therefore, prevention of PIP contractures becomes of paramount importance. Even if orthosis management and therapy resolve the volar restrictions causing the contracture, the adverse dorsal mechanics of length or dorsal adhesion may prevent the maintenance of the improved extension.

Loss of PIP PROM in flexion can result from many of the factors described earlier. In the presence of a functioning FDP, most PIPs eventually flex. One notable exception is a fracture or dislocation (especially one that is immobilized too long) that results in significant scarring at the joint. This extra tissue can create a physical block to motion that only surgical excision of the scar tissue can improve (Cannon, 2011; Means et al., 2011). Functional exercise orthoses can be helpful as part of a home program to improve joint AROM and tendon gliding (Fig. 15–37A–H).

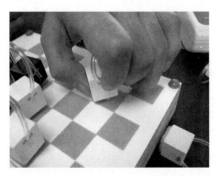

FIGURE 15–36 Note the natural position of flexion with this functional prehensile activity.

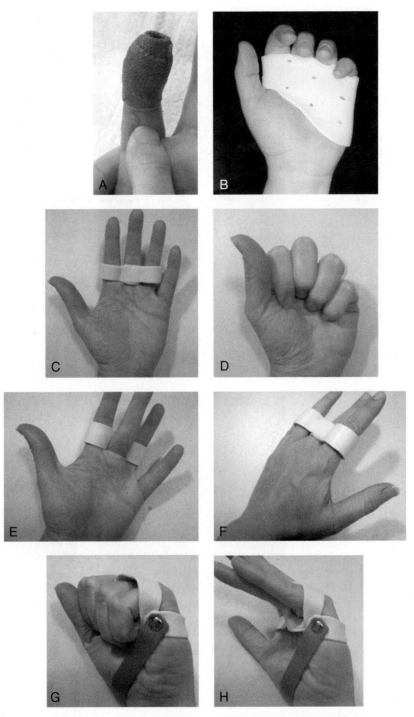

FIGURE 15–37 **Exercise orthoses to encourage PIP joint AROM. A,** DIP cast fabricated from Orficast™ to direct active efforts to the PIP joint with active flexion. **B,** Blocking the MCP joints into extension can provide a means to actively stretch the intrinsics as well as prevent the compensation of overly flexing the MCP joints with efforts to bend distally. **C and D,** Fabricating a nonarticular "yoke" style orthosis with the affected digit in relative extension compared to the adjacent digits will provide a block at the proximal phalanx, encouraging flexion distally. This can be worn during functional activities to promote active flexion. **E and F,** The reverse of the previous orthosis, molded with the affected digit in relative flexion at the MCP joint to provide pressure over the proximal phalanx with active PIP extension efforts. This prevents the patient from hyperextending the MCP joint. These orthoses **(C–F)** can be modified for any digit; including three totals within the orthosis design. **G and H,** Due to the difficulty controlling for MCP hyperextension when addressing the small finger, consider fabricating an MCP extension restriction orthosis (similar to one for ulnar nerve palsy) to promote active PIP extension during functional use. Notice the riveted strapping system which helps prevent migration.

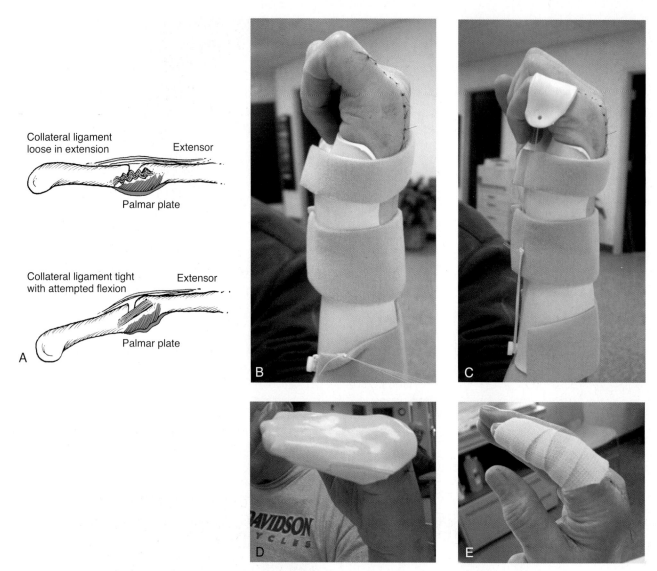

FIGURE 15–38 **A and B,** Small finger (SF) MCP joint extension contracture. This patient underwent an extensor tenolysis. **C,** SF MCP flexion mobilization orthosis, dynamic approach. Note clearance of the fifth volar MCP crease, which is important to achieve full MCP flexion. **D,** Digit extension orthosis ("flipper") used as an exercise device to encourage active flexion at the MCP joints. This directs the force of flexion to the MCP joints, preventing the common compensatory flexion distally. **E,** To address an individual digit, consider using a circumferentially designed orthosis to block motion distally during active MCP flexion.

Finger Metacarpophalangeal Joint

Problems at the finger MCP joint rarely result in loss of extension. Even when the joint has been held in flexion for years by Dupuytren's fascial contracture, surgical release of the fascia most often readily returns the joint to extension. Injuries involving the soft tissue crossing the MCP crease at a 90° angle or involving most soft tissue in this location (e.g., burns, degloving injuries, and palmar skin graft) create loss of extension. However, restoration of soft tissue length restores normal motion. With rheumatic disease, the patient may lose passive MCP extension owing to multiple factors, including loss of joint capsule and ligament integrity, intrinsic tightness, and ulnar subluxation of the EDC (Alter, Feldon, & Terrono, 2011; Melvin, 1989).

The bane of the hand specialist's existence at the MCP joint is the extension contracture (Fig. 15–38A–E). Diagnoses associated with this problem are any injury causing generalized edema of the hand, intrinsic paralysis, crush injury, metacarpal and proximal phalanx fractures, dorsal or circumferential burns, and a zone V extensor tendon injury that is not mobilized properly. Each of these injuries results in the sustained extension of the MCP joint, often in the presence of edema, inflammation, and scar formation. The MCP joint's unique anatomy predisposes it to the extension contracture.

The collateral ligaments of the MCP joint are slack in extension and taut in flexion (Chase, 1989; Rosenthal & Elhassan, 2011). When the ligaments are allowed to remain slack, especially in the presence of inflammation and scar formation, they can fall prey to the accordion phenomenon, adaptive shortening, or both. Like the volar plate of the PIP, these collateral ligaments are dense and recalcitrant to lengthening. A well-established MCP extension contracture may require 23 to 24 hours a day of end range time to change length and increase PROM.

Thumb MP Joint

Trauma to the thumb often causes stiffness at the MP joint. The diagnoses of fracture—collateral ligament injury, tendon injury, and nerve injury—all frequently present with loss of MP flexion (Fig. 15–39). The problem with restoring thumb MP flexion mirrors those of contracture at the finger but does not have the same primary cause. The collateral ligaments of the thumb have a different architecture than those of the finger MCPs (Imaeda, An, & Cooney, 1992; Kapandji, 1982; Melone, Beldner, & Basuk, 2000). The loss of flexion seems to originate with joint swelling, which may be worsened by dorsal adhesions.

The thumb MP may lose extension with the loss of extensor pollicis brevis (EPB) continuity and a concomitant rent in the extensor expansion. This imbalance creates a dynamic similar to that of the finger boutonniere deformity. Left untreated, the IP joint of the thumb loses flexion and assumes a hyperextended position. Over time, a fixed deformity can result. A grade 3 tear of either the ulnar or the radial collateral ligament of the thumb MP can lead to MP joint

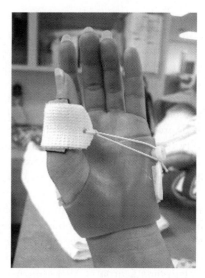

FIGURE 15–39 Thumb MP flexion mobilization orthosis; notice neoprene beneath the QuickCast 2 sling to improve comfort.

instability with subsequent subluxation and the creation of a flexion contracture.

Rheumatic disease can create various thumb contractures. Rheumatoid arthritis, lupus, and similar diseases can create the Nalebuff type 1 thumb, characterized by MP flexion and IP hyperextension (Fig. 15–40A–D). The appearance is similar to the boutonniere deformity of the finger. This

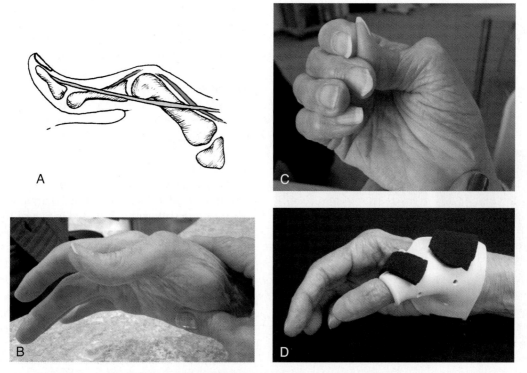

FIGURE 15–40 A and B, The Nalebuff type 1 thumb: MP flexion and IP hyperextension. **C,** This deformity is further exacerbated by lateral pinch. **D,** A thumb immobilization orthosis aides in positioning the MP in extension, which rebalances the thumb IP for a more efficient pinch.

occurs as a result of chronic synovitis of the thumb MP joint, intrinsic muscle tightness, weakening or attenuation of the EPB, and ulnovolar displacement of the EPL (Melvin, 1989). The joint deformities are further emphasized by the natural tendency to use the thumb for pinch as noted in Figure 15–40C. Clinicians most commonly use orthoses to prevent this deformity. However, aggressive disease or late treatment may present the clinician with the need to address this deformity. Goga-Eppenstein, Hill, Seifert, and Yasukawa (1999) describe a casting technique used successfully for a patient with juvenile rheumatoid arthritis. The casting was followed up with a program of static orthotic intervention and electrical stimulation to the thumb extrinsic extensors.

In contrast, the stiffness problem commonly associated with osteoarthritis is the Nalebuff type 2 thumb (Fig. 15–41A–C). The condition associated with this classification is carpometacarpal (CMC) synovitis of the joint, which stretches the joint capsule and allows the joint to sublux or dislocate in adduction. This adducted posture results in shortening of the adductor pollicis muscles and web space. MP hyperextension develops with attempts to abduct the contracted first metacarpal (Melvin, 1989). Once this deformity exists, an orthosis will not improve it. A thumb MP extension restriction orthosis minimizes the hyperextension and may prevent it from getting worse (Fig. 15–42). Such an orthosis may also help distribute forces in a biomechanically sound way that will unload the CMC joint. The main role for orthosis management for MP hyperextension secondary to CMC instability is prevention.

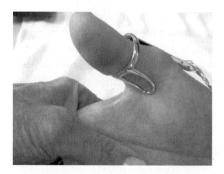

FIGURE 15–42 SIRIS™ Stable Thumb Orthosis with proximal volar extension (PVX); this splint stabilizes the MP joint dorsal and volar to prevent hyperextension and flexion. It is used for MP hyperextension when there are significant joint changes at the CMC joint. A bracelet keeps the orthosis from migrating. Available through the Silver Ring Splint Company, Charlottesville, VA.

Thumb Carpometacarpal Joint

The CMC joint of the thumb has a unique saddle architecture that renders it highly mobile (Kapandji, 1982). The thumb is critical to hand function and is a frequently used and overused joint. Many people experience thumb CMC arthritis as a result of overuse, trauma, or a multijoint disease. Pelligrini, Olcott, and Hollenberg (1993) hypothesized that over time, overuse or trauma compromises the ligament system supporting the joint. This allows the joint surfaces to lose congruency, which leads to friction that wears away the cartilage, creating CMC arthritis. Clinical experience shows that osteoarthritis often first presents at the basal joint of the thumb. This disease has an insidious onset, and the cause and the cure are as yet unknown. Refer to Chapter 17 Arthritis for greater detail on this patient population.

Joint incongruity, weakness, and pain all lead to loss of motion at the thumb CMC. As the cartilage loses integrity, the joint becomes painful and inflamed. The joint receptors send a signal to the spinal cord to inhibit efferent signals. The patient experiences loss of coordination and strength and has trouble performing ADLs. The condition leads to loss of motion, inflammation, and pain.

No matter the cause, at the end stage of thumb CMC arthritis (stage 4 disease), the metacarpal dislocates from the trapezium altogether as noted in Figure 15–41A,B (Alter et al., 2011; Eaton & Glickel, 1987). This dislocation usually occurs ulnarly. With such joint compromise, the thumb abductors are no longer able to function and the first metacarpal remains in an adducted position. Over time, the thumb adductor shortens. Even when the patient undergoes CMC arthroplasty to restore joint kinematics, the shortened adductor prevents normal thumb motion and function. Although orthotic intervention and exercise to restore the width of the first web space can increase ROM, experience has shown that it does not restore normal abduction. It is critical that the patient be aware of this and undergo a joint reconstruction before adduction contracture occurs.

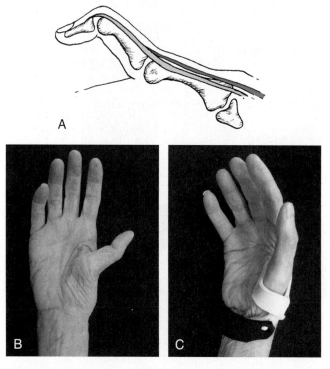

A

B   C

FIGURE 15–41 **A and B,** The Nalebuff type 2 thumb: MP hyperextension and IP flexion. **C,** This patient was passively correctable by stabilizing the first CMC joint with this very simple counterforce orthosis.

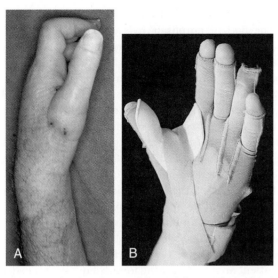

FIGURE 15–43 The thumb is unable to abduct with median inner-vated thumb musculature paralysis. **A,** Without orthosis interven-tion, a first web space contracture will result. **B,** A thumb abduction mobilization orthosis using a serial static approach. Note use of com-pressive glove for edema.

As with other stiff structures, orthotic intervention may be able to improve web space width or may stabilize the joint and improve comfort and function; however, the only real solution at the current level of technology is surgery (Means et al., 2011).

With the loss of the median innervated thumb muscu-lature, the thumb is unable to abduct in the palmar plane. Without the ability to lengthen the thumb adductor, the muscle shortens, producing a first web space contracture (Fig. 15–43). In the case of combined ulnar and median paralysis, the ulnar innervated thumb adductor ceases to function and often becomes fibrotic. This speeds up the for-mation of a first web space contracture. Clinicians use web space orthosis intervention to protect the length and width of this web space (Brandsma, 1993).

Wrist Joint

Unlike the joints discussed so far, the wrist is not generally predisposed to any particular patterns of motion loss. The wrist consists of a complex of joints and contains multiple articulations. As with other joints, stiffness here can arise from intra-articular or extra-articular pathology. Some causes of stiffness at this level are unique to this joint (Saffar, 1997):

- Certain types of idiopathic arthritis (gout)
- Avascular necrosis of the lunate
- Volkmann ischemic contracture (produces wrist flexion)
- Ligamentous injury and carpal instability, including carpal collapse
- Carpal nonunion, especially of the scaphoid

Trauma and its sequelae are the most commonly causes of lost wrist PROM. Saffar (1997) states that carpal instability causes 70% of chronic wrist stiffness. He describes post-traumatic osteoarthritis secondary to carpal joint injuries as a frequent cause of wrist stiffness. The position of the wrist during immobilization often predetermines the direction of stiffness.

The most common type of wrist fracture, the Colles, requires reduction of the wrist in a flexed, ulnarly deviated, and pronated position to align the dorsally displaced distal fragment with the proximal radius (Frykman & Kropp, 1995). The patient remains in the cast for many weeks and often cannot attain a neutral wrist or forearm even after weeks out of the cast. The direction of wrist stiffness is always the oppo-site of the position in which the patient was casted. Thus for the common Colles fracture, the patient lacks extension, radial deviation, and supination (Fig. 15–44A–C).

According to P. LaStayo (personal communication, 2000), the greater the distal radius malunion, the more opportunity exists for what appears to be an ulnar shift of the proximal row. This ulnar shift can occur if the radial inclination is lost and there is a distal radioulnar joint (DRUJ) disruption. The ulnar shift limits radial deviation; without radial deviation, normal wrist extension can never be achieved.

Soft tissue scarring in the forearm can also limit wrist PROM as noted in Figures 15–23A,B. When extrinsic flexor and/or extensor muscle–tendon units become adherent to either bone or surrounding less mobile soft tissue, wrist PROM suffers (Fig. 15–45A,B). In the case of predominantly dorsal extensor scarring, wrist flexion decreases. When volar flexor scarring occurs, the wrist loses extension. It is impor-tant to note that if these extrinsic problems can be addressed early and if the wrist is spared involvement in inflammation

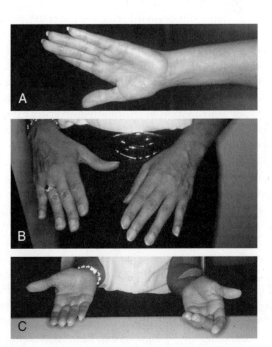

FIGURE 15–44 Note the lack of motion on the patient's left side with wrist extension **(A)**, radial deviation **(B)**, and forearm supination **(C)**.

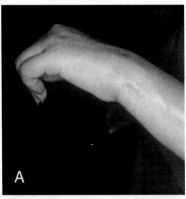

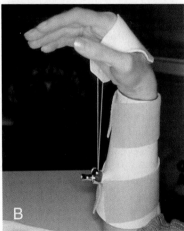

FIGURE 15–45 **A,** Loss of wrist flexion. **B,** A wrist flexion mobilization orthosis using a static progressive stretch provided by a MERiT™ component.

and scar formation, then the wrist complex itself remains healthy and true stiffness of the joint will not result. However, in the case of long-standing extrinsic adhesions, especially if the inflammatory process of the injury involves the radiocarpal joint or the carpal complex, the wrist may become stiff. The clinician has many choices available for mobilization of the stiff wrist and/or tight extrinsic tendons (Fig. 15–46A–E).

Loss of wrist motion in rheumatoid arthritis has multifactorial origins (Alter et al., 2011; Garcia-Elias, 1997). The presence of significant synovitis alone can take up so much space that the wrist cannot achieve normal ROM. Loss of articular cartilage and supporting ligaments causes the wrist to shift in a characteristic manner. Usually, the adult with rheumatoid arthritis experiences carpal volar subluxation and an ulnar shift of the carpus rotating the hand radially on the forearm. With juvenile rheumatoid arthritis, volar subluxation of the carpus occurs; however, frequently, the carpus shifts radially, creating an ulnar deviation deformity at the wrist (Melvin, 1989). See Chapter 17 Arthritis for more information.

Overt (visible and palpable) and occult (by MRI or differential diagnosis) ganglions can limit wrist ROM much in the same way that edema does (Angelides, 1988). The soft mass takes up space and limits normal tissue excursion and

extensibility. When ganglions affect nerves, they cause pain, and the patient purposely restricts ROM. If the ganglion remains over a long period of time, wrist ROM can suffer, largely from adaptive shortening. More often, however, ganglion-related stiffness results from operative treatment.

Ganglions can present volarly or dorsally. In these authors' experience, the dorsal ganglion is more common. When surgically excised, it frequently results in a loss of wrist flexion that is recalcitrant to active and passive exercise and scar-modification techniques. This scenario indicates the need for a wrist flexion mobilization orthosis (Fig. 15–45B and 15–46B). Managing the wrist with an orthosis in flexion is a foreign concept for many therapists. Most clinicians focus on wrist extension for function. Placing the wrist in a flexion orthosis for sustained periods leads to concerns about median nerve compression. Certainly, it is important to instruct the patient about monitoring for median nerve sensory status; however, the main author has successfully used wrist flexion orthosis management after dorsal ganglion excision to restore normal PROM in flexion without median nerve compromise and without loss of wrist extension. Likewise, patients who have lost passive wrist extension after volar ganglion excision can benefit from a mobilizing orthosis for wrist extension (Fig. 15–46A&D).

The patient with carpal instability may undergo surgery—for example, partial fusion, ligament repair, or wrist capsulodesis—to restore stability and decrease pain. In this case, wrist stiffness is iatrogenically introduced; the patient trades some motion to have a stable, pain-free wrist. However, these patients remain immobilized postoperatively for a long duration and frequently come out of the cast with little or no motion. When diligent therapy, including a thorough home program, fails to result in adequate increases in PROM, a dilemma arises. Opinions diverge about treatment indications (Levine, 1992).

Some clinicians believe that the stiffness will resolve somewhat over a very long period of time, perhaps of 1 year or more. They also believe that passive approaches to increasing motion are contraindicated because these methods compromise the surgically induced stiffness and ultimately may produce instability and pain. Other clinicians introduce guarded passive exercise and carefully monitored mobilization orthoses to improve PROM. They use guidelines from several studies on cadavers that underwent partial fusion to limit the goals of motion (Gellman, Kauffman, Lenihan, & Botte, 1988; Ruby, Cooney, An, Linscheid, & Chao, 1988). These clinicians do not seek to restore full motion; the goal is the amount of motion the studies suggest as safe. Although the concerns of the more conservative clinicians warrant consideration, waiting a year or more to regain functional motion may not be an option for all patients. In addition, surgically induced stiffness can produce pain in and of itself. The careful and strategic application of passive treatment, including orthotic mobilization after surgery to restore carpal stability, can result in a more rapid return to motion and function that is both safe and comfortable.

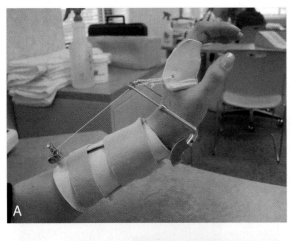
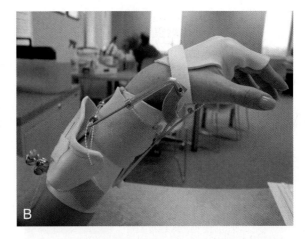
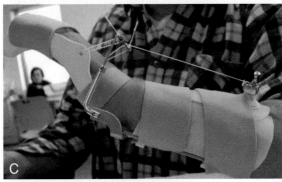
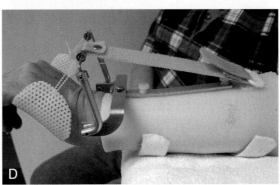
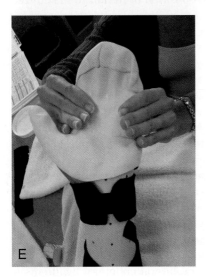

FIGURE 15–46 A, Wrist extension mobilization orthosis: static progressive approach. **B,** Wrist flexion mobilization orthosis: dynamic approach (note this orthosis combines both wrist flexion and extension). **C,** Simultaneous wrist and digit/thumb extension mobilization orthosis: static progressive approach. **D,** Wrist extension mobilization orthosis: static progressive approach using simple hook and loop. **E,** Serial static digit extension piece being applied over a wrist immobilization orthosis to prevent further extrinsic flexor tightness and resolve digit flexion and thumb web contractures.

Forearm

As for the wrist, a common cause of lost forearm PROM is trauma, and the position of the forearm in the cast usually dictates the direction of stiffness. Because wrist and forearm fractures are often reduced in pronation, loss of supination is more common than the loss of pronation (Fig. 15–44C). However, clinical experience shows that with severe forearm fractures and complex fractures of the DRUJ or the proximal radioulnar joint (PRUJ), the patient often loses rotation in both directions. Reduction of the radius that produces a less-than-optimum DRUJ relationship reliably decreases forearm rotation. Saffar (1997) states that radiocarpal joint stiffness is associated with decreased pronosupination. The formation of exostosis is associated with forearm fractures. A bony bridge between the radius and ulna fuses the two bones together. Exostosis is easily diagnosed on radiographs and represents a contraindication to PROM exercise and the use of mobilizing orthoses. Only surgical excision resolves the PROM loss (Raney et al., 1971).

Although fractures commonly cause loss of forearm motion, soft tissue injury (with or without fracture) can also cause PROM limitation. Injury to the triangular fibrocartilage

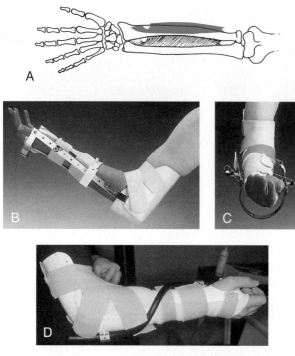

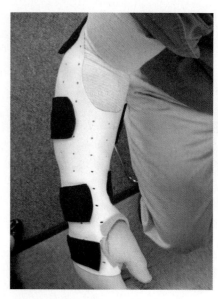

FIGURE 15–48 This orthosis allows nearly a full plane of elbow flexion and extension but limits forearm rotation.

FIGURE 15–47 **A,** The dense interosseus ligament joins and stabilizes the radius and ulna along their entire course. **B and C,** MERiT™ SPS Forearm Rotation Orthosis. **D,** Rolyan® forearm rotation orthosis.

complex (TFCC) limits rotation and tends to affect supination more than pronation. Adaptive shortening or scarring of the interosseus ligament prevents the normal rotation of the radius (Fig. 15–47A–D) (J. Stanley, 1997). Injury to other periarticular soft tissues, such as the supinator muscle or either of the pronator muscles, can limit forearm rotation. In particular, the pronator quadratus has been implicated in restriction of supination (P. Dell, personal communication, 2000).

Rheumatoid arthritis affects both the DRUJ and the PRUJ. Bone and cartilage erosions, ligament instability, and joint effusions all contribute to forearm PROM loss.

Elbow Joint

Although fractures are the most common injuries that result in post-traumatic stiffness, other conditions such as central nervous system dysfunction, osteoarthrosis, burns, infection, and hemophilia can also lead to elbow contractures (E. B. Evans, Larson, & Yates, 1968; Figgie, Inglis, Mow, & Figgie, 1989; Josefsson, Gentz, Johnell, & Wendeberg, 1989; Jupiter, Neff, Holzach, & Allgower, 1985; Millard & Ortiz, 1965; Morrey & Nirschl, 2000; Sherk, 1977). Many factors contribute to elbow stiffness after trauma. Delay in instituting active motion contributes to stiffness, especially in the elbow; therefore, if early on, the injury can be managed with a restriction-type orthosis, this is preferable (Fig. 15–48) (Morrey, 2000). These orthoses can be designed to allow a safe degree of motion yet stabilize the intended area as to minimize stiffness (Morrey, 2000).

Elbow stiffness also comes from mechanical causes. Galley, Richards, and O'Driscoll (1993) studied the effect of intra-articular effusions to explain the early development of flexion contracture from trauma. This condition causes the joint to assume a position of flexion to maximize capacity and minimize pressure. Hotchkiss (1995) describes how the uninjured elbow joint has a thin and usually transparent capsule that leaves adequate clearance for full flexion and extension. However, after trauma, the capsule thickens and limits both flexion and extension as a doorstop and a tether (Fig. 15–49A–D). Loss of motion can also occur owing to a fracture that has fallen apart because of failed internal fixation or a persistently dislocated elbow (Jupiter et al., 1985). A static progressive or serial static approach is often used with dense, long-standing contractures.

Weiss and Sachar (1994) address a wide range of elbow PROM problems and describe a loss of terminal extension as a result of olecranon fracture and complete joint ankylosis as a result of high-energy injuries. They describe the unique way the soft tissue structure surrounding the elbow joint responds to trauma.

The medial and lateral collateral ligaments are often injured in elbow fractures and have a propensity toward calcification (Thompson & Garcia, 1967). The brachialis muscle is broad and lies directly on the capsule as it crosses the elbow joint. It is highly vascular, has no tendinous portion at this point, and thus bleeds in response to trauma. Hematoma has been implicated as an inciting cause of heterotopic ossification and subsequent capsular contracture (Glynn & Neibauer, 1976; Husband & Hastings, 1990; Urbaniak, Hansen, Beissinger, & Aitken, 1985). Both the anterior and the posterior capsule often contract. Heterotopic ossification is not amenable to orthotic management.

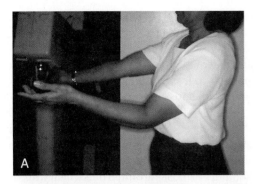

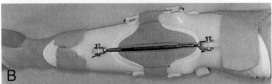

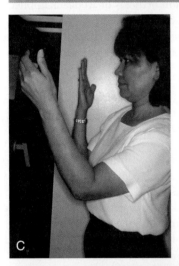

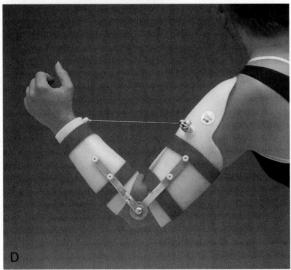

FIGURE 15–49 After trauma, the elbow capsule thickens and limits both flexion and extension. **A,** Note the elbow flexion contracture. **B,** An elbow extension mobilization orthosis using a turnbuckle for static progressive positioning. **C,** Elbow extension contracture. **D,** An elbow flexion mobilization orthosis using the Phoenix elbow hinge and a MERiT™ component to exert a static progressive force.

Ectopic ossification about the elbow can result from various local or systemic insults, including direct injury, neural axis trauma, burns, and genetic disorders (Viola & Hasting, 2000). The most common cause of elbow ectopic ossification is direct elbow trauma (Green & McCoy, 1979). Pathologic bone formation at the elbow level forms an unyielding block to motion and is generally not amenable to orthosis management and ROM treatment. As stated earlier, ectopic ossification is a contraindication for a mobilization orthosis.

Rheumatic disease at the elbow can affect the synovial lining at both the humeroradioulnar joint and the PRUJ. Pain encourages the patient to position the arm in flexion and pronation, which can lead to contracture caused by prolonged positioning (Beasley, 2011; Melvin, 1989). A conservative approach using a serial static orthosis at comfortable end range and soft orthoses that limit flexion during sleep may help minimize flexion contractures (Fig. 15–6D) (Beasley, 2011; D. Stanley, 2011). Prevention of deformity provides the best results.

Morrey (1965) proposed a classification system for posttraumatic elbow stiffness that helps plan treatment and influences prognosis. Morrey (1965) categorizes stiffness as caused either by intrinsic factors (intra-articular adhesions) or extrinsic factors (capsular contractures). In addition, stiffness may have a mixed origin, which is associated with increased morbidity.

Shoulder Joint

Like the wrist, the shoulder is a complex joint made up of several articulations: glenohumeral joint, acromioclavicular joint, scapulothoracic joint, and sternoclavicular joint. According to Copeland (1997), trauma is the primary cause of shoulder stiffness with osteoarthritis, and rheumatoid arthritis is a close second. Other rarer inflammatory arthropathies can contribute to shoulder motion problems. Soft tissue inflammation, especially rotator cuff tendonitis with impingement and subacromial bursitis, may result in permanent motion loss.

Common extrinsic factors related to regaining shoulder motion are the health and balance of the cervical and thoracic spine and rib cage; these complexes cannot be ignored when working with shoulder motion loss. Compromise of brachial plexus function often affects shoulder movement. Clinical experience shows that myofascial dysfunction affects shoulder complex motion more frequently than any other upper extremity joint. Shoulder stiffness has some causes unique to the glenohumeral complex. Primary frozen shoulder, or adhesive capsulitis, has no known cause. Copeland (1997) emphasizes the need for a general systemic assessment as part of the comprehensive shoulder stiffness examination to rule out contributions from remote sites, including Pancoast tumor, myocardial infarction, esophagitis, subphrenic abscess, cholecystitis, and gastric ulcer. Shoulder PROM loss may also result from shoulder immobilization. This immobilization may occur as treatment for primary shoulder pathology or may happen as the result of sling immobilization or self-treatment during recovery from injury to

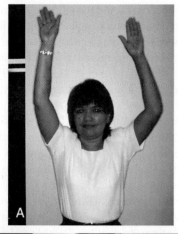

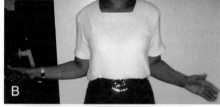

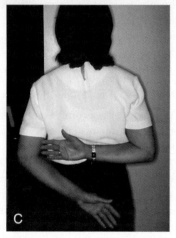

FIGURE 15–50 Capsular pattern in the patient's left shoulder after sling immobilization with loss of elevation (**A**), external rotation (**B**), and internal rotation (**C**).

the distal joints. Copeland (1997) notes that of all the upper extremity joints, the shoulder most frequently responds to decreased movement with rapid onset of stiffness.

The shoulder demonstrates patterns of motion limitation. Impingement syndrome usually results in loss of elevation, abduction, and horizontal abduction. Cyriax (1978) described the capsular pattern, with loss of elevation and external rotation greater than internal rotation. The clinician frequently encounters this capsular pattern after sling immobilization (Fig. 15–50).

Because shoulder orthoses are often bulky, heavy, and difficult to fabricate and fit, clinicians and patients rarely chose a shoulder orthosis as the first line of treatment. Because a large shoulder orthosis renders the entire extremity nonfunctional, compliance is predictably poor. The diagnosis of axillary burn and rotator cuff repair are notable exceptions, and the shoulder abduction orthosis or wedge is applied at the earliest possible moment. Compliance in such instances improves significantly because of the acuity of the problem and prophylactic nature of the device.

Conclusion

The stiff joint continues to be one of the great challenges in hand surgery and rehabilitation. With unique anatomy, each joint presents its patterns of response to injury and disease. Understanding the tendencies for a joint to respond to trauma and disease in a certain way helps the therapist predict problems with stiffness and often provides the opportunity to prevent loss of motion. To work toward the goals of either preventing stiffness or minimizing the duration of stiffness, therapists must continue to study the nature of stiffness at the molecular, histologic, and joint complex levels.

CASE STUDY
S E C T I O N

The case studies presented here are meant as a teaching guideline only. Treatment and orthosis protocols vary greatly from surgeon to surgeon and from therapist to therapist. The therapist should check with the referring physicians and colleagues to define the preferred treatment and appropriate orthotic intervention.

CASE STUDY 1: Hand Crush Injury

MM is a 27-year-old right-dominant male baker who sustained a crush injury to his right hand when it went into a baguette-making machine. His index finger (IF) and middle finger (MF) were crushed up to the proximal phalanx and his thumb was crushed up to the CMC joint. His ring and small fingers were generally unaffected. He had small superficial lacerations on the affected fingers and thumb that were healing well.

He was referred 10 days postinjury with a diagnosis of right crush injury with MF and thumb distal phalanx tuft fractures and a chip fracture of the MF middle phalanx. He presented with moderate edema and hematoma under the nails of the IF, MF, and thumb. He was generally hypersensitive and unwilling to move his hand, apparently owing to pain. His hand postured with his affected fingers in MCP extension, PIP flexion, and DIP in neutral. His thumb MP postured in hyperflexion with the IP joint in slight hyperextension. This thumb posture suggested an undiagnosed soft tissue injury at his thumb MP joint that would affect active and passive MP extension. This concern was shared with the treating physician and patient. A subsequent radiograph revealed a mild subluxation of the thumb MP joint, confirming the diagnosis of a grade 2 to 3 sprain and extensor mechanism compromise.

The therapist discussed the treatment priorities with MM and the rationale for them. MM was told that most physicians and patients prioritize regaining finger IP flexion. However, the therapist's clinical experience supported prioritizing extension. The patient did demonstrate FDP function, and so prognosis for gaining flexion was excellent. MM learned that if the extensor mechanism was left attenuated over the flexed IP joint, it would almost certainly be permanently lengthened and would never be able to provide full extension again. This would sentence MM to lifelong PIP flexion contractures. MM agreed to the plan.

MM's initial orthosis focused on providing a safe position, with the finger MCPs in maximum tolerable flexion and the IPs in maximum tolerable extension (Fig. 15–51). The thumb was placed in maximum tolerable abduction with the MP in maximum tolerable extension and the IP neutral. The patient received a custom, volar, hand-based orthosis made of ⅛" combination rubber and plastic material. This type of thermoplastic provides a rigid orthosis owing to its plastic content while allowing for easier modification because of the rubber content. In conjunction with his orthosis program, the patient was provided with a comprehensive home program of edema control, gentle ROM to the fingers and thumb IP, and

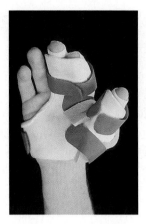

FIGURE 15–51 Hand-based IF, MF, and thumb immobilization orthosis in the safe position.

desensitization. The orthosis was progressed at each subsequent treatment session to achieve the goal of 75° finger MCP flexion, 0° IP extension, 50° thumb abduction, and 0° thumb MP extension. He rapidly achieved his finger MCP flexion and thumb abduction goals. He progressed in finger PIP and thumb MP extension.

Once the diagnosis of thumb soft tissue injury was confirmed, the patient was placed in a circumferential, hand-based thumb orthosis made of 1" QuickCast 2 tape without a liner to allow MM to bathe and wash his hands (Fig. 15–52). When fabricating such a cast without a liner, extreme care must be taken to keep all parts of the cast smooth and all edges trimmed or folded back on themselves.

For the PIPs, MM received custom gutter orthoses fabricated of ¹⁄₁₆" thermoplastic with a 1" strap directly over the PIPs (Fig. 15–52). The contours of the gutter orthoses were straight volarly at the PIP, and the patient was instructed to tighten the loop strap gradually until the finger met the orthosis. The patient was also provided with a prefabricated PIP extension mobilization orthosis to be used intermittently as tolerated (Fig. 15–53). MM achieved neutral PIPs 1 week after receiving the new PIP orthosis regimen. It is important to note that during the 7 to

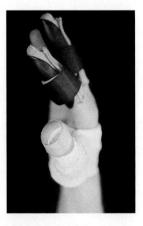

FIGURE 15–52 Hand-based QuickCast 2 thumb cast and with custom gutter orthoses and 1" strap directly over the PIP joints.

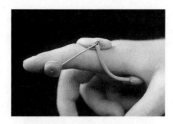

FIGURE 15–53 Prefabricated PIP extension mobilization orthosis. The dynamic force is applied through the spring-loaded design of this orthosis. The patient was taught how to adjust the tension.

10 days of therapy, MM would not have tolerated the extension forces he was able to tolerate when switched to the gutter/spring orthosis combination.

After achieving neutral extension at the PIPs, the patient received a flexion glove (Fig. 15–54). The therapist replaced the rubber bands with static line to allow MM to use a static progressive approach to stretch composite flexion of the fingers. MM was instructed to focus on flexion but to return to the gutter

orthoses intermittently if he began to lose extension; 2 days later, the patient had increased his flexion by 40° at the PIPs. He could still extend fully.

The thumb cast was changed every other day until the MP reached neutral, for a total of three casts. It should be noted that significant pressure had to be applied to achieve maximum thumb MP extension. Initially, the patient would not have tolerated this degree of force. It should also be noted that after application of each thumb cast, the thumb tip turned a deep red. The patient was asked to remain in the clinic until the color normalized, which it did for every cast.

MM was then placed in a final QuickCast 2 thumb cast that included a rigid dorsal stay made of QuickCast 2; it positioned the thumb MP in anatomical neutral. This orthosis remained in place for 6 weeks, at which time the thumb extensor mechanism was evaluated for competence and a radiograph was taken to confirm anatomical alignment..

Additional case studies can be found on the companion web site on thePoint.

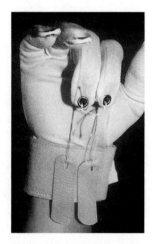

FIGURE 15–54 Static lines provide a static progressive approach to composite flexion of the fingers. Commercially purchased flexion gloves come packaged with rubber bands; however, static line can easily be substituted.

Chapter Review Questions

1. Describe three reasons why the upper extremity may become stiff.

2. Give one example of a diagnosis with the most appropriate mobilization orthosis choice and the rationale for use.

3. Briefly describe casting motion to mobilize stiffness (CMMS) and offer an example of when a clinician would consider this treatment.

4. Give an example of three types of different mobilization orthoses (offer an appropriate diagnosis for each type of device).

5. Describe what low-load, prolonged stress (LLPS) is and why this is important clinically.

Fractures

Jennifer Stephens Chisar, MS, PT, CHT
Nancy Chee, OTR/L, CHT*

Chapter Objectives

After study of this chapter, the reader should be able to:

- Describe the upper extremity fractures hand therapists commonly treat.
- Understand the importance of properly positioning joints acutely to prevent contractures often seen in the later healing stages.
- Appreciate the issues and complications related to fracture management of the nonoperative and postoperative patient.

- Give examples and indications for the various materials and closure systems used to fabricate fractures orthoses.
- Understand the options and design choices for managing this population.

Key Terms

Barton's fracture
Bennett's fracture
Boxer's fracture
Chauffeur's fracture
Colles' fracture
Distal radius fractures
Essex-Lopresti injuries

Galeazzi fracture
Gamekeeper's thumb
Humeral fractures
Metacarpal fractures
Monteggia fracture
Phalanx fractures
Pilon fractures

PIP joint fractures or dislocations
Radial head fractures
Rolando's fracture
Scaphoid fractures
Skier's thumb
Smith's fracture
Terrible triad

Introduction

The use of an orthotic device can play an important role in the aftercare of an acute fracture by providing protection, proper positioning to prevent deformities, and patient comfort during the healing process. In recent years, the increased use of open reduction and internal fixation (ORIF) techniques to address upper extremity fractures has changed the timing and duration of orthotic application, but the aforementioned goals remain the same. The proper application of an orthosis during the initial fracture healing phase protects the fracture while allowing at least partial mobility of adjacent structures. Typical conservative practice for fractures is to immobilize the joints proximal and distal to the involved bone. In some situations, a fracture brace may replace traditional

*This chapter is based on the first edition chapter written by Kristina E. Maniello, MS, OTR/L, CHT

cast immobilization. The materials used in custom and prefabricated upper extremity orthoses are usually lighter in weight than those used with casting, promoting patient comfort. Additionally, the low-temperature thermoplastic materials used for custom devices can conform around small areas of the upper extremity, such as the metacarpals (MCs), and be easily modified to maintain proper fit as edema resolves or healing progresses, requiring less restriction in motion.

This chapter reviews the use of orthoses in the intervention of acute upper extremity fractures sequentially, from the shoulder complex through to the distal phalanx. Tables present a quick reference of recommended styles of orthoses for the types of fractures discussed. The devices, joint positioning, and timeline recommendations outlined in this chapter are meant as general guidelines only. Each fracture is unique, and therapeutic intervention must be individualized according to the clinical presentation and healing of each patient. However, a given fracture is described or classified by the physician; when it comes to the therapist's orthotic intervention and rehabilitation strategies, the most important elements to ascertain from the treating physician are the following:

1. Is the fracture extra-articular or intra-articular?
2. Is the fracture stable or unstable?
3. Are the surrounding joints stable or unstable?
4. After reduction or surgical intervention, was the anatomy restored?

Fracture Description and Treatment

Fractures are generally described by the anatomical location (base, neck, or shaft) and the direction of the break line (longitudinal, transverse, or spiral) (Fig. 16–1). They are further categorized by whether they are linear (two fragments) or comminuted (several fragments) (Fig. 16–2) and open (tissue disrupted; fragment exposed to environment) or closed (soft tissue intact) (Harkess & Ramsey, 1991). Table 16–1 highlights definitions of other frequently used fracture terms.

The treatment of fractures includes a closed, immobilization approach, which involves manipulation of the bone fragments to reduce the fracture, followed by casting, traction, or use of an orthosis to hold the bones in the corrected position. Traditional methods immobilize the joints proximal and distal to the fracture site. Functional fracture bracing immobilizes the fracture site only (Latta, Peng, Sarmiento, & Tarr, 1980). The physician directs the type of immobilization method to be used. Operative treatment is performed when closed reduction efforts are unsuccessful or may be the primary method of treatment for some types of fractures based on outcome evidence in the medical literature. Surgical techniques for fracture management include external fixation, percutaneous pinning, tension bands, and plate and screw fixation (Schutz & Ruedi, 2010).

Scapula Fractures

Scapula fractures occur infrequently, accounting for only 1% of fractures (Lapner, Uhthoff, & Papp, 2008). This is likely due to the fact that the scapula is well protected because

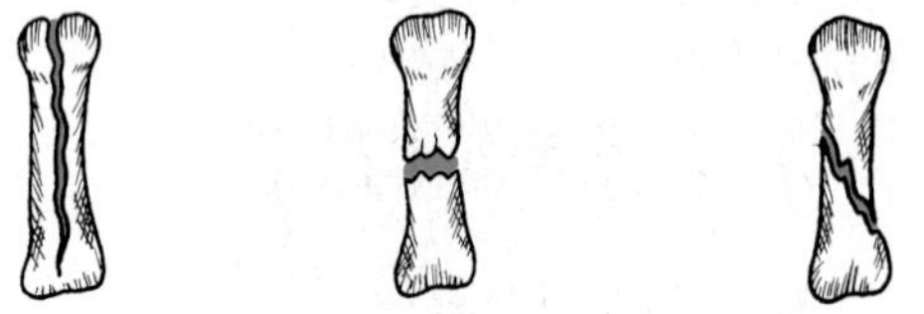

Longitudinal fracture   Transverse fracture   Spiral fracture

FIGURE 16–1 Fractures can be classified by the direction of the fracture.

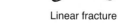

Linear fracture   Comminuted fracture

FIGURE 16–2 Linear fractures produce two fragments; comminuted fractures produce more than two fragments.

TABLE 16–1

Common Upper Extremity Fracture Definitions

Fracture	Definition
Avulsion	Occurs when a tendon or ligament attachment tears away from the bone with a fragment attached
Comminuted	More than two bone fragments result
Complicated	May involve injury to nerves, arteries, viscera, or other soft tissue
Compound	Associated with an open wound; susceptible to infection if not properly treated
Greenstick	Impacted or buckling from bony cortex; associated with the pediatric population
Osteochondral	Involves the articular cartilage of the bone

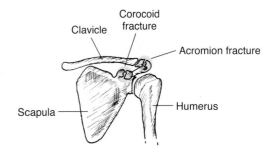

FIGURE 16–4 Fractures of the acromion and coracoid process.

it is enveloped by muscles and is in close proximity to the rib cage (Fig. 16–3). The scapula body is fractured mainly in cases of direct, high-energy trauma such as with motor vehicle accidents and falls from elevation. Acromion and coracoid fractures are usually isolated injuries caused by a direct blow to the area (Fig. 16–4). Often, scapula fractures can be managed nonoperatively and heal without complication (Jeong & Zuckerman, 2005). A systematic review by Zlowodzki, Bhandari, Zelle, Kregor, and Cole (2006) concluded that 99% of isolated scapula body fractures were treated nonoperatively with 106 or 123 achieving good to excellent results. Surgical intervention is indicated for displaced glenoid, neck, and body fractures (Jeong & Zuckerman, 2005).

Standard management of scapula fractures includes ice and immobilization of the shoulder for 3 to 4 weeks with a sling or sling and swathe (Fig. 16–5) (McKoy, Bensen, & Hartsock, 2000). The patient should be instructed in donning the sling, positioning the strap across the lateral aspect of the contralateral clavicle to avoid undue stress across the neck. The involved shoulder girdle should rest as close to anatomical position as tolerated to limit scapular protraction. Education regarding edema control, activity limitations, and range of motion (ROM) exercises for the uninvolved distal joints to prevent contracture is indicated initially postinjury. As pain subsides, pendulum exercises, progressive ROM for the shoulder, and pulley exercises are introduced as tolerated. Strengthening exercises are deferred until the fracture is healed at approximately 6 weeks (Barei, Taitsman, & Nork, 2006).

Fractures of the Clavicle

The clavicle serves as a strut between the shoulder girdle and the axial skeleton, provides attachment for several muscles of the shoulder girdle, and protects the brachial plexus and subclavian vessels as they enter the upper extremity. The ends of the clavicle are held firmly in place to the adjacent sternum and acromion by the sternoclavicular and the acromioclavicular ligaments, respectively. The sternoclavicular joint is further reinforced by the interclavicular and costoclavicular ligaments, whereas the acromioclavicular joint obtains further stability from the coracoclavicular ligament.

Fractures of the clavicle typically occur from a direct fall or blow to the shoulder but may also occur indirectly

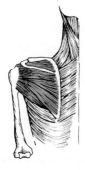

FIGURE 16–3 Scapula fractures are rare, owing to the large number of muscles that surround the bone.

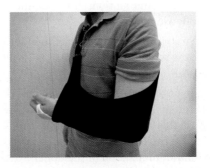

FIGURE 16–5 An arm sling can be used for many diagnoses, including injuries to the scapula, clavicle, humerus, and elbow.

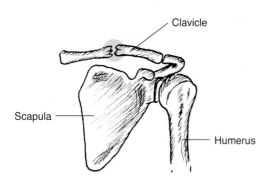

FIGURE 16–6 The middle third of the clavicle is the most common area of the clavicle to be injured.

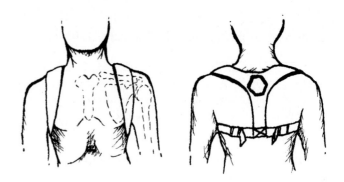

FIGURE 16–7 The Figure-8 strap places the shoulder in a retracted and upright position.

from a fall onto an outstretched hand (Kubiak, Koval, & Zuckerman, 2005). The bending and torsional forces transmitted through the clavicle are highest in the midportion of the diaphysis, making this region the most susceptible to injury (Fig. 16–6) (Preston & Egol, 2009). Displacement is also common in midclavicle fractures due to the unopposed pull of the sternocleidomastoid muscle, which draws the medial fragment superiorly while the weight of the arm displaces the lateral fragment inferiorly. A prominence and/or skin tenting may result.

Historically, clavicular fractures have been described by the classification system introduced by Allman in 1967 and expanded upon by Neer in 1968. Allman's system divided fractures into three groups:

- *Group 1*: midshaft fractures
- *Group 2*: lateral third fractures
- *Group 3*: medial third fractures

In 1968, Neer further classified group 2 fractures into stable or undisplaced fractures (type 1) and displaced fractures (type 2). Type 2 fractures were subdivided according to the coracoclavicular ligaments being (1) intact or (2) disrupted (Allman, 1967; Neer, 1968).

More recently, the "Edinburgh system" has appeared in the literature and been used in outcome studies (Robinson, 1998). This system serves to describe clavicular fractures by four characteristics: anatomical location, whether there is articular involvement, whether there is displacement, and whether there is comminution. This classification system defines the following types:

- *Type 1*: fractures are the medial fifth of the clavicle
- *Type 2*: the middle three-fifths
- *Type 3*: the lateral fifth of the clavicle

Each type have further subdivisions according to the other characteristics noted earlier. Note how the numerical designations in this system differ from Allman's.

Most clavicle fractures continue to be managed nonoperatively with immobilization of the upper extremity. ORIF may be indicated in situations of neurovascular compromise, or to restore anatomy with significantly displaced,

comminuted, or angulated bone fragments (Preston & Egol, 2009).

Immobilization options for patients with a clavicle fracture are a sling, a sling and swathe, or a Figure-8 strap (Figs. 16–5 and 16–7). The Figure-8 strap, sometimes recommended for midshaft fractures, requires patient education in properly positioning and adjusting the strap tension as edema resolves. If the straps are too tight, discomfort and compression of the neurovascular structures in the axilla or skin irritation may result. The broad arm sling is appropriate for all types of clavicle fractures when used alone or in conjunction with a Figure-8 strap. Andersen, Jensen, and Lauritzen (1987) compared the use of the Figure-8 bandage versus a sling and concluded the sling was more comfortable with fewer clinical complications. A more recent literature review concluded that there is insufficient evidence to determine which conservative method is most effective (Lenza, Belloti, Andriolo, Gomes Dos Santos, & Faloppa, 2009).

Immobilization is typically full time for 2 weeks then weaned over 2 to 6 weeks postinjury as guided by pain, clinical presentation, and physician preference. ROM of the uninvolved joints is begun immediately with passive shoulder motion beginning as pain allows, 7 to 14 days postinjury. Shoulder flexion should be limited to 90° initially to minimize rotation of the clavicle, which may stress the healing fracture site (Kubiak et al., 2005).

Humeral Fractures

The humerus is a long bone that articulates with the glenoid fossa of the scapula proximally and the trochlear notch of the ulna and radial head of the radius distally, connecting the shoulder girdle with the forearm. **Humeral fractures** are caused by various insults including, but not limited to, falls, motor vehicle accidents, gunshot wounds, or other direct trauma to the humerus (Biangini, 1991; Tejwani & Metha, 2007). Commonly fractured sites of the humerus are the surgical neck, greater and lesser tuberosities, anatomical neck, humeral shaft, and distal humerus about the condyles (Fig. 16–8) (Beredjiklian, 2011; Brown, 1983).

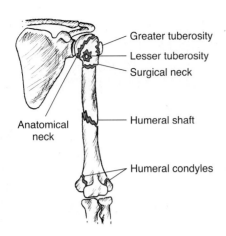

FIGURE 16-8 Areas of the humerus susceptible to fracture.

Proximal fractures—involving the surgical neck, humeral head, or greater or lesser tuberosities—that are stable may be managed with a sling or sling and swathe (Fig. 16–5) (McKoy et al., 2000). Humerus shaft fractures may be successfully managed conservatively using a functional humeral fracture orthosis or brace (Fig. 16–9) (Sarmiento, Horowitch, Aboulafia, & Vangsness, 1990; Sarmiento, Zagorski, Zych, Latta, & Capps, 2000). As a singular long bone, enveloped by soft tissue, the humeral shaft is ideal for fracture bracing. The functional brace design is a circumferential orthosis that works by soft tissue compression of the fracture while restricting movement of the bony fragments, even when the muscles are actively contracting. The pressure from the orthosis stabilizes the fracture, and the gravity-assisted weight of the arm can help reduce minor angulation deformities (Sarmiento, et al., 2000; Sarmiento & Latte, 1999, 2006). Fracture braces are available commercially or can be cus-

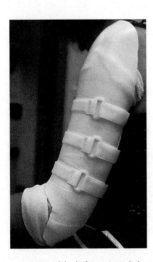

FIGURE 16-9 A custom-molded functional humeral brace (nonarticular humeral orthosis) that allows partial shoulder and elbow ROM. Notice the use of D-rings to allow adjustments to the amount of compression.

tom fabricated by the therapist. The primary benefit of this nonarticular orthotic intervention is the freedom of motion afforded to the adjacent joints, whereas slings or casts usually immobilize the joints proximal and distal to the fracture site (Beredjiklian, 2011; Sarmiento, Kinman, Galvin, Schmitt, & Phillips, 1977). Patients should be instructed in proper donning of the fracture brace for skin care and hygiene. Leaning on the elbow is discouraged during healing because this may contribute to fracture angulation (Sarmiento et al., 2000). Shoulder pendulum exercises and ROM for elbow, forearm, wrist, and hand are initiated as early as safely possible to maximize motion without compromising the stability of the fracture.

Patients with humeral shaft fractures may have an associated radial nerve injury because the nerve wraps around the humerus in the spiral groove at this level. In cases where the radial nerve has been lacerated or tractioned, additional orthotic intervention should be provided to support the wrist and digits (refer to Chapter 19, Peripheral Nerve Injuries for further details). This provides improved patient comfort, positions the hand for light activities of daily living (ADLs), and prevents elongation of the extensors and shortening of the flexors. Depending on the needs of the patient, a wrist immobilization orthosis may be adequate initially and progressed to a tenodesis or a forearm-based dynamic digit extension orthosis.

Functional fracture bracing has also been found to be effective for distal humerus fractures. Sarmiento et al. (1990, 2006) demonstrated a 96% union rate in a study performed on 85 patients with extra-articular comminuted fractures. For these fractures, the humeral cuff may be extended distally and molded around the lateral and medial condyles for additional support. In some cases, the addition of a circumferential forearm cuff attached with a hinge device may be desired to reduce varus and valgus forces at the elbow (Fig. 16–10A) (Beredjiklian, 2011; Colditz, 2011). Careful attention must be paid to align the hinge with elbow axis of rotation.

Orthotic intervention for humeral head and shaft fractures managed surgically may include the use of a sling or functional fracture bracing. Distal humeral fractures managed surgically may be supported and protected by use of a sling, a posterior elbow immobilization orthosis, (Fig. 16–11), a humeral fracture brace with or without a hinge (Fig. 16–10A), or a prefabricated hinged elbow orthoses (Fig. 16–10B). Table 16–2 summarizes management of fractures in the shoulder region.

Elbow Fractures

The elbow joint is inherently stable due to its bony anatomy and design. The articulations of the humeroulnar, humeroradial, and proximal radioulnar joints provide stability with additional support from the joint capsule, annular, and collateral ligaments. One of the complexities in rehabilitation of the elbow is that all three of these articulations are within

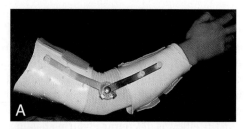

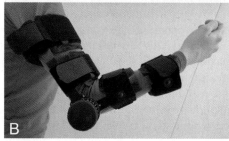

FIGURE 16–10 **A,** An elbow restriction orthosis using the Phoenix elbow hinge that permits protected elbow ROM. Note that the hinge is set to restrict elbow extension while allowing full flexion. **B,** A prefabricated elbow restriction hinge orthosis allowing for a selected arc of motion while restricting varus and valgus forces during fracture healing (shown is the Mayo Clinic Elbow Brace available from DJO Global, Vista, CA).

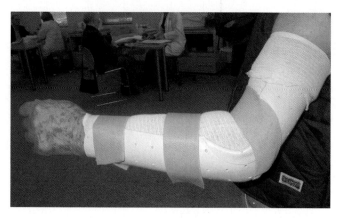

FIGURE 16–11 A posterior elbow immobilization orthosis; notice the rolling away of material about the lateral epicondyle region.

a single joint capsule. Early motion following elbow fractures is always a goal because prolonged immobilization can result in fibrosis and limit ROM in any or all of these articulations (Davila, 2011). When freely mobile, the combined actions of these joints allow for effective placement of the hand for function with elbow flexion and extension and forearm pronation and supination without movement of the shoulder.

A fall on an outstretched hand (FOOSH) with the elbow partially flexed and pronated can result in a **radial head fracture** because the radial head absorbs as much as 60% of the axial load transmitted through the elbow (Ring & Jupiter, 1998a). These injuries account for 33% of all elbow fractures (Beredjiklian, 2011; Tejwani & Metha, 2007; Van Riet, Van Glabbeck, & Morrey, 2009). Radial head fractures are divided into three types:

- *Type 1*: small fragment that does not interfere with ROM (Fig. 16–12)

TABLE 16–2

Management of Shoulder Girdle, Clavicle, and Humeral Fractures[a]

Fracture	Orthosis Options	Time Frame
Shoulder girdle		
Scapula	• Arm sling, sling and swathe	3–4 weeks
Clavicle		
Midshaft	• Figure-8 strap, arm sling, sling and swathe	2 weeks full time, wean as pain resolves until healed at 6–8 weeks
Lateral	• Arm sling, sling and swathe	2–6 weeks, wean as pain resolves until healed
Humerus		
Surgical neck or greater tuberosity	• Sling, humeral fracture brace with proximal extension	Variable depending on healing
Shaft	• Humeral fracture brace with or without sling	6+ weeks until healed
Distal	• Humeral fracture brace with or without elbow hinge, arm sling, posterior elbow and wrist immobilization orthosis, hinged elbow orthosis	Dependent on healing

[a]Note that the orthosis options and time frames depend on the individual patient. Obtain clear orders from the referring physician before providing the patient with any therapy intervention.

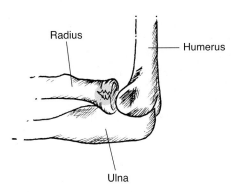

FIGURE 16–12 Type 1 radial head fracture.

- *Type 2*: fragment with greater than 2 mm of displacement that may result in limitations of movement
- *Type 3*: severely comminuted radial head or neck fractures (Adams & Steinmann, 2009; Ring & Jupiter, 1998a, 1998b)

Type 1 fractures can be managed conservatively with reduction under anesthesia and protected by use of a sling (Fig. 16–5), hinged elbow orthosis (Fig. 16–10), or posterior elbow immobilization orthosis (Fig. 16–11). Early ROM should be initiated (Bano & Kahlon, 2006). Type 2 and 3 fractures require surgical fixation to achieve articular congruity and stability to the joint.

Radial head fractures may be further complicated by a concurrent coronoid fracture and dislocation of the humeroulnar joint, known as the "**terrible triad**" (Seijas et al., 2009). Following surgical reduction, fixation, and stabilization, a posterior elbow and wrist immobilization orthosis with the elbow in 80 to 90° flexion and the wrist in neutral is applied (Fig. 16–13). The position of the forearm will be according to the reconstruction performed at the elbow: pronation when the lateral collateral ligament (LCL) is repaired, supination when the medial collateral ligament (MCL) is repaired, and neutral rotation if both ligaments are repaired (Pipicelli, Chinchalkar, Grewal, & Athwal, 2011). Carefully supervised early ROM exercises may be performed, maintaining the appropriate forearm positioning.

Olecranon fractures account for 10% of elbow fractures and often occur from a direct impact to the posterior elbow, from direct high energy loading of the joint from a fall, or from forceful hyperextension of the elbow (Adams & Steinmann, 2009). Although not as common, a fall on a partially flexed elbow may avulse the triceps tendon from the olecranon with a bony fragment (Fig. 16–14A), affecting the dynamic stability of the elbow (Adams & Steinmann, 2009; Ring & Jupiter, 1998b). When applying an orthosis to the elbow after an olecranon avulsion fracture, the therapist must appreciate the degree of elbow flexion in relation to the tension on the triceps repair. Positioning the elbow in more extension places less tension on the healing structures (Fig. 16–14B).

Although literature presents limited information on orthotic intervention for fractures of the elbow, goals for are the same as for other fractures: to protect healing structures, to maintain stability, and to encourage protected mobility and optimal healing with minimal residual stiffness or

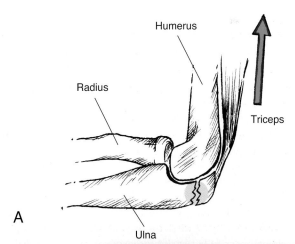

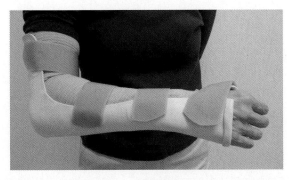

FIGURE 16–13 A posterior elbow/wrist immobilization orthosis is often used after radial head injuries and repairs. The wrist is included to restrict forearm rotation.

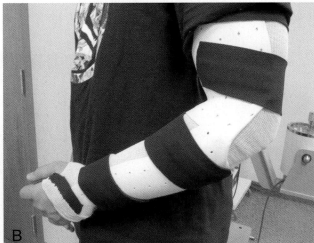

FIGURE 16–14 **A,** With an olecranon avulsion fracture, the triceps tendon pulls proximally with a fragment of bone. **B,** Inclusion of the wrist in an elbow orthosis may be needed to restrict forearm rotation and for the comfort of the patient. Notice the anterior/posterior design in this orthosis to unload pressure at the fracture site.

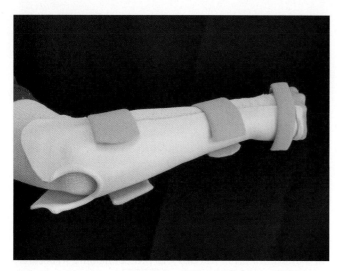

FIGURE 16–15 A Muenster-style orthosis supports the wrist and forearm and extends around the medial and lateral epicondyles of the humerus, allowing for elbow flexion and extension but limiting forearm rotation.

contractures (Davila, 2011). Initially, a sling or orthosis is applied to protect the elbow, whether managed conservatively or surgically. Slings may be applied for type 1 radial head injuries with early ROM indicated once cleared by a physician (Fig. 16–5). A posterior elbow immobilization orthosis may be fabricated for immobilization and protection of a stable reduced fracture or after surgical repair (Figs. 16–11 and 16–13). When early mobility is indicated, orthoses allowing for controlled elbow flexion and extension and restricted supination and pronation such as a Muenster (Fig. 16–15), sugar tong (Fig. 16–16A,B), or prefabricated hinged elbow brace (Fig. 16–10B) may be used. Therapists should be aware that neither the sugar tong nor the Muenster-style orthoses fully restrict forearm rotation. A study by Slaughter, Miles, Fleming, and McPhail (2010) suggests that

if the patient is cued to respect sensory feedback provided by the orthosis, then an arc of approximately 31° rotation is available. However, if the patient is not compliant and forces to the limits of the orthosis, significantly more rotation can be achieved: 71° for the sugar tong and 92° for the Muenster-style orthoses. Table 16–3 summarizes orthotic management of fractures in the elbow region.

Forearm Fractures

Fractures in the forearm include isolated and concurrent fractures of the radius and ulna and more complex injuries with associated dislocations of the proximal or distal radio-ulnar joints (DRUJs). Singular ulna shaft fractures usually result from a direct blow to the forearm, for example, when the arm is raised to protect one's head or face from an attack or falling object. In cases where displacement is less than 50% of the width of the bone and angulation is less than 10°, cast immobilization or functional forearm fracture bracing is indicated (Fig. 16–17) (Chow & Leung, 2010; Osterman, Ekkernkamp, Henry, & Muhr, 1994). This concept is similar to functional humeral fracture bracing previously described. A circumferential custom or prefabricated orthosis is fit over the fracture site, placing pressure along the interosseous membrane to provide soft tissue compression between the radius and ulna. This will effectively limit end range supination and pronation but allow free forearm rotation through the midrange and early motion of the uninvolved joints. The brace is used full time until fracture healing is noted on x-ray at approximately 8 to 10 weeks. Research suggests functional fracture bracing provides greater patient satisfaction, earlier return to work, and improved ROM over immobilization in a long arm cast for these injuries (Gebuhr et al., 1992; Latta et al, 1980; Sarmiento & Latta, 2006; Sarmiento, Latta, Zych, McKeever, & Zagorski, 1998).

Fractures of both bones often result from a motor vehicle accident, direct blow, gunshot wound, or other high-energy

FIGURE 16–16 **A,** A sugar tong–style orthosis allows for limited elbow flexion and extension while restricting forearm rotation. **B,** This design allows for fluctuation in forearm edema. Notice the use of elasticized stockinette beneath for edema management.

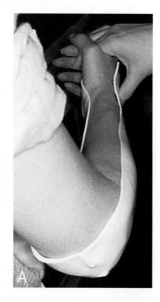

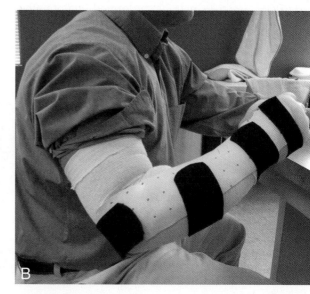

TABLE 16–3

Management of Radius and Ulna Fractures[a]

Fracture	Orthosis Options	Position	Time Frame
Elbow			
Radial head	• Posterior elbow immobilization orthosis	Elbow: 90°; forearm: neutral	2 weeks (removed for exercise)
	• Hinged elbow orthosis, sling	Variable	

"Terrible triad"
 	
LCL repair
MCL repair
LCL & MCL repair
	• Posterior elbow/wrist immobilization orthosis	Elbow: 80–90°; wrist: neutral
		Forearm:
		  Pronated
		  Supinated
		  Neutral
			Depending on healing and joint stability

Olecranon	• Posterior elbow (wrist) immobilization orthosis	Elbow: 45–70°; forearm: neutral	3–4+ weeks depending on bone healing
	• Hinged elbow orthosis	Wrist: neutral if needed	
With triceps avulsion	• Posterior elbow (wrist) immobilization orthosis	Elbow: 40°; forearm: neutral	4+ weeks depending on bone healing
	• Hinged elbow orthosis	Wrist: neutral if needed	
Coronoid	• Posterior elbow immobilization orthosis	Variable depending on associate injuries	2–3 weeks depending on bone healing
	• Hinged elbow orthosis for nonoperative intervention		
Forearm			
Ulna, midshaft	• Posterior elbow immobilization orthosis	Elbow: 90°; forearm: neutral	Variable
	• Forearm fracture brace	Forearm: neutral	
Radius, midshaft	• Posterior elbow immobilization orthosis (after surgical repair)	Elbow: 90°; forearm: neutral	Variable
	• Forearm fracture brace (after surgical repair)		
Galeazzi	• Sugar-tong orthosis	Forearm: neutral	4–6 weeks
	• Posterior elbow/wrist immobilization orthosis or cast	Elbow: 90°; forearm: supinated	
	• Muenster	Forearm: neutral	
Monteggia	• Posterior elbow/wrist immobilization orthosis or cast	Elbow: 70–100°; forearm: neutral	4–6 weeks
Essex-Lopresti	• Posterior elbow/wrist immobilization orthosis	Elbow: 70–90° Forearm: supinated Wrist: neutral	3–4 weeks
Distal radius			
Colles', Smith's, or Barton's	• Long arm then short arm cast	Variable depending on radiograph	2–3 weeks then 2–4 weeks
	• Wrist immobilization orthosis	Wrist: in slight extension unless specified by MD	2–4 weeks after cast removal 3–6 weeks (ORIF)

[a]Note that the orthosis options and time frames depend on the individual patient. Obtain clear orders from the referring physician before providing the patient with any therapy intervention.

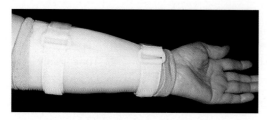

FIGURE 16–17 A custom-fabricated, functional forearm fracture brace indicated for stable, nondisplaced ulna fractures or for additional support following ORIF.

traumatic event (Chow & Leung, 2010; Geissler, Valdes, & Kaiser, 2010). ORIF is the current standard of care. Depending on the alignment achieved and the integrity of the fixation, a cast or orthosis may or may not be required.

Examples of more complex conditions of the forearm that include fractures with associated soft tissue trauma and joint dislocation include Galeazzi, Monteggia, and Essex-Lopresti injuries. A **Galeazzi fracture** (Fig. 16–18) is a fracture of the lower third of the radial shaft, resulting in DRUJ disruption, often caused by a FOOSH with forearm pronation (Ring, 2006). These fractures usually require ORIF to restore forearm and DRUJ stability. An elbow and wrist immobilization orthosis with the forearm in supination (Fig. 16–19) is indicated when DRUJ instability persists postoperatively for 4 to 6 weeks (Giannoulis & Sotereanos, 2007; Ring, 2006). Galeazzi fractures may also be managed with a Muenster (Fig. 16–15) or sugar-tong (Fig. 16–16A,B) orthosis to restrict DRUJ motion but allow early elbow flexion and extension when the DRUJ is pinned and/or stable postoperatively.

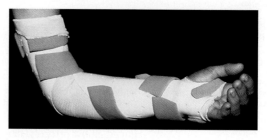

FIGURE 16–19 An elbow/wrist immobilization orthosis made from thermoplastic material to maintain fracture reduction. Note the unique spiral design to facilitate supination positioning. This positioning maybe indicated to promote DRUJ stability in Galeazzi and Essex-Lopresti lesions.

A **Monteggia fracture** (Fig. 16–20) involves the proximal third of the ulna with radial head dislocation caused by high-energy injuries (Earhiraju, Mudgal, & Jupiter, 2007). Dislocation of the radial head may cause traction to the posterior interosseous nerve (PIN), resulting in a concurrent PIN palsy (Chow & Leung, 2010). Monteggia fractures are classified into four types (Bado, 1967; Chow & Leung, 2010; Earhiraju et al., 2007):

- *Type 1*: anterior dislocation of the radial head with anterior angulation of the fracture of the ulna diaphysis
- *Type 2*: posteriolateral dislocation of the radial head with posterior angulation of the fracture of the ulna diaphysis
- *Type 3*: lateral or anterolateral dislocation of the radial head with fracture of the ulna metaphysis
- *Type 4*: anterior dislocation of the radial head with fracture of the proximal third of the radius and ulna

These complex fracture dislocations are managed surgically with the goal of restoring anatomy and forearm stability for immediate motion. Postoperatively, a removable posterior elbow immobilization orthosis is appropriate for protection between ROM exercise sessions (Fig. 16–11).

Essex-Lopresti injuries involve concurrent fractures of the radial head with soft tissue disruption of the interosseous membrane and the DRUJ. Due to the injury to the interosseous membrane and possible forearm instability, they are often clustered with forearm fractures. These high-velocity complex injuries are typically treated surgically and

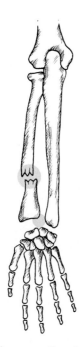

FIGURE 16–18 Galeazzi fractures affect the lower third of the radial shaft, resulting in distal radioulnar disruption.

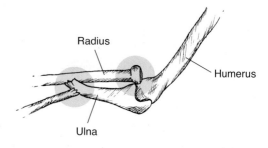

Radius

Humerus

Ulna

FIGURE 16–20 Monteggia fractures affect the proximal third of the ulna, resulting in radial head dislocation. These fractures often require ORIF.

stabilized postoperatively in a long arm cast or posterior elbow and wrist immobilization orthosis in elbow flexion with supination for 3 to 4 weeks (Fig. 16–19) (Chow & Leung, 2010; Dodds, Yen, & Slade, 2008).

Distal Radius Fractures

There is a plethora of published classification systems for **distal radius fractures** documented and used in the literature, including those of Frykman, Melone, the Mayo Clinic, and the Association for Study of Internal Fixation (AO), just to name a few (Fernandez & Wolfe, 2005; Laseter & Carter, 1996; Medoff, 2011). Most of these systems define and group fractures at the distal radius as either extra-articular or intra-articular, and the AO classification system adds a third category of complex articular fractures. Within these categories are additional subsets of the fracture types. The Fernandez classification system classifies injuries according to the mechanism of injury: bending, shearing, compression, avulsion, or combined high-energy injuries (Ilyas & Jupiter, 2010). These classification systems are well described in the medical literature.

In spite of efforts to scientifically classify all fracture patterns of the distal radius, physicians still may opt to note eponyms on prescriptions; thus, it is important for the therapist to be familiar with these common terms. A **Colles' fracture** is a distal radius fracture with dorsal angulation and displacement and radial shortening (Fig. 16–21A). This type of distal radius fracture is frequently sustained by a FOOSH (Fernandez & Wolfe 2005; Laseter & Carter, 1996; Michlovitz & Festa, 2011; Medoff, 2011).

A **Smith's fracture**, also known as a reverse Colles' fracture, is a fracture of the distal radius with volar displacement of the distal fragment and usually results from a fall on the dorsum of the hand (Fig. 16–21B). A **Barton's fracture** is an unstable, displaced intra-articular fracture of the distal radius resulting in subluxation of the carpus, typically sustained from a fall on an extended and pronated wrist (Fig. 16–21C). A **Chauffeur's fracture** is an intra-articular fracture of the radial styloid that may result in displacement of the carpus (Fernandez & Wolfe, 2005).

Conservative treatment via closed reduction and cast immobilization remains a widely accepted option for distal radius fractures. A sugar tong or long arm cast may be applied for a 2- to 3-week period initially and then replaced with a short arm circumferential cast for an additional 2 to 4 weeks. Colles' fractures may be placed in slight wrist flexion and pronation initially to promote reduction of the dorsally angulated fragments, whereas Smith's fractures may be positioned in mild wrist extension and supination (Jiuliano & Jupiter, 2006). In cases where the fracture is determined to be unstable, the duration of a long arm cast may be extended or the patient may require a more invasive intervention for fracture stabilization with percutaneous pinning, placement of an external fixator, or ORIF.

Once the cast is removed, a custom or prefabricated forearm-based wrist immobilization orthosis is appropriate intermittently for 2 to 4 weeks to provide comfort and

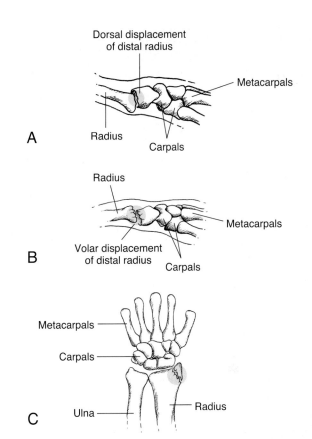

FIGURE 16–21 **A,** Colles' fracture with dorsal displacement. **B,** Smith's fracture with volar displacement. **C,** A Barton's fracture is a displaced, unstable articular fracture.

support with easy donning and doffing as wrist motion and upper extremity function is restored (Fig. 16–22A). The device should allow for full metacarpophalangeal (MCP) motion of the fingers. To enhance wrist stabilization, a dorsal piece can be added to a volar-based orthosis (clamshell), or a circumferential design may be implemented (Fig. 16–22B,C).

Over the past decade, with the improvement in designs of volar plating systems, the use of ORIF has become more common in the management of distal radius fractures (Michlovitz & Festa, 2011). The benefits to this procedure include better restoration of the original bone and joint anatomy and earlier implementation of ROM to the wrist joint (Ruch & McQueen, 2010). Use of a removable custom or prefabricated wrist immobilization orthosis postoperatively allows for early wound care, edema control, ROM exercise, and proper hand hygiene. The orthosis is weaned gradually over 3 to 6 weeks following surgery depending on the patient's pain complaints, clinical presentation, and visible callus formation on x-ray (Fig. 16–22A–C).

Use of external fixation for distal radius fractures is becoming rare. When applied, the external fixator is drilled into the radial shaft and the second MC. Tension across the device results in traction across the fracture and ligamentotaxis (distracting tension on ligaments), bringing the fracture fragments into alignment and preserving the length of the

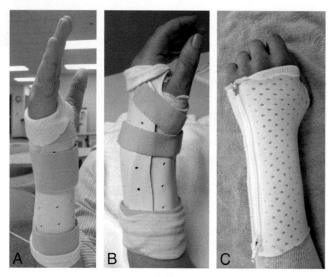

FIGURE 16-22 A, A wrist immobilization orthosis including two-thirds of the length of the forearm for maximal comfort. **B,** A dorsal clamshell piece added to a wrist immobilization orthosis provides stability at the fracture site. The dorsal ½" overlapping piece of thermoplastic material is applied after the volar piece has been fabricated and is fully set. Manual pressure along the edges creates an interlocking groove. **C,** A circumferential design of a wrist immobilization orthosis. This precut zipper design can be effective in promoting compliance with pediatric patients by using a zip tie to "lock" the zipper (shown is the Rolyan® AquaForm™ Zippered Wrist Splint available through Patterson Medical, Warrenville, IL).

radius. Adjustments can be made to the device during the healing process to correct angulation and/or reduction of the bony fragments. A bulky dressing is typically applied postoperatively, which may be replaced by an ulnar-based wrist orthosis for support, protection, and patient comfort (Fig. 16–23). One of the reasons this fixation technique has

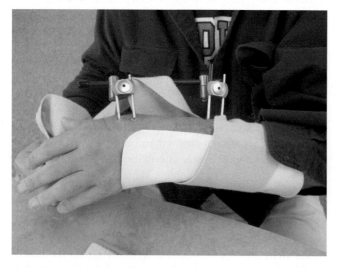

FIGURE 16-23 This ulnar-based immobilization orthosis is held in place with an elasticized wrap and can provide the patient with an external fixator comfort and support.

fallen from favor are the reported complications. Some of these complications include index finger (IF) MCP joint stiffness, first web space contractures, superficial radial nerve irritation or injury, chronic regional pain syndrome, and pin tract infections (Ruch & McQueen, 2010).

Carpal Fractures

The wrist is an intricately balanced structure, consisting of eight small bones bound by multiple ligaments that allow the motions of wrist flexion, extension, ulnar and radial deviation, and intercarpal rotation. Fracturing one of these bones can disrupt wrist kinematics and result in an alteration of wrist stability or mobility impairing hand and upper extremity function.

The most frequently fractured carpal bone is the scaphoid, accounting for 60% to 70% of all carpal fractures and 11% of all hand fractures (Fig. 16–24) (Hove, 1999; Suh, Benson, Faber, MacDermid, & Grewal, 2010). A FOOSH or a high-velocity impact into forced wrist extension with radial or ulnar deviation is common mechanism of injury (Mayfield, 1980; Weber & Chao, 1978). Most **scaphoid fractures** occur through the waist of the bone (75%), followed by the proximal pole (20%) and the tubercle (5%) (Knoll & Trumble, 2006). Due to the vascular anatomy, the blood supply to the proximal pole is more tenuous, resulting in slower healing, requiring longer immobilization when treated conservatively (Adams & Steinmann, 2010). Nonoperative management requires immobilization with a long or short arm thumb spica cast until osseous healing is confirmed, which may take as long as 3 to 6 months. A review of the literature suggests there is insufficient evidence to support which immobilization technique is most effective (Yin, Zhang, Kan, & Wang, 2007).

Indications for surgical intervention include displaced, comminuted, and proximal pole fractures or when diagnosis of the scaphoid fracture has been delayed (Knoll & Trumble, 2006). Conservative and operative treatment options for scaphoid fractures are well represented in the literature; however, it remains unclear which approach is most effective (Suh et al., 2010).

When referred for treatment, a forearm-based wrist and thumb immobilization orthosis may be fabricated for

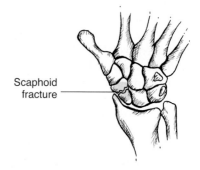

Scaphoid fracture

FIGURE 16-24 Scaphoid fractures are the most common carpal fracture and often occur from a FOOSH.

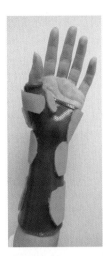

FIGURE 16-25 A wrist/thumb immobilization orthosis with the IP joint free is a management option for scaphoid, trapezium, and Bennett's fractures.

continued protection during healing and remobilization of the wrist and hand (Fig. 16–25). If included initially, the interphalangeal (IP) and MP joints may later be freed for thumb mobility to decrease joint stiffness. A dorsal clamshell piece can be added to a volar orthosis, or a circumferential design may be used to provide further stabilization of the wrist.

The therapist's involvement in managing other carpal bone fractures typically occurs following cast immobilization when remobilization of the wrist is indicated. Most carpal fractures can be managed with a wrist or a wrist and thumb immobilization orthosis for 4 to 6 weeks. Then therapy is directed at controlling residual edema, addressing joint stiffness to increase ROM and progressing upper extremity strength to restore ADL function. Knowing mechanisms of injuries and concurrent injuries associated with fractures of the other carpal bones can be helpful in designing rehabilitation programs.

Lunate fractures can occur acutely from a FOOSH but are more frequently associated with pathologic changes in the bone from avascular necrosis of the lunate known as Kienböck's disease (Dell, Dell, & Griggs, 2011). Cast immobilization is recommended for 4 to 6 weeks for minimally displaced stable fractures, but immobilization may be prolonged if healing is delayed (Papp, 2010). Surgery may be performed if the fracture is unstable or if restoration of the joint congruity is needed. In cases of avascular necrosis, procedures to unload forces transmitted through the lunate such as a radial shortening osteotomy or salvage procedures such as a proximal row carpectomy or wrist arthrodesis may be performed (Dell et al., 2011).

Fractures of the triquetrum may occur from a hyperflexion injury avulsing the dorsal intercarpal or radiocarpal ligament or from a shearing mechanism with wrist flexion and ulnar deviation impingement of the triquetrum between the hamate and distal ulna. These fractures affecting the dorsal ridge are typically stable and can be addressed with wrist

immobilization for 4 to 6 weeks (Dell et al., 2011). Triquetral body fractures are rare but when seen tend to occur with other significant injuries to the carpus such as perilunate dislocations.

Pisiform fractures can result from direct trauma or from forceful avulsion of the flexor carpi ulnaris (FCU). They may be addressed with wrist immobilization for 2 to 4 weeks or with excision of the bone (Dell et al., 2011). Following surgical excision, an orthosis lined with silicone gel may offer protection and support to the hypothenar eminence area.

Trapezium fractures can result from a blow to the abducted thumb or trauma, resulting a forceful wrist extension and radial deviation (Prosser & Herbert, 1996). Stable and minimally displaced fractures can be conservatively addressed with wrist and thumb cast immobilization for 4 to 6 weeks, whereas ORIF is recommended if the fracture is displaced greater than 2 mm to restore the intra-articular anatomy of the first carpometacarpal (CMC) joint (Papp, 2010).

Fractures of the trapezoid bone are rare, resulting from high-velocity trauma that forces the second MC into the trapezoid. Frequently, there is an associated fracture and/or dislocation of the second MC (Brach & Goitz, 2003). Cast immobilization for 4 to 6 weeks is the standard of care.

Fractures of the capitate are caused by an impact to the second and third MCs, with the wrist flexed and radially deviated (Papp, 2010). The therapist should be aware of other associated injuries such as scaphoid fractures, lunotriquetral ligament injuries, or other perilunate dislocations (Seng & Blazar, 2006). Proximal pole fractures are sometimes associated with late onset avascular necrosis. Depending on the nature of the fracture, it may be treated with 4 to 6 weeks of cast immobilization, closed reduction and pinning, or ORIF.

Hook of the hamate fractures is often associated with sports that use a club, bat, or racquet. Injury can occur either from a direct blow, for example when the club is inadvertently driven into the ground, or indirectly from strong muscle contraction while grasping the racquet or bat with wrist in extension and ulnar deviation as the ball makes contact resulting in an avulsion injury. Hamate body fractures may present with concurrent MC base fractures of the ring and little fingers (Dell et al., 2011). Minimally displaced fractures of the hamate (hook or body) can be immobilized with a cast for 4 to 6 weeks, whereas displaced fractures may be addressed with fixation or excision. A wrist immobilization orthosis may be used during the remobilization phase (Fig. 16–22A). In addition to ROM, intervention for scar management and hypersensitivity may be indicated postsurgery. Table 16–4 summarizes orthotic management for carpal fractures.

Metacarpal Fractures

Finger Metacarpal Fractures

Proximally, the MC bones are anchored into the carpal arch by interosseous ligaments with more stability in the index and middle CMC joints and more joint mobility in the ring, small, and thumb CMC joints. MC fractures account for

TABLE 16–4

Carpal Fracture Management[a]

Fracture	Orthosis Options	Position	Time Frame
Scaphoid	• Long to short arm cast • Wrist/thumb immobilization orthosis	Wrist: extension	6+ weeks depending on radiograph
		Thumb: midpalmar/radial abduction	6+ weeks depending on radiograph
Trapezium	• Wrist/thumb immobilization orthosis or cast	Wrist: extension	4–6 weeks
		Thumb: midpalmar/radial abduction	
Trapezoid	• Wrist immobilization orthosis or cast	Wrist: extension	4–6 weeks
Capitate	• Wrist immobilization orthosis or cast	Wrist: extension	4–6+ weeks (may be prolonged depending on radiograph)
Hamate			
Hook excision	• Soft orthosis (after excision, if needed)		
Body/hook conservative	• Wrist immobilization orthosis or cast	Wrist: extension	4–6+ weeks (depending on radiograph)
Triquetrum	• Wrist immobilization orthosis or cast	Wrist: extension	4–6 weeks
Pisiform	• Wrist immobilization orthosis	Wrist: neutral	2–4 weeks
Excision	• Soft orthosis as needed		
Lunate	• Wrist immobilization orthosis or cast		4–6+ weeks may be prolonged depending on radiograph

[a]Note that the orthosis options and time frames depend on the individual patient. Obtain clear orders from the referring physician before providing the patient with any therapy intervention.

40% of hand fractures and are classified according to their anatomical location: base, shaft, neck, or head (Markiewitz, 2003). Metacarpal base fractures may be associated with carpal fractures and occur from direct axial loading. These fractures can be either intra-articular or extra-articular but tend to be stable. Base extra-articular fractures are frequently managed with closed reduction and acute MC fracture bracing. Intra-articular fractures, like a reversed Bennett's fracture with dislocation at the fifth MC and hamate joint, may require surgical repair due to forces of the FCU and extensor carpi ulnaris (ECU) tendon on the ulnar portion of the small finger MC (Gallagher & Blackmore, 2011; Markiewitz, 2003).

Metacarpal shaft fractures appear as transverse, oblique, or spiral and occur with axial loading through the MC or by direct blows onto the dorsum of the hand. Transverse fractures may result in dorsal angulations at the fracture apex due to forces from the volar interosseous muscles. This angulation may leave an aesthetically unpleasing "bump" but is rarely functionally disabling (Jones, 1996). Oblique and spiral fractures may be affected by rotational torsion forces

on the MC leading to rotational deformities with overlap or scissoring of digits with finger flexion. These may require closed reduction with pinning or ORIF (McNemar, Howell, & Chang, 2003).

The neck is the area of transition between the shaft and head of the MC. When excessive forces from the hand impacting an object or person transfer to the metacarpal neck, this may result in fracturing the ring or small MCs. This is known as a **boxer's fracture** (Fig. 16–26). Interventions range from no treatment for nondisplaced fractures to surgical repair.

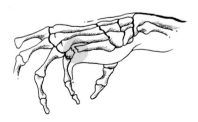

FIGURE 16–26 A boxer's or fighter's fracture involves the fifth MC neck and often presents with apex dorsal angulation.

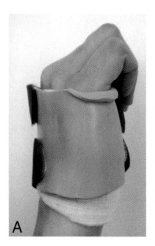 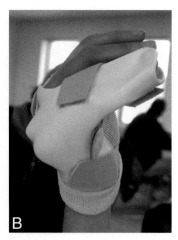

FIGURE 16–27 **A,** A nonarticular MC orthosis (fracture brace) can be used to support stable MC shaft fractures with early unrestricted motion of the digits and wrist. **B,** Ulnar-based MCP/IP immobilization orthosis; notice dorsal pins are protected by forming a protective "bubble" around this region.

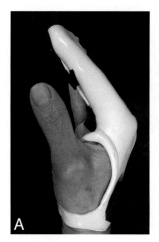 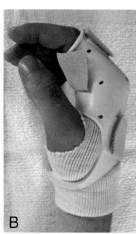

FIGURE 16–28 **A,** A hand-based radial gutter orthosis for a second MC fracture with the IP joints included. **B,** A radial MCP immobilization orthosis for an index MC neck fracture.

Metacarpal head fractures are less common and occur from direct impact with a clenched fist (McNemar et al., 2003).

MC fractures can be protected using functional MC fracture bracing or more traditional immobilization methods such as a hand-based radial or ulnar-based orthosis (Figs. 16–27A,B and 16–28A,B). The following recommendations may be used as a guideline to select the appropriate orthosis for surgical and nonsurgical patients. Base and shaft fractures usually include the wrist for proper immobilization. Traditional management of the index, middle, ring, and small finger MC fractures involves an immobilization orthosis using an ulnar- or radial-based design with the MCP joints at 60 to 70° of flexion. The proximal interphalangeal (PIP) and distal interphalangeal (DIP) joints may be immobilized for comfort or to prevent movement of the fracture, or if stable, they may be left free to prevent stiffness of unaffected joints. It is important to hold these digits in the described position to prevent MCP joint extension contractures and maintain fracture stability (Freiberg, Pollard, MacDonald, & Duncan, 2006).

In more progressive treatment, Colditz (2011) recommends that all MC shaft fractures be immobilized in a hand-based orthosis (ulnar or radial design) with buddy taping of the injured finger to the adjacent fingers. For added protection from external forces in shaft or neck fractures, the proximal phalanx should be included in the orthosis with the MCP joints in flexion and the IP joints free. This allows for functional ROM and can help prevent extensor tendon adherence to the fracture site. Table 16–5 summarizes orthotic intervention for MC fractures of the fingers.

TABLE 16–5

Metacarpal Fracture Management[a]

Fracture	Orthosis Options	Position	Time Frame
Base	• Wrist immobilization orthosis	Wrist: neutral; MCP: free	3–4 weeks
Shaft	• Radial/ulnar forearm-based wrist/digit immobilization orthosis • MC fracture brace	Wrist extension MCP: 60–70°, PIP: 0° or free; with or without buddy taping	3–4 weeks
Neck	• Radial/ulnar hand-based digit immobilization orthosis	MCP: 60–70°, PIP/DIP: 0° or free	3–4 weeks
Head	• Radial/ulnar hand-based digit immobilization orthosis	MCP: 60–70°, PIP/DIP: 0°; immobilize involved finger or with adjacent finger; include adjacent MC for stability	3–4 weeks

[a]Note that the orthosis options and time frames depend on the individual patient. Obtain clear orders from the referring physician before providing the patient with any therapy intervention.

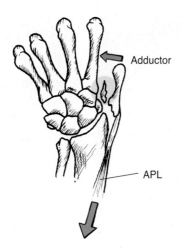

FIGURE 16–29 With a Bennett's fracture, the fractured fragment separates from the MC shaft, which is further displaced by the pull of the APL tendon dorsally and radially.

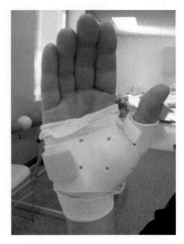

FIGURE 16–30 This thumb MP immobilization orthosis is appropriate for an adult, it may be modified when addressing small hands to include the thumb IP joint and further protect the healing UCL.

Thumb Metacarpal Fractures

Thumb MC fractures also occur at the base, shaft, and head. A **Bennett's fracture**, occurring at the base, results from an axial blow with dislocation of the first MC and CMC joint. This may also be associated with avulsion of the palmar oblique ligament or displacement by the pull of the abductor pollicis longus (APL) tendon dorsal and radially (Fig. 16–29). A greater axial load may result in a **Rolando's fracture**, a comminuted intra-articular fracture with fragments in "Y" or "T" configuration. Management of these fractures may require surgery to reestablish contours of the CMC joint. Extra-articular fractures may be transverse or oblique. With stable reduction, transverse fractures may only require immobilization; however, oblique fractures are usually repaired via percutaneous pinning (McNemar et al., 2003).

Shaft fractures of the thumb are rare as the mobility of the thumb allows forces to dissipate proximally. More common are first MC **head** fractures with bony avulsion of the ulnar collateral ligament (UCL) from the MC head, referred to as a

gamekeeper's or **skier's thumb** injury (Freeland, 2000). This injury may be managed conservatively or surgically depending on the severity of the ligament disruption. A hand-based design including the ulnar side of the hand is necessary to prevent any deviation stress on the healing UCL (Fig. 16–30).

Thumb MC fractures require the wrist and thumb to be immobilized (except in the case of a UCL injury as noted earlier). The thumb is positioned in midpalmar and radial abduction to preserve the first web space. The IP may be immobilized initially or free if the MC fracture is stable. However, once there is evidence of bone healing, the IP joint should be freed to minimize joint stiffness (Fig. 16–25). Table 16–6 summarizes orthotic management of thumb MC fractures.

Phalangeal Fractures

Proximal, Middle, and Distal Phalanx Fractures

The therapist frequently fabricates orthoses for finger fractures acutely. Goals for intervention include maintaining fracture stability, preventing joint stiffness, and minimizing

---

TABLE 16–6

Thumb Fracture Management[a]

Fracture	Orthosis Options	Position	Time Frame
Metacarpal	• Wrist/thumb immobilization orthosis or cast	Wrist: neutral; thumb CMC: midpalmar and radial abduction	4–6+ weeks depending on healing
Proximal phalanx	• Thumb immobilization orthosis	MP: slight flexion MP: 10–20° flexion; IP: 0°; CMC: midpalmar and radial abduction	4–6+ weeks
Distal phalanx	• Thumb immobilization orthosis	IP: 0–5° hyperextension	3+ weeks

[a]Note that the orthosis options and time frames depend on the individual patient. Obtain clear orders from the referring physician before providing the patient with any therapy intervention.

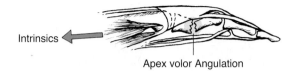

Intrinsics

Apex volor Angulation

FIGURE 16–31 A proximal phalanx fracture with apex volar angulation. Note pull of intrinsic muscles.

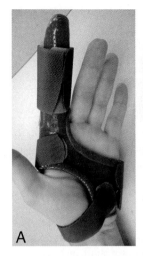
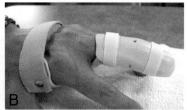
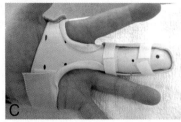

FIGURE 16–33 **A,** A hand-based volar digit immobilization orthosis for a proximal phalanx fracture. **B and C,** Hand-based design with protective dorsal "clamshell" segment to offer additional protection.

adhesions of tendons during the healing process. **Proximal** and middle phalanx fractures mainly involve the neck and the shaft. Shaft fractures may be transverse, spiral, oblique, or comminuted. Simple fractures may be treated with reduction and with or without fixation. However, due to the anatomical relationship of the soft tissue surrounding these bones, injury and treatment may become more complex. Unstable proximal phalanx fractures often produce an apex volar angulation, owing to the pull of the interossei muscles on the base of the proximal phalanx (Fig. 16–31). Unstable middle phalanx fractures also present with volar angulation of the neck caused by the strong pull of the flexor digitorum superficialis (FDS) tendon on the proximal side of the fracture. If the base of the middle phalanx is fractured, a dorsal angulation will likely occur (Fig. 16–32) (Henry, 2010). Surgical interventions may include ORIF with placement of K-wires, mini screws, or plates (Freeland & Orbay, 2006). Management of these injuries can be made more difficult because they are highly susceptible to tendon adherence of the extensor mechanism to the fracture site resulting in decreased extensor glide (Freeland, Hardy, & Singletary, 2003; Gutow, Slade, & Mahoney, 2003). Orthoses are used after surgical intervention to protect the fracture repairs and allow for safe mobility of tendons and joints (Freeland et al., 2003; Gutow et al., 2003). However, adhesions may still occur, and these patients may be candidates for a surgical tenolysis after the initial stages of healing are complete.

For proximal **phalanx fractures**, hand-based digit immobilization orthoses are often used with the MCP joints generally positioned at 60 to 70° of flexion to keep the collateral ligaments at length, preventing MCP joint extension contractures. The PIP and DIP joints may be placed in near to full extension to prevent potential flexion contractures (Fig. 16–33A–C). Some therapists include the wrist positioned in 30° of extension with the MCP joints flexed and the IP joints at 0° for additional protection or for patient

comfort. Nonarticular functional fracture bracing may also be used for stable proximal phalanx fractures because it provides the immobilization necessary for the healing fracture yet allows tendon gliding and motion of uninvolved joints (Gutow et al., 2003; Oxford & Hidreth, 1996).

Middle phalangeal fractures can be successfully managed with a digit-based orthosis (Fig. 16–34A). However, a hand-based design may be fabricated to provide additional support, protection, and rest as in the pediatric population, postoperatively, or when other structures and/or multiple digits are involved (Fig. 16–34B).

Distal phalangeal fractures commonly result from a crush injury and generally can heal without complicated treatment (Kaplan, 1940). These injuries occur frequently with a finger becoming caught between two objects such as a door and a door jam. According to Kaplan (1940), distal phalanx fractures are described as tuft, shaft, or base fractures. Tuft fractures do not necessarily require immobilization; however, concurrent nail bed injuries may require an

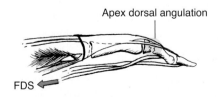

Apex dorsal angulation

FDS

FIGURE 16–32 A middle phalanx fracture can produce apex dorsal angulation. Note the pull of the FDS tendon.

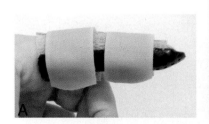
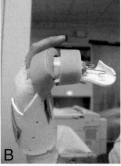

FIGURE 16–34 **A,** A digit immobilization orthosis for a middle phalanx fracture. **B,** This hand-based digit immobilization orthosis extends distally to provide protection for extruding pins. Notice the foam overlying the PIP joints to encourage PIP extension.

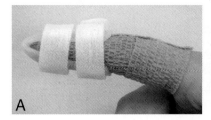
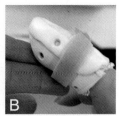

FIGURE 16–35 A, A volar/dorsal style DIP joint immobilization orthosis may be used to manage distal phalanx fractures and mallet finger injuries. **B,** This clamshell design can assist in protecting associated nail bed injuries.

orthosis for protection and comfort. A clamshell design can be used to provide further protection for a hypersensitive fingertip (Fig. 16–35A,B). Distal phalanx shaft or base fractures may require surgical repair, usually with K-wire fixation. When providing a protective orthosis, the PIP joint may be incorporated to improve stability and prevent the device from migrating distally off the finger (Fig. 16–36). This can be modified later to free the PIP joint as healing progresses.

Phalangeal Fracture/Dislocations

Proximal Interphalangeal Joint

PIP joint fractures or dislocations occur more commonly because they are more vulnerable to injury during normal functional, occupational, and athletic activities. Because they are often diagnosed as sprains, proper and timely intervention may be delayed. According to Kiefhaber (1996), there are three categories of these injuries. Dorsal lip fracture dislocations are hyperflexion injuries with volar dislocation of the PIP joint causing an avulsion-type fracture of the central tendon. If nondisplaced, the PIP joint can be immobilized in extension for 6 weeks with a clamshell or circumferential orthosis with the DIP joint left free for active ROM (AROM) (Fig. 16–37A,B). Displaced fractures most often require ORIF and may be immobilized with MCP in flexion, PIP extended, and DIP free (Fig. 16–37C,D) (Chinchalkar & Gan, 2003; Freiberg et al., 2006).

Volar lip fracture dislocations involve hyperextension injuries with dorsal forces dislocating the PIP joint, resulting in volar plate avulsion and injury to collateral ligaments. They may be classified based on stability with stress testing: type 1

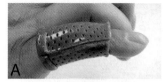
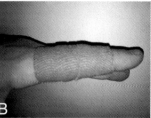
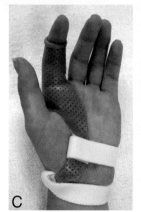
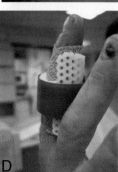

FIGURE 16–37 A, Finger-based circumferential PIP immobilization orthosis for nondisplaced PIP joint fracture dislocation injuries, allowing for DIP ROM exercises. As edema and pain resolves, the orthosis can be serially remolded to increase extension at the PIP joint. **B,** Orficast™ material circumferentially applied to maximally distribute pressure and immobilize the PIP joint, allowing MCP and DIP motion. **C,** A hand-based PIP joint immobilization orthosis to protect a repaired dorsal lip fracture dislocations of the PIP joint, leaving DIP joint free for motion. **D,** If a circumferential design is not appropriate due to fluctuating edema, a volar PIP immobilization orthosis with elasticized wrap beneath may be indicated.

(stable), type 2 (tenuous), and type 3 (unstable) fractures (Kiefhaber & Stern, 1998). Type 1 and 2 fractures may be protected with a PIP extension restriction orthosis or with buddy taping of the affected finger to adjacent fingers (Fig. 16–38). Early movement is highly encouraged for these injuries to minimize joint stiffness and tendon adhesions. Type 3 fractures require surgical intervention and a postoperative hand-based orthosis to protect repairs.

Pilon fractures result from high-energy axial force with the finger in full extension. This causes a severe, centrally impacted comminuted fracture of the middle phalanx and collapse of soft tissue surrounding the PIP joint. Often, these difficult intra-articular fractures are treated with dynamic traction orthoses (Fig. 16–39) to regain length of tissue surrounding the joint (ligamentotaxis) and to provide early passive motion (Gallagher & Blackmore, 2011; Schenck, 1994). In some cases, the traction assists in stabilizing the fracture, and passive motion would not be used immediately.

Distal Interphalangeal Joint

Tension and compression forces can produce DIP joint fracture and dislocations. For example, sudden forced flexion of the DIP joint while the finger is actively extended may result in avulsion of the terminal tendon with a bone

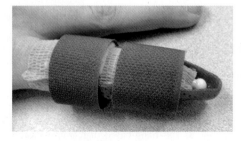

FIGURE 16–36 A digit immobilization orthosis may be applied for a distal phalanx fracture repaired with K-wire fixation.

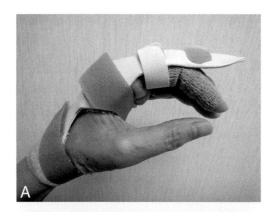

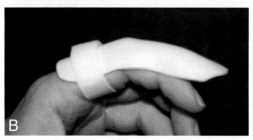

FIGURE 16–38 **A,** A hand-based dorsal PIP extension restriction orthosis used for a PIP joint volar lip fracture dislocation to allow early protected flexion but to restrict end range extension. **B,** Finger-based design may allow for greater function of unaffected digits.

fragment of distal phalanx. This is known as a bony mallet finger injury (Fig. 16–40). Conservative management for these injuries includes wearing a protective DIP immobilization orthosis positioned in extension continuously for 6 to 8 weeks until the bone appears healed (Fig. 16–41A,B) (Cannon, 2003). If surgical repair is performed, an orthosis is made to protect the fixation (Fig. 16–41C). Refer to Chapter 18, Tendon Injuries for details.

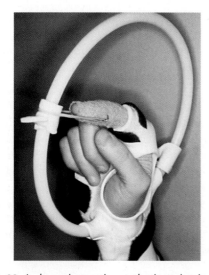

FIGURE 16–39 A dynamic traction orthosis maintains ligamento-taxis throughout a specific ROM.

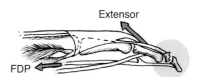

FIGURE 16–40 Distal phalanx avulsion fracture. Note the pull of the flexor and extensor tendon attachments and the resulting deformity.

Injuries to the DIP joint also may appear as a volar margin fracture with flexor digitorum profundus (FDP) rupture, a palmar plate avulsion fracture (hyperextension force with dorsal DIP joint dislocation), or impaction shear fractures (when fingertip is slightly flexed with force) (Kiefhaber, 1996). In the case of a fracture involving the FDP tendon, a dorsal blocking orthosis is made to include the wrist, and treatment would be initiated as per post-flexor tendon repair guidelines. Refer to Chapter 18 Tendon Injuries for details.

Options for orthotic management to address phalangeal fractures vary greatly owing to differing physician preferences. The therapist may need to modify the orthosis repeatedly as the fracture heals to maintain support as edema decreases, to modify joint positioning as motion improves, or to free joints from the orthosis as healing progresses. A material that can withstand being repeatedly reheated is the material of choice for managing these injuries. Therefore, an elastic or rubber material is preferable for convenience as well as cost-effectiveness. Table 16–7 summarizes orthotic management of hand fractures.

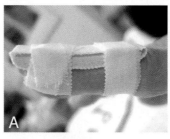

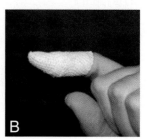

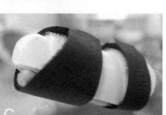

FIGURE 16–41 **A,** Dorsally applied AlumaFoam® positioning the DIP joint in slight hyperextension. **B,** QuickCast 2 applied circumferentially maximally distributes the pressure, minimizing incidence of irritation dorsally at DIP joint. **C,** Dorsal-based DIP immobilization orthosis extended distally to protect pins.

TABLE 16–7

Phalangeal Fracture Management[a]

Fracture	Orthosis Options	Position	Time Frame
Phalangeal			
Proximal	• Volar hand-based digit immobilization orthosis	MCP: 60–70°; PIP: 0–15°; DIP: 0–10°	2–4 weeks
Middle	• Digit immobilization orthosis	MCP: free, PIP: 0°; DIP: 0°	3+ weeks
Distal	• Stax splint	Prefabricated	4–6 weeks
	• DIP immobilization orthosis	DIP: 0°	4–6 weeks
Fracture or dislocation of PIP joint			
Dorsal lip			
Nondisplaced	• Digit immobilization orthosis	PIP: 0° as tolerated DIP: 0° or free	6 weeks
Displaced	• Hand-based digit immobilization orthosis after surgical repair	MCP: 60–70° PIP: 0°; DIP free	6 weeks
Volar lip			
Type 1 and 2	• PIP extension restriction orthosis (hand based or finger based) • Buddy taping	PIP flexed per physician recommendation (increase extension by 10° each week until full extension achieved) To adjacent digit	6 weeks
Type 3	• Digit- or hand-based immobilization orthosis • Traction orthosis	MCP: 60–70°; PIP: 0° Per physician: Wrist extension MCP: 60–70°; PIP: per physician	Variable 6+ weeks
Pilon	• Digit- or hand-based immobilization orthosis • Traction orthosis	MCP: 60–70°; PIP: 0° Per physician: Wrist extension MCP: 60–70°; PIP: per physician	Variable
Fracture or dislocation of the DIP joint			
Volar margin with FDP rupture	• Wrist/hand extension restriction orthosis (dorsal blocking orthosis)	Wrist: 0–45° depending per physician flexion; MCP: 45–60° flexion; PIP/DIP: 0°	4–6 weeks based on healing
Volar plate avulsion	• Digit immobilization orthosis	PIP/DIP: 0°	4 weeks
Bony mallet finger	• Digit immobilization orthosis	DIP: 0°	6–8 weeks

[a]Note that the orthosis options and time frames depend on the individual patient. Obtain clear orders from the referring physician before providing the patient with any therapy intervention.

Conclusion

This chapter reviewed orthotic intervention for common upper extremity fractures. The appropriate selection and judicious use of orthoses can aid in managing fractures early while maximizing functional use of uninjured structures. Orthoses applied immediately postinjury or postsurgery can offer excellent conformability for secure fracture stabilization while allowing joint mobility and gliding of surrounding soft tissue structures. Orthoses used during the remobilization phase of rehabilitation provide continued protection and help guard against reinjury during the patient's return to activity. Close communication with the physician regarding fracture stability and proper joint positioning within the orthosis is essential to prevent secondary problems such as joint or soft tissue contracture, tendon adherence, or chronic instability.

CASE STUDY SECTION

The case studies presented here are meant as a teaching guideline only. Treatment and orthosis protocols vary greatly from surgeon to surgeon and from therapist to therapist. The therapist should check with the referring physicians and colleagues to define the preferred treatment and appropriate orthotic intervention.

CASE STUDY 1: Small Finger Metacarpal Head Fracture

AM is a 27-year-old man who fell onto a clenched fist while trying to catch a football and sustained a right small finger MC head fracture. ORIF with placement of two screws through the MC head was performed. AM was followed by the medical doctor (MD); however, referral for outpatient hand therapy was delayed until 4 weeks postsurgery. Upon evaluation, AM's wound was healed, but he was noted to have thick scarring and joint stiffness with severe limitation in ROM throughout the small finger. He was unable to grip or lift using his left hand.

Initially, a hand-based, ulnar-based orthosis was fabricated to protect the small finger and adjacent ring finger at night and with daily activity to limit stress on the healing MC head fracture for an additional 2 weeks per MD orders (Fig. 16–42). The MCP joints were placed in end range flexion as tolerated with the IP joints in extension. AM was instructed to wear this orthosis at night and for heavier ADLs during the day. On follow-up visit, an ulnar-based MCP protective orthosis was made for only the small finger, allowing AM to better incorporate his right hand for grasping light objects and full use of unaffected fingers for ADLs.

Passive/active/active assistive ROM (PROM/AROM/AAROM) exercises were initiated including tendon gliding exercises and blocking exercises for isolated movements of PIP and DIP joints. He was instructed in methods to increase scar mobility and to decrease edema around the small finger. At 6 weeks postoperative, AM was weaned from the daytime MCP protection orthosis and instructed in use of buddy straps, allowing full use of his right hand for ADLs. Passive intrinsic plus and minus stretching as well as grip and pinch strengthening exercises were introduced.

Despite his diligence in following his home program, AM had developed scar adhesions of the small finger, limiting full active

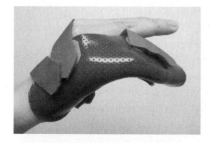

FIGURE 16–42 An ulnar-based digit immobilization orthosis for MC head fracture of the small finger.

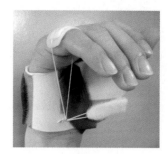

FIGURE 16–43 Static progressive MCP mobilization orthosis to improve MCP joint flexion of the small finger.

MCP extension ($-25°$). A night extension orthosis was made to rest the small finger in full extension at night, and active MCP extension exercises with skin mobilization were emphasized. He continued to have limited passive MCP flexion of 40°. A dynamic MCP flexion orthosis was fabricated, and he was instructed to wear it intermittently during day (4 to 6 times per day, beginning with 15 minutes and increasing as tolerated to 30 minutes). The tension on the dynamic orthosis was checked and adjusted. As his ROM progress slowed, the dynamic component of the orthosis was changed to a static progressive force (Fig. 16–43).

At 8 weeks postsurgery, AM had returned back to most light to moderate ADLs using his right dominant hand and, after follow-up with MD, was cleared for full weight bearing and lifting as tolerated. His grip strength was 60% of his left nondominant hand and with near tight grip. PROM of his small finger MCP extension/flexion was 0/70° with AROM of $-10/65°$ and with full ROM of PIP and DIP joints. By 10 weeks postsurgery, AM's right grip strength had improved to 75% of the left, and his MCP joint PROM was 0/80°; AROM was 0/75°. He had returned to performing most ADLs including workout activities and was discharged from therapy with a home exercise program of ROM, stretching, and strengthening exercises.

Additional case studies can be found on the companion web site on thePoint.

Chapter Review Questions

1. Name three common hand fractures that a hand therapist would treat and manage with an orthosis.

2. What is the importance of properly positioning joints acutely?

3. Describe a minimum of two design choices for orthotic management of a distal radius fracture.

4. What position should the thumb MP be placed in after a skier's injury? Why is this position so important?

5. Describe the three common locations a metacarpal bone tends to fracture and the proper orthotic management and position for each fracture location.

17 | Arthritis

MaryLynn Jacobs, MS, OTR/L, CHT
Shrikant Chinchalkar, M.Th.O, B.Sc.OT, OTR, CHT, OT Reg. (ONT)
Joey Pipicelli, M.Sc.OT, CHT, OT Reg. (ONT)

Chapter Objectives

After study of this chapter, the reader should be able to:

- Understand the disease process and general characteristics of osteoarthritis and rheumatoid arthritis of the elbow, wrist, and all joints of the hand.
- Explain the general goals and precautions for the use of orthoses in the arthritic upper extremity.
- Understand the rationale and evidence-based information for orthotic management of the nonsurgical

and postsurgical osteoarthritic or rheumatoid elbow, wrist, and hand.
- Explain the specific differences of immobilization, mobilization, restriction, or prefabricated orthoses for use with this patient population.

Key Terms

Arthritis
Arthrodesis
Arthroplasty
Arthroscopic debridement
Articular cartilage
Basal joint complex
Bouchard's nodes
Boutonniere deformity
Caput ulnae syndrome
Crepitation
DeQuervain's tenosynovitis
Dorsal Chamay repair
First carpometacarpal joint
Grind test

Heberden's nodes
Interposition arthroplasty
Juvenile rheumatoid arthritis
Low-load prolonged stress
Mannerfelt's syndrome
Mucus cysts
Osteoarthritis
Osteophytes
Pannus
Psoriatic arthritis
Rheumatoid arthritis
Scleroderma
Stenosing tenosynovitis
Swan-neck deformity

Synovectomy
Synovial fluid
Synovial membrane
Synovitis
Systemic lupus erythematosus
Systemic sclerosis
Tenolysis
Tenosynovectomy
Tenosynovitis
Trapeziometacarpal joint
Vaughan-Jackson syndrome
Zigzag deformity

Introduction

The word ***arthritis*** is derived from the Greek word *arthros* (joint) and *itis* (inflammation). Arthritis encompasses approximately 100 rheumatic diseases, all of which have joint disease as a prominent manifestation. In addition to joint involvement, the adjacent bones, tendons, and muscles can also be involved. The two most common rheumatic diseases are **osteoarthritis (OA)** and **rheumatoid arthritis (RA)**. Less common but often encountered by the hand therapist are **juvenile rheumatoid arthritis (JRA)** also known as juvenile idiopathic arthritis, **systemic lupus erythematosus (SLE)**, **psoriatic arthritis (PA)**, and **scleroderma**, also known as **systemic sclerosis (SS)** (Beasley, 2011). For most kinds of arthritis, there is as yet no cure; therefore, the main goals for treating these diseases are to minimize pain, control the inflammatory process, preserve joint structures, minimize progression of deformities, and maintain as much functional independence as possible.

The patient with arthritis of the upper extremity is best served by a supportive team approach including the primary care physician; rheumatologist; hand, orthopedic, or plastic surgeon; physical therapist; occupational therapist; and family members. The therapist is uniquely qualified to educate the patient regarding joint protection, energy conservation, exercise programs, and orthotic management (Beasley, 2011; Bernstein et al., 2010; Crepeau & Schell, 2009; Estes, Bochenek, & Fasler, 2000; Henry & Kramer, 2009; Kelley & Ramsey, 2000; Kozin, 1999; Kozin & Michlovitz, 2000; Poole & Pellegrini, 2000).

This chapter reviews joint disease, patient assessment, general characteristics of OA and RA, common surgical procedures, and the value of orthoses for these conditions. Threaded throughout this chapter are evidence-based highlights related to historically applied orthoses for the management of common arthritic conditions. Specific rehabilitation techniques, therapeutic modalities, medical management, related inflammatory diseases, and detailed surgical procedures are not reviewed; see "Suggested Readings" section of this chapter for further study.

Goals for the Use of Orthoses

Initial conservative management of OA and RA may include an orthosis, often in combination with patient education, anti-inflammatory medication, and/or a local steroid injection. Controversy in the literature exists regarding the efficacy of orthotic interventions for the nonsurgical patient with arthritis, although there is agreement among experts in the field of hand therapy and surgery that orthoses can play a role in protecting the joints and retarding the joint and soft tissue degeneration, pain relief, edema management, and functional performance (Barron, Glickel, & Eaton, 2000; Beasley, 2011; Fess, Gettle, Philips, & Janson, 2005; Kozin et al., 2000; Melvin, 1982; Philips, 1995; Seeger & Furst, 1987; Stern et al., 1997; Swigart, Eaton, Glickel, & Johnson, 1999; Valdes, 2012; Weiss, LaStayo, Mills, & Bramlet, 2000). Immobilization orthoses can be custom molded with thermoplastics or neoprene material or purchased prefabricated. The type of postsurgical orthosis is determined by many factors, including the procedure performed and the integrity of the patient's tissue. Commonly, there is some type of orthosis that is introduced after the postoperative dressing is removed (Bernstein et al., 2010; Fess et al., 2005; Kozin et al., 2000; Melvin, 1982; Philips, 1995; Seeger et al., 1987; Stern et al., 1997; Swigart et al., 1999; Tomaino, 2011; Weiss et al., 2000). General management of orthoses for each joint

of the wrist and hand, as well as the elbow, will be discussed in this chapter.

Goals for the Use of Orthoses in Patients with Arthritis

Use of orthoses in patients with arthritis includes the following (Fess et al., 2005; Jacobs, 2003; Melvin, 1982; Philips, 1995; Weiss et al., 2000):

- Reduce pain and inflammation of the involved joints
- Rest and support the weakened structures
- Position the involved joints as close to proper alignment as possible
- Help prevent, minimize, and/or retard joint deformity
- Provide external support (increase stability) to improve functional use of the hand
- Position healing structures appropriately after postoperative procedures

Joint Assessment

Components of a Normal Joint

Before discussing the diseased joint, normal joint anatomy must be understood. A joint is composed of many parts, each of which has a definite role and function (Fig. 17–1).

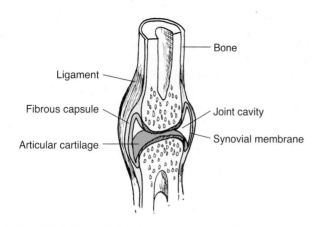

FIGURE 17–1 Normal joint anatomy and surrounding structures.

Altogether, in a carefully orchestrated sequence, they provide smooth, fluid, and pain-free joint motion. The main components and functions of a joint are described in the following text.

Bone

Bone is living tissue that provides the framework of the body. This hard porous material is composed of osteocytes that secrete a dense fibrous ground substance. This ground substance then calcifies into a strong and stiff material. Bone is considered the hardest structure in the body except for parts of the teeth. Bones have a blood and nerve supply and are constantly being remodeled.

Articular Cartilage

Articular cartilage is a tough connective tissue that covers the ends of the bones and functions as a cushion and shock absorber by lowering forces on adjacent bone. Cartilage goes through specific changes when the joint is loaded and possesses the ability to deform and reform many times. Cartilage has traditionally been thought to be incapable of regrowth, although recent research may prove that cartilage has regenerative capacity.

Fibrous Joint Capsule

The fibrous joint capsule is composed of two layers: stratum fibrosum and stratum synovium. The stratum fibrosum is a relatively dense layer of tissue that envelops the joint and maintains the integrity of the joint structure. The capsule consists of sheets of collagen, which supply stability and strength, and the protein elastin, which gives the capsule its ability to stretch and return to its previous state. This elastic capability plays a significant role in joint mobility. Besides its elastic nature, this structure is highly innervated, giving continuous feedback to the central nervous system.

The stratum synovium contains a **synovial membrane**, which lines the joint just beneath the capsule and produces **synovial fluid**, which nourishes and lubricates the joint.

It also provides the mechanism by which fluid is removed from the joint, which plays an important role in the rheumatoid patient. The stratum synovium is a highly vascular structure.

Ligaments

Ligaments are strong fibrous bands that connect the bones together, reinforcing the joint position and providing static stability. Ligaments are composed of dense longitudinal connective tissue bundles with little ground substance.

Muscles

Muscles are the contractile tissue that provides joint motion. They attach to the bones on either side of the joint via cordlike tendons. This "team" is often referred to as the muscle–tendon or muscular–tendinous unit. Muscles provide dynamic stability to the joint.

Joint Disease and Inflammation

The disruption of any normal component of a joint, either through injury or a disease process, affects the quality of joint motion. This change in motion may significantly limit a person's ability to perform even the simplest of daily tasks. OA is a noninflammatory joint disease that occurs with advancing age and specifically at the articular cartilage. The cartilage deteriorates over time as bony osteophytes simultaneously proliferate at the borders of the involved joint(s) (Bernstein et al., 2010; Melvin, 1982; Poole et al., 2000; Swanson, 1995a). RA is an inflammatory joint disease localized to the synovial lining. As the disease progresses, the synovial membrane stretches and fluid herniates from the fibrous capsule, causing damage to the capsule and supporting structures (Fig. 17–2) (Bernstein et al., 2010; Melvin, 1982; Swanson, 1995a).

Clinicians working with patients who have arthritis use their fundamental knowledge of normal joint anatomy and the consequences of joint disease to develop an effective therapeutic regime.

Osteoarthritis

Characteristics

Osteoarthritis is referred to as degenerative joint disease (DJD). It affects approximately 27 million people in the United States, usually between 40 and 50 years of age. Generally, women are more often affected than men. There are usually no systemic features; it occurs as a chronic, noninflammatory disease that causes cartilage destruction and reactive changes about the periphery of joints and in subchondral bone. The cause of the disease may be genetic factors, trauma (via work or sports), mechanical problems, metabolic issues, and/or age.

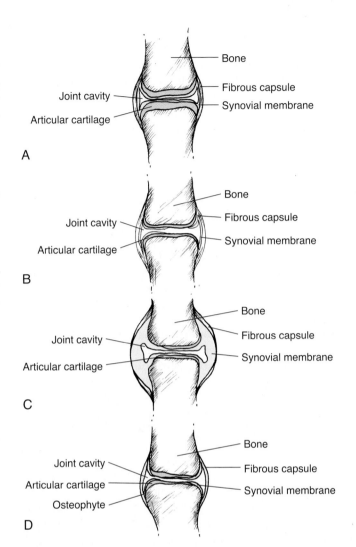

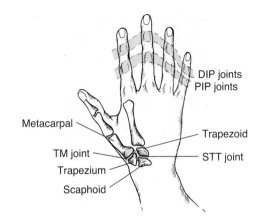

FIGURE 17–3 Joints commonly affected by osteoarthritis.

FIGURE 17–2 Healthy joint surfaces (A). Changes owing to OA and RA: early inflammation (B), advanced inflammation with herniation of synovial fluid and bone and cartilage destruction (C), and non-inflammatory disease with cartilage breakdown and osteophyte formation (D).

The most common sites are the weight-bearing joints (e.g., hips, knees, feet, and spine), and it may affect only one side or one part of the body such as *only* the hands or one thumb. The joints of the hand and wrist that are most involved are the distal interphalangeal (DIP) joints; the basal joint of the thumb; specifically, the first carpometacarpal (CMC) joint, also known as the trapeziometacarpal (TM) joint; the proximal interphalangeal (PIP) joints; the metacarpophalangeal (MCP) joints; and the scaphotrapeziotrapezoid (STT) joint (Fig. 17–3) (Barron et al., 2000; Bernstein et al., 2010; Melvin, 1982; Poole et al., 2000; Swanson, 1995a; Tomaino, 2011). To increase clarity and consistency for the reader of this chapter, the authors will use the term *first CMC* throughout this chapter. It is important to note that the term *TM joint* is widely used in clinical practice and in the literature.

General Signs and Symptoms

Initially, patients may present with one or more of the clinical symptoms discussed in the following text. Over time, radiographs may reveal asymmetric joint space narrowing with actual joint damage; however, the degree of radiologic involvement may not always correspond with the patient's complaints (Bernstein et al., 2010).

Pain

Joint pain with motion subsiding with rest is one of the first symptoms. Patients often complain of aching in cold weather. As the disease progresses, pain is noted during motion and rest, sometimes accompanied by muscle spasm.

Stiffness

Stiffness of the involved joints may occur, especially after an extended rest period. Active range of motion (AROM) and gross functional use of the involved joint may be limited and painful. As the disease progresses, strength may also diminish due to pain or disuse.

Crepitation

Crepitation may be noted in the joint or along the tendons as motion is performed. This is distinguished by a crunching sensation or sound produced as the joint or tendon moves.

Osteophytes

Bone spurs, or **osteophytes**, are common in the OA disease process, forming at the borders of the PIP and/or DIP joints of the fingers (Buckland-Wright, Macfarland, & Lynch, 1991; Swanson, 1995a) (Fig. 17–2D). These bony enlargements can appear gradually over time or have a rapid onset. Discomfort resulting from bone spurs varies. Some patients describe a functional hindrance (e.g., putting on rings), whereas others describe episodes of pain (Buckland-Wright et al., 1991; Burkholder, 2000; Estes et al., 2000; Melvin, 1982). Osteophytes at the DIP joints are called **Heberden's nodes**; those at the PIP joints are referred to as **Bouchard's nodes** (Fig. 17–4) (Burkholder, 2000; Melvin, 1982).

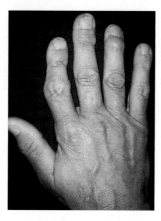

FIGURE 17–4 Note the Heberden's and Bouchard's nodules at the PIP and DIP joints, respectively.

Mucus Cysts

Mucus cysts tend to appear in the fifth to seventh decade of life. They are firm, nontender, painless cysts in the vicinity of the dorsum of the DIP joint and are often indicative of DIP joint OA (Cassidy & Green, 2011). The first symptoms may be a subtle variety of nail deformities (grooving, splitting). If left untreated, some may progress to cyst rupture (Bernstein et al., 2010).

Orthotic Management

Early referral to therapy is paramount. Conservative management for patients with OA may consist of supportive, protective, and preventive orthoses; anti-inflammatory medications; exercise programs; and instruction in joint protection and activity modification. Patient education is imperative for providing information on compensatory techniques in all activities of daily living (ADLs) and life's tasks (vocational and recreational) in order to decrease external forces on joints. If this is not addressed, continued joint stress may contribute to further deformity and/or pain (Estes et al., 2000; Kelley et al., 2000; Kozin, 1999; Poole et al., 2000). Providing information on adaptive equipment and/or custom-fabricating adaptations for ADLs may be extremely helpful in maintaining functional use of the hand (e.g., increasing the size of grips on a utensil, changing a round door knobs for a lever handle, adapting a steering wheel, modifying a grip on a golf club).

Orthoses made with thermoplastic materials may not always be well tolerated by some patients because of the following:

- Pressure felt at bony prominences
- Fragility of the patient's skin
- The weight/heaviness of the orthosis is too much
- Restrictive nature of the orthosis limits necessary use
- Bilateral involvement may limit strength and/or dexterity to apply the device

Some patients may prefer a softer, more conforming orthosis for immobilization. Chapter 14 dedicates a section with many examples to custom neoprene orthoses for this patient population.

Whether custom or prefabricated, when applied early in the DJD process, an orthosis can assist in stabilizing the involved joint(s) during at-risk activities (situations that stress the involved joint), minimize further joint damage, and decrease pain during activity (Barron et al., 2000; Colditz, 2000; Jacobs, 2003; Weiss et al., 2000).

Material Selection

Thermoplastics

Thermoplastic materials for the patient with OA should be carefully chosen. The selection ranges from heavyweight to lightweight materials, and the choice depends on the purpose of the orthosis and the patient's skin tolerance and joint integrity. An orthosis intended to provide gentle pressure for adequate joint stabilization might need to be more rigid than one used to position an inflamed joint (Austin, 2003; Colditz, 2000). Materials should easily contour about bony prominences such as the ulnar styloid and the dorsal metacarpal heads. Because bony changes may occur over time in OA, consideration should be given to a material that can be reheated and reshaped repeatedly such as an elastic-based material (see Chapter 5).

Another consideration is material flexibility. Materials that are thin (1/16") and/or highly perforated tend to be more flexible than traditional (1/8") solid materials (see Chapter 5 for further details) (Austin, 2003). However, a highly perforated material may irritate the fragile skin, owing to the friction of the perforations on the skin's surface. Cotton stockinette worn under the orthosis can minimize this irritation. Meticulous placement of straps with properly placed foam padding over or around bony prominences can minimize mobility within the orthosis, which in turn will additionally aid in decreasing friction on the skin's surface.

Materials may need to be "popped" apart to allow the orthosis to pass over an enlarged area and/or joint. This can be done by using coated thermoplastic (nonsticky) or by placing a wet paper towel or hand lotion between overlapping pieces of thermoplastic material. This is often referred to the patient as making them a "trap door" to allow for fluctuations in edema and easy donning and doffing. Not only does this provide a way for the patient to slip in and out of the orthosis, but it also provides a sense of security for the patient who may be worried about getting stuck in the orthosis. An excellent example involves an orthosis of the thumb MP joint. In some patients, the interphalangeal (IP) joint can be significantly wider than the proximal phalanx, making removal of a thumb orthosis difficult unless it can be popped open (Fig. 17–5A,B).

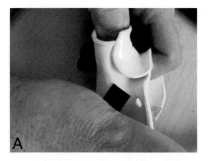
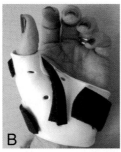

FIGURE 17–5 Enlargement of the IP joint of the thumb with OA can make removal of an orthosis difficult. **A and B,** By lightly and carefully overlapping the material during molding, a "trap door" can be made as shown here. This type of design provides for an expansion during application and removal and may also provide a sense of security to the patient that may feel "trapped" in the device.

Strapping

When securing straps onto the orthosis, consideration should be given to where the straps are going to traverse. Is the skin under the strap fragile? Are there bony prominences? Are Bouchard's or Heberden's nodes and/or mucous cysts present? If so, are they tender and will straps irritate them? Strapping considerations for the extremity with arthritis should include soft, conforming, and flexible material. Straps can be lined with foam to soften the contact around bony areas. Consider soft 2″ foam straps for night use and less bulky elasticized straps for day use (such as thin neoprene material). Both soft and elasticized strapping systems are comfortable, durable, and, when applied correctly, contribute to minimizing shear and compression stress on tissue (see Chapter 4 for details) (Fig. 17–6).

Prefabricated Orthoses

Prefabricated orthoses can be used for many patients with OA. Soft prefabricated wrist and thumb orthoses are a

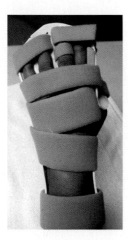

FIGURE 17–6 Soft strapping should be considered when applying an orthosis to this patient population, who often have thin fragile skin.

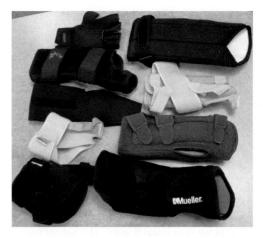

FIGURE 17–7 Various prefabricated orthoses are available and widely used to manage the early intermittent symptoms of arthritis. These are all orthoses that one patient purchased while trying to seek relief from first CMC OA.

popular choice with physicians (Fig. 17–7) (Boozer, 1993; Murphy, 1996; Pagnotta, Baron, & Korner-Bitensky, 1998; Stern, Ytterberg, Krug, & Mahowald, 1996). Most patients initially do well with these orthoses. However, many of these prefabricated designs are meant to fit the population at large and may not provide the exacting support the patient or referring professional is seeking. For instance, a prefabricated thumb first CMC stabilization orthosis may not fully immobilize this joint; allowing too much motion within the device, which in turn, continues to contribute to pain during use. Prefabricated orthoses have a role when fit by a skilled clinician. If appropriate fit is not achieved and/or joint/bony changes begin to alter the shape of the wrist and/or thumb, a more customized design may be necessary.

PIP and DIP Joints with Osteoarthritis

Osteoarthritis of the PIP and DIP joints can result in pain, edema, decreased digital AROM, and difficulty in tasks requiring gripping and pinching. The alterations in physical appearance that osteophytes can cause may be disturbing to some patients (Estes et al., 2000; Melvin, 1982). Such patients may see their fingers as becoming deformed, and they have great difficulty putting rings on because of the bony changes and swelling. Although osteophytes and cysts are not always painful, they can be episodically tender (Burkholder, 2000; Cassidy & Green, 2011; Estes et al., 2000). Pain is reported as localized specifically to the involved joints during functional activities. The intensity of the pain does not necessarily indicate the amount of joint destruction or deformity as seen on a radiograph. Surprisingly, there are patients with minimal pain who have significant joint destruction on the radiograph (Estes et al., 2000).

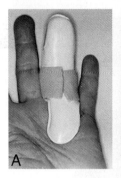
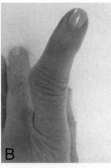
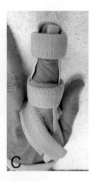

FIGURE 17–8 **A,** A volar RF digit immobilization orthosis that extends proximally to include the MP joint. This extension provides a longer lever arm for increased stability and comfort, especially for patients with small hands or digits. **B and C,** This patient had significant radial deviation at the PIP joint, and the use of the longer orthosis combined with the precise strapping placed this joint back into anatomical alignment.

Nonsurgical Orthotic Management Guidelines

Fitting an orthosis is usually reserved for the acutely painful PIP or DIP joint. Lightweight volar immobilization orthoses can be supportive, especially to prevent lateral movements of the PIP and DIP joints. (Fig. 17–8A–C) (Cassidy & Green, 2011). The orthoses place the joints in comfortable extension and are worn mostly at night. Gel-lined products (such as the Silopad mesh digital cap or silicone-lined thermoplastic materials) may provide an absorbent cushion and layer of warmth to a painful joint (Fig. 17–9). A piece of silicone gel can be incorporated into an orthosis for added protection and cushioning (Austin, 2003).

Postsurgical Orthotic Management Guidelines

DIP Joint Arthrodesis

There are few surgical options for the patient with DIP joint osteoarthritis, with the exception of DIP joint arthrodesis (fusion); because for this small but important joint, stability takes priority over mobility (Bernstein et al., 2010; Cassidy & Green, 2011; Estes et al., 2000; Melvin, 1982; Pelligrini & Burton, 1990). An arthrodesis can provide this stability, along with decreasing intractable pain and enhancing cosmetic

appearance (Bernstein et al., 2010; Cassidy & Green, 2011; Pelligrini & Burton, 1990).

The DIP joint is protected after **arthrodesis** for 6 to 8 weeks until sufficient osseous healing has occurred when evaluated radiographically (Cassidy & Green, 2011; Pelligrini & Burton, 1990). Postsurgically, the patient can be placed in a DIP immobilization orthosis, which supports and protects the arthrodesis. The distal tip should be fully protected by the orthosis so that the patient cannot bump against a possible external K-wire(s) or a sensitive tip where a compression screw may have been placed. For added length and support, the orthosis can include the hand and/or the PIP joint and can later be modified to include only the DIP joint once the patient is comfortably able to exercise and use the PIP joint (Fig. 17–10A,B) (Cassidy & Green, 2011; Rizio et al., 1995).

PIP Joint Arthrodesis

PIP joint arthrodesis is considered for patients who use their hand for activities that require a forceful grip, such as in meat cutting or construction work. Surgical fusion has been recommended for the index finger (IF) when ulnarly directed force via the thumb is necessary (Bernstein et al., 2010). Other situations to consider PIP arthrodesis include to provide increased functional use of the hand when the soft tissues in the joint cannot support an implant, when stability is more important than mobility, and to provide for a pain-free joint. The postoperative orthosis should protect the PIP joint in the fused position for 6 to 8 weeks or until the arthrodesis has sufficiently healed, which is evaluated radiographically.

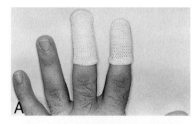

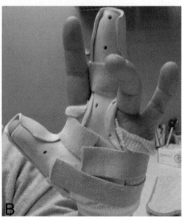

FIGURE 17–10 **A,** QuickCast 2 used to fabricate DIP immobilization orthoses for protecting recent DIP joint fusions. **B,** This patient underwent MF DIP and thumb IP joint fusion and is being protected postsurgically with this "clamshell" designed orthosis.

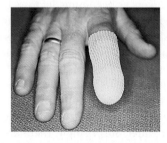

FIGURE 17–9 A mesh digital silicone lined cap used to provide warmth and pain relief to a patient with OA of the IF DIP joint.

Initially, the orthosis should include both the PIP and DIP joint for pain control and, as mentioned for DIP arthrodesis, should envelop any exposed hardware as shown in Figure 17–10B. In the latter weeks, the DIP joint may be cut free, or a second orthosis could be fabricated leaving the DIP joint free, permitting FDP tendon glide to prevent tendon adherence and DIP stiffness (Estes et al., 2000; Rizio & Belsky, 1995). Lightweight thermoplastics or casting materials can be used as shown in Figure 17–8 or 17–10A.

The position of fusion for the PIP or DIP joint is based on which digit is involved and the function/demands of that particular joint as determined by preoperative discussion with the patient (Cassidy & Green, 2011; Estes et al., 2000). In normal hand function, the IF and middle finger (MF) are used mostly for prehension and do not require as much flexion as the ring finger (RF) and small finger (SF) PIP joints. The RF and SF require greater flexion, especially at the DIP joints, because they contribute greatly to grip strength (Estes et al., 2000; Rizio et al., 1995).

PIP Joint Arthroplasty

PIP joint arthroplasty can be considered to restore motion, alleviate pain, and enhance PIP joint stability. An arc of motion of 0 to 70° can be expected at the PIP joint (Bernstein et al., 2010; Goldfarb, 2011; Kozin, 1999; Pelligrini & Burton, 1990; Rizio & Belsky, 1995; Swanson, Swanson, & Leonard, 1995). Exercise protocols vary and depend on the surgical approach and procedure, implant, and intraoperative joint stability (Feldscher, 2010). Therefore, postoperative rehabilitation and orthosis application depends on close communication between the surgeon and therapist. Common surgical approaches to PIP joint arthroplasty include the central slip sparing technique, palmar approach, lateral approach, and **dorsal Chamay repair**, which typically all permit immediate early active flexion and extension of the effected digit. They do not require the application of a mobilization orthosis (dynamic) for movement (Bechenbaugh & Linscheid, 1993; Chamay, 1988; Feldscher, 2010; Lipscomb, 1967; Schneider, 1991). Another common surgical approach is the central slip splitting technique, which often delays mobilization for 2 to 4 weeks and uses an extension mobilization orthosis (dynamic) during the day to facilitate active PIP joint flexion with a gentle, "dynamic," passive assist into extension (Swanson, Maupin, Gajjar, & Swanson, 1985).

Therapeutic management should take into account other surgical procedures that may have been performed at the same time, such as tenolysis, extensor tendon reconstruction, or volar plate release. In general, AROM exercises are initiated between 2 and 7 days postoperatively. A recommended exercise schedule is 5- to 10-minute sessions, 4 to 6 times a day.

A postoperative hand-based PIP extension immobilization orthosis is fabricated and worn at all times for 4 to 6 weeks; it is removed only for hygiene and exercise sessions (Fig. 17–11A). The MCP joint is usually included, at least initially, for improved purchase and comfort. If the patient had a swan-neck deformity (PIP hyperextension, DIP flex-

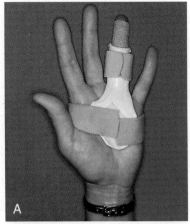

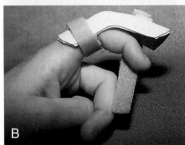

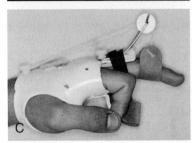

FIGURE 17–11 PIP orthoses used after arthroplasty. **A,** This MP/PIP immobilization orthosis allows gentle DIP motion in order to facilitate tendon gliding. It can be removed for short periods of exercise per physician protocol. **B,** With this digit extension restriction orthosis, the patient is instructed to exercise into flexion from the dorsal block of the device. **C,** A PIP extension mobilization orthosis (using a Phoenix Outrigger) may be indicated to allow frequent motion of PIP joint.

ion) before surgical implant, then consider positioning the involved joints in some degree of PIP flexion (approximately 10 to 30°) within the orthosis. This may help prevent the tendency for the PIP joint to rebound into hyperextension (Fig. 17–11B). Extension mobilization orthoses are an alternative postoperative management option (Fig. 17–11C). These orthoses are fabricated to position the PIP gently in extension yet allow gentle active flexion exercise against rubber band traction.

Regardless of whether immobilization, restriction, or mobilization orthoses are used postoperatively, the orthoses should protect the joint from lateral stress and facilitate the encapsulation process (Estes et al., 2000). Immobilization and restriction orthoses should have sufficient depth for lateral protection and allow the ability for the patient

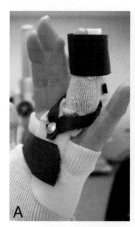
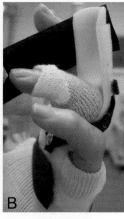

FIGURE 17–12 **A and B,** Postoperative PIP joint arthroplasty. This uniquely designed restriction orthosis allows for simple strap removal for hourly gentle exercises in flexion and extension within the confines of the orthosis the confines of the orthosis.

to easily perform the home exercise program prescribed (Fig. 17–12A,B). Mobilization orthoses should maintain the line of pull centrally over the middle phalanx and avoid any undesired rotation or lateral deviation stresses. It is important to recognize any tendon adherence, extension lag, and prolonged inflammation.

Thumb with Osteoarthritis

The thumb has a large arc of motion allowing opposition to all the digits. Through the aging process, an active person's first CMC joint can be subjected to a large amount of stress. The cumulative impact of these stresses may exceed the load tolerance of the tissues including the articular cartilage, joint capsule, and ligaments. It is believed that ligamentous laxity and instability, either through the aging process or demands placed on the joint, are the initiators of OA at the first CMC joint (Barron et al., 2000; Boozer, 1993; Estes et al., 2000; Freedman, Eaton, & Glickel, 2000; Kelley& Ramsey, 2000; Pelligrini & Burton, 1990; Poole et al., 2000). Additional predisposing factors to first CMC joint OA (Katarincic, 2001; Pellegrini & Burton, 1991) include the following:

- Subtle joint anatomical abnormalities, which lead to an increase in contact stress on the articular structures
- Periarticular soft tissue trauma
- Base fractures of the first metacarpal
- Thinning of the articular cartilage combined with incongruency of the joint
- Excessive capsular laxity associated with hormonal changes

Clinical Examination

The diagnosis of first CMC joint OA is made primarily through a comprehensive physical examination followed by

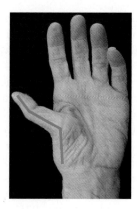

FIGURE 17–13 Note the subluxation of the TM joint, first metacarpal adduction, and MP joint hyperextension in this patient with advancing first CMC OA.

radiographic confirmation. Generally, patients complain of pain, pinch weakness, and/or crepitus at the TM joint. The typical patient notes pain during functional activities, such as opening jars, brushing teeth, and turning a doorknob. Pain is generalized to the thenar eminence but may also be noted proximal and distal to the involved joint. Palpation may reveal tenderness over the volar aspect of the first CMC joint, and in approximately half the population, concurrent pain is appreciated at the STT joint (Glickel, Kornstein, & Eaton, 1992; Kozin, 1999; Poole et al., 2000). The patient may have a positive **grind test**—pain elicited when the examiner imparts gentle compression and rotation of the head of the first metacarpal into the trapezium (Bernstein et al., 2010; Estes et al., 2000). In the earlier stages of the disease, gross appearance may be normal. Progression of the disease often results in subluxation of the TM joint; this positive "shoulder sign" may be seen at the base of the first CMC (Fig. 17–13). As the disease progresses, motion at the first CMC joint diminishes. Patients often develop an adduction contracture as well as a loss of radial abduction and exaggerated IP flexion. Compensatory thumb MCP joint hyperextension may develop leading to a "Z" or swan-neck deformity of the thumb. This classic deformity is the hallmark of advanced stage first CMC joint arthritis (Fig. 17–14).

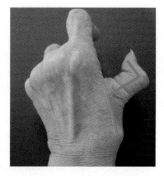

FIGURE 17–14 Advanced first CMC disease with significant thumb IP flexion. Thumb mechanics are greatly altered.

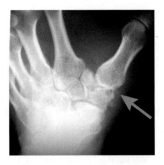

FIGURE 17–15 Stage IV radiograph of the basal joint of the thumb with significant sclerosis and joint destruction.

Radiographic examination will confirm as well as determine the extent of osteoarthritic change present at the first CMC joint (Fig. 17–15). The radiologic severity of first CMC OA may be graded according to the well-accepted staging system described by many surgeons. Refer to Table 17–1.

Pathomechanics of First Carpometacarpal Osteoarthritis

The first CMC joint is the key articulation responsible for imparting mobility to the thumb. The trapezium also articulates with the scaphoid, trapezoid, and the index metacarpal. This complex of articulations is also commonly referred to as the **basal joint complex**. Osteoarthritis of the basal joint is due to a placement of greater loads on the trapezium by the first metacarpal during grasp and pinch. The trapezium is inherently unstable due to its anatomical location and relatively poor ligamentous stability. Because of these two factors, it is believed that the first CMC joint, over time,

develops excessive axial and cantilever bending forces during thumb use. The trapezium then begins to tilt radially, causing the base of the metacarpal to slide in a dorsoradial direction. Consequently, the adductor pollicis pulls the metacarpal medially, increasing the tension on the abductor pollicis longus (APL) tendon, contributing to the zigzag collapse of the TM joint. This in turn results in attenuation or failure of the anterior oblique ligament (AOL) of the first CMC joint leading to osteoarthritis (Katarincic, 2001). Also considered part of the basal thumb complex and often involved in later stages of first CMC OA are the scaphotrapezial, scaphotrapezoid, and trapeziotrapezoid joints (Bernstein et al., 2010).

Nonsurgical Orthotic Management Guidelines

Orthosis application is the mainstay of conservative (nonsurgical) management of first CMC joint OA. However, other common methods of conservative treatment include pain control, principles of joint protection teaching, exercise, dynamic stability training (as described by O'Brien & Giveans, 2013) thermal modalities, nonsteroidal anti-inflammatory medications, and corticosteroid injections. The overall objectives of an orthosis is to stabilize the first CMC joint, provide pain control, and prevent adduction contracture (Barron et al., 2000; Colditz, 1995, 2000; Jacobs, 2003; O'Brien & Giveans, 2013; Poole & Pellegrini, 2000; Weiss et al., 2000). The designs of orthoses can vary, and many options are available. Common to most of these designs is the maintenance of a wide first web space because as the disease process advances, adduction and subluxation of the first metacarpal may occur, causing a contracture and/or narrowing of the first web space (Bernstein et al., 2010; Colditz, 2000; Diaz, 1994; Melvin, 1982, 1995; Poole et al., 2000; Swigart et al., 1999; Tomaino, 2011; Wajon, 2000; Weiss et al., 2000). Ideal orthotic management for first CMC joint arthritis involves positioning the thumb in palmar abduction and approximately 30° of MP flexion (Bernstein et al., 2010; Colditz, 1995; Jacobs, 2003; O'Brien & Giveans, 2012; Poole & Pellegrini, 2000; Weiss et al., 2000). The orthosis can be custom made from thermoplastic material or neoprene material (see Chapter 14), or a clinician can choose a prefabricated design. There are many prefabricated designs, discussed in Chapter 11, which may work very well for this population. Proper fit is key for any of the orthoses chosen.

For a custom design, it may help to extend the orthosis border proximally on the radial aspect just beyond the STT joint to secure the thumb column. A conforming, lightweight material (e.g., ³⁄₃₂″ Aquaplast, Polyform light, Polyflex light, or TailorSplint) is an excellent choice for fabricating this orthosis (Austin, 2003). Unfortunately, the material's thinness can make fabrication challenging to a novice fabricator, and it may not offer the strength necessary to stabilize the first metacarpal (Fig. 17–16) (Austin, 2003; Colditz, 2000). These orthoses are used during daily activities to promote pain-free function. Unfortunately, dosage for precise wearing time of an orthosis has yet to be established. In these authors' experience, orthoses are most likely to be beneficial

TABLE 17–1	
Stages of Carpometacarpal Joint Osteoarthritis (Barron, 1998, 2000; Tomaino, 2011)	
Stage I:	Appears normal on radiographic exam; there may be no degenerative joint changes to minimal changes or widened joint space secondary to synovitis.
Stage II:	May present with a reduction of joint space and possible appearance of sclerosis and osteophytes less than 2 mm in diameter; STT joint is normal.
Stage III:	More dramatic joint space narrowing and notable subchondral sclerosis as well as sclerosis and/or osteophytes measuring more than 2 mm in diameter
Stage IV:	Characterized by advanced degenerative changes involving the first CMC and the ST joint and could involve neighboring joints as well (Fig. 17–15)

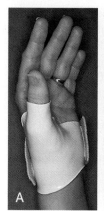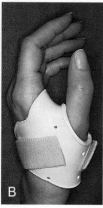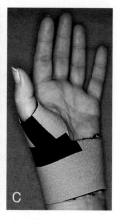

FIGURE 17–16 A, Hand-based first CMC immobilization orthosis to limit motion at the thumb first metacarpal and to place the thumb column in a position of function. Note the intimate contouring of the material about the proximal orthosis border. **B,** This orthosis (described by Colditz, 2000) places an extension force to the volar/ulnar aspect of the distal metacarpal with counterpressure to the dorsal/radial portion of the metacarpal base. **C,** A custom orthosis fabricated from neoprene (or prefabricated) may be appropriate when a nonrigid support is recommended.

in patients who suffer from stages I to III of first CMC joint OA. Refer to Table 17–1 for reference.

It is generally accepted that people with severe stage IV degenerative stages will be less likely to respond to conservative management and should be referred for surgical consultation. Some physicians request that the daytime orthoses be complemented with a more substantial resting orthoses for night use (Jacobs, 2003; Weiss et al., 2000). Forearm-based night orthoses can be fabricated to immobilize a wider and/or

longer surface area, incorporating proximal and distal structures to achieve a greater degree of immobilization (Austin, 2003; Colditz, 2000; Fess et al., 2005; Jacobs, 2003; Leonard, 1995; Simmons, Nutting, & Bernstein, 1996; Weiss et al., 2000). Therapists may find that patients become concerned about wearing an orthosis too much, possibly leading to joint stiffness and/or weakness. In some cases, stiffness may be the desired outcome because a decrease in joint motion may also produce a decrease in pain. If pain persists without relief from orthotic intervention (use a trial period of 4 to 6 weeks), other modalities such as injection or surgical consult should be considered (Barron et al., 2000; Estes et al., 2000; Kozin et al., 2000).

Postsurgical Orthotic Management Guidelines

Surgical intervention may be an option for patients with painful, progressive OA of the thumb. In these advanced cases, there usually has been first CMC subluxation and/or dislocation. Managing this disease with an orthosis is likely to be of little help (Fig. 17–17) (Ataker, 2012; Bernstein et al., 2010; Colditz, 1995). Several surgical procedures (and variations of these procedures) for ligament reconstruction of the first CMC joint have been described (Ataker, 2012; Bernstein et al., 2010; Estes et al., 2000; Freedman et al., 2000; Kozin, 1999; Poole & Pellegrini, 2000; Rozental & Bora, 2000; Tomaino & King, 2000; Tomaino, Pelligrini, & Burton, 1990; Trumble et al., 2000; Varitimidis, Fox, King, Taras, & Soreranes, 2000). All have the primary goals of pain relief: reestablishing the thumb/IF web space to provide a stable post for the digits to pinch against and preventing further joint destruction. One such procedure uses a tendon interposition graft with a slip of the flexor carpi radialis (FCR) lon-

---

BOX 17–1

Evidence-Informed Orthotic Management: Thumb Osteoarthritis

Therapeutic interventions for persons with osteoarthritis commonly involve the use of orthoses. To date, there have been few systematic reviews on the effectiveness of orthotic application in the patient with osteoarthritis. Orthotic management in persons suffering from OA has been most studied when applied to the thumb. Positioning with an orthosis is the mainstay of conservative management of the osteoarthritic thumb. The success of an orthosis positioning program is determined by the reduction in pain and improved hand function along with dynamic thumb stability training/strengthening (O'Brien, 2013). A review of the literature has shown only limited evidence on the effectiveness of static orthosis positioning for persons with varying stages of CMC joint OA of the thumb (Beasley, 2011; Buurke & Baten, 1999; Sillem, Backman, Miller, & Li, 2011; Swigart et al., 1999; Weiss et al., 2000, 2004).

Three types of orthoses are commonly used in the treatment of first CMC joint OA. They are the following:

1. A wrist/thumb immobilization orthosis (Fig. 17–18A,B)
2. A hand-based thumb immobilization orthosis; various designs are described in chapters 11 and 14 (Figs. 17–5B and 17–16A,B)
3. A custom or prefabricated soft/neoprene orthosis (Figs. 17–6C and 17–66)

A review of the literature provides some evidence that orthosis application for first CMC joint can improve hand function and decrease pain (Valdes & Marik., 2010). There is no evidence that one type of orthotic design is more effective than another (Egan et al., 2003). There is evidence that rigid custom orthoses provide better pain reduction compared to soft prefabricated neoprene orthoses; however, patients may prefer the neoprene designs (Sillem et al., 2011; Weiss et al., 2004). These findings suggest that therapists should be patient centered when providing orthoses to meet the individual needs of patients.

To the knowledge of the authors of this chapter, orthosis application to digits with osteoarthritis in either the PIP or DIP joints to date have not been studied in the literature. Furthermore, orthosis application following an operative procedure to the osteoarthritic hand or wrist has not been studied in the literature. Managing osteoarthritis with an orthosis, in these instances, is based on expert opinion and the clinical experience of the authors of this chapter.

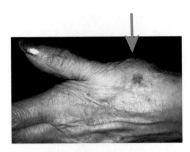

FIGURE 17–17 This patient presented with exquisite, unrelenting joint pain with even the lightest of activity. This patient was considered a candidate for first CMC joint arthroplasty.

gus tendon with excision of the trapezium (Poole et al., 2000; Tomaino et al., 1995; Tomaino et al., 2011). The successful outcome of ligament reconstruction of the thumb requires stabilization of the base of the thumb metacarpal and simultaneous adjustment of distal deformity (Ataker, 2012; Colditz, 1995; Estes et al., 2000; Poole et al., 2000; Tomaino et al., 1995; Tomaino et al., 2011).

Ligament reconstruction procedures of the first CMC joint normally require a short period of cast immobilization, which is followed by transition into an orthosis during the first 2 to 4 weeks postsurgery; however, protocols vary from surgeon to surgeon (Fig. 17–18A,B) (Ataker, et al., 2012; Bernstein et al., 2010; Colditz, 1995; Kozin, 1999; Poole et al., 2000; Tomaino, 2011; Tomaino et al., 1995; Tomaino et al., 2011; Weiss et al., 2000). From the cast, commonly a forearm-based wrist/thumb immobilization orthosis is fabricated that allows the IP joint to move freely. The orthosis is typically worn full time during the first 6 weeks postoperatively and is gradually weaned as tolerated by the patient. Some surgeons prefer to shorten the orthosis after 6 to 8 weeks to allow wrist motion. After approximately 12 weeks, the orthosis can be discontinued or worn only at night, if necessary (Jacobs, 2003; Poole et al., 2000). The therapist must appreciate that depending on the type of ligament reconstruction

used and the preference of the surgeons post operative rehabilitation protocol may influence the type and duration of orthosis wear. Some patients may prefer to use a soft custom or prefabricated orthosis for added comfort and stability during the first 3 to 6 months postoperatively (see Chapters 11 and 14).

Wrist with Osteoarthritis

Osteoarthritis of the wrist presents most often at the STT joint. Confusion can exist between STT arthritis and first CMC joint arthritis; the literature has clearly outlined clinical distinctions of each (Kozin et al., 2000; Poole et al., 2000) Refer to Figure 17–13.

STT Joint versus First CMC Joint Osteoarthritis: What Is the Difference?

Patients with *STT joint arthritis* may exhibit pain with radial deviation (e.g., using scissors, pulling up socks), a decrease in active radial deviation, tenderness with palpation over the STT area, a positive grind test, joint space narrowing on radiograph, pain with the scaphoid shift test, and only occasional first CMC joint changes.

Patients with *first CMC joint arthritis* may demonstrate difficulty with fine motor tasks (using clothespins, writing, doing needlepoint, turning a car key), a positive grind test, and subluxation of the first CMC joint with possible MP hyperextension. Approximately half of patients with first CMC joint OA show STT joint space narrowing with possible osteophyte formation on radiographs (Bernstein et al., 2010; Kozin, 1999; Kozin et al., 2000; Poole et al., 2000; Weiss et al., 2000).

Nonsurgical Orthotic Management Guidelines

Patients with STT arthritis may find some temporary relief from such interventions as cortisone injection, pain-modulating modalities, activity modification, and orthosis use (Kozin & Michlovitz, 2000). A recommended orthosis design is a wrist/thumb immobilization orthosis with the thumb IP free (Fig. 17–18A,B). Wrist immobilization orthoses may also be successful in controlling pain and permitting limited hand use. Circumferential wrist orthoses (such as the Rolyan® AquaForm™ Zippered Wrist orthosis) may be more appropriate for heavy labor workers, whereas a lightweight volar wrist immobilization orthosis will likely suffice for a person with less functional demands. There are several prefabricated orthosis designs that can work well for this population that are well described in Chapter 11 (Boozer, 1993; Stern et al., 1997; Stern, Ytterberg, Krug, & Mahowald, 1996; Trumble et al., 2000).

Postsurgical Orthotic Management Guidelines

Several procedures have been described for managing OA of the wrist, including scaphoid excision with four-corner

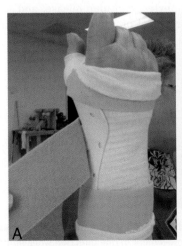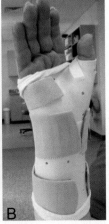

FIGURE 17–18 A and B, A wrist/thumb immobilization orthosis is often used after first CMC joint arthroplasty.

fusion, proximal row carpectomy, wrist arthrodesis, arthrodesis of the distal radioulnar joint, arthrodesis of the STT joint, and distal ulna resection (Beer & Turner, 1997; Bernstein et al., 2010; Cross & Baratz, 2011; Feinberg, 1999; Kozin, 1999; Michlovitz, 1999; Shapiro, 1996; Swanson, 1995b; Tijhuis, Vliet Vlieland, Zwinderman, & Hazes, 1998; van Vugt, van Jaarsveld, Hofman, Helders, & Bijlsma, 1999; Watson & Ballet, 1984; Watson, Weinzweig, Guidera, Zeppieri, & Ashmead, 1999; R. Wilson & Fredick, 1994). Common to these surgical procedures is the judicious postoperative orthosis intervention. Orthoses are used after bulky dressing removal to further stabilize and protect the surgical site. Position of the wrist and the length of time the orthosis is worn may depend on the exact procedure performed. A wrist/thumb immobilization orthosis with the IP joint free may be used 6 to 8 weeks after STT fusion (Fig. 17–18A,B). Once satisfactory radiographic union is observed, gentle motion of the wrist is often initiated (Cross & Baratz, 2011; Kozin, 1999).

Elbow with Osteoarthritis

Primary OA of the elbow is a relatively rare condition that comprises only 1% to 2% of patients with elbow arthritis (Morrey, 1992). It almost exclusively affects males and has a strong association with strenuous use of the arm in activities ranging from operating heavy machinery, throwing athletes, to aggressive weight training. The pattern of pain in patients suffering from primary elbow OA is very different than that of patients suffering from the rheumatoid elbow. Patients with elbow OA classically complain of impingement pain at the extremes of motion. Unlike OA of other joints, elbow OA is characterized by the relative preservation of articular cartilage and the maintenance of joint space but with hypertrophic osteophyte formation and capsular contracture. Osteophytes may be present in the olecranon fossa and on the olecranon, which may cause pain in maximal extension. Osteophyte formation may also occur in the coronoid process or the trochlea, which may cause impingement pain in full flexion. As the disease progresses, patients may complain of pain throughout the arc of ulnohumeral motion. This is most often present typically in advanced stage disease. Classically, patients will complain of pain while carrying heavy objects at the side of the body with the elbow in extension. They often complain of painful catching or locking, which may represent the presence of a loose body or a synovialized osteocartilaginous fragment, which can be found in approximately 50% of patients (Antuna, Morrey, Adams, & O'Driscoll, 2002; Forster, Clark, & Lunn, 2001; Morrey, 1992; Oka, 2000). The extension/flexion arc of ulnohumeral joint motion is often limited and patients may have up to a 30° flexion contracture (Antuna et al., 2002; Oka, Ohta, & Saitoh, 1998; Wada, Isogai, Ishii, & Yamashita, 2004).

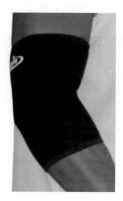

FIGURE 17–19 Soft conforming neoprene-type orthoses are available in many sizes and lengths.

Nonsurgical Orthotic Management Guidelines

Conservative management for the painful elbow with OA consists of rest, anti-inflammatory medication, long-term activity modification, referral to physical/occupational therapy, and orthotic management. A soft neoprene orthosis that provides soft tissue compression, warmth, and protection can provide patients with symptom improvement during aggravating activities (Fig. 17–19) (McAuliffe & Miller, 2000). A hinged elbow orthosis that limits full extension and flexion may be trialed to prevent anterior and posterior ulnohumeral impingement (Fig. 17–20). These can be custom made as shown or prefabricated as well (described in Chapter 11).

Postsurgical Orthotic Management Guidelines

Current surgical treatment options for elbow OA include **arthroscopic debridement**, open debridement with ulnohumeral arthroplasty, distraction **interposition arthroplasty**, and total elbow arthroplasty (Cheung, Adams, & Morrey, 2008). Orthosis application will vary based on the surgical procedure and physician preference.

An arthroscopic debridement involves decompression of the impinging osteophytes, capsular release, and joint debridement with the removal of any loose bodies within

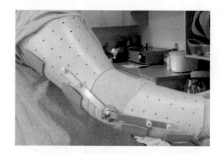

FIGURE 17–20 A custom-fabricated extension restriction orthosis can be fabricated to allow movement in one direction while limiting movement in another (Phoenix elbow hinge shown here).

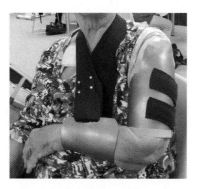

FIGURE 17–21 Custom-modified, "collar and cuff" designed orthosis for a patient who underwent an elbow debridement and, a few days later, sustained a nondisplaced humerus fracture.

the joint. Advantages of this approach include less postoperative pain and decreased intraoperative bleeding, which allows for early gains in range of motion (ROM; O'Driscoll, 1995). Following such procedures, patients are often placed simply in a "collar and cuff" or some type of sling during the day to assist with pain control (Fig. 17–21). In addition, patients are instructed in frequent ROM exercises to prevent stiffness. A night static progressive extension orthosis is often applied to maintain any extension achievements made during the operative procedure. This is preferably applied the same day as the operative procedure and can be progressively remolded as edema decreases and extension improves. This orthosis can be either custom fabricated or obtained through commercial sources. If custom fabricated, the orthosis can be either applied anteriorly or posteriorly. The authors' preference is a custom-fit anterior design with the forearm positioned in supination or neutral (Fig. 17–22). The distal portion of the orthosis must be flared to prevent irritation to the dorsal sensory branch of the radial nerve.

If more extensive procedures are performed, then patients should be placed in an elbow immobilization orthosis or restriction orthosis similar to those used following rheumatoid elbow

procedures. The patient must be instructed in edema management and a carefully guided exercise program to prevent stiffness. The precise exercise regime will be dependent on the surgical procedure performed and surgeon preference, all of which require close communication between the patient, therapist, and surgeon.

Rheumatoid Arthritis

Characteristics

RA is an unpredictable, systemic, chronic, autoimmune, potentially debilitating disease of the synovial tissue of joints. It affects roughly 2.1 million people in the United States, touching the lives of women more than men in a 3:1 ratio. The disease process is inflammatory and may be characterized by exacerbations and remissions that occur over the course of time. If the inflammation remains unchecked, the disease process may eventually cause severe joint destruction, attenuation or rupture of tendons, ligament laxity, joint deformity, and a generalized decrease in function (Bernstein et al., 2010; Fess et al., 2005; Kozin, 1999; Massarotti, 1996; Melvin, 1982; Poole et al., 2000; Swanson, 1995a, 1995b). Advancements in anti-inflammatory medications and disease-modifying drugs have greatly influenced the goals of reducing pain, inflammation, and retarding joint damage.

Early onset is often seen in the shoulders, wrists, and knees but may then involve other joints of the upper and lower extremities including the MCP and PIP joints of the hand (Fig. 17–23). RA is a systemic disease, and patients may also complain of intermittent fevers, weight loss, fatigue, muscle atrophy, and prolonged morning stiffness (Swanson, 1995a, 1995b).

In the early stages of the disease, orthotic management and medical management may be all that is required. As the disease progresses, surgical intervention such as joint replacement and tendon transfer may be considered, depending on the degree of functional impairment (Poole & Pellegrini, 2000;

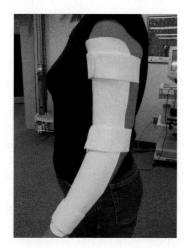

FIGURE 17–22 Custom anterior design with forearm in neutral.

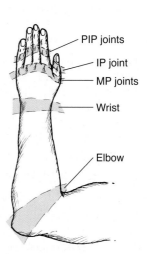

PIP joints
IP joint
MP joints
Wrist
Elbow

FIGURE 17–23 Upper extremity joints commonly affected by RA.

CHAPTER 17

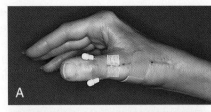

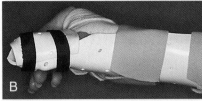

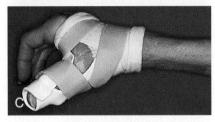

FIGURE 17–24 First CMC joint arthroplasty with MP joint fusion. **A,** Note that pins secure the fusion during healing. **B,** At 6 days postsurgery, the patient was placed in a wrist/thumb immobilization orthosis with a protective cover for the pins. **C,** At 4 to 5 weeks postsurgery, the orthosis was modified to allow wrist motion per physician.

Shapiro, 1996). A generally accepted operative sequence usually involves initially stabilizing the affected proximal structures (R. Wilson & Fredick, 1994). For example, procedures would commence at the wrist (arthrodesis) followed by the MCP joints (arthroplasty). Some procedures can be performed simultaneously, such as a wrist and thumb MP fusion or a first CMC arthroplasty and thumb MP arthrodesis (Fig. 17–24) (R. Wilson & Fredick, 1994). When surgical intervention is planned, the hand dominance and ambulatory status of the patient must also be considered. If the patient is presently using a cane or crutches, he or she should be instructed in the use of platform crutches before surgery to allow ambulation without placing undue stress on the surgically repaired structures.

General Signs and Symptoms

RA is characterized by joint redness, inflammation, and tenderness over involved areas on gentle palpation (Fess et al., 2005; Massarotti, 1996; Melvin, 1982; Swanson, 1995b). The involved joint(s) may be warm and swollen, with a decrease in joint ROM. Unlike the normal healing process in which the inflammation subsides and the patient progresses through the stages of healing, patients with RA often remain in an extended inflammatory phase, which results in damage and deformity to the joints, pain, and impaired function (Swanson, 1995a; Terrono, Feldon, & Kimball, 2011).

Pain

Joint pain can occur during rest and may indicate acute inflammation (Melvin, 1982). Gentle pressure at the lateral

aspects of an inflamed joint can cause some degree of pain, depending on the severity of the inflammation and joint damage. The joint(s) involved are generally described as sore with a notable decrease in AROM and functional use.

Stiffness and Decreased Function

Fluctuations in AROM can be related to joint pain and the extent of joint damage. Most patients with RA describe an increase in joint stiffness in the morning, after prolonged inactivity, and during periods of exacerbation when pain limits functional use (Fess et al., 2005; Melvin, 1982).

Synovitis

Synovitis, inflammation of the joint lining (synovium), occurs slowly in the patient with RA. There are biochemical and autoimmune responses that cause changes in the synovium (Swanson, 1995a). Inflammatory cells and enzymes attack the synovial lining of the joints, and the synovial tissues can eventually become fibrotic and form a scar tissue–like substance (pannus), which may invade tendons and ligaments (Fig. 17–2B). This process is progressive; continued swelling causes greater thickening of the synovium, capsular stretching, pain, and eventually destruction of the cartilage and bone (Fig. 17–2C) (Blank & Cassidy, 1996).

The synovitis associated with RA may be divided into three phases: acute, subacute, and chronic active (Melvin, 1982). Each phase has the same symptoms of pain, tenderness, warmth, and limited ROM. The disease is most active in the acute phase, which leads to joint destruction. The symptoms begin to subside as the subacute phase is entered. The disease may be considered to be in the chronic active phase if the symptoms persist over a long period of time. The course of the disease varies and is unique to each patient; not all progress through these phases (Melvin, 1982; Swanson, 1995a).

Tenosynovitis

Tenosynovitis is an inflammation of the synovial lining of the tendon sheaths. In patients with RA, tenosynovitis usually occurs at the level of the flexor tendons, as they traverse the wrist (under the flexor retinaculum), and at the dorsum of the wrist, deep to the extensor retinaculum (Leslie, 1999; R. Wilson & Fredick, 1994). These tunnels are lined with the same synovial fluid that surrounds the joints. If left untreated, the lining becomes thickened, and plaques and nodules may form, disrupting normal tendon excursion (Alter, Feldon, & Terrono, 2011; Leslie, 1999).

Tenosynovitis in a *digit* usually appears as a sausage-type swelling in which the entire digit may be enlarged and tender to palpation. Digital flexion can be significantly impaired by even a small amount of tenosynovitis (Leslie, 1999). Pain, mild triggering, and/or crepitation may be noted with attempted ROM (Ferlic, 1996; Melvin, 1982; Valdes, 2012).

Tenosynovitis in the *volar wrist* can present with median nerve irritation or carpal tunnel syndrome. The group of thickened, enlarged flexor tendons within the small carpal canal secondarily place pressure on the median nerve as it passes through the shared carpal tunnel (Ferlic, 1996; Leslie, 1999).

Tenosynovitis in the *dorsal wrist* is quite evident by swelling, which can occur in one or all six dorsal compartments. Dorsal tenosynovitis can be distinguished from dorsal wrist synovitis by observing movement of the distended tenosynovium with active digital flexion and extension (Leslie, 1999; R. Wilson & Fredick, 1994).

DEQUERVAIN'S TENOSYNOVITIS

DeQuervain's tenosynovitis is inflammation of the extensor pollicis brevis (EPB) and the APL tendons within the first dorsal wrist compartment. Tenderness, thickening, and crepitation are often present over the radial styloid. Pain may radiate proximally and dorsally with active wrist radial/ulnar deviation (Kirkpatrick & Lisser, 1995).

STENOSING TENOSYNOVITIS

Stenosing tenosynovitis, also known as *trigger finger*, commonly occurs at the RF and/or MF but can also occur in the thumb and other digits. Stenosing tenosynovitis is the result of swelling and thickening of the flexor tendon proximal to the A1 pulley (Ferlic, 1996; Kirkpatrick & Lisser, 1995; Valdes, 2012). As the tendon attempts to traverse through the pulley, it catches, holding the digit in a flexed position that has to be manually released by the patient. Attempted movement and direct palpation over the A1 pulley can be painful. Oftentimes, the patient will complain of simultaneous dorsal PIP joint pain. This is at least in part due to the extensor mechanism working to overcome the resistance from the "stuck" flexor tendon. Custom orthosis intervention has been shown effective in the early management of stenosing tenosynovitis (<6 months), with reports of the subjective reduction of pain and objective increase in functional use (Valdes, 2012).

Tendon Ruptures and Repairs

Tendon ruptures can occur when tendons are invaded by inflamed synovium or when tendons rub on a rough edge of a bone (Alter et al., 2011; Leslie, 1999). These rough edges or bony spurs are most likely the result of joint inflammation that has led to joint damage (Fig. 17–25) (Ferlic,

1996; Shapiro, 1996; Swanson, 1995b; R. Wilson & Fredick, 1994). Tendon ruptures in the hand occur most commonly at prominent bony sites, such as the scaphoid waist, the distal ulna, and Lister's tubercle on the dorsal radius. As a result, most common ruptures are of the flexor pollicis longus (FPL), index flexor digitorum profundus (FDP), the extensor digiti quinti (EDQ), and the extensor pollicis longus (EPL) tendons (Ferlic, 1996; Katz & Moore, 2000; Leslie, 1999; Shapiro, 1996; Swanson, 1995b; R. Wilson & Fredick, 1994).

Pathomechanics of Deformities in Rheumatoid Arthritis

As mentioned earlier, RA is the most common connective tissue disorder. It is a systemic disease that produces a joint inflammation. This is as a result of immunologic response occurring from the synovial tissue. The pathogenesis in RA causes synovitis and the synovium produces a **pannus**, which infiltrates cartilage, tendon, and ligaments. This pannus eventually produces significant stress on the joint capsule causing it to attenuate and the cartilage and subchondral bone to erode. Subsequently, there is often ligamentous disruption that affects the way the tendon(s) glide and eventually the way the joints ultimately move. Over time, as the hand and/or wrist are used, abnormal stressors continue to produce a significant load on tendons and other tendon-supporting structures. Because of instability and derangement of the joint–tendon relationship, patients often have pain. Alteration of joint motion, along with the abnormal tendinous pull, often produces crepitus associated with swelling and pain. The hand pathomechanics in RA is unfortunately progressive in nature. Pathogenesis of deformities of the wrist and hand is divided into four stages; see Table 17–2 for the typical characteristics of each of the stages.

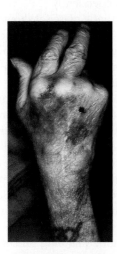

FIGURE 17–25 Rupture of the EDQ and extensor digitorum communis (EDC) tendons of the RF and SF in a patient with RA.

TABLE 17–2

Stages of Rheumatoid Arthritis

Stage I:	Synovitis of the joints and tendons, pain and swelling, impaired tendon gliding associated with crepitus, and no obvious deformity
Stage II:	Synovitis of the joint and tendon continues; with use, the wrist and hand joints may demonstrate a tendency for subluxation and/or dislocation because of joint laxity. The deformity is apparent at the joints; however, it is passively correctable.
Stage III:	Deformities become fixed. The joints may demonstrate minimal or no joint destruction.
Stage IV:	Evidence of joint destruction and presence of soft tissue disturbance associated with multiple wrist and hand deformities

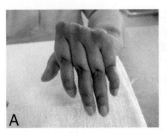
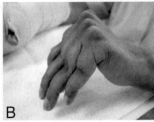

FIGURE 17–26 **A and B,** A patient with severe RA of the wrist and digits; note the ulnar deviation, MP subluxation, and swan-neck deformities.

The entire upper extremity is a kinematic chain supported and/or stabilized by various ligaments and joint capsules controlled by the musculotendinous units. The degree and amplitude of joint motion is dependent on the precise functioning of the neuromuscular structures. The articulation of various joints may depend on the skeletal configuration and are either classified as stable or inherently unstable. Once the ligamentous and capsular stability is lost, along with tenosynovitis due to the disease process, sequential disturbance in the affected joint(s) follows. The distal joint position is a consequence of the altered musculotendinous vectors, causing progression of the deformities (Fig. 17–26A,B). In addition, an abnormal compressive load placed on the joints, due to the aforementioned factors, contributes to joint degenerative changes. For instance, looking at the various stages of pathogenesis of RA deformities, derangement occurring at the radioulnar joint subsequently will produce changes at the wrist followed by changes at the digital levels. Imbalance occurring at the digital level thus will produce changes at the proximal joints.

Therefore, it is critical to assess *both* the rheumatoid wrist and hand together when applying an orthoses because altered mechanics at the proximal level will affect the distal levels and vice versa.

Nonsurgical Orthotic Management Guidelines

A combination of rest (with an immobilization orthosis) and medical management can aid in reducing the symptoms of RA (Fig. 17–27A,B). Postsurgical patients should

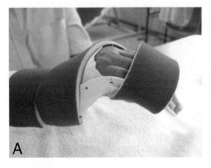
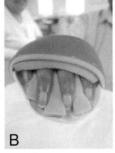

FIGURE 17–27 **A,** Soft straps aid in proper anatomical positioning of the digits into the orthosis. **B,** Digit dividers are added by using high-density foam wedges to align and separate digits.

be instructed in digital motion to decrease the chance of adhesions and maximize movement. Gentle, early ROM and blocking exercises aid in optimizing tendon excursion and intrinsic tightness. The therapist should teach the patient adaptations to ADLs and other techniques for joint protection and energy conservation because these tips help the patient cope with arthritis on a daily basis (Colditz, 2000; Fess et al., 2005; Massarotti, 1996; Poole et al., 2000; Simmons et al., 1996; Terrono, Nalebuff, & Philips, 1995).

Although orthosis application is a treatment component, it is rarely used alone. Other interventions should be integrated into the treatment plan. Thermal agents can be useful adjuncts in preparing the joints for exercise and reducing pain (e.g., paraffin, hot packs, and ultrasound) (Katz & Moore, 2000). A well-instructed home exercise program can aid in maintaining joint flexibility and daily function. Physicians should be encouraged to refer patients early for therapy, patient education, joint protection, and orthotic management. When used soon after diagnosis, orthoses can support weak structures around a joint, reduce stress to the joint capsule, decrease pain during use, and perhaps retard soft tissue damage (Blank & Cassidy, 1996; Jacobs, 2003).

Material Selection

THERMOPLASTICS

The need for and type of orthosis may change as the disease process evolves. The therapist must use his or her skill and experience to create the most appropriate orthosis and orthosis regime. For example, a wrist/hand immobilization orthosis (resting hand orthosis) may be ordered for a patient, but lifestyle and daily demands may require at least some use of the hand. An option may be to fabricate a wrist immobilization orthosis for day use (digits and thumb free) and a wrist/hand immobilization orthosis for night use (Simmons et al., 1996). Before fabrication, consideration must be given to the acuteness of the disease, material choice for skin type, wearing schedules, patient's lifestyle, and ability to don and doff the orthosis independently.

The choice of orthotic material should take into account conformability and weight. Orthoses should be lightweight and allow for fluctuating edema and synovitis whenever possible. Materials that are highly conforming (minimal resistance to stretch, such as plastic-based material) may not be the best choice if joint swelling fluctuates or if frequent adjustments are anticipated to accommodate joint and soft tissue changes. Materials that are more rigid (high resistance to stretch, such as a rubber-based material) tend not to fit as intimately to the contours of the body part and may be a better choice for this patient population (Austin, 2003). These materials provide joint support, are more forgiving than highly conforming materials, and may better accommodate fluctuations in edema.

During the orthotic planning process, a clinician must take into account the likelihood of the patient having varying levels of edema/synovitis and then account for this

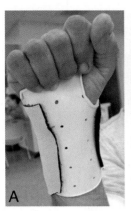
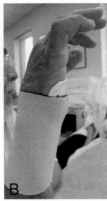

FIGURE 17–28 **A and B,** A custom cut wide neoprene strap/wrap is used to compliment this wrist orthosis. This wide ⅛″ thick neoprene material provides an even dorsal pressure distribution as well as warmth to the underlying tissue.

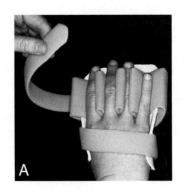
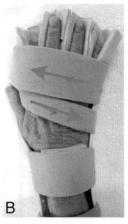

FIGURE 17–30 **A,** Soft straps are used for a liner as well as light and comfortable digit separators. **B,** Straps placed judiciously can be extremely effective in gently directing joints to a more anatomically correct position and can prevent undue stress on vulnerable joints during sleep.

as they are fabricating the orthosis. Several options such as (1) layering cotton stockinette, (2) using elastic wrap over the intended body segment, (3) choosing a material with flexibility such as a ³⁄₃₂″ highly perforated material, and/or (4) incorporating a softer material into the design such as a neoprene/thermoplastic combination (Fig. 17–28A,B).

The therapist must also keep in mind that an orthosis worn for a specific problem may aggravate a proximal or distal condition. For example, a wrist immobilization orthosis may work well to stabilize the wrist, but during functional use, the forces may transfer proximally to the elbow, irritating existing elbow inflammation or distally increasing forces to the MCP joints.

STRAPPING

The strapping design of the orthosis should allow for easy independent donning and doffing. Straps should be wide, soft, and conforming because patients with RA often have thin, fragile skin owing to their age, medications, or the disease process. Straps can be fabricated to allow extra

length or loops on the end of the strap for easy application and removal (Fig. 17–29).

Soft strapping material can also be used as digit dividers on wrist/hand immobilization orthoses. These dividers can aid in alignment and prevent maceration between the digits (Fig. 17–30A). Care should be taken to place straps advantageously. They can be used as an aid in gently redirecting joints into an antideformity position (Fig. 17–30B). Straps can successfully provide light joint positioning (Fig. 17–31A,B).

PREFABRICATED ORTHOSES

As previously mentioned in this chapter, commercially purchased neoprene orthoses can often work well to provide intermittent light support to joints during times of symptom exacerbation (Fig. 17–7). For some patients, these orthoses are easy to apply and care for. Chapter 11 reviews these options in more detail.

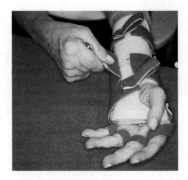

FIGURE 17–29 A patient with severe RA of the wrist and digits uses a custom-made strapping system to don and doff this orthosis by combining soft strap closures with loop attachments.

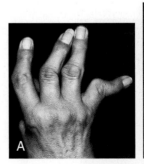
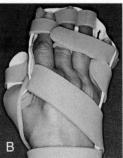

FIGURE 17–31 **A,** A patient with psoriatic arthritis. **B,** A night resting orthosis with soft straps strategically placed to help improve joint alignment and prevent joint contracture.

Elbow with Rheumatoid Arthritis

RA in the elbow can manifest itself similarly as it does in other joints (Bernstein et al., 2010). Elbow involvement in the patient with RA can be noted as joint synovitis and, occasionally, the presence of subcutaneous nodules at the posterior aspect of the elbow joint (Fig. 17–32). Chronic synovitis can lead to elbow flexion and extension contractures and to limitations in forearm rotation. These contractures tend to develop because of reduced motion secondary to joint pain and patient guarding. Ulnar nerve irritation may occur owing to tension on the nerve resulting from local trauma, static posturing, joint inflammation, osteophyte formation, or pressure from a subcutaneous nodule (McAuliffe & Miller, 2000). As with other joints in RA, disease-modifying drugs have made a big difference in managing the disease progression. However, should pain and joint destruction continue, surgical options such as **synovectomy** and **arthroplasty** are recommended (Stanley, 2011).

Nonsurgical Orthotic Management Guidelines

Conservative management of the painful rheumatoid elbow typically consists of anti-inflammatory or disease-modifying antirheumatoid medications, referral to physical/occupational therapy, activity modifications, and orthotic management (Bernstein et al., 2010; McAuliffe et al., 2000; Nirschl & Morrey, 1993). Orthoses at the elbow joint should be used cautiously because of the high risk of joint contracture (Morrey, 2000b). Soft devices can be used as an option in the early stages of the disease to provide protection and support to the painful elbow. Commercially or custom-fabricated available elbow sleeves or protectors can limit full range of flexion and extension and protect tender nodules or skin ulcerations (Fig. 17–33). A custom-made donut design fabricated from foam padding, silicone gel sheeting, neoprene, or a combination of these can absorb shock, protect a painful nodule/bursa, cushion the ulnar nerve, or decrease pressure about painful sore tissue (Fig. 17–34A–C). Neoprene orthoses produce gentle soft tissue compression and have the added

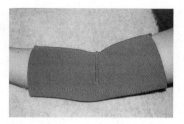

FIGURE 17–33 Custom-made or prefabricated protection about the elbow.

benefit of neutral warmth and insulation (see Chapter 14) (McAuliffe et al., 2000).

When greater support is needed, an anterior or posterior orthosis can be applied. An anterior elbow immobilization orthosis is recommended if nodules are present on the posterior elbow; it can be used during sleeping because it allows the arm to relax on the bed rather than against hard material (Figs. 17–22 and 17–35) (McAuliffe et al., 2000). The anterior design may be less complicated to fit because there are fewer bony prominences and less potential for pressure areas. The anterior approach also allows for gravity-assisted application with precise conformability.

When posterior orthoses are used, the wrist should be considered in the design. Patients with elbow arthritis may be more comfortable with the wrist included in the orthosis to control forearm rotation and excess motion. Posterior orthoses should be cautiously molded and, if necessary, well padded about the condyles, ulnar styloid, and the olecranon process (Austin, 2003).

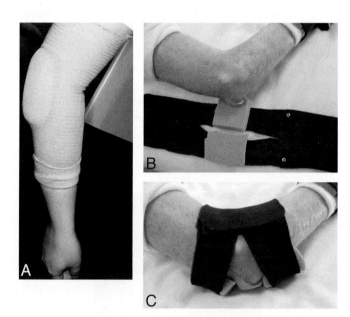

FIGURE 17–34 A, Protection using foam padding for a tender subcutaneous nodule is secured with an elasticized sleeve. **B and C,** This patient with a right elbow ulceration from advanced scleroderma receives comfort with this custom-made orthosis from neoprene and Tee foam padding. The orthosis allows her to rest her elbow without direct pressure on tender, sore tissues.

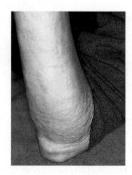

FIGURE 17–32 Subcutaneous rheumatoid nodules are often seen about the posterior elbow of a patient with RA.

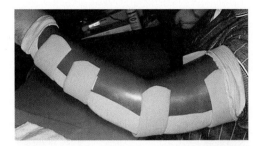

FIGURE 17–35 An anterior elbow extension immobilization orthosis. A wider or a criss cross designed strap at the posterior elbow may enhance fit of this orthosis.

Contractures of the elbow can cause devastating limitations in all ADLs and all of life's tasks. The development of an elbow flexion contracture is a common sequela following elbow trauma as well as postsurgery. When noted early, contractures can be managed with gentle serial static or static progressive mobilization via an orthosis in the desired direction of correction.

Postsurgical Orthotic Management Guidelines

An elbow joint synovectomy can be performed to alleviate pain and increase functional joint ROM in the early stages of the disease, with or without a radial head resection (Varitimidis, Plakseychuk, & Sotereanos, 1999). Orthosis application following synovectomy is based on surgeon preference and is used with caution. If the surgery was relatively simple due to mild synovitis, the patient can easily use a sling and remove frequently for active ROM. If more extensive dissection is undertaken, the forearm is often positioned in neutral rotation with the elbow comfortably positioned at approximately 90° of flexion within an orthosis. The orthosis is typically worn for 2 to 4 weeks postoperatively, removing frequently for ROM.

Elbow joint arthroplasty is reserved for the severely involved joint. Pain, joint instability, ulnar nerve involvement, and the inability to perform simple ADLs may lead a patient to this decision. Several procedures have been described (Bryan & Morrey, 1982; Ferlic, 1999; Gill & Morrey, 1998; Morrey, 2000a; Wright, Froimson, & Stewart, 1993). Regardless of the procedure, early orthosis application and postoperative therapy play significant roles in achieving maximal results (Ferlic, 1999; Gill & Morrey, 1998; Melvin, 1982; Morrey, 2000b; Nirschl & Morrey, 1993; Wolf, 2000). After arthroplasty, elbow immobilization or restriction orthoses are used cautiously and in combination with a carefully guided exercise and edema management program (Brach, 1999; Edmond, 1993; Wolf, 2000). The position of the elbow depends on the procedure(s) performed. The capsule of the elbow is at its greatest capacity at approximately 80° of flexion (Johansson, 1962). Therefore, positioning the elbow in approximately 80 to 90° of flexion reduces pressure within the joint, making this position quite comfortable for the patient. The position of the forearm within the orthoses will depend

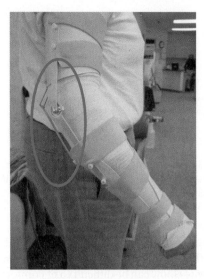

FIGURE 17–36 This patient had a custom elbow flexion restriction orthosis (Phoenix elbow hinge) with the forearm in neutral. Note the "dynamic" extension assists to aid in triceps extension and the flexion block positioned on the center of the hinge. As the surgeon's protocol allows, the flexion arc can be increased by moving the block counterclockwise.

on whether ligamentous reconstruction was performed (Szekeres & King, 2006). The forearm is placed in supination if the medial collateral ligament was repaired, pronation if the lateral collateral ligamentous complex was repaired, and in neutral if both were repaired in surgery (Szekeres & King, 2006). Furthermore, the position of the elbow will depend on the status of the triceps tendon. For example, if the triceps tendon is detached and reattached as part of the joint replacement, the elbow may be positioned in some degree of extension, which is based on the intraoperative tension observed on the repair and surgeon preference (Fig. 17–36).

The anterior or posterior elbow resting orthosis should be removed four to eight times a day for ROM exercises. The orthosis can be prefabricated or custom made. However, the precise exercise regime is dependent on close communication between the surgeon and therapist, type of prosthesis, surgical procedure, condition of the ulnar nerve, triceps status, collateral ligament status, and overall stability of the elbow joint. The prolonged use of an immobilization orthosis carries the risk of joint contractures, as previously emphasized (Edmond, 1993; Wolf, 2000). Circumferentially wrapping the orthosis on the arm (e.g., using an elasticized bandage) instead of using straps may aid in postoperative edema management and prevent orthosis migration as the edema subsides. Orthotic fabrication over the midpoint of the olecranon, medial and lateral epicondyles, and the bony grooves of the cubital tunnel require particular care because these areas are prone to irritation from direct pressure (Fig. 17–37). A hinged orthosis (mobilization or restriction) may be prescribed versus an immobilization orthosis following elbow arthroplasty. This will allow for a precise controlled amount of flexion and extension and can facilitate joint and tendon glide, increase

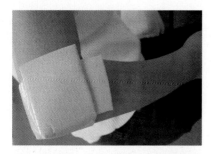

FIGURE 17–37 Pre-padding the condyles and/or posterior elbow may aid in decreasing direct pressure over bony prominences while custom molding.

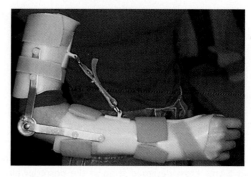

FIGURE 17–39 At 12 weeks after elbow arthroplasty, this patient was unable to gain functional elbow flexion. Thus, a static progressive elbow flexion mobilization orthosis with a Phoenix elbow hinge was prescribed. Note the D-rings and loop strapping materials that provide the static progressive mobilization force. Including the wrist in this design prevents forearm rotation.

blood flow and nutrition to the repair site, and aid in preventing joint stiffness while healing (Fig. 17–38A). However, hinge orthoses at the elbow can be difficult to fit comfortably. There are few contours about the elbow that contribute to a congruent fit. Obtaining a secure mechanical hold of the orthosis in the proper position (axis of the elbow hinge lined up with the elbow's joint axis) may warrant fabrication of some type of shoulder harness to prevent migration as the forearm moves (Fig. 17–38B).

Orthotic interventions that apply a mobilization force in the latter healing stages can elongate soft tissue in the event that a joint flexion or extension contracture has developed (Fig. 17–39). These orthoses can be custom fabricated or purchased/rented commercially. This form of orthotic intervention is not used until at least 6 to 8 weeks postoperatively and is only used if the patient is not making adequate gains in ROM with his or her prescribed exercise program (Szkeres & King, 2006). The rationale behind this form of orthotic intervention is based on **low-load prolonged stress (LLPS)** to mobilize a stiff joint (Flowers & LaStayo, 2012; Hepburn,

1987; Light, Nuzik, Personius, & Barstrom, 1984) (refer to Chapter 15 for further details). These mobilization orthoses are used to apply LLPS to the stiff elbow through the mobilization device to hold the joint at the end of available ROM for a long period of time so the tissue can adapt to the stress. It is critical to ensure that minimal lateral force is being applied in order to protect the collateral ligaments of the elbow joint (McAuliffe et al., 2000; Morrey, 2000a, 2000b).

Wrist with Rheumatoid Arthritis

Wrist and hand deformities caused by RA are often the first noticed because these typically are the first joints affected in the upper extremity (Colville, Nicholson, & Belcher, 1999; Melvin, 1982; Swanson, 1995a, 1995b; Vamos, White, & Caughey, 1990; R. Wilson & Fredick, 1994). Deformity results from a combination of ligamentous laxity and the location of the synovitis. The patient with acute RA presents with diffusely swollen and red appearance of the involved joints (Fess et al., 2005). Any attempt to move the wrist or fingers may be exquisitely painful. On palpation, the wrist and hand may be warm, owing to a combination of joint and tendon inflammation. Rest (orthosis) is one of the first treatment choices that may be prescribed (Blank & Cassidy, 1996; Fess et al., 2005; Kozin, 1999; Melvin, 1982; Stirrat, 1996).

The wrist is a complex joint with multiple ligamentous connections on both the volar and dorsal surfaces. Many combinations of deformities may occur, depending on the location of the inflammation and the ligaments that have been affected. The three most common patterns of deformity are subluxation of the distal radioulnar joint, volar subluxation/supination of the carpus at the radiocarpal joint, and radial deviation of the wrist (Feinberg, 1999; Michlovitz, 1999; Rizio et al., 1995; Shapiro, 1996; Swanson, 1995b; Talesnick, 1989; van Vugt et al., 1999; R. Wilson, 1986; R. Wilson & Fredick, 1994).

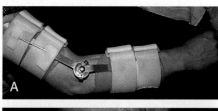

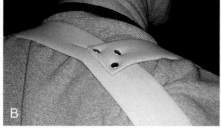

FIGURE 17–38 **A,** This Phoenix elbow hinged orthosis used after elbow reconstruction restricts elbow AROM and prevents lateral stress. **B,** A custom made shoulder harness can be custom fabricated to secure the proximal portion of an elbow hinged orthosis in order to prevent distal migration and maintain proper hinge alignment.

The triangular fibrocartilage complex (TFCC) stabilizes the distal radioulnar joint. If synovitis invades the TFCC, it can weaken and damage the supporting ligaments. As a result, the radius subluxates volarly, making the ulnar head prominent dorsally. This is typically called **caput ulnae syndrome** (Shapiro, 1996; Swanson, 1995b). This deformity may be seen on radiographs or noted on simple palpation and visualization of a notably prominent distal ulna. The patient is likely to present with pain during active forearm rotation and the motion of the wrist joint.

Synovitis in the radiocarpal joint also weakens the ligamentous structures surrounding it. There is often attenuation and laxity of the radioscapholunate and radiocapitate ligaments volarly and dorsal radiocarpal and intercarpal ligaments. This laxity, in combination with the natural volar inclination of the radius, may facilitate volar carpal subluxation. The direction of force of the extensor carpi ulnaris (ECU) tendon shifts from extension to flexion. Volar subluxation can contribute to carpal supination, ulnar translocation of the carpus, and ulnar shift of the metacarpals; all of these changes can decrease support to wrist extension and weaken the digital extensor tendons (Fig. 17–40) (Shapiro, 1996; Swanson, 1995b; R. Wilson & Fredick, 1994).

Disturbance of radioulnar alignment subsequently produces instability of the radiocarpal joint and progressively produces proximal carpal row and midcarpal instability. This instability occurring at the wrist joint eventually leads to the deforming forces produced by the digital flexors and extensors affecting the MCP and IP joints. Altered orientation of the flexors and extensor tendons at the level of the wrist as well as at the MCP joints causes failure of the sagittal bands dorsally and the fibroosseous sheath volarly, contributing to the ulnarly directed forces at the MCP joints (Fig. 17–41). The extensor tendons fall in the ulnar valley between the MCP joints, eventually causing an extensor lag at the MCP joints. This contributes to various secondary deformities at the distal joints. Besides, an alteration in radioulnar, radiocarpal, and midcarpal kinematics increases the gliding resistance (friction) to the extensor tendons, leading to potential tendon ruptures.

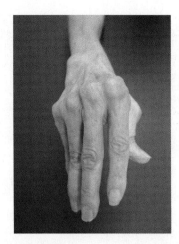

FIGURE 17–41 Note the ulnarly oriented extensor digitorum communis (EDC) of the MF & RF over the MP joints. This in turn will influence ulnar migration of the digits and volar subluxation of the proximal phalanges.

Radial deviation of the wrist is mainly caused by an ulnar translocation of the carpus with ulnar shift of the metacarpals. The bones may displace in any number of directions. This shifting of the carpal bones can contribute secondarily to ulnar deviation of the digits, commonly referred to as **zigzag deformity**. In the normal resting hand, the wrist is positioned in about 10° of ulnar deviation, causing the radius to align with the IF (Leslie, 1999; Swanson, 1995b). In the zigzag deformity, the body seems to attempt to re-create this balance (Fig. 17–42).

Nonsurgical Orthotic Management Guidelines

Orthosis options for RA of the wrist are similar even when the pathology is different. A wrist immobilization orthosis is often the treatment of choice for the patient with wrist inflammation (Blank & Cassidy, 1996; Fess et al., 2005; Kozin, 1999; Melvin, 1982; Stirrat, 1996). A lightweight, rubber-based material may be a good option for these immobilization orthoses (Orthoplast or Ezeform). To avoid

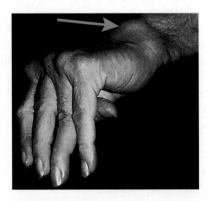

FIGURE 17–40 Synovitis in the radiocarpal joint weakens the surrounding ligamentous structures.

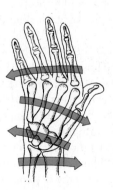

FIGURE 17–42 Typical deforming forces: The wrist deviates radially, the carpal bones deviate ulnarly, the metacarpals deviate radially, and the proximal phalanges deviate ulnarly and often sublux volarly as well.

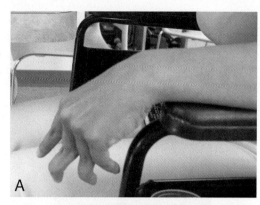

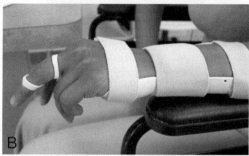

FIGURE 17–43 **A and B,** Note the position of the distal digits once an orthosis has been applied to stabilize the wrist. The middle digit had a long-standing swan-neck deformity that was not corrected with wrist positioning; therefore, a simple, functional PIP extension restriction orthosis was fabricated.

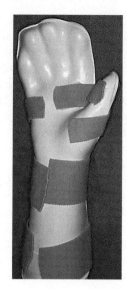

FIGURE 17–44 A (mitten design) wrist/hand/thumb immobilization orthosis is generally worn at night to provide volar support to the wrist and MP joints to properly align inflamed structures. Note the use of a plastic based thermoplastic material that has excellent comfortability about the volar aspect of the digits.

increased pressure on the median nerve, the suggested wrist position is neutral to 10° of extension if the deformity allows (Fig. 17–43A,B) (Melvin, 1982).

Rigid orthoses that immobilize the wrist and hand may be initially recommended for night use because full-time wear can greatly limit any function of the hand(s) during the day (Leonard, 1995). It is important to incorporate volar support within the orthosis at the distal ulna and MCP joints (Philips, 1995). This support helps protect against carpal and MP joint subluxation and MCP joint ulnar deviation. A wrist/hand/thumb immobilization (resting hand) orthosis can provide this position for night use (Fig. 17–44). This design is selected because it positions the thumb comfortably between midpalmar and radial abduction while supporting the wrist and digits. Suggested positions include the wrist at neutral to 10° extension, MCP joints at 25 to 30° of flexion, and IP joints in a gentle, relaxed flexion (Fess et al., 2005; Melvin, 1982). The MCP joints should be in no more than 30° of flexion because any greater flexion could force the joints into a position of deformity: volar subluxation of the MCP joints and strained IP joint extension (Philips, 1995; Shapiro, 1996; R. Wilson & Fredick, 1994). Positioning the IP joints in full extension with the MCP joints flexed may contribute to intrinsic muscle spasm and IP stiffness, which is difficult to overcome.

RA is often bilateral and symmetrical, requiring the patient to wear immobilization orthoses for both hands.

Without assistance at home, it can be challenging to don or doff bilateral orthoses. Consider alternating the use of right and left orthosis each night. Wearing schedules depend on the presenting condition. If only wrist synovitis is present, the wrist orthosis may be worn as necessary. However, patients often present with coexisting MCP joint synovitis, so immobilizing the wrist alone could place increased stress on the MCP joints (Melvin, 1982; Philips, 1995). If MCP pain and/or swelling become an issue, consideration should be given to alternating the orthosis regime (wrist orthosis for functional day use, wrist/hand orthosis for night).

Prefabricated wrist orthoses with a removable metal stay can be an option for daytime activities that contribute to wrist pain (Leonard, 1995; Murphy, 1996; Pagnotta et al., 1998; Stern et al., 1997; Stern et al., 1996b; Tijhuis et al., 1998; Veehof, Taal, Heijnsdijk-Rouwenhorst, & Van de Laar, 2008). The metal stay can be removed, allowing a small amount of wrist motion when necessary, which may decrease the forces placed on the MCP joints. Neoprene wrist orthoses may also help provide a light support while allowing some degree of motion. Neoprene may provide some pain relief owing to its neutral warmth properties. Careful fitting of soft prefabricated orthoses is paramount. Not all of these orthoses fit well because of the often encountered alteration in bony anatomy and size of the forearm in relationship to the wrist (Leonard, 1995). A neoprene orthosis can be custom fabricated to accommodate bony changes (Fig. 17–45A,B). Thermoplastic materials can be added to neoprene to provide additional reinforcement and support (see Chapter 14).

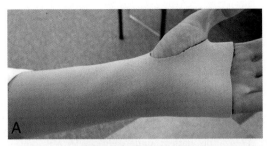

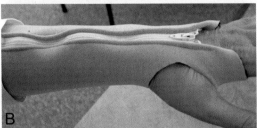

FIGURE 17–45 A and B, Custom neoprene orthoses, such as this wrist-based zipper design, can be considered as an alternative to hard thermoplastic materials.

Postsurgical Orthotic Management Guidelines

There are many surgical procedures that have been described for managing pain, increasing stability, improving functional use, and minimizing deformity of the wrist with RA (Blank & Cassidy, 1996; Colville et al., 1999; Linscheid, 2000; Nalebuff, 1990; Shapiro, 1996; Stirrat, 1996; Talesnick, 1989; Terrono, Feldon, et al., 2011; van Vugt et al., 1999; Watson & Ballet, 1984; Watson et al., 1999; R. Wilson, 1986). Relevant surgical procedures include synovectomy, tenosynovectomy, tendon repair or transfer, arthroplasty, and arthrodesis (Shapiro, 1996).

Synovectomy or Tenosynovectomy

Wrist synovectomy or **tenosynovectomy** is designed to decrease pain, increase function, prevent tendon rupture, and improve appearance. Synovectomy is not usually performed when there is advanced bony erosion, subluxation of the carpus, ruptured tendons, or flexion contractures (R. Wilson & Fredick, 1994). Orthoses are used to position the wrist joint after the postoperative dressing is removed. If tenosynovectomy has been performed in combination with wrist synovectomy, the orthotic protocol should protect the tendons as well (Fig. 17–46). Carefully instructed exercise sessions are essential for preventing tendon adherence postoperatively. The following are suggested positioning guidelines; however, the referring surgeon should recommend the positions of the involved joints (Fess et al., 2005; Leonard, 1995; Melvin, 1982; Philips, 1995).

- Wrist synovectomy: wrist positioned in neutral.
- Dorsal wrist tenosynovectomy: wrist positioned in gentle extension with the MCP joints in 35 to 40° of flexion.
- Volar wrist tenosynovectomy: wrist positioned in neutral to 25° extension.
- Digital flexor tenosynovectomy: If wrist is included, wrist positioned in approximately 20° of extension, and MCPs in 30° flexion. For a hand-based orthosis, MCPs blocked at approximately 30° of flexion.

Tendon Ruptures and Tendon Repairs

The cause of **tendon rupture** in patients with RA is relatively common in the hand and wrist. Tendon rupture is typically the result of attrition as the tendon becomes abraded by a rough bone or osteophyte as the tendon crosses over it during active motion and normal daily use

---

BOX 17–2

Evidence-Informed Orthotic Management: Rheumatoid Wrist

Wrist orthoses are mainly prescribed for pain reduction in persons who suffer from RA. Prefabricated, off-the-shelf type wrist orthoses have been found to be effective in reducing wrist pain (Kjeken, Møller, & Kvien, 1995; Nordenskiold, 1990; Pagnotta et al., 1998; Pagnotta, Mazer, Baron, & Wood-Dauphinee, 2005; Veehof et al., 2008). With regards to improvement in grip strength, the literature is conflicting because some studies found an improvement, whereas others found no effect or a reduction in grip strength (Anderson & Maas, 1987; Kjeken et al., 1995; Nordenskiold, 1990; Stern et al., 1996). These findings suggest that off-the-shelf orthoses may provide a positive reduction in pain relief, which may enhance overall function with their use. Precise dosage or wearing regimes have not been determined.

Wrist/hand immobilization orthoses are one of the most widely used orthosis applications in persons who suffer from RA. These orthoses are generally worn at night to provide volar support to the wrist and MP joints and aid in proper aligning of inflamed structures. These are prescribed to both newly diagnosed as well as for persons who suffer chronic RA. To date, studies indicate that hand immobilization orthoses provide no beneficial effect in improving hand function in patients with early RA. Thus, current evidence to support immobilization orthoses is lacking (Adams, Burridge, Mullee, Hammond, & Cooper, 2008; Egan et al., 2003; Steultjens et al., 2004; Steultjens, Dekker, Bouter, Leemrijse, & van den Ende, 2005). Clinicians have been providing these orthoses for decades based on expert opinion. RA is a chronic, systemic, autoimmune disorder that orthosis application likely has some effect on in delaying the progression of hand deformity, pain, and dysfunction. However, orthoses in conjunction with patient education and pharmacologic management may assist with short-term pain relief, especially in the event of a flare. This is based on expert opinion; orthosis application remains a rational biomechanical form of treatment that likely has a positive effect on the mechanics of joint motion and musculoskeletal function.

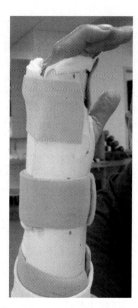

FIGURE 17–46 This orthosis supports the wrist and MP joints in comfortable extension postoperatively. It also places the tendons that were involved in the synovectomy in a stress-free, protected position.

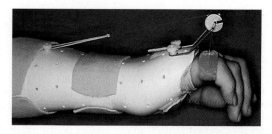

FIGURE 17–47 This patient underwent an SF MP joint implant arthroplasty and carpal tunnel release (CTR). The MP extension mobilization orthosis (with a Phoenix Outrigger) positions the wrist appropriately for the CTR and supports the MP joint arthroplasty, allowing gentle ROM via rubber band traction.

(Ferlic, 1996; Leslie, 1999; Michlovitz, 1999; Shapiro, 1996; R. Wilson & Fredick, 1994). Furthermore, the destructive effects of chronic tenosynovitis may weaken the tendon, leading to eventual rupture. The common sites for tendon rupture include the following:

- The tendons of the fourth, fifth, and occasionally sixth dorsal extensor compartment. This is often referred to as **caput ulnae** or **Vaughan-Jackson syndrome** (Vaughan-Jackson, 1948).
- The FPL and FDP to the index and long fingers may be abraded by a spur formed at the level of the scaphotra-pezial joint. This is often referred to as **Mannerfelt's syndrome** (Mannerfelt & Norman, 1969).

Tendon ruptures in patients with RA are rarely repaired primarily. Surgical reconstruction is typically done through the use of tendon transfers or grafts. Before undergoing tendon reconstruction, the status of the MCP joints and wrist must be assessed thoroughly via physical and radiographic examination. Any reconstructive wrist procedures should be carried out simultaneously at the time of tendon reconstruction. Orthotic management guidelines for tendon repairs and tendon transfers are similar to those described in detail in Chapters 18 and 19; however, due to the slower healing rates with this population, the rehabilitation program will likely need to be adjusted. The therapist must keep in mind the extent of surgical intervention and whether other procedures were done at the same time of the repair such as tenosynovectomy or arthroplasty (Fig. 17–47). Management of the tendon-repaired hand greatly depends on the extent of disease and surgical procedure; close communication with the referring surgeon is essential. Some physicians prefer complete cast immobilization for several weeks, whereas others prefer restrictive mobilization through a carefully guided orthosis program and therapy regime.

Arthroplasty

There are several indications for partial or total wrist arthroplasty: significant articular cartilage degeneration, pain, increasing difficulty with simple ADL tasks, and wrist deformity. The main goal is to preserve some painless wrist motion. After the postoperative dressing is removed, a wrist immobilization orthosis can be applied, including the MCP joints per physician protocol (Fig. 17–46). This orthosis can be removed for carefully guided exercises. AROM is generally initiated within 1 to 6 weeks postoperatively, depending on soft tissue integrity, prosthetic fit and stability, and surgical preference (M. Anderson & Adams, 2005; Kozin, 1999; Michlovitz, 1999). The therapist's goal for flexion and extension arc should be approximately 60° (Feinberg, 1999; Michlovitz, 1999).

Arthrodesis

A limited or total wrist arthrodesis sacrifices motion for stability but provides maximal function of the distal and proximal joints for the severely arthritic wrist (Hayden & Jebson, 2005; Kozin & Michlovitz, 2000). This procedure is usually considered for patients with exquisite wrist pain, rupture of tendons, poor bone stock, and significant wrist deformity (Hayden & Jebson, 2005; Shapiro, 1996; Watson et al., 1999). It is often performed after other options have failed. A circumferential orthosis is sometimes used preoperatively to simulate the outcome of a wrist arthrodesis. Often, this same orthosis can be reheated and adjusted as a postoperative support (Fig. 17–48A–C). Whether the arthrodesis is partial or total, postoperative orthotic management is essentially the same. In general, the cast is removed 1 to 2 weeks after arthrodesis, and the patient is placed in a wrist immobilization orthosis. Digital tendon gliding exercises are performed to prevent tendon adherence over the fusion site. The orthosis is generally worn until the fusion site is considered well healed, which is evaluated radiographically or by CT scan (6 to 8 weeks postoperatively) (Feinberg, 1999).

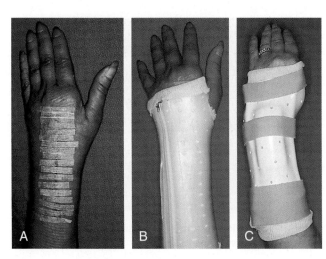

FIGURE 17–48 A, A patient 2 weeks after undergoing a wrist arthrodesis. **B,** The same patient wearing a Rolyan® Aquaform™ Zippered Wrist orthosis. The elastic material allows for easy remolding and refitting, and the circumferential design ensures secure immobilization. **C,** A clamshell orthosis fabricated for a woman who underwent a wrist synovectomy and limited arthrodesis; she was exquisitely tender over the surgical site and slow to heal. The design allows the patient to remove the dorsal piece easily for wound care and dressing changes.

Thumb with Rheumatoid Arthritis

As with any chronic synovitis, the thumb may develop many different deformity patterns well described in the literature (Nalebuff, 1968; Stein & Terrono, 1996). In 1968, a classification system for thumb deformities in RA was devised by Nalebuff. Any or all of the thumb joints may be involved to some degree. Management of the thumb with RA is based on the pattern of deformity and the functional needs of the patient. Orthosis application, used early in the disease process, can enhance function and reduce pain of the thumb by stabilizing the joint(s) involved during hand use. Orthosis application is used as a conservative measure but can also be used to manage postoperative thumb procedures.

The **boutonniere deformity** of the thumb is commonly seen in RA and is characterized by MP flexion and IP hyperextension (Fig. 17–49A–C) (Gellman, Statson, Brumfield, Costigan, & Kuschner, 1997; Rizio et al., 1995; Tomaino et al., 1995). Prolonged synovitis at the MP joint causes attenuation of the extensor mechanism made up of the EPB and EPL tendons. This results in EPL tendon subluxation volarly and ulnarward. In turn, the proximal phalanx assumes a flexed position and often subluxates volarly. Early on, the patient may maintain passive MP joint extension but may not be able to extend the joint actively. As a compensatory mechanism, the patient radially abducts the first metacarpal and hyperextends the IP joint. Accentuation of this hyperextension occurs when pinch forces are applied. With progression of the disease, this deformity often becomes fixed and can no longer be corrected passively.

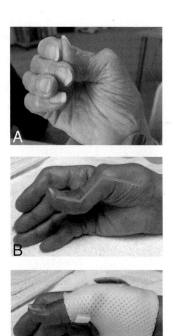

FIGURE 17–49 A, A patient with advanced rheumatoid disease. The boutonniere deformity of the thumb is exacerbated by tasks requiring pinch. **B and C,** This patient had psoriatic arthritis and was able to function well with the use of a thumb immobilization orthosis supporting the MP joint, preventing further collapse.

Swan-neck deformity of the thumb is also frequently seen in the RA population (Stein & Terrono, 1996). This deformity is characterized by metacarpal adduction, MP joint hyperextension, and IP joint flexion (Fig. 17–14). The deformity is initiated by synovitis of the first CMC joint, which results in attenuation of the joint capsule and leads to radial subluxation of the base of the first metacarpal. This imbalance of forces progresses to the development of an adduction contracture of the first CMC joint. As the deformity progresses, the volar plate of the MP joint becomes lax, allowing the joint to go into hyperextension. Dorsal and radial shift of the first metacarpal progresses which further contributes to the imbalance of the extensor forces. This leads to CMC adduction with MP joint hyperextension and IP joint flexion (Stein & Terrono, 1996; Swanson, 1995b).

Deformity of the thumb MP joint can occur without first CMC involvement (Stein & Terrono, 1996). Synovitis at the MP joint can result in attenuation of the ulnar collateral ligament (UCL) and volar plate. UCL attenuation allows the proximal phalanx to deviate radially. This in turn may cause the first dorsal interossei and the adductor muscles to become shortened and the web space contracted. With volar plate involvement, the MP joint hyperextends and the IP joint flexes. The pattern of thumb deformity is varied and may occur in different patterns and combinations. The goal of both conservative and operative treatment is restoration of pain-free balance and stability (Glickel et al., 1992; Stein & Terrono, 1996).

Nonsurgical Orthotic Management Guidelines

Orthoses can be used conservatively to protect the passively correctable joints from increased damage and to slow the progression of a fixed contracture (Stein & Terrono, 1996). In thumb boutonniere and swan-neck deformities, the goal is stabilization of the thumb in gentle abduction to prevent adduction contracture of the first web space, to provide pain relief, and to protect during rest and activity. A hand-based orthosis can allow for functional use, permitting full wrist mobility while performing ADLs (Figs. 17–49C and 17–50A,B). For advanced thumb boutonniere deformity—in which the IP joint significantly hyperextends—an orthosis that stabilizes the MP in slight flexion and provides a dorsal block to IP hyperextension may be of value for light use (Fig. 17–51). A forearm-based wrist/thumb immobilization orthosis is recommended for all other times to reduce pain and properly stabilize the CMC joint (Fig. 17–18B) (Colditz, 1995; Terrono et al., 1995). Patients should be encouraged to wear this orthosis at night.

To address isolated thumb MP joint deformity, the joint should be positioned as close to full extension as possible and the web space maintained, even if there is no pain (Colditz, 1995). The orthosis supplies the external stability to maintain the MP in extension and allows IP flexion; little motion is needed at the MP joint for good function. Various orthotic designs can be used, depending on the preference of the surgeon or therapist, similar to and variations of (Figs. 17–5B and 17–16A). Thinner materials (³⁄₃₂″) are recommended for fabrication if the deformity is easily passively correctable. If there are tight volar structures, a more rigid material should be considered to provide adequate support (⅛″).

Protection can also be given to the thumb IP joint if instability occurs (Philips, 1995; Terrono et al., 1995). A small

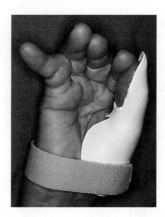

FIGURE 17–51 A dorsally applied orthosis holds the MP in slight flexion and prevents IP hyperextension.

dorsal thermoplastic orthosis can be fabricated or commercially available orthotics (e.g., Silver Ring™ orthoses from Silver Ring™ Company, Charlottesville, VA) can be ordered to provide lateral support, prevent hyperextension, and provide stability for functional use or while awaiting surgical intervention (Fig. 17–52).

Postsurgical Orthotic Management Guidelines

The goals of surgery for the patient with RA of the thumb depend on which joints are involved and how much the disease has progressed. The stability of each joint depends on the forces applied to it during use and the direction of the tendon forces that act on it (Stein & Terrono, 1996).

Thumb Interphalangeal Joint

Surgical intervention at the IP joint may consist of extrinsic tendon reconstruction if tendon integrity allows. Extensor tendon repairs should be positioned in an orthosis for at least 5 weeks in wrist extension, thumb radial abduction and extension, and MP/IP extension (Stein & Terrono, 1996). After flexor tendon repair, the patient is positioned in a safe degree of wrist flexion, thumb midpalmar/radial abduction, and slight MP/IP flexion (see Chapter 18 for details).

IP arthrodesis is reserved for the unstable, painful joint, providing there is minimal involvement of the first CMC,

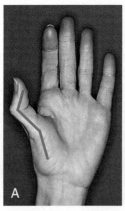 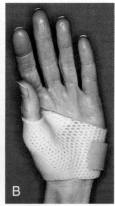

FIGURE 17–50 A, Note the metacarpal adduction with MP joint hyperextension and IP flexion in this patient with a swan-neck deformity of the thumb. The initial stage of this deformity is CMC subluxation. **B,** This hand-based orthosis applies gentle three-point pressure to correct the CMC subluxation passively, which in turn aids in realignment of the MP and IP joints. The device design allows the patient to perform light ADLs.

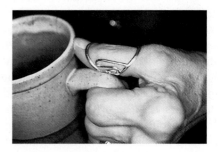

FIGURE 17–52 A thumb orthosis (SIRIS™ Lateral Support Splint) to prevent IP hyperextension and provide lateral joint stability. Ring-type orthoses can be custom fit and are durable, attractive, and low profile. Photo courtesy of Silver Ring™ Splint Company, Charlottesville, VA.

STT, and MP joints (Nalebuff, 1968). This procedure provides a stable joint for the digits to pinch against. A small thermoplastic orthosis can be applied to protect the IP joint during the healing phase.

Thumb Metacarpophalangeal Joint

Surgical intervention for the thumb MP joint may include synovectomy, arthrodesis, relocation of EPL, capsulodesis, and arthroplasty (Chung, Kowalski, Myra, & Kazmers, 2000; Rizio et al., 1995; Terrono et al., 1995). **Synovectomy** is reserved for patients who have had chronic synovitis for 6 months or more (Chung et al., 2000). Orthotic positioning in extension is typically the postoperative position to prevent MP flexion contracture (Fig. 17–53A,B).

For severe instability and articular damage of the thumb MP, surgical options include MP joint arthrodesis or arthroplasty. The decision is influenced by vocational and avocational demands, the integrity of the MP joint, the condition of the bordering first CMC and IP joints, and the anticipated future activity level (Chung et al., 2000; Colditz, 1995; Rizio et al., 1995). Some protocols limit the use of implant arthroplasty at the MP level to only those with flexion deformity (Chung et al., 2000; Terrono et al., 1995).

Thumb MP joint arthroplasty is done when the joint is painful, unstable, or shows articular destruction. If the thumb IP joint necessitates fusion, attempts may be made to preserve some motion of the MP joint through arthroplasty. The goal of the procedure is to gain stability with some motion, 10 to 35° of flexion (Chung et al., 2000; Swanson et al., 1995). Patients are positioned in an orthosis close to full extension for 4 to 5 weeks at which time AROM is begun (Chung et al., 2000).

The goal of thumb MP joint arthrodesis is to provide for thumb stability. The postoperative orthotic intervention program is based on the surgeon's protocol. In general, after the initial postoperative immobilization phase, the patient is placed in a hand-based protective orthosis that maintains the fused position and protects it from injury while allowing use

of the proximal and distal joints as shown in Figures 17–16A, 17–49C, and 17–50B. Importance is placed on early IP joint motion to decrease the risk of extensor tendon adherence over the surgical site.

Digit MCP Joints with Rheumatoid Arthritis

The digit MCP joints of the hand are frequently involved in patients with RA. Chronic inflammation with aggressive synovial proliferation may damage the surrounding structures (Flatt, 1996; Gellman et al., 1997; Nalebuff, 1968; Rothwell, Cragg, & O'Neil, 1997; Stirrat, 1996; Terrono, Feldon, et al., 2011). Reasons for applying an orthosis to the MCP joints include to rest the acutely inflamed hand, minimize deformity, and provide pain relief. Orthoses are also applied following operative procedures to the MCP joints such as arthroplasty or joint fusion (Boozer, 1993; Murphy, 1996; Rennie, 1996; Theisen, 1993).

The two major deformities that occur at the digit MCP joints are ulnar drift and MCP volar subluxation/dislocation (Fig. 17–54). They may occur as a result of several factors (Rizio & Belsky, 1995; Shapiro, 1996; Stirrat, 1996; Swanson, 1995b; Swanson et al., 1995; R. Wilson & Fredick, 1994):

- The flexor tendons approach the MCP joints from the ulnar side and, therefore, exert a stronger ulnar pull with muscular contraction.
- Most functional activities involving MCP function (prehension) increase ulnar and palmar displacement of the flexor tendons across the MCP joint.
- The shape of the metacarpal heads influences ulnar drift. The ulnar side of the metacarpal is shorter than the radial side, inducing the proximal phalanx to favor an ulnar-oriented position during flexion. Any ligamentous laxity allows the joint to slip to the ulnar side.
- Chronic synovitis weakens all of the soft tissues about the MCP joint. Ulnarward tendon drift is a result of this weakening, distention of the capsular structures, laxity of the radial and UCLs, and laxity of the radial sagittal bands.
- Wrist involvement can ultimately influence ulnar deviation of the digits. Often seen in early RA, the wrist radially deviates, and the digits position themselves ulnarly (Figs. 17–42 and 17–55).

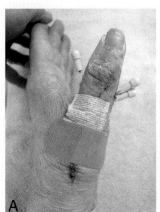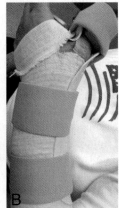

FIGURE 17–53 **A,** Thumb MP joint fusion increases stability and improves the ability to pinch. **B,** Used after the postoperative immobilization period, this MP immobilization orthosis further protects the MP joint fusion during functional use.

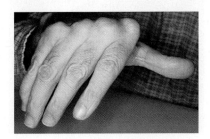

FIGURE 17–54 Volar MP subluxation and ulnar deviation of the proximal phalanxes.

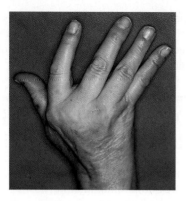

FIGURE 17–55 Zigzag deformity with radial deviation at the wrist and ulnar deviation at the MP joints. Note the tenosynovitis over the dorsal MP joints.

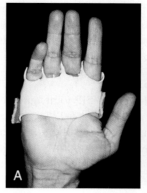
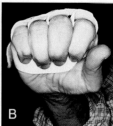

FIGURE 17–57 At 4 to 6 weeks after MP joint arthroplasty, a small, hand-based orthosis can be used for light functional tasks: digit extension (**A**) and flexion (**B**).

Nonsurgical Orthotic Management Guidelines

During periods of exacerbation, the wrist should be included when applying an orthosis to the MCP joints to prevent or minimize any zigzag deformity (Stirrat, 1996). The optimal position of the orthosis includes wrist in 10 to 15° of extension and 10° of ulnar deviation and MCP joints in full extension (Stirrat, 1996). The MCP joints should be positioned in extension to support weakened structures, prevent volar subluxation, minimize reflex intrinsic muscle contracture, and correct for ulnar drift (Boozer, 1993; Fess et al., 2005; Melvin, 1982; Murphy, 1996; Rennie, 1996). The orthosis is generally worn at night (Fig. 17–56). Carefully positioned straps can be the key to guiding the wrist and MCPs gently into an antideformity position. A strap that attaches to the inside of the orthosis (just beneath the second metacarpal

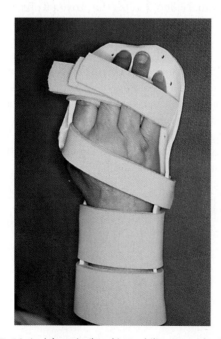

FIGURE 17–56 A night wrist/hand immobilization orthosis that uses straps to enhance the antideformity position of the wrist and digits.

head) and traverses obliquely toward the fifth metacarpal can aid in gently directing the wrist and digits into the antideformity position (Boozer, 1993; Flatt, 1996; Melvin, 1982; Philips, 1995).

Daytime functional orthosis application for ulnar drift can be challenging to fabricate, especially for a novice therapist. This is due in part to the necessity of molding the material between each digital web space and at the same time having to account for adequate digital flexion/extension. Also to consider is how easily the MCP joints passively move into extension. This determines the resistance and/or friction the digits will encounter against the thermoplastic material. For these few reasons alone, one can appreciate the skill needed to make this type of orthosis comfortable, effective, and cosmetically acceptable to the wearer (Fig. 17–57A,B). Various forms of prefabricated orthoses can be tried to aid in support and alignment (Fig.17–58A,B) (Flatt, 1996; Rennie, 1996).

Postsurgical Orthotic Management Guidelines

A surgical option for advanced MP joint arthritis is an **MCP joint implant** arthroplasty (Fig. 17–59A). Indications for this procedure include ulnar drift not amenable to soft tissue repair alone, pain, subluxation or dislocation that severely limits function, and displeasing appearance (Flatt, 1996; Gellman et al., 1997; Melvin, 1982; Nalebuff, 1968; Rennie, 1996; Rizio et al., 1995; Rothwell et al., 1997; Terrono, Feldon, et al., 2011; Theisen, 1993; R. Wilson & Carlblom, 1989). MCP arthroplasty involves resection of inflamed soft tissue, the metacarpal head, and the base of the proximal phalanx. A silastic implant is typically used as a spacer between these bones. During the healing process, a capsule typically forms about the new joint; this is referred to as encapsulation (Philips, 1995; Stirrat, 1996; Swanson, 1995a; Tomaino et al., 1995).

The therapist's role is critical in the postoperative management of these patients (Swanson et al., 1995; Terrono, Feldon, et al., 2011). A typical protocol would include the use of a daytime forearm-based MCP extension mobilization

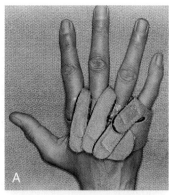
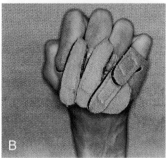

FIGURE 17–58 Neoprene supports tend to work well for some patients and allow for excellent ROM with continued light protection of the surgical procedure: digit extension **(A)** and flexion **(B)** These supports assist in preventing further deforming forces of ulnar deviation and MCP subluxation.

orthosis, allowing controlled and limited active MCP flexion to facilitate the encapsulation process (Fig. 17–59B) (Melvin, 1982; Stirrat, 1996; Theisen, 1993; R. Wilson & Carlblom, 1989). If there has been reconstruction of the radial collateral ligament of the IF MCP joint, a radial outrigger is used to prevent pronation and support the MCP in slight radial deviation (overcorrection). The MCP of the SF should be allowed unrestricted flexion, which may require removal from the extension component (sling) to that finger during exercise sessions (Stirrat, 1996). SF MCP flexion can be inadequate because of the significant instability preoperatively or owing to weakness resulting from surgical release of the ulnar-sided intrinsic muscles (Rizio & Belsky, 1995). If not carefully fit, the sling may actually position the SF in MCP hyperextension. The clinician may consider casting the SF PIP and DIP joints into extension then applying the sling over the cast to better target forces of flexion (during active movement) to the MCP joint (Terrono, Feldon, et al., 2011) (Fig. 17–59C). The mobilization orthosis is normally worn during the day for a period of 4 to 6 weeks. The expected arc of flexion at the MCP joints is approximately 40 to 60° (Kozin, 1999; Rizio et al., 1995; Stirrat, 1996; Terrono, Feldon, et al., 2011). This dynamic mobilization orthosis is often prescribed in combination with a night wrist/hand immobilization orthosis (Fig. 17–60) (Michlovitz, 1999; Stirrat, 1996; Theisen, 1993; Terrono, Feldon, et al., 2011). The immobilization orthosis maintains the wrist in slight extension while the MCPs

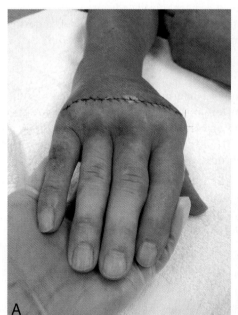
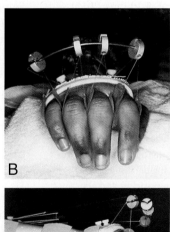
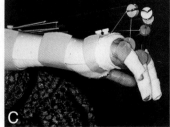
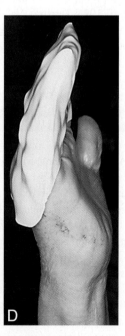

FIGURE 17–59 **A,** Postoperative view of an IF-SF MP joint arthroplasty with reconstruction of all radial collateral ligaments of the MP joints. **B,** Dynamic MP extension mobilization orthosis applied 5 days postoperatively using Phoenix Outrigger kit. Note the slight radial pull at the proximal phalanges to protect the reconstructed MP joint radial collateral ligaments. **C,** Active MP flexion: caution not to place too much tension through the rubber bands; use just enough to hold the MPs in extension while allowing gentle gliding in flexion. PIP extension casts were added 2 weeks after surgery to gently direct greater flexion force to the MP joints during exercise. **D,** As healing allows, a composite PIP/DIP extension immobilization orthosis can be fabricated to concentrate the flexion forces uniformly to the MP joints during exercise.

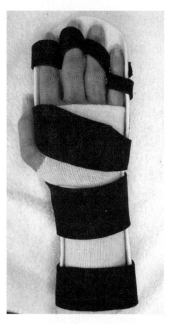

FIGURE 17–60 Volar forearm-based wrist and hand immobilization orthosis used post operatively for a IF - SF MCP implant arthroplasty. Such orthoses are used to maintain MP extension alignment. Note the soft neoprene straps forming comfortable troughs for the digits to rest in.

are slightly flexed to approximately 10° with the IPs gently extended. The immobilization orthosis is worn for 3 or more months postoperatively to maintain good MCP alignment (Terrono et al., 1995; Terrono, Nalebuff, & Philips, 2011).

A hand-based orthosis can be fabricated from thermoplastic material 4 to 6 weeks postoperatively for intermittent

---

BOX 17–3

Evidence-Informed Orthotic Management: Postoperative MCP and PIP Joint Arthroplasty

Application of an orthosis following MP and PIP joint arthroplasty is an important component of postoperative management. The purpose of the dynamic or mobilization orthosis is to allow for ROM while controlling the position and alignment of the reconstructed joint(s). However, many papers fail to discuss this orthosis application process within the rehabilitation program in any detail (Burr, Pratt, & Smith, 2002; Hansraj, Ashworth, & Ebramzadeh, 1997; Jensen, Boeckstyns, & Kristiansen, 1986; Mannerfelt & Andersson, 1975; Massy-Westropp, Johnston, & Hill, 2008; Nicolle & Gilbert, 1979; Pereira & Belcher, 2001; Y. Wilson, Sykes, & Niranjan, 1993). It is difficult to compare outcome studies for the application of an extension mobilization orthosis (which allows controlled active flexion and dynamically assisted extension) compared to an immobilization orthosis, which is removed by the patient to perform *active* flexion and extension. Therefore, immobilization (static) versus mobilization (dynamic) orthosis application following MP and PIP joint arthroplasty should be based on physician preference and expert opinion.

---

light activity (Flatt, 1996; Kozin, 1999; Rennie, 1996; Rizio et al., 1995; Stirrat, 1996). This small orthosis can provide external support for continued MCP extension, preventing ulnar deviation, especially when the thumb attempts pinch against the IF. Care must be taken to decrease bulk and rough edges between the fingers, which can lead to discomfort and impaired function (Fig. 17–57A,B). Soft neoprene orthoses can also be used postoperatively to provide some volar MCP support, guide against ulnar deviation, and increase ease of digital function (Fig. 17–58A,B).

PIP and DIP Joints with Rheumatoid Arthritis

Finger deformities as a result of RA impair function and appearance (Rizio & Belsky, 1995; Swanson et al., 1995). They can be difficult to treat because of the critical involvement of the extensor mechanism at this level. Synovitis of these small joints may cause pain, chronic edema, and stiffness (R. Wilson & Fredick, 1994). Swan-neck and boutonniere deformities of the rheumatoid hand are the most common finger pathologies. Implant arthroplasty or arthrodesis can be considered for the rheumatoid PIP or DIP joint and managed in the same way as discussed for OA earlier in this chapter. Orthotic intervention in the early stages of the disease process can be used as an external support to place joints in a mechanically advantageous position to enhance function. Orthoses can also be used as a postoperative tool to support and protect surgical procedures.

Swan-Neck Deformity

Swan-neck deformity in the digit presents as PIP joint hyperextension and DIP flexion, as noted in Figure 17–43A. An anatomical classification of swan-neck deformity of the fingers was first introduced by Zancolli (1979), whereas clinical classification was added by Nalebuff (1989). Refer to Table 17–3.

TABLE 17–3

Swan-Neck Deformity (Nalebuff, 1989)

Stage I:	Joints are supple and mobile. Preventing hyperextension at the PIP joint corrects the flexion of the DIP joint.
Stage II:	Presence of mild interosseous contracture is often seen.
Stage III:	Retraction of tendons, dorsal joint capsule, and interosseous contracture is profound. Surgical management should be considered.
Stage IV:	Deformity is more profound with articular destruction

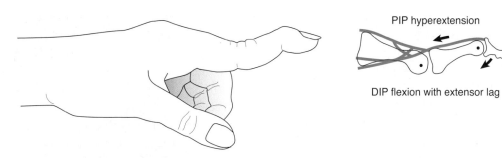

FIGURE 17–61 Swan-neck deformity. Adapted with permission from American Society for Surgery of the Hand. (1990). *The hand: Examination and diagnosis* (3rd ed.). New York, NY: Churchill Livingstone.

The first two stages of the Nalebuff classification are responsive to orthotic management, and the latter two should be considered for surgical intervention. The intrinsic/extrinsic muscle imbalance in the rheumatoid hand may occur from synovitis about the wrist, MCP, PIP, or DIP joint(s) or along the flexor tendon sheath (Eckhaus, 1993; Rizio et al., 1995; Swanson, 1995b; R. Wilson & Fredick, 1994). The most common cause is synovitis at the MCP joint, which can lead to extensor tendon subluxation (ulnarward) as a result of radial-sided sagittal band attenuation. This subluxation eventually produces an extensor lag leading to MCP joint subluxation, accentuating the swan-neck deformity (Chinchalkar & Pitts, 2006). Chronic synovitis appears to cause a reflex intrinsic muscle contracture. This contracture pulls on the PIP joint extensors, leading to volar plate laxity, PIP hyperextension, attenuation of the transverse fibers of the retinacular ligaments, dorsal subluxation of the lateral tendons, and attenuation of the oblique retinacular ligament (ORL) distally (Swanson, 1995b). The DIP tends to flex secondarily to the proximal pathology (Melvin, 1982; Swanson, 1995b).

Swelling of the DIP joint may cause attenuation or a rupture in the terminal extensor tendon with resultant DIP flexion. The harmony of the entire extensor mechanism is disrupted, producing hyperextension at the PIP joint. Synovitis of the PIP joint itself may lead to stretching of the volar ligaments with a resultant dorsal migration of the lateral bands (Fig. 17–61). Early management may consist of joint injections and corrective "anti–swan-neck" orthoses (Figs. 17–43B and 17–62A–C) (Rizio et al., 1995).

Nonsurgical Orthotic Management Guidelines

The primary goal of fitting an orthosis for swan-neck deformity is to reduce and/or minimize the progression of the deforming stages. The goal of the orthosis application to a passively correctable swan-neck deformity is to allow near to full flexion of the PIP joint while preventing PIP

BOX 17–4

Evidence-Informed Orthotic Management: Swan-Neck Deformity

The swan-neck deformity is a common finger deformity associated with RA, and orthoses are often prescribed for newly diagnosed patients as well as for patients who suffer from chronic RA. Studies indicate that Silver Ring™ orthoses or similar, prefabricated orthoses, and custom-made orthoses can improve dexterity and reduce pain (Schegget & Knipping, 2000; Zijlstra, Heijnsdijk-Rouwenhorst, & Rasker, 2004). All of these orthoses have been found beneficial. Some studies have reported that patients prefer Silver Ring™ orthoses versus custom-made orthoses due to the small thin ring design and attractive appearance (Schegget & Knipping, 2000).

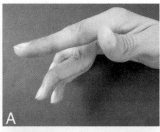
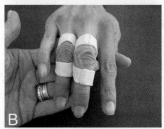
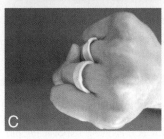

FIGURE 17–62 **A,** Swan-neck deformity with hyperextension at PIP and flexion at DIP joint. **B and C,** This deformity be managed with an extension restriction orthosis (Figure-8 design) that allows near full digital flexion yet limits PIP joint hyperextension.

joint hyperextension (Eckhaus, 1993). A supple swan-neck deformity can be managed with an extension restriction orthosis (Fig. 17–62B,C). These small orthoses can be beneficial for short-term solutions. More permanent orthoses can be purchased from various companies and/or catalogs that may be less bulky and work well for some patients. These tend to be more durable, fit well, and cosmetically pleasing (Fig. 17–52).

Postsurgical Orthotic Management Guidelines

Surgical restoration of the hyperextended PIP joint may involve the use of a tendon transfer, such as a superficialis tendon. In some situations, DIP joint pin fixation in 0° is warranted. Postoperative orthosis application depends on individual physician preferences; however, most include early fabrication of an orthosis, which positions the wrist in neutral to slight extension, slight MCP flexion, PIP flexion of 20 to 30°, and the DIP in neutral. If the PIP joint is pinned in flexion, the orthosis should support this position. This orthosis is generally worn for 2 to 3 weeks. The patient can then use a hand- or finger-based extension restriction orthosis. At approximately 6 weeks, gently increase the amount of allowable extension at the PIP joint. The orthosis should carefully accommodate these gradual changes per healing constraints (Fig. 17–63A–D).

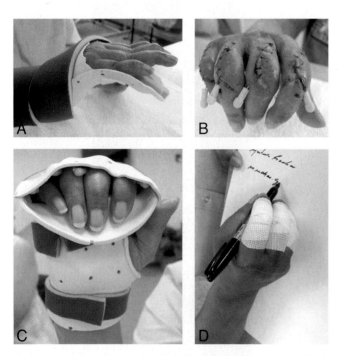

FIGURE 17–63 Severe swan-neck deformities in this 26-year-old college grad student preoperatively **(A)**, postoperatively **(B)**, hand-based protective orthosis **(C)**, allowing removal for pin care and gentle AROM on noninvolved structures, small digits casts were used at 6 weeks to continue to support the fusions while she began to use her hand for all ADLs **(D)**.

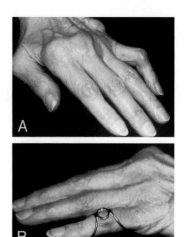

FIGURE 17–64 A, Boutonniere deformity with flexion at the PIP joint. This deformity may be managed with a PIP extension orthosis on a long-term basis. Many patients find a ring-type orthosis **(B)** to be more cosmetically appealing than a thermoplastic PIP extension restriction orthosis (SIRIS Boutonniere Splint shown). Photo courtesy of Silver Ring™ Splint Company.

Boutonniere Deformity

Boutonniere deformities of the digits are characterized by PIP flexion and DIP hyperextension (Fig. 17–64A,B). Similar to the swan-neck classification, boutonniere deformity is also classified based on clinical stages (Tubiana, 1981). Refer to Table 17–4.

In the first three stages of boutonniere deformity, MCP joint hyperextension during digital motion is observed, whereas in stage IV, fixed hyperextension of the MP joint may be an aggravating factor. The most common cause of this deformity in the rheumatoid hand is chronic PIP joint synovitis (Eddington-Valdata, 1993; Nalebuff & Millender, 1975; Rizio et al., 1995; Swanson et al., 1985; R. Wilson & Fredick,

TABLE 17–4

Boutonniere Deformity (Tubiana, 1981)

Stage I:	Minimal deficiency of less than 30° of extension is noted.
Stage II:	Mild flexion contracture of the PIP joint along with volar subluxation of the lateral bands; hyperextension of DIP joint and a negative retinacular test are also present.
Stage III:	Presentation of contracture of the retinacular ligaments; enabling passive extension of the PIP joint with associated positive retinacular test
Stage IV:	Deformity exhibits a fixed contracture of the PIP and DIP joints.

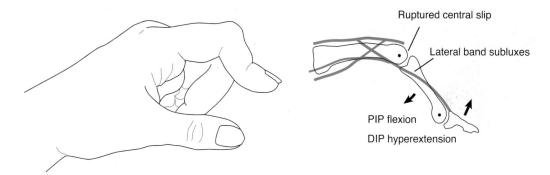

FIGURE 17–65 Boutonniere deformity. Adapted with permission from American Society for Surgery of the Hand. (1990). *The hand: Examination and diagnosis* (3rd ed.). New York, NY: Churchill Livingstone.

1994). The synovitis migrates dorsally between the lateral bands, displacing them laterally and volarly (Swanson, 1995b). This, in turn, creates lengthening of the central tendon. The lateral bands eventually orient themselves below the axis of the PIP joint, becoming PIP joint flexors instead of extensors. This places a secondary pull on the DIP joint in extension. Left untreated, the ORL shortens, causing the DIP joint to become tight in extension (Fig. 17–65).

Nonsurgical Orthotic Management Guidelines

Applying an orthosis for a passively correctable boutonniere deformity is best achieved with a twofold process. The patient should have a digit immobilization orthosis for night use, which keeps the PIP joint in full extension (Fig. 17–66A) (Glickel et al., 1992). An effective option for daytime orthotic application includes the use of a custom-made PIP extension immobilization orthosis that allows full MCP and DIP motion. If the deformity is the result of an attritional rupture of the central tendon, uninterrupted PIP extension must be maintained for approximately 6 weeks before motion is allowed (Eddington-Valdata, 1993). In these authors' opinion, the best way to achieve uninterrupted motion is to apply a circumferential nonremovable orthosis (Fig. 17–66B). Gentle isolated DIP active motion or joint-blocking exercises can help maintain the length of the extensor mechanism,

ORL, and mobility of the lateral bands (Poole et al., 2000; R. Wilson & Fredick, 1994).

If the patient presents with a fixed flexion contracture of the PIP joint, a gentle serial static extension mobilization approach may be implemented until full PIP extension is achieved (Eddington-Valdata, 1993). Full PIP extension is critical to achieve before the patient is considered for surgical intervention, such as a flexible implant arthroplasty (Nalebuff & Millender, 1975). Once fully extended, the PIP is held in extension for an additional 4 to 6 weeks (Eddington-Valdata, 1993). If, at that time, the patient cannot maintain extension, surgical intervention should be considered.

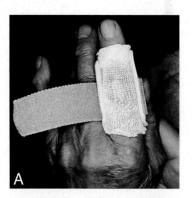

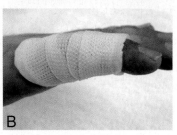

FIGURE 17–66 **A,** Orthosis fabrication for night extension is important for reducing the possibility of a PIP flexion contracture. **B,** A circumferential cast is used for uninterrupted PIP motion to allow for better compliance and assured healing.

BOX 17–5

Evidence-Informed Orthotic Management: Boutonniere Deformity

To date, there have been no randomized control trials on the effectiveness of orthosis application to correct this deformity. Studies are needed to determine the clinical effectiveness. In the authors' expert opinion, orthosis application can be of benefit with passively correctable deformities in the compliant patient who follows the prescribed orthosis regime carefully.

CHAPTER 17

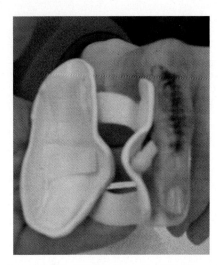

FIGURE 17–67 A protective orthosis used after PIP joint reconstruction. Note how the pin was incorporated into this small "clamshell-type" design. This design protects the repair yet allows for easy removal for wound care and gentle, guarded DIP exercises as dictated by the surgeon.

Postsurgical Orthotic Management Guidelines

Surgical intervention may be considered to reestablish PIP extension if conservative management has failed. Postoperative management varies depending on the exact procedure or combination of procedures performed, such as pinning, **tenolysis**, and/or volar plate release (Eddington-Valdata, 1993; Nalebuff & Millender, 1975; Rizio et al., 1995). The PIP joint is most often positioned in extension for approximately 4 weeks, after which, gentle active exercises are introduced (Fig. 17–67). Cautious active DIP joint flexion exercises should begin as soon as possible postoperatively to aid in advancing the extensor mechanism, allowing for lateral band glide and the prevention of tendon adherence (the PIP joint should be held in extension during this exercise) (Eddington-Valdata, 1993; Nalebuff & Millender, 1975; R. Wilson & Fredick, 1994).

Conclusion

Although medical options and surgical advances have combined to aid in the prevention and further progression of joint deformity in the patient with rheumatic disease, fabricating an orthosis remains both a valuable early modality and an important postoperative adjunct. Knowledge of the disease process, joint anatomy and function, and the patient's desired functional goals is crucial to providing effective and appropriate therapy interventions.

CASE STUDY SECTION

The case studies presented here are meant as a teaching guideline only. Treatment and orthosis protocols vary greatly from surgeon to surgeon and from therapist to therapist. The therapist should check with the referring physicians and colleagues to define the preferred treatment and appropriate orthotic intervention.

CASE STUDY 1: Osteoarthritis: Thumb Carpometacarpal Joint

LS, a 45-year-old physically active and fit right-handed woman was diagnosed with bilateral first CMC joint OA. She was referred to therapy for evaluation and treatment. She presented with bilateral thumb pain that was localized to the thenar eminences and reported pain with all functional activities involving grasp and pinch.

Clinical examination revealed bilateral tenderness on palpation and thickening at the first CMC joints. No acute swelling was noted. She had a positive grind test bilaterally. AROM was equal in both hands, with thumb opposition to the SF MCP joint. Grip strength was bilaterally equal. Pinch strengths (lateral, tip, and three-point) were decreased and associated with pain.

LS was referred to therapy with a prescription for bilateral hand- and forearm-based thumb immobilization orthoses. The hand-based orthoses were to be used for days, and the forearm-based orthoses were to provide further joint rest, support, and protection while sleeping. The day orthoses were fabricated from $^1/_{16}$" Aquaplast (Fig. 17–16A). This elastic-based thermoplastic material provided the right amount of stretch and conformability to fit the first web space intimately and stabilize the first CMC joint. The night orthoses were made out of a perforated $^1/_8$" plastic-based material (Fig. 17–18A,B).

LS wore the orthoses with some pain relief at home and work. However, the intensity of her thumb pain increased to the point that even with these devices, she had consistent, unrelenting pain day and night. After 5 years of conservative management, LS opted for surgical intervention of her nondominant hand first. Her surgeon performed a ligament reconstruction with a tendon interposition graft (LRTI).

The postsurgical wrist/thumb immobilization cast was worn for 4 weeks. At the time of cast removal, a wrist/thumb immobilization orthosis was applied and gentle wrist/thumb AROM was begun. The orthosis was the same night orthosis she had worn with adjustments made for postsurgical edema and dressings (Fig. 17–18A,B). This orthosis was worn at all times except for hygiene and exercise sessions. The same device was cut down to a hand-based design at 6 weeks, and a decrease in the wearing schedule was begun (Fig. 17–5B). At 8 weeks, therapy focused on grip and light thenar/pinch strengthening with orthosis use for only at-risk activities.

LS was instructed in joint protection principles and activity modifications to provide ways to decrease external stress on the

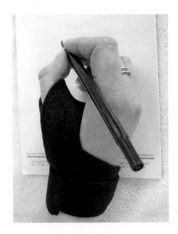

FIGURE 17–68 A custom-fabricated neoprene orthosis is used for ongoing support for ADL and vocational and recreational activities. See Chapter 14 for more information and orthotic designs with neoprene materials.

thumb with ADLs. She was made a custom neoprene orthosis, which allowed her to comfortably transition from guarded use of her hand to having a light external support to aid in protection. She used this device when she engaged in activities that required repetitive wrist and thumb use. This orthosis worked well for returning to work and recreational activities (Fig. 17–68). When last seen, 12 weeks after surgery, LS was able to do her normal activities with little discomfort and was scheduling this same surgery for her dominant hand.

Additional case studies can be found on the companion web site on thePoint.

Chapter Review Questions

1. Describe the general difference between osteoarthritis (OA) and rheumatoid arthritis (RA), including all joints that are commonly affected.

2. What are the general indications for use of immobilization and mobilization orthoses in both populations? Give an example of each.

3. What are the considerations for material choice in this patient population and why is it so important?

4. What is the conservative orthotic management of first CMC OA? What are the choices described in this chapter?

5. What is the difference between a swan-neck deformity and a boutonniere deformity, and how does the orthotic management differ? What material choices would one consider?

CHAPTER 17

Tendon Injuries

Alexandra MacKenzie OTR/L, CHT*

Chapter Objectives

After study of this chapter, the reader should be able to:

- Identify the flexor and extensor tendon anatomy.
- Describe the three phases of wound healing and how they impact the healing tendon.
- Determine the appropriate therapeutic management and orthotic intervention for each tendon injury.
- Understand common surgical techniques and various types of tendon repairs.
- Appreciate the important role of communication between patient, therapist, and surgeon.

Key Terms

Annular pulleys
Boutonniere
Camper's chiasm
Cruciform pulleys
Duran and Houser
Early active mobilization (EAM) protocol
Early passive mobilization
Early *protected* mobilization
Extrinsics
Flexor retinaculum
Four-strand tendon repair
Immediate Active Tension

Immediate Controlled Acitve Motion (ICAM)
Intrinsics
Jersey Finger
Juncturae tendinum
Kleinert
Lateral bands
Modified Duran
No man's land
Norwich Regime
Oblique retinacular ligament
Pyramid of Progressive Force
Quadriga

Sagittal bands
Short arc of motion (SAM) protocol
Strickland and Cannon
Swan neck
Synovial sheath
tendon adhesion
tendon gap
Terminal tendon
Vincula system
Washington/Chow
Yoke orthosis

Introduction

Tendon injuries can be devastating to the function of the hand and can be daunting to treat. Therapy plays a critical role in the recovery process. The tendon anatomy is complicated, and scar tissue can wreak havoc with the intricate motions required of the hand. Historically, tendon repair has gone through many incarnations. Prior to the 1960s, it was not felt that tendons could be successfully repaired without having to use tendon grafts (Riboh & Leversedge, 2011; Seiler, 2011). As surgical techniques improved, repaired tendons were initially immobilized in casts because the suture techniques of the time could not withstand the forces of early

---

*This chapter is based on the first edition chapter written by Lisa Cyr OTR/L, CHT.

motion. It soon became evident that immobilization resulted in a very stiff digit, and changes were made in the postoperative care of these injuries. For all of the advances that have occurred, the issues remain the same as they were 50 years ago: tendon adhesions, **tendon gapping**, risk of rupture, and loss of motion.

In addition to surgical advances, rehabilitation protocols and orthotic management have also gone through an evolutionary process. Orthosis application postoperatively went from being fairly simple (casts, dorsal blocking orthoses) to the addition of rubber bands, springs, hinges, and hooks glued to fingernails. As surgical techniques have improved over the years, it has allowed the orthotic management and rehabilitation process to become more streamlined, with better results for the patient. The four-strand flexor tendon repair has changed how we treat tendons postoperatively.

The first part of this chapter will focus on flexor tendon anatomy and treatment, with the latter section addressing extensor tendons. The goal of this chapter is to give the reader a thorough understanding of tendon anatomy, the healing process, common protocols, the type and timing of orthotic intervention, and how to integrate this knowledge for the most appropriate clinical decision making in this patient population.

Flexor Tendons: Anatomy

Extrinsic Tendons

Extrinsic tendons originate outside of the hand and insert within the hand. There are nine extrinsic digital flexor tendons (Fig. 18–1): the flexor pollicis longus (FPL), flexor digitorum superficialis (FDS) to digits two to five (approximately 20% of the population does not have FDS to the fifth digit) (Austin, Leslie, & Ruby, 1989), and flexor digitorum profundus (FDP) to digits two to five (Fig. 18–2). The FDS is innervated by the median nerve, the FPL and FDP to index and middle fingers are innervated by the anterior interosseous branch of the median nerve, and the FDP to the ring and small fingers are innervated by the ulnar nerve. There are two extrinsic wrist flexors: flexor carpi radialis (FCR) and flexor carpi ulnaris (FCU) (the palmaris longus is not considered in this discussion because of its relative insignificance).

The FDP and FPL form the deep muscle layer in the flexor compartment of the forearm (Fig. 18–1C). The FDP originates on the anterior surface of the shaft of the midulna, the interosseous membrane, and occasionally the proximal radius. Typically, the muscle belly of the FDP separates into a radial and ulnar bundle in the midforearm. The radial bundle becomes the tendon to the index finger (IF), and the ulnar bundle forms the tendons to the middle finger (MF), ring finger (RF), and small finger (SF). The muscle bellies transition to tendons in the distal forearm. These four tendons traverse the carpal tunnel, occupying its floor, and then diverge to their respective digits in the palm. They enter the particular flexor sheaths at the level of the metacarpophalangeal

(MCP) joints and insert on the palmar base of the distal phalanx of each finger. Their primary function is to flex the distal joint of the fingers.

The FPL originates from the proximal radius and the interosseous membrane. The tendon also lies on the floor of the carpal tunnel and then enters the flexor sheath of the thumb and inserts on the proximal volar surface of the distal phalanx. Its primary function is to flex the IP joint of the thumb.

The FDS occupies the intermediate layer of the flexor compartment superficial to the FDP and FPL (Fig. 18–1B). Proximally, two separate heads originate from the elbow region. The humeroulnar head arises from the medial epicondyle of the humerus and the coronoid process of the ulna; the radial head originates from the proximal shaft of the radius. The FDS evolves into four distinct muscle bellies as it traverses distally in the midforearm and becomes four individual tendons in the distal forearm. The tendons travel through the carpal tunnel, with the tendons to the MF and RF, superficial and central to those of the IF and SF. The FDS enters the flexor sheath at the level of the MP joint with the FDP tendon. At the level of the midproximal phalanx, the FDS tendon bifurcates, and the radial and ulnar slips insert into the proximal aspect of the middle phalanx (Fig. 18–2). This bifurcation, referred to as **Camper's chiasm**, allows the FDP tendon to pass through on its course to the distal phalanx. When the digit is flexed, the bifurcation migrates proximally, making the FDP extremely vulnerable to injury in this position (Kleinert, Schepel, & Gill, 1981). The primary function of the FDS is to flex the proximal interphalangeal (PIP) joints of the fingers; the FDP flexes the dorsal interphalangeal (DIP) joints.

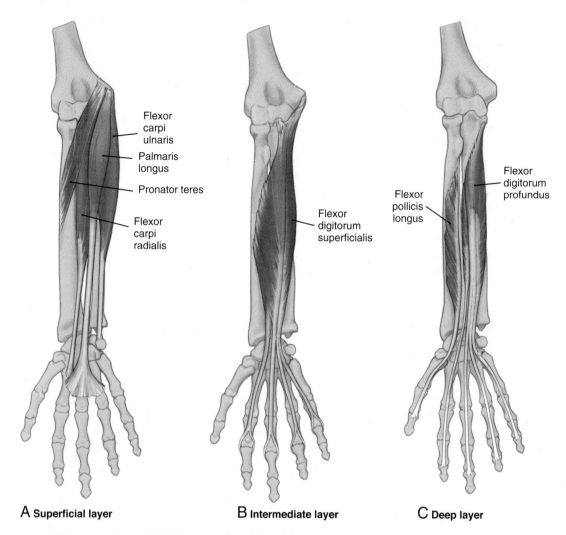

FIGURE 18–1 Superficial **(A)**, intermediate **(B)**, and deep **(C)** layers of the flexor muscles of the forearm (volar view). Reprinted with permission from Clemente, C. D. (2011). *Anatomy: A regional atlas of the human body* (6th ed.). Baltimore, MD: Lippincott Williams & Wilkins.

The FCR and FCU are part of the superficial layer of the flexor surface (Fig. 18–1A). The FCR inserts proximally with the common flexor tendon at the medial epicondyle. Distally, the tendon passes through the **flexor retinaculum** to insert on the base of the second metacarpal. The FCU has two sites of origin: the humeral head arises from the common flexor tendon, and the second head originates from the medial border of the olecranon and the upper two-thirds of the posterior ulna border. Distally, it inserts on the pisiform, the hook of the hamate, and the base of the fifth metacarpal. The FCR and FCU are the primary wrist flexors.

Synovial Sheath

There is a **synovial sheath** system (or fibroosseous tunnel) in the hand that serves several functions: provides a better gliding system, supplies nutrition to the tendons, and contributes to biomechanical efficiency of the tendons during flexion. The sheaths to digits two to four originate at the level of the volar metacarpal phalangeal (MCP) joint, whereas the sheaths to the thumb and small fingers extend into the carpal tunnel, becoming the radial and ulnar bursae (Doyle, 1988). The digital tendon sheath has two layers. The outer layer (parietal layer) attaches to the fibrous part of the sheath (i.e., the pulley system), whereas the inner layer (visceral layer) is attached to the tendon.

Pulley System

The pulley system in zone II is complex. There are **annular pulleys**, which are thicker and whose fibers lay perpendicular to the tendon fibers, as well as thinner, more flexible **cruciform pulleys**, which form an "X" over the tendons. From a biomechanical standpoint, the pulleys help hold the tendon close to the surface of the bone as the finger flexes. Without the intricate pulley system, the tendon would bowstring and that phenomenon would compromise both strength and

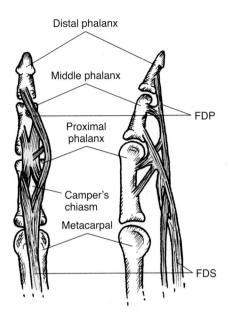

FIGURE 18–2 The bifurcation of the FDS tendon is also referred to as Camper's chiasm. The radial and ulnar slips insert into the proximal aspect of the middle phalanx and permit the FDP tendon to pass through.

motion (if the tendon takes the shortest path possible, the muscle fibers may reach a state of full contraction before the tendon can pull the finger through its full range of motion [ROM]). The A1, A3, and A5 pulleys originate from the volar plates of the MCP, PIP, and DIP joints. The pulleys are numbered proximal to distal, with odd numbers over the joints, whereas the tendon zones are numbered distal to proximal. The A2 and A4 pulleys originate from the bases of the proximal phalanx and middle phalanx (Fig. 18–3A,B) (Seiler, 2011). These are the two most structurally important pulleys. The surgeon may elect to repair these pulleys if they were also injured. A pulley ring may be indicated to further protect the repair (Fig. 18–4).

There are three pulleys over the FPL (Fig. 18–3). The A1 pulley arises from the volar plate of the MP joint and the A2 pulley arises from the volar plate of the IP joint. The oblique pulley (the most important pulley in the thumb) lies diagonally in between the A1 and A2 pulleys, originating from fibers of the adductor pollicis.

Tendon Nutrition

Tendon nutrition plays a large role in how well the tendons heal. Tendons do not have a vast vascular supply, especially in zone II. Tendons receive nutrition through vascular infusion as well as synovial diffusion. The tendon receives blood supply from the bone at the site of tendon insertion. There is also a **vincula system**, vascular "highways" leading directly from the bone to the dorsal surface of the tendon. Each FDS and FDP tendon has a brevis and profundus vincula.

The pulley system plays an important role in the nutrition of the tendons; the mechanical action of the pulleys "pumps" nutrition via diffusion into the volar surface of the tendons. In addition to nutritional benefits, this action aids in creating a better environment for the gliding of the tendon ("motion is lotion"). Active flexion of the finger creates a high pressure system within the pulleys to push the nutrients into the tendon (this may be part of why patients performing early protected active mobilization tend to have better results and is something to consider when choosing a rehabilitation protocol) (Amadio, Jaeger, & Hunter, 1990).

Tendon Healing: Intrinsic versus Extrinsic

There are two theories as to how tendon healing occurs: intrinsically and extrinsically. Extrinsic healing occurs through factors that are external to the tendon tissue: scar tissue and adhesions, which are necessary for the tendon to heal. Adhesions bring blood supply to the healing tendon as well as the fibroblasts needed for collagen production. But they also prevent the tendon from moving through surrounding tissue. Intrinsic healing occurs within the tendon itself, from tendon end to tendon end. This theory allows early mobilization to occur to prevent tendinous adhesions. The common belief today is that it is necessary for both extrinsic and intrinsic healing to occur.

An early study in an animal model from 1941 showed that the ends of the repaired tendon start to soften between postoperative days 5 and 9, so the tendon actually gets weaker before it gets stronger (Mason & Allen, 1941). However, later studies have shown that this does not happen when the tendon is mobilized early and that early mobilization also limits adhesion formation (Hitchcock et al., 1987; Strickland & Glogovac, 1980). Gapping at the repair site has also been associated with increased adhesions. Advances in suture techniques allow for the prevention of gap formation as well as increased strength through the recovery process (Boyer, Goldfarb, & Gelberman, 2005). In a study by Duran, Houser, Coleman, and Postlewaite (1976), it was noted that adhesions could be minimized if the tendon was allowed 3 mm of excursion (Duran et al., 1976). With the wrist held in flexion and the digits passively flexed, the tendon undergoes not only the least amount of load but also the least amount of excursion (1.7 mm). Passive finger flexion/extension in combination with synergistic wrist motion (tenodesis) produces the most excursion (3.5 mm) with a minimal load (Lieber, Amiel, Kaufman, Whitney, & Gelberman, 1996). The goal with tendon rehabilitation should be to minimize the load the tendon receives while maximizing the excursion necessary to prevent adhesions.

Wound Healing

In treating tendon injuries, it is important to be aware of the basic concepts of tissue/wound healing. Review of Chapter 3

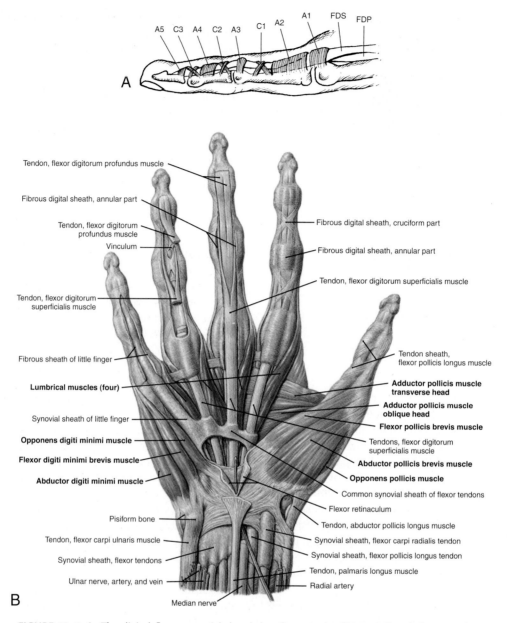

FIGURE 18–3 A, The digital flexor synovial sheath has five annular (A1 to A5) and three cruciate (C1 to C3) pulleys surrounding it. Note the relative size of the A2 and A4 pulleys; biomechanically, they contribute greatly to maximizing tendon function. **B,** Dissection of hand showing the digital synovial sheath system. Reprinted with permission from Clemente, C. D. (2011). *Anatomy: A regional atlas of the human body* (6th ed.). Baltimore, MD: Lippincott Williams & Wilkins.

and further reading in this area is recommended. Having an understanding of the concepts of healing will help guide the therapist in the clinical decision-making process. Not only is the tendon undergoing healing but also all of the surrounding tissues. There are three phases that all overlap as the body moves from one phase to the next. The first phase is the inflammatory phase; this is the body's immediate response to a traumatic event (surgery can also be considered a traumatic event) (Fig. 18–5A). This phase can last anywhere from 3 to 7 days postoperatively. The second phase is called the fibroblastic or proliferative phase. In this phase, fibroblasts

start the production of collagen fibers (Fig. 18–5B). Early collagen fibers are weak, disorganized, and have little tensile strength, but they begin to lay the foundation for stronger collagen fibers that will be produced in the later phase. The fibroblastic phase lasts from around day 5 to day 21. The third and longest phase is the remodeling or maturation phase. Early collagen fibers begin to become more differentiated and more linear, and the tendon gains tensile strength (Fig. 18–5C). The early collagen fibers are broken down (lysis) and newer, stronger, more mature fibers are produced. In the earlier phases of scar production, collagen fibers are dense

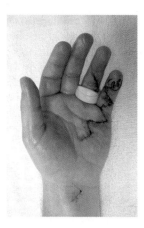

FIGURE 18–4 Nonarticular proximal phalanx orthosis (pulley ring) fabricated to protect pulley repair in zone II injury.

and disorganized, but over time, the collagen fibers lie in a more parallel orientation (e.g., cooked spaghetti in a pot vs. spaghetti in the box). Collagen fibers that are more parallel take up less room and do a better job of gliding through surrounding tissue. This phase can last anywhere from 3 weeks postoperatively to well over a year. Externally, we can watch the scar and determine how well it will respond to therapeutic techniques. A pink-red scar is metabolically active and is still undergoing the remodeling phase, whereas a scar that has faded to a color paler than the surrounding skin is no longer active and is less likely to respond to efforts aimed at changing scar tissue properties.

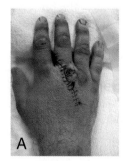
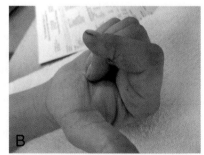
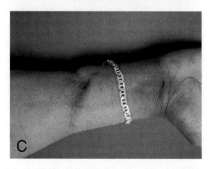

FIGURE 18–5 Stages of wound healing. A, Inflammatory stage shown after saw injury 2 days postoperatively. **B,** Attempts at active flexion during proliferative stage during the height of collagen synthesis. **C,** Scar maturation phase noted by fading of scar and dense adhesion formation during active digital extension.

It is important to watch for signs of infection during the postoperative course of recovery. Infection may interfere with the stages of wound healing and prolong the healing process as well as create more scar tissue.

Surgical Repair

Advances in repair techniques over the past few decades have led to improvements in postoperative functional outcomes. Ultimately, the goal is a repair that will not attenuate or rupture and will glide smoothly, resulting in functional ROM. Despite years of research and modification of surgical repair and rehabilitation techniques, we still face the same challenges that were faced decades ago. As early as 1941, it was noted that early motion and stress created a stronger repair; however, at that time, it was felt that the risks of early motion were too great (Mason & Allen, 1941). Further studies have shown that **early *protected mobilization*** has beneficial effects on healing tendon, leading to increased tensile strength and increased ability for tendon gliding to occur (Buckwalter & Grodzinsky, 1999; Fong et al., 2005; Gelberman, Woo, Lothringer, Akeson, & Amiel, 1982). In order for the tendon to withstand the forces required of it during early protected mobilization, the repair itself must be strong but not so bulky as to be unable to glide through the surrounding tissue.

Surgically, there have been changes in suture material used and in suture technique (how many strands cross the site of repair, where the loops and knots are placed at repair, etc). Early surgical techniques with a two-strand core suture have been shown to create a repair that does not gain strength until 3 weeks postoperatively (Hatanaka, Zhang, & Manske, 2000). A high-strength, low-friction repair technique is optimal. The epitenon is fragile, and too much handling intraoperatively may lead to more adhesions. The **four-strand tendon repair** involves a single suture crossing the repair site four times with a cross in the middle (Fig. 18–6). Increased strength of the tendon repair is

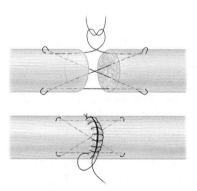

FIGURE 18–6 Four-strand cruciate repair with epitenon stitch. Reprinted with permission from Hunt, T. R. (2011). Operative techniques. In *Hand, wrist and forearm surgery* (p. 466). Baltimore, MD: Lippincott Williams & Wilkins.

achieved if the epitenon is repaired as well, which has been shown to lead to decreased gapping at the repair site (Dy, Hernandez-Soria, Ma, Roberts, & Daluiski, 2012; Mashadi & Amis, 1992). An eight-strand repair has been shown to be even stronger (Winters et al., 1998). Ideally, it is best to repair the tendon shortly after injury. Delaying repair may lead to increased scar tissue and contracted muscles. If the tendon has retracted into the palm (which may occur if the finger was flexed at time of injury), there is additional trauma to the tendon due to the greater chance of vincula disruption as well as increased handling of peritendinous structures during tendon retrieval. The surgical incision is typically a zig-zag (Bruner's) incision, which allows for maximal exposure of the tendon. Alternately, a surgeon may elect to place the incision on the lateral border of the finger, with the hopes that this will lead to less scarring and increased ROM. This is a technically more difficult approach because care must be taken to avoid the digital nerve branches and the vascular supply to the digit. There have been early promising results in research with the addition of surface lubricants applied to the tendon at time of repair to improve tendon glide (Kim et al., 2010).

Postoperative Treatment

Therapy Evaluation

Treatment of flexor tendon injuries requires a team approach: a skilled surgeon, an experienced hand therapist, and a patient who can follow through with the home exercise program (HEP). Ideally, the patient should be seen for therapy within the first 3 days postoperatively. The longer it takes to initiate therapy, the more likely limiting adhesions will form along with joint stiffness. Therefore, greater stress is being placed on a newly repaired tendon when initiating an early active ROM (AROM) or passive ROM (PROM) program. Communication with the referring surgeon is essential. Refer to Box 18–1 for important questions the therapist should ask the referring hand surgeon.

BOX 18–1

Physician Questions

Note: These are only a few of the many questions a clinician should discuss with the referring surgeon.

- What was the condition of the tendon?
- Were there any other structures involved? Nerves, arteries, pulleys?
- What is the strength of the repair? How many strands was the tendon repaired with?
- Will the patient be able to tolerate an early AROM program?

Choosing the right treatment approach will depend on several factors; a thorough history must be taken at the initial visit. Information gathered should include the following (Tan et al., 2010; van Adrichem, Hovius, van Strik, & van der Meulen, 1992):

- Mechanism of injury
- Past medical history (conditions such as diabetes and arthritis may have a negative impact on healing potential)
- Medications (a recent study by Tan et al. in 2010 demonstrated that NSAIDs appear to reduce flexor tendon adhesions)
- Social habits such as smoking or drinking (van Adrichem et al. in 1992 demonstrated that cigarette smoke negatively impacts microcirculation after surgery)
- Any preexisting injuries to the affected hand that would lead to a decrease in ROM
- Concomitant injuries may prevent early mobilization; these can include fracture, nerve or vascular repair, skin grafts, and a tenuous repair that is unable to withstand the forces necessary that occur during mobilization.
- Age plays a factor in clinical decision making. The patient must be cognizant and able to understand the precautions and exercise program. Patients who are too young may not be able to participate in an early mobilization postoperative program. Older patients may have a decreased capacity for healing.

Other factors may hinder therapy, such as that the patient may not have insurance (or limited insurance with high co-pays/deductibles) or the patient may need to travel from far away to come to therapy. For these reasons and more, education is paramount. An overeager patient may exercise too much, potentially leading to increased swelling, scar tissue, gapping, and/or rupture. A patient who does not understand the importance of or comply with the home program may be overly fearful and more likely to develop stiffness and limiting adhesions. All measurements (e.g., PROM, edema, sensation) that are safe to document should be taken at the initial visit and at regular intervals throughout the course of therapy.

A smooth and freely gliding tendon that is able to produce a functional ROM is always the goal. As the tendon passes through the soft tissue structures of the hand, a certain amount of normal "drag" is encountered. However, in an injured hand, drag may be heightened by postinjury and postoperative edema, sutures, scar tissue, and/or a dressing that is bulky or on too tight. Edema, adhesions, and other injured tissues can create biologic resistance. In addition, a newly repaired tendon is only as strong as the sutures that bind it. The tendon cannot withstand the forces required to actively pull the finger into flexion. Tendon rupture, gapping, or attenuation at the repair site are consequences that could occur if the tendon is moved too forcefully. It is difficult to assess if gapping has occurred, but it can lead to problems such as increased scar formation, a weaker tendon, and an insufficient excursion of the digit (a tendon that is too long, causing an inability to fully flex).

Other factors that may have an impact on prognosis and tendon healing include the following:

- Level of injury (zone)
- Type of injury
- Other structures involved
- Clean laceration versus a crush injury (The more trauma there is to the tissue at time of injury, the greater the potential for scar tissue.) (Pettengill & Van Strien, 2011.)
- Tendon sheath integrity
- Surgical technique (careful handling of the tendon will minimize scar tissue and risk for adhesions)
- Suture strength (number of core strands crossing the repair site, combined with circumferential epitendinous running stitch repair)
- Timing of repair (after 2 weeks, the ends tend to scar down to surrounding tissue)

Flexor Tendon Protocols

Protocols have been developed to help provide timelines for when to progress the patient in the therapy program. In current practice, the patients can be treated based on one of three postoperative protocols: immobilization, early PROM, and early AROM. Research has shown that early mobilization leads to improved ability for the tendon to glide as well as increased strength of the repair. However, early mobilization may not be appropriate for every patient.

Immobilization

Despite advances in knowledge of tendon healing and tendon repair, there may be situations where immobilization postoperatively is the best choice. A patient who is too young, cognitively unable, or unwilling to participate in an early mobilization program is best suited for this protocol. When a tendon is immobilized, it loses strength after initial repair (when the ends of the tendon soften) until the second week postoperatively before strength builds up again. This loss of strength must be taken into consideration during the rehabilitation process.

Orthosis/Cast

A wrist and hand extension restriction orthosis, historically named a dorsal blocking splint (DBS) or cast, is used with the wrist at 10 to 30° of flexion, MCP joints at 40 to 60° of flexion, and IP joints in full extension when possible (Fig. 18–7A,B).

Exercise

0 to 3 or 4 weeks: The patient is allowed to move any joint not protected by the orthosis (elbow, shoulder).

3 to 4 weeks: The wrist is brought to neutral in the orthosis and the patient can initiate an exercise program: PROM to each joint, followed by active tendon gliding exercises.

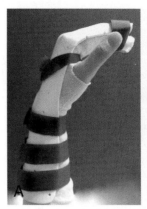
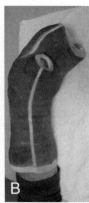

FIGURE 18–7 A, Wrist and hand extension restriction orthosis for flexor tendon repair. **B,** Cast for immobilization protocol. The amount of wrist and MCP flexion depends on the protocol used.

The orthosis can be removed for bathing and exercise but should be on at all other times.

4 to 6 weeks: Orthosis is discontinued. Exercises are progressed to include joint blocking. At this time, if flexion contractures have developed or extrinsic flexor tightness, then gentle extension mobilization with an orthosis may be initiated at night.

Early Passive Mobilization

Early passive mobilization (EPM) protocols came into use in the 1970s. These protocols are rarely used in isolation, but it is important to see the progression in which these protocols developed. They are based on the work of Kleinert, Kutz, Ashbell, and Martinez (1967) and **Duran and Houser** (1975), which showed that early mobilization of the tendons allowed better gliding of the tendon and produced better outcomes. Passive motion allows for some tendon glide without the force required of active motion. Further studies showed that for every 10° of DIP flexion, the FDP had 1 to 2 mm of excursion, whereas PIP flexion produced 1.5 mm of glide. These numbers are for unrepaired tendons. The amount of excursion goes down significantly in repaired tendons, presumably due to edema and tendon bulk from the sutures (Strickland, 2000). Each protocol has specific cookbook style guidelines, but in practice, most therapists using early PROM protocols use a combination of the different protocols. EPM is a good option in situations where the surgeon was only able to do a two-strand repair (or if it is unknown the type of repair, this is a safer option).

Duran and Houser

In their research, it was observed that 3 to 5 mm of glide was sufficient to prevent adhesions. Patient is positioned in a wrist and hand extension restriction orthosis, wrist in 20° of flexion, MCP joints in relaxed flexion, and IP joints held in flexion with dynamic traction (such as a rubber band). Isolated PIP and DIP PROM is performed with wrist and MCP joints held in flexion, six to eight repetitions, two times

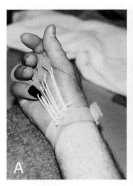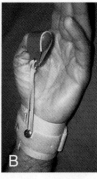

FIGURE 18-8 A wristlet is worn during the intermediate phase of treatment with the modified Duran protocol. **A,** The force can be secured distal to the proximal phalanx directly to the nail (SF) or applied via a sling on the proximal phalanges (IF, MF, and RF). **B,** FPL repairs can be managed in a similar fashion with a passive thumb IP flexion cuff.

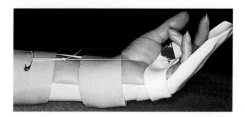

FIGURE 18-10 Rubber band traction is used for gentle digital flexion in an EPM program (shown is a modified splint with palmar pulley).

per day. After 4.5 weeks, the orthosis is discontinued and a wristlet is placed with a rubber band attached from wrist strap to the fingernail to allow for finger flexion/extension to occur with tenodesis (Fig. 18-8A,B). Resisted flexion does not begin until 8 weeks.

Modified Duran

For the **modified Duran** protocol, the orthosis is applied as mentioned earlier; however, the IP joints are held in extension in the orthosis between exercise sessions. Passive flexion and extension exercises are performed as outlined earlier. The patient is also allowed to *actively* extend IP joints to the extension block of the orthosis, which is the component that makes this the "modified" Duran protocol (Fig. 18-9A,B).

Kleinert

The original **Kleinert** protocol placed the wrist in 45° of flexion and the MCP joints in 10 to 20° of flexion. However, the original protocol is rarely, if ever, used; therefore, wrist and MCP joint position is no longer recommended. Kleinert's research showed that extension against resistance actually quieted the activity of the flexors (based on electromyography [EMG] findings), so he used the rubber band from the Duran protocol to actively resist extension and allowing the tension of the

rubber band to pull the finger back into flexion. The Kleinert protocol also uses a palmar pulley for the rubber band to pass through to allow for more DIP flexion. Exercise includes active extension to the extension block of the orthosis, completed 10 times every waking hour. Gentle active flexion is initiated at 3 to 6 weeks and resistance at 6 to 8 weeks.

Washington/Chow

This protocol combines the passive flexion recommended by Duran and Houser, with the controlled active extension/passive rubber band flexion recommended by Kleinert along with a pulley in the palm for increased DIP flexion (Fig. 18-10). Active flexion is not begun until week 4, the wrist position in the orthosis is brought to neutral at week 5, and the orthosis is generally discontinued at week 6 (Dovelle & Heeter, 1989).

Early Active Mobilization

With EPM protocols, the tendon achieves some glide, but the tendency is for the tendon to be compressed or "bunched up" rather than actually to glide through the sheath. True gliding has better potential to help prevent adhesions. A study by Trumble and colleagues (2010) showed that patients have better outcomes (increased active flexion and decreased flexion contractures) with an **early active mobilization (EAM) protocol** than with EPM protocols (Trumble et al., 2010). Studies have also shown that the repair site is stronger with early active motion, particularly when there is some tension as well as motion occurring at the repair site (Kubota, Manske, Mitsuhiro, Pruitt, & Larson, 1996). Regardless of protocol, studies have shown differing opinions on when to initiate early motion. Several studies (Halikis, Manske,

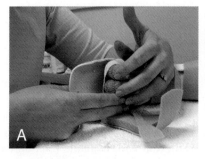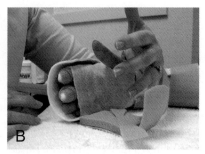

FIGURE 18-9 Modified Duran protocol: passive digit flexion performed in clinic under supervision **(A)** with active digit extension to the confines of the orthosis **(B)**.

Kubota, & Aoki, 1997; Zhao et al., 2004) found that the tendon encounters the least amount of work when motion is initiated anywhere from 3 to 7 days postoperatively (compared to initiating motion days 0 to 2 postoperatively). The first few days after surgery, the tendon is presented with a lot of resistance (due to newly traumatized tissue), and more force is required of the tendon to achieve motion. Waiting a few days allows the tissue to rest and inflammation to go down.

There are various early AROM protocols in the literature demonstrating that tendon rehabilitation is not an exact science (Pettengill, 2005; Pettengill & Van Strien, 2011). Most important is the experience of the therapist and surgeon as well as good communication between the two, along with choosing the appropriate patient who can follow the protocol. Protocols coming out of Europe are based on studies where patients are hospitalized initially, ensuring adherence to the protocol and exercise compliance.

Belfast and Sheffield

One protocol that came out of the United Kingdom, originally proposed by studies from Belfast and Sheffield, and subsequently modified (Gratton, 1993), recommends a wrist and hand extension restriction orthosis with the wrist in 10° of flexion, MCP joints at 80 to 90° of flexion, and IP joints extended fully. For exercise, the patient places the uninjured hand perpendicular in the palm with the small finger along the distal palmar crease. The patient then actively flexes to the index finger. Each week, one fewer finger is placed in the palm so that the patient gradually gets more active flexion. The orthosis is discontinued at 4 to 6 weeks depending on how the tendon is gliding (the patient is left in an orthosis longer if the tendon is gliding very well).

Strickland and Cannon

A commonly used EAM protocol proposed by Strickland (1993) and Cannon (1993) is based on the tensile forces placed on the tendon during AROM. It has been shown that by placing the wrist in slight extension, the forces on the tendon are further decreased (Savage, 1988). When the wrist is slightly extended, the flexors do not need to pull as much against the passive tension of the extrinsic extensors. Zhao and colleagues (2002) showed that synergistic wrist and finger motion achieve the goal of tendon excursion with low force to the tendons. It has also been shown that the tendons get the most excursion with early AROM when all four digits are mobilized together (Korstanje et al., 2012; Silfverskiold, May, & Oden, 1993).

Based on this information, **Strickland and Cannon** advocate an early place/hold protocol, where the wrist is placed in slight extension, the fingers are placed in flexion, and then the patient gently actively holds this position (the patient can practice the gentle hold with the contralateral hand first). For this protocol, two orthoses are used. When not exercising, the patient is in a wrist and hand extension restriction orthosis that holds the wrist at 20° of flexion and the MCP joints at 50° of flexion. The exercise orthosis is hinged at the wrist and blocks wrist extension at 30°, which is where the

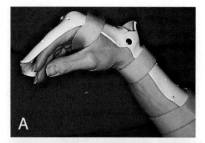
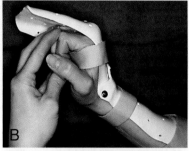
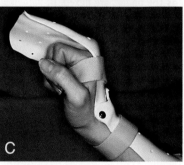

FIGURE 18–11 This tenodesis splint allows full flexion of the wrist but blocks extension at 30°. **A,** Wrist flexion with digit extension. **B,** Passive digit flexion with wrist extension. **C,** Active digit flexion hold. The orthosis shown is one of many design options for this protocol.

place/hold exercise occurs (Fig. 18–11A–C). In the interest of saving time/resources, the exercise orthosis alone can be fabricated, but with a removable block placing the wrist in 20° of flexion to be worn between exercise sessions. In this protocol, modified Duran exercises followed by active place/hold exercises are performed hourly. At 4 weeks, the exercise orthosis is discontinued and the patient is allowed to initiate active flexion in a tenodesis fashion (active wrist extension with finger flexion, followed by active wrist flexion, finger extension). At 7 to 8 weeks, the extension restriction orthosis is discontinued and resistive exercises are initiated.

Gallagher in 2006 modified the place and hold protocol to simplify it (Gallagher, 2006b). A traditional extension restriction orthosis is fabricated as described earlier. After performing PROM exercises to warm up the joints, the patient comes out of the orthosis for place and hold tenodesis exercises. The patient is shown where approximately 30° of wrist extension is and told to gently hold fingers in a composite fist (starting with holding in midrange, as if holding a feather) (Fig. 18–12A,B). If, by the second or third week, the patient is having difficulty achieving flexion at the DIP joint, the patient can be shown

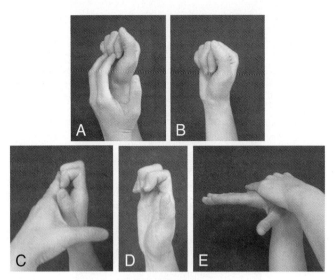

FIGURE 18–12 **A,** Early active place/hold ROM: Passively bring wrist into extension as the fingers are flexed. **B,** Patient is instructed to hold fingers in a gentle fist for 3 to 5 seconds. **C,** Place/hold hook fist: Fingers are passively brought into a hook fist. **D,** Patient is asked to gently hold the hook fist. This position encourages differential gliding between FDS and FDP. **E,** The place and hold motions are followed by wrist flexion with active finger extension.

gentle place and hold hook fist (Fig. 18–12C,D). This minimizes the activity of the lumbricals and focuses the attention on the extrinsic flexors. With tenodesis wrist motion, it is important to try to get as much active IP extension as possible to allow the tendon to glide distally and to help minimize flexion contractures (Fig. 18–12E).

With any early AROM protocol, it is the *quality* of motion achieved that is important: The exercises should be performed correctly in order to achieve the most glide with the lowest load. Increasing the frequency will not have an impact on adhesion formation if the tendon is not gliding. In addition, overexercising may incite an inflammatory response, which may lead to more adhesions.

Zones of Injury

The flexor tendons are divided into zones, depending on the location of injury (Fig. 18–13) (Table 18–1). There are different anatomical considerations in each zone. An injury in one zone may recover quite differently than an injury to the same tendon in a different zone.

Zone I

With injuries in this zone, only the FDP tendon is affected. The patient loses the ability to flex the DIP joint. In zone I injuries, if there is not enough of a tendon stump left for repair, the surgeon may elect to either use a bone anchor or to place suture material through the bone and attach

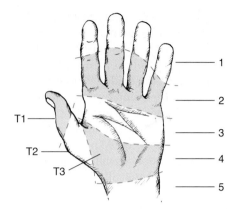

FIGURE 18–13 The flexor tendon zones.

a button on the fingernail to hold the suture in place (Fig. 18–14).

Jersey Finger

Jersey finger is an injury that occurs in zone I. The FDP is avulsed off the bone (it is so named because it can happen to football players when the tip of the finger gets caught in the

TABLE 18–1
Flexor Tendon Zones of Injury

Note: Zones are described distal to proximal.

Zone I:	Distal tips of digits to just proximal to the DIP joint crease. This zone contains the insertion of the FDP.
Zone II:	Starts from middle of middle phalanx and goes to distal palmar crease. This zone contains the insertion of FDS on the base of the middle phalanx. Also known as "no man's land" because of complications arising from injury in this zone. Most rehabilitation protocols are based on injuries within this zone.
Zone III:	Distal palmar crease to flexor retinaculum (carpal tunnel).
Zone IV:	Flexor retinaculum. As the nine tendons enter the carpal tunnel, they are oriented in the following way: the FDS of middle and ring fingers are the most superficial, with the FDS of index and small fingers just underneath. The four FDP tendons and the FPL are in the deepest layer.
Zone V:	Proximal to volar wrist crease to the musculotendinous junction.
Zone TI:	Distal phalanx of thumb.
Zone TII:	Proximal phalanx of thumb.
Zone TIII:	Thenar muscles.

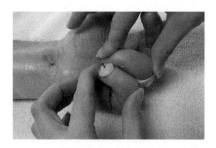

FIGURE 18–14 Button (pull out suture) in place during the initial stages of healing to keep distal repair secure.

jersey of another player). Sometimes, it may even take a part of the bone, which prevents the FDP from retracting too far proximally. The ring and middle fingers are the most commonly involved. Oftentimes, this injury may go undiagnosed or be misdiagnosed as "finger sprain."

Quadriga

Quadriga is a syndrome that occurs when the FDP tendon is repaired too tightly (if it needs to be advanced greater than 1 cm). This shortening of the FDP can lead to flexion contractures of the affected digit. Because the FDP to the middle, ring, and small fingers share the same muscle belly, the tendons to these three digits need to be tensioned equally to ensure full flexion. If one is shorter, muscle contraction will bend that finger first and the other unaffected digits will be unable to flex completely. The FDP does not have a lot of glide in this zone, which means that there is not a lot of room to shorten the repair without secondary consequences.

Zone II

This area is referred to as **no man's land** because, historically, injuries in this zone have the poorest prognosis. Both the FDS and FDP can be injured in this zone. Camper's chiasm is located here; this is the area where the FDS splits into two slips, which rotate 180° around and under the FDP, inserting on the base of the middle phalanx. Care must be taken to avoid injury to the pulley system during repair, particularly the A2 and A4 pulleys. Sometimes, the surgeon may elect to only repair one slip of the FDS tendon if repairing both will make the tendon too bulky to smoothly glide through the pulley system.

Zone III

Injuries in this zone are not within the fibroosseous tendon sheath, and scar tissue may not be as functionally limiting as injuries in zones II and IV. Repairs in this zone using early AROM protocol have been found to have good to excellent results (Al-Qattan, 2011).

Zone IV

Injuries in this zone are within the carpal tunnel and are not as frequent. The median nerve lies superficial to the tendons, so there may be an associated median nerve injury as well.

For tendon repairs in this zone, the flexor retinaculum is often not repaired (as in a standard carpal tunnel release), and the wrist should be positioned in neutral in the orthosis to prevent bowstringing of the tendons. **Tendon adhesion** can be a problem in this zone because there is a synovial sheath in the carpal tunnel and the tendons lie in a very constricted space.

Zone V

Injuries in this zone may include other structures in addition to the finger flexors, such as nerves, vessels, and wrist flexors. Prognosis tends to be better for injuries in this zone. Tendon adherence occurs but does not generally lead to function loss at this level because the overlying tissue is loose and mobile.

Zones TI through TIII

The FPL tendon lies alone in its sheath and it only crosses one IP joint. However, this tendon is more likely to retract proximally because there is only one vinculum and no lumbrical muscle attached (as there is in the FDP). This may lead to increased tendon adhesions with injuries to this tendon.

Rehabilitation and orthosis management for FPL repair is more complicated. There are limited research studies following FPL repair. Most protocols are based on research to FDS and FDP tendons. Brown and McGrouther (1984) found that most FPL glide occurs when the thumb MP is held in extension while the IP is passively flexed (as opposed to passive composite flexion). FPLs are more prone to scar formation as they are more likely to retract after laceration. Muscle shortening makes tendon retrieval challenging and IP flexion contractures are common.

There is no formal FPL protocol. Therefore, the clinician must apply knowledge about tendon rehabilitation for FDS and FDP laceration/repair and apply it to the FPL tendon. The four-strand repairs have been shown to better tolerate early motion, with lower rupture rates (Elliot, Moiemen, Flemming, Harris, & Foster, 1994; Elliot & Southgate, 2005).

In general, the orthosis for FPL injuries should position the wrist in slight flexion and the thumb in palmar abduction with the IP straight (Fig. 18–15). The fingers are left free; however, the patient should be cautioned against gripping or attempting to use the hand functionally due to intertendinous connections between the FDP of the IF and the FPL. This orthosis can be used with either EPM or EAM tendon protocols.

Clinical Decision Making

The therapist will need to evaluate when the patient can be advanced through the next stages of therapy or when the patient needs to be held back. Some people tend to produce more scar than others; therefore, it is necessary to

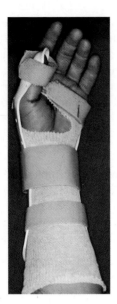

FIGURE 18–15 Extension restriction orthosis for FPL repair. The thumb should be positioned between palmar and radial abduction.

individually tailor each therapy program. A patient may need to be progressed a little sooner if they are particularly stiff or held back a little longer if the patient is moving too well.

The therapist must watch for several potential issues during the course of rehabilitation because there are several complications that can occur. Prevention is the best approach because it can be difficult to deal with the issues later on down the road. The most common problem is the formation of limiting adhesions. Another complication that can occur is flexion contractures, especially at the PIP joint. This can occur with any protocol because the natural tendency is for the PIP to rest in slight flexion when there is edema. Volar suture placement and scar tissue can further contribute to the flexion contracture. The PIP joint is particularly vulnerable when the finger is held in dynamic flexion with a rubber band. The therapist needs to be able to evaluate if the patient is developing a contracture and modify the exercises and add a digit extension mobilization orthosis or strategically placed foam within the restriction orthosis to provide a gentle extension stretch. This should be cleared by the physician to be sure there is no contraindication in providing this extension positioning such as a nerve repair or a tendon repair on tension.

Pyramid of Progressive Force (Gail Groth)

In 2004, Groth proposed a theoretical guideline to help therapists and surgeons decide how to progress the rehabilitation of the injured flexor tendon. Traditional flexor tendon protocols (as outlined earlier) are based on a chronologic timeline (based on where the patient is in the course of the

TABLE 18–2
Tendon Adhesion Grading System

- **Absent:** Greater than or equal to 5° discrepancy between digital active and passive flexion

- **Responsive:** Greater than or equal to 10% resolution of active lag between therapy sessions

- **Unresponsive:** Less than 10% resolution of active lag between therapy sessions

wound healing process) and do not accommodate individual healing differences from patient to patient. The information in the Groth article is used more for clinical judgment making rather than a precise protocol. As such, it can be used in conjunction with other early mobilization protocols.

A tendon adhesion grading system helps to guide the progression of exercise. This grading system allows the therapist to assess how great of a difference there is between active and passive motions and also their response to the exercise program. A tendon that is adherent not only prevents full flexion of the joint but it can also limit extension as that tendon is tethered down to adjacent tissue (Table 18–2).

This pyramid outlining progression of exercise was developed based on knowledge of tendon excursion and amount of force encountered per motion. The least amount of force is at the bottom of the pyramid, increasing as it gets closer to the top. Frequency of exercise is the most at the base of the pyramid, decreasing toward the top as the force increases. The pyramid allows the therapist to advance the exercises based on how the tendon is performing (Fig. 18–16).

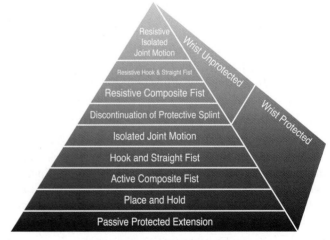

Pyramid of Progressive Force Application

FIGURE 18–16 Pyramid of progressive force exercises to the injured flexor tendon. Reprinted with permission from Groth, G. N. (2004). Pyramid of progressive force exercises to the injured flexor tendon. *Journal of Hand Therapy, 17*, 31–42.

Pyramid description

- **Base level:** At the bottom of the pyramid is protected passive finger extension (based on Duran, Houser, and Kleinert protocols).
- **Second level:** Patient performs protected place and hold loose fist initiated at first postoperative visit. This exercise is best initiated early on in the postoperative period before scar tissue has had a chance to form, creating more resistance for the tendon. This exercise is performed three to five times per day. If it is determined (at third or fourth postoperative visit) that there is an unresponsive lag, the patient is progressed to the third level.
- **Third level:** Active composite fist. The wrist is held protected in 20° of extension.
- **Fourth level:** Active hook and straight fist. The wrist is held at neutral to provide even stress to the tendon. If there is an unresponsive lag, the patient is progressed to joint blocking (isolated joint motion). With all exercises, it is important to maintain the ability to extend fully between each repetition. This aids in gliding the tendon distally as well as in maintaining full joint ROM.
- **Fifth level:** Discussions around discontinuing the protective orthosis. Initially, when the orthosis is discontinued, no new exercises are added while the patient adjusts to the new stresses of being orthosis free (the patient can be weaned from the orthosis gradually over the course of 1 to 2 weeks).
- **Final levels:** Progress as the earlier levels: resisted composite fist, followed by resisted hook and straight fists, to finally resisted isolated joint motion. Varying the positions of the proximal joints can increase the amount of resistance the tendon receives.

In order to progress the patient along the proposed pyramid, the therapist must be able to evaluate the tendon's response to exercise. If there is no flexion lag (i.e., the patient has full motion with place and hold), the patient is maintained on the lowest level of the pyramid over the course of 12 weeks (unless there is a change in tendon status earlier). This is fairly uncommon. If the tendon is responsive to the current level of stress on the pyramid level, the patient is maintained at that level. If the tendon is unresponsive, then the patient is progressed to the next level on the pyramid. Progression to the next level occurs at the rate of one level per visit (if the patient attends therapy one to two times per week).

Orthosis Considerations

Several issues must be taken into consideration when fabricating an extension restriction orthosis. It may be helpful to position the patient's arm on a foam ramp or on a homemade hand rest, preferably with a towel roll under the arm and the digits draped over the edge (Fig. 18–17A,B).

Wrist Position

It is most comfortable for the patient to be in no more than 10 to 20° of flexion, and this position is less likely to compromise the median nerve at the carpal tunnel. Ten degrees of wrist flexion should still provide sufficient protection to the healing tendon(s). Padding placed over the ulnar styloid prior to orthosis fabrication will increase comfort and prevent skin breakdown (Fig. 18–18A,B).

MCP Joints

Full MCP flexion may not be comfortable for the patient, especially if the wound extends into the palm. Too little MCP flexion, however, may not be sufficient enough to put slack on the repair. MCP flexion to 50 to 60° gives a landmark for the orthosis to rest and helps to prevent distal migration of the orthosis. To maintain position of the orthosis, it should conform to the MCP joints (but watch for potential areas of pressure), and the palmar strap should securely hold the patient up into the hood of the orthosis (Fig. 18–19A). The orthosis itself can be contoured adequately, but if the strap across the palm is not sufficiently holding the dorsum of the hand against the orthosis, the patient can unknowingly rest in too much MCP extension, potentially putting the tendon repair at risk (Fig. 18–19B).

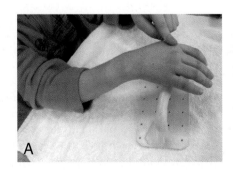
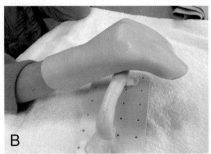

FIGURE 18–17 A and B, Homemade thermoplastic hand stand used to prevent flattening of forearm musculature during the molding process as seen when using foam supports. This also allows for easy adjustments of wrist and MCP joint angles.

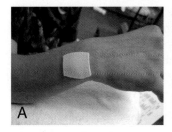 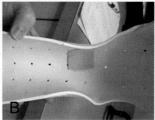

FIGURE 18–18 **A,** Prepad the distal ulna and **(B)** invert the foam into the orthosis for a permanent solution to prevent bony irritation.

IP Joints

There should be sufficient room for the interphalangeal (IP) joints to extend fully to the roof of the orthosis, even if the IP joints have not yet achieved full extension. During fabrication, it is important that the roof of the orthosis is made to allow for full IP joint extension. This may be challenging to ensure that the MCP joints are flexed to the right angle while keeping the IP joints straight, but this is crucial. Not only does full IP extension in the orthosis help prevent PIP flexion contractures but it also allows the tendon to glide distally when actively extending to the orthosis, helping to prevent adhesions (Fig. 18–20A–C). Note: if there is an associated nerve repair, the surgeon may request restricting full extension at the PIP joint for the first few weeks. Adding a small foam wedge dorsally at the middle phalanx will allow for this restriction of motion and can be altered as the weeks progress to provide greater available extension.

Orthoses to Address Postoperative Complications

Early in the postoperative course, the orthosis is a protective mechanism. Over time, as the patient progresses and no longer needs the same level of protection, motion deficits may become apparent. A new orthosis can be fabricated to help gain motion and facilitate exercises. Or perhaps the

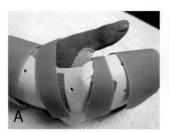 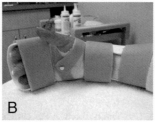

FIGURE 18–19 **A,** When molding about the MCP joints, use a strategy such as this cut/overlap technique to obtain contour about this bony area (dorsal 2nd MCP). **B,** Riveting a strap that contours around the thumb carpometacarpal (CMC) joint secures the orthosis on the arm, preventing migration.

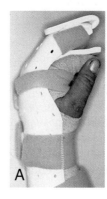 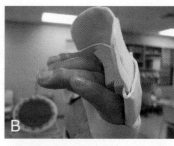
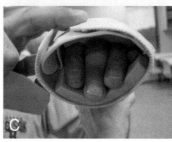

FIGURE 18–20 **A,** An AlumaFoam® insert positions the IF MCP joint in flexion, facilitating active PIP extension with exercise and allowing the PIP to be safely strapped into extension to prevent PIP flexion contracture. **B and C,** Applying foam dorsally over the proximal phalanges and volarly on the distal strap can be another way to achieve greater PIP extension within the orthosis.

old orthosis can be reconfigured into a new design to save money.

Flexion Contractures

Flexion contractures are a common complication in zone II injuries. Scar tissue tends to contract the PIP joint, and the extensor tendons are not strong enough to overcome the power of the contractile force of scar tissue. This can also occur from too much time spent in dynamic traction or from the hood of the orthosis not molded in a fully extended position combined with the swollen PIP joint preferring a position of slight flexion at rest. Early in the course of therapy, a digit extension orthosis can be fabricated for the patient to wear inside the forearm-based orthosis. Once the long orthosis is discontinued, an extension mobilization orthosis can be fabricated to promote finger extension (Fig. 18–21A,B).

Scar Remodeling

Silicone gel dressings applied under an orthosis may assist in preventing the formation of excessive scar tissue. Silicone sheeting (sold by various manufacturers) is thought to prevent moisture from entering the scar area. If moisture at the scar area is lessened, blood flow in turn is reduced, leading to less collagen formation at the scar area. By reducing collagen at the targeted area, the scar becomes paler and less visible, without the red and purple skin tone that scars often become (Fig. 18–22A). Scar remodeling materials can be incorporated into the orthosis for gentle compression to the scar during resting hours. The compression properties that

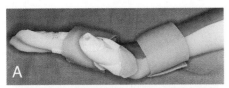

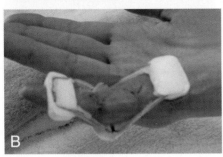

FIGURE 18–21 **A,** A serial static wrist/hand/thumb extension mobilization splint for extrinsic flexor tightness is remolded as the tissues gently elongate. Note the use of QuickCast 2 serial static digit extension splints to direct corrective force to the extrinsic flexors (Patterson Medical, Warrenville, IL). **B,** Digit PIP extension mobilization orthosis used to stretch contracted volar structures (LMB Spring Finger Extension Assist Splint, DeRoyal, Powell, TN). *Note: the therapist should consult with the physician prior to using any mobilization orthosis that may place stress on a healing tendon.*

are applied by using these materials under an orthosis contributes to desensitizing a hypersensitive scar and assists in remodeling dense, thick, ropelike scars (Fig. 18–22B,C).

Exercise Orthoses

Differential gliding can be difficult to achieve because of tendinous adhesions. For 6 weeks, the patient has been held in a position of intrinsic plus. This position facilitates the lumbricals. Because the lumbricals originate on the FDP tendons, DIP joint flexion is compromised. The normal cascade of motion is affected: when the patient attempts to initiate DIP joint flexion, they may initiate with the lumbricals instead of initiating at the DIP joint. To promote DIP flexion and differential tendon glide, the lumbricals need to be deactivated. An MCP joint blocking orthosis holds the MCP joints in full extension while the IP joints are left free (Fig. 18–23A). This helps to guide the hook fist while

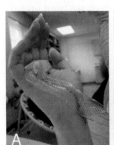
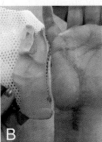
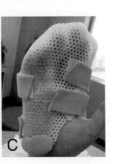

FIGURE 18–22 **A,** Silicone gel applied to a healing incision and **(B and C)** elastomer mold incorporated into a night orthosis.

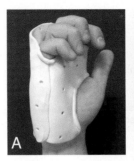
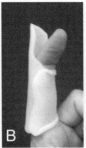
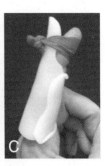

FIGURE 18–23 **Exercise orthoses. A,** MCP blocking orthosis: This is worn for exercise sessions to encourage IP joint motion and differential tendon glide. **B,** PIP blocking orthosis to encourage FDP glide. **C,** The addition of an exercise band adds resistance to the exercise once the patient is cleared for heavier activities. This puts a lot of stress on the FDP and should be used cautiously.

preventing the lumbricals from kicking in and taking over. A PIP joint blocking orthosis (cylinder orthosis holding the PIP joint in extension with the DIP joint free) helps to encourage DIP flexion. If the dorsal portion of the orthosis extends to the fingertip, a rubber band can be added to give resistance to the FDP (when it is safe to add resistive exercises) (Fig. 18–23B,C).

Extensor Tendons

Anatomy and Function

The extensor tendon system is engineered for finesse, not power. For this reason, it can be more complicated to conceptualize than the flexor tendon system. The flexor system is muscle to tendon to bone, where each muscle acts primarily on one joint (secondarily contributing to flexion at each joint it crosses). Much of the extensor system is not so straightforward. Both extrinsic and intrinsic muscles work together to extend the fingers, and the muscles are smaller in mass than the flexors. Fibrous bands arising from the tendons contribute greatly to finger extension. The extensor tendons balance out the power of the flexor tendons and play a large role in fine motor control (Fig. 18–24).

Extensor Tendons: Digits

There are nine extrinsic extensors that are relevant for orthotic fabrication: three each for the wrist, fingers, and thumb. Similar to the extrinsic flexors, these muscles all originate in the forearm and insert distal to the wrist to elicit motion at the designated joint(s). At the level of the wrist, the tendons traverse the extensor retinaculum. This is a fibroosseous tunnel system that is partitioned into six dorsal compartments (A–F) (Fig. 18–25). In addition to acting as a source of nutrition, the extensor retinaculum acts as a pulley to give biomechanical advantage and prevent bowstringing of the extensor tendons. There is great potential for scar and adhesions to

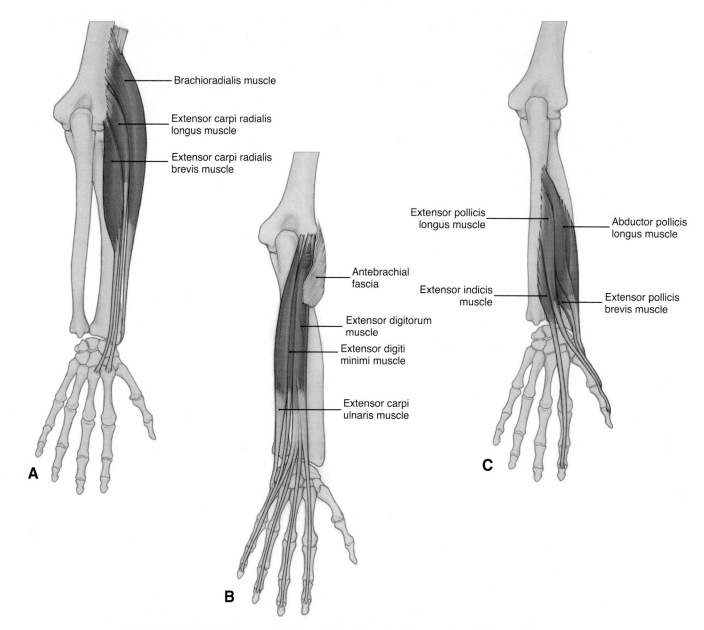

FIGURE 18–24 Radial **(A)**, superficial dorsal **(B)**, and intermediate and deep **(C)** layers of the extensor compartment (dorsal view). Reprinted with permission from Clemente, C. D. (2011). *Anatomy: A regional atlas of the human body* (6th ed.). Baltimore, MD: Lippincott Williams & Wilkins.

develop within the peritendinous fascia and within the synovial retinaculum with injury to the extensor tendons (Rosenthal & Elhassan, 2011). The digital extensors distal to the wrist fan out into broad and flat tendons. They receive nutrition from vascular mesotendon fibers (similar to vinculae), from the peritendinous fascia that surrounds the tendons, and via synovial diffusion from the extensor retinaculum (at the wrist). The extrinsic digital extensors are the extensor digitorum communis (EDC), the extensor indicis proprius (EIP), and the extensor digiti minimi (EDM). These three muscles extend the MCP joints while the EIP and the EDM allow for independent extension of the index and small fingers. The EDC has tendons to the index, middle, and ring fingers, but not everyone has

an EDC to the small finger. In addition, people can maintain independent function of the index finger even without an EIP because of an independent EDC muscle belly to the index finger (Moore, Weiland, & Valdata, 1987). The EDC extends the MCP joints of digits two to five via soft tissue connections: the **juncturae tendinum** on the dorsum of the hand as well as the sagittal bands at the MCP joints (Fig. 18–25). The EDC does not insert on the base of the proximal phalanx; instead, MCP extension occurs as muscle contraction of EDC leads to tensioning of the fibers of the **sagittal bands**, causing MCP extension (van Sint Jan, Rooze, van Auderkerke, & Vico, 1996). If the MCP joints are not hyperextended, the EDC can also secondarily assist with IP extension. The prime muscles acting

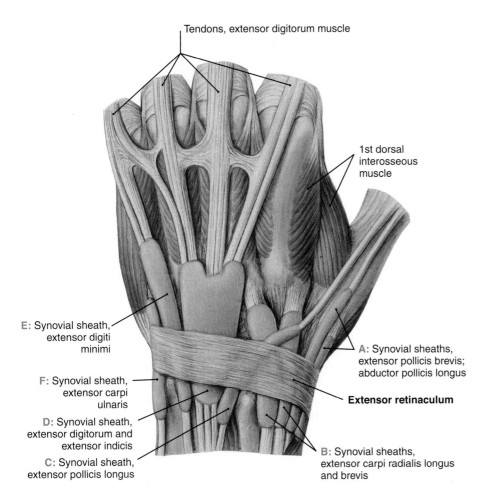

Tendons, extensor digitorum muscle

1st dorsal interosseous muscle

E: Synovial sheath, extensor digiti minimi

F: Synovial sheath, extensor carpi ulnaris

D: Synovial sheath, extensor digitorum and extensor indicis

C: Synovial sheath, extensor pollicis longus

A: Synovial sheaths, extensor pollicis brevis; abductor pollicis longus

Extensor retinaculum

B: Synovial sheaths, extensor carpi radialis longus and brevis

FIGURE 18–25 **A,** Synovial sheaths of extensor tendons of the hand. **B,** The six dorsal compartments of the extensor tendons. *A,* abductor pollicis longus and extensor pollicis brevis; *B,* extensor carpi radialis longus and extensor carpi radialis brevis; *C,* extensor pollicis longus; *D,* extensor digitorum communis; *E,* extensor digiti minimi; *F,* extensor carpi ulnaris; *1–4,* dorsal interossei. Reprinted with permission from Clemente, C. D. (2011). *Anatomy: A regional atlas of the human body* (6th ed.). Baltimore, MD: Lippincott Williams & Wilkins.

CHAPTER 18

on IP extension are the intrinsic muscles. The lumbricals are the primary IP extensors, whereas the dorsal and palmar interossei act secondarily as extensors.

MCP Joints

The dorsal hood is a broad fibrous structure at the MCP joint, which is composed of fibers from the EDC, the juncturae tendinum, and the sagittal bands. The juncturae tendinum are bands arising from the ring finger EDC, which branch out to the EDC of the small, middle, and occasionally the index finger as well as to the EDM. They also send fibers to the sagittal bands. As the fingers flex, the juncturae become more transverse and help in stabilizing the EDC tendons. The juncturae help provide uniform extension of the fingers. If a tendon is lacerated proximal to the juncturae, tension through this structure can provide extension to the injured finger (thereby masking whether the tendon is actually lacerated). If a tendon is lacerated distal to the juncturae, those fibers help prevent proximal migration of the tendon.

The sagittal bands are ligamentous structures at the MCP joints. Their vertical fibers surround the MCP joint to insert on the volar plate and intermetacarpal ligaments. They serve two functions: (1) to centralize the EDC over the MCP joints and (2) to transmit forces from the EDC to provide MCP extension. When the finger is fully flexed, the sagittal band is distal to the MCP joint. Injury to the sagittal bands (either through rupture or laceration) will result in subluxation of the EDC off the MCP joint (usually in an ulnar direction) (Fig. 18–25).

IP Joints

The lumbrical muscles originate on the FDP tendons and insert radially onto the fibers of the dorsal hood (Fig. 18–26). The lumbricals act primarily as IP extensors and secondarily as MCP flexors. If the FDP is contracted, the lumbricals are on slack and the IPs will not extend (the opposite is also true: if the lumbricals are contracted, the FDP relaxes).

The interossei muscles originate along the metacarpals and send fibers to insert on the bases of the proximal phalanges (for finger abduction and adduction and MCP flexion), but they also send fibers to the dorsal apparatus to secondarily contribute to IP extension (if the MCP joints are extended). The EDC can assist in extending the IP joints if the MCP joints are flexed.

The fibers on the dorsal hood at the MCP joint continue on to the proximal phalanx and combine with fibers from the intrinsic hand muscles to form the dorsal apparatus (Fig. 18–26). These fibers contribute to both flexion and extension of the MCP joint. The more proximal vertical fibers contribute to MCP flexion, whereas the more oblique distal fibers contribute to IP extension.

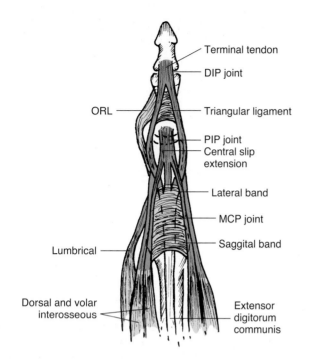

- Terminal tendon
- DIP joint
- ORL
- Triangular ligament
- PIP joint
- Central slip extension
- Lateral band
- MCP joint
- Lumbrical
- Saggital band
- Dorsal and volar interosseous
- Extensor digitorum communis

FIGURE 18–26 The intricate extensor apparatus. *DIP*, distal interphalangeal; *ORL*, oblique retinacular ligament.

Central fibers from the extrinsic tendon continue past the MCP joint and are joined by fibers from the intrinsic muscles to form the central slip, which inserts at the base of the middle phalanx (Fig. 18–26). The lateral fibers from the extrinsic tendon combine with fibers from the intrinsic tendons to form the **lateral bands**. The lateral bands lay dorsal to the axis of PIP joint motion during extension and migrate volarly during PIP flexion.

The lateral bands come together over the middle phalanx to form the **terminal tendon**, which inserts on the base of the distal phalanx (Fig. 18–26). Too much volar or dorsal migration of the lateral bands can lead to deformity (**boutonniere** or **swan neck**). The PIP joint has fibers in similar orientation as the sagittal bands. These fibers arise from the flexor tendon sheath and encircle the joint to help stabilize the lateral bands. Dorsal to the lateral bands, these fibers are called the triangular ligament and help centralize the lateral bands over the middle phalanx. The triangular ligament prevents palmar subluxation of the lateral bands as the PIP flexes. The fibers below the lateral bands form the transverse retinacular ligament, which prevents subluxation of the lateral bands as the PIP extends.

The **oblique retinacular ligament** (ORL; also known as Landsmeer's ligament) arises volarly from the flexor sheath and crosses obliquely over the middle phalanx to blend with fibers from the terminal tendon (Fig. 18–26). The ORL likely does not contribute to active DIP extension; however, tightness of this ligament can contribute to decreased DIP flexion, particularly if the PIP joint is extended (Shrewsbury, 1977). In the normally functioning hand, extension of the PIP and DIP joints occurs together; the joints cannot extend independently.

Extensor Tendons: Thumb

There are three extrinsic tendons for the thumb: the extensor pollicis brevis (EPB), abductor pollicis longus (APL), and the extensor pollicis longus (EPL). In the thumb, there is one muscle per joint for extension (Fig. 18–24 and Fig. 18–25).

Extensor Tendon Protocols

To mobilize or not to mobilize a repaired extensor tendon is one of the biggest controversies in tendon management. Extensor tendon injuries tolerate early motion well in all zones except for zone I. The risks of rupture or tendon attenuation from an early mobilization program do not seem to be as great with extensor tendons as with flexor tendons (Evans, 2012; Newport & Tucker, 2005; Griffin et al., 2012). Ruptures that occur may be caused by the powerful force of flexion rather than via forced extension. The extensors are simply not as powerful as the flexors. There is research that shows how early loading of healing tissue does help strengthen material properties of the tissue (Buckwalter & Grodzinsky, 1999; Fong et al., 2005; Gelberman et al., 1982). Most research on properties of tendon healing has been on flexor tendons with a synovial sheath or on animal models. Knowledge of flexor tendon healing properties can be applied to extensor tendon healing, as the principles and timelines of wound healing should be similar.

Early Mobilization Protocols

If an early mobilization protocol is chosen, should it be early active or early controlled passive mobilization with a dynamic orthosis? Multiple studies have shown favorable outcomes with early mobilization (Chow, Dovelle, Thomes, Ho, & Saldana, 1989; Howell, Merritt, & Robinson, 2005; Ip & Chow, 1997; Russell, Jones, & Grobbelaar, 2003; Sameem, Wood, Ignacy, Thoma, & Strumas, 2011; Sylaidis, Youatt, & Logan, 1997). However, there are only two studies that compared early active with early controlled dynamic mobilization (Chester, Beale, Beveridge, Nancarrow, & Titley, 2002; Khandwala, Webb, Harris, Foster, & Elliot, 2000). Both studies showed no long-term differences between the two protocols, although Chester et al. (2002) found that ROM was better at 4 weeks in the dynamic orthosis group (however, by week 12, the differences were insignificant). Eissens, Schut, and van der Sluis (2007) recommend adding protected wrist motion to the dynamic orthosis for zones V to VII, although there is no evidence to show this as being more effective than other early mobilization protocols. Newport and Shukla (1992) found that in a dynamic orthosis, it is unlikely that the extension is truly passive and that some degree of active extension is occurring.

Conversely, there is evidence that these injuries seem to tolerate immobilization as well, although the recovery process will take longer. Multiple studies have looked at injuries in zones V to VIII and compared early mobilization (either active or controlled dynamic passive motion) with immobilization. They have shown that although patients performing an early mobilization protocol have more motion at week 4, in the long term, there are no functional differences between the protocols (Bulstrode, Burr, Pratt, & Brobbelaar, 2005; Talsma, de Haart, Beelen, & Nollet, 2008). One study found that by 6 months, there were no significant differences in grip strength between the immobilized and mobilized groups (Mowlavi, Burns, & Brown, 2005). Purcell, Eadie, Murugan, O'Donnell, and Lawless (2000) found 95% good or excellent results with the use of an immobilization orthosis at 4 months postoperatively. With early mobilization, patients may return to previous level of function sooner; however, not every patient may be appropriate for an early mobilization protocol. The exercise regime is more complicated and the orthosis, if dynamic, is more cumbersome for daily life, both of which may reduce overall compliance.

Another consideration with any tendon injury is that frequently, there are concomitant injuries (fractures, nerves repairs, etc.), and those injures may dictate the postoperative course of treatment. The more bony and/or soft tissue damage there is, the greater the likelihood for the formation of adhesions. Tendon adhesions can cause loss of motion in both flexion and extension. Loss of flexion and decreased grip strength both have a greater impact on function than an extensor lag. Postoperatively, the repaired tendon should be positioned in slack to prevent a lag because a lag is much more difficult to treat than soft tissue tightness.

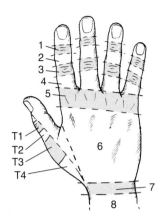

FIGURE 18–27 The extensor tendon zones.

Zones of Injury

The extensor tendons are separated into eight zones of injury. Treatment of extensor tendon injuries varies greatly depending on the zone of injury. All of the odd-numbered zones are over joints. Zone I is over the DIP joint, III is over the PIP joint, V is over the MCP joint, and VII is over the wrist. The zones are numbered distal to proximal (as in the flexor tendon zones) (Fig. 18–27) (Table 18–3).

TABLE 18–3	
Extensor Tendon Zones of Injury	

Note: Zones are described distal to proximal. All of the odd-numbered zones are over joints.

Zone I:	Over the DIP joint. This zone includes the terminal tendon.
Zone II:	Over the middle phalanx.
Zone III:	Over the PIP joint. This zone contains the central slip and the lateral bands.
Zone IV:	Over the proximal phalanx. There is a large amount of contact between the tendon and bone in this zone, which can lead to significant adherence to the bone.
Zone V:	Over the MCP joint. This zone contains the sagittal bands.
Zone VI:	Over the dorsum of the hand. This zone contains the juncturae tendinum, where the tendons are broad and flat.
Zone VII:	Over the wrist. This zone contains the extensor retinaculum, which is synovial and may lead to increased scarring in this zone. Without the retinaculum, the tendons will have a tendency to bowstring, which will decrease excursion and strength.
Zone VIII:	Dorsal forearm just proximal to the extensor retinaculum. Includes the musculotendinous junctions of the digital and wrist extensors.
Zone TI:	At the thumb IP joint. This is where the EPL inserts.
Zone TII:	Over the proximal phalanx.
Zone TIII:	Over the thumb MP joint. In addition to the EPL passing through here, this is where the EPB inserts.
Zone TIV:	At the level of the first metacarpal.
Zone TV:	At the level of the wrist. This includes the extensor retinaculum, which is synovial and may lead to increased scar tissue formation in this zone.

Zones I and II

Zone I lies over the DIP joint and is commonly referred to as a mallet finger. The structure of importance in this zone is the terminal tendon. Injury can occur through rupture, laceration, avulsion fracture of the bone where the tendon inserts, or through crush injury (Fig. 18–28A,B). Mucous cysts from osteoarthritis at the DIP joint can also secondarily lead to a mallet finger. Even if the terminal tendon is completely lacerated, the DIP joint will not assume a fully flexed position; rather, it will rest in approximately 45° of flexion. This is because of the action of the collateral ligaments and the ORL.

Regardless of the mechanism of injury, the mallet finger is treated by immobilizing the DIP joint in extension and maintaining that position for 6 to 8 weeks, followed by 2 to 4 weeks of night immobilization and with strenuous activity to prevent

an extension lag (Fig. 18–28C,D) (Griffin, et al., 2012). If the DIP joint is allowed to flex at any point in the initial 6 to 8 weeks, the integrity of the healing process is interrupted and the immobilization regimen must start again. The PIP joint is left free in the orthosis, but if the patient has a hypermobile PIP, it is recommended that a separate PIP extension restriction orthosis be made, which allows PIP flexion but not hyperextension (Fig. 18–28E). The mallet orthosis can be challenging to fabricate. Volarly, the orthosis must be long enough to provide sufficient support for DIP extension, but it must not be so long that it blocks PIP flexion or causes the orthosis to migrate distally as the PIP flexes. The small finger is the toughest finger to achieve this balance because of the shortened lever arms (see Chapter 7 for detailed instructions and helpful hints). Prior to orthosis fabrication, it may be helpful to place paper tape or

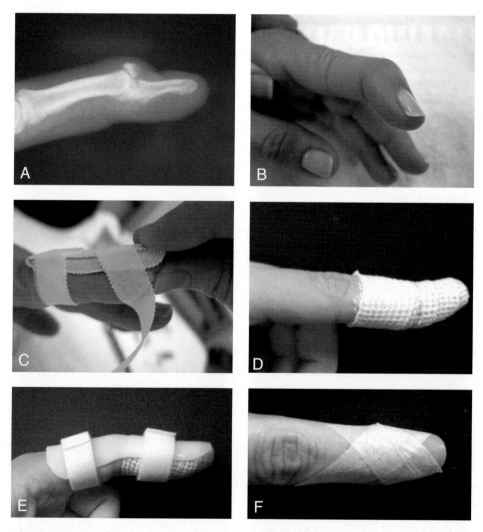

FIGURE 18–28 A and B, Zone I extensor tendon injury (mallet finger) with bony avulsion. **C,** AlumaFoam® applied dorsally—note placement of tape at an angle to contour at tip. **D,** Orthosis fabricated using Quick-Cast 2 (Patterson Medical). The DIP is positioned in slight hyperextension and there is enough clearance to allow for PIP flexion. **E,** A dorsal orthosis can be helpful if the patient has a tendency to hyperextend at the PIP (to discourage the potential for developing a swan-neck deformity). This is worn between PIP blocking exercises. **F,** Paper tape placed in Figure-8 fashion to help encourage DIP hyperextension within the orthosis.

elastic therapeutic tape (such as Balance Tex™ or Kinesio® Tex) to hold the DIP in extension. This can give added security in the orthosis (Fig. 18–28F). Custom orthoses have been shown to have more favorable outcomes when compared to prefabricated or aluminum foam–type orthoses (O'Brien & Bailey, 2011). An untreated mallet finger may lead to a swan-neck deformity over time as the fibers from the ORL are stretched for a prolonged period of time (Griffin, et al., 2012).

Zone II lies over the middle phalanx. Injuries here are usually the result of laceration. After the tendon is repaired, treatment is the same as it is for zone I injuries.

Zones III and IV

Zone III lies over the PIP joint and contains the central slip as well as the lateral bands and transverse retinacular ligaments. Zone IV lies over the proximal phalanx. Injuries in either zone are treated the same. The central slip is the portion of the tendon that can initiate PIP extension from a flexed position. The lateral bands can maintain extension once the joint is extended and if they lie dorsal to the axis of joint motion (Rosenthal & Elhassan, 2011). Injury to the central slip and triangular ligament can lead to a boutonniere deformity, where the PIP joint assumes a flexed posture and the DIP is hyperextended. The lateral bands, untethered from the triangular ligament, are allowed to migrate volarly. This shortens the connection to the terminal tendon, pulling the DIP into hyperextension. The FDS, which is now unopposed, further pulls the PIP into flexion, accentuating the deformity. The lateral bands also act as flexors of the PIP joint when they are volar to the axis of motion. Over time, tissues shorten and the deformity becomes fixed. If this is the case, then the flexion contracture must be treated before the tendon injury. Injury in this zone can be either closed or open.

Closed Injuries

A closed boutonniere is treated conservatively: the PIP joint is immobilized at 0° for 6 weeks (Fig. 18–29A–D). Flexion exercises are introduced gradually, with the focus on maintaining active extension. The orthosis is worn between exercise sessions for another 2 to 4 weeks. A circumferential orthosis is commonly the best immobilization option; the pressure aids in reducing swelling, and the circumferential nature of the design maximizes the pressure distribution making the orthosis comfortable for the patient. A volar- or dorsal-based orthosis often is unable to maintain the PIP joint in full extension and pressure problems often arise. The orthosis can be made out of thin thermoplastic, QuickCast 2, Orficast™ Tapes, or plaster of paris. The DIP is left free and the patient is instructed in active DIP exercises. This allows the lateral bands to advance and the ORLs to stretch, which will further prevent the boutonniere deformity. Frequently, a patient, coach/trainer, or family member may assume this injury is a "finger sprain" and will wait to see if it heals on its own before seeking medical attention. Commonly, the PIP will develop a flexion contracture caused by adhesions forming in the volar plate with a swollen, inflamed PIP joint that is allowed to rest in a flexed position. The contracture must be treated first (via a serial static extension mobilization orthosis). Once the PIP reaches full passive extension, the 6-week immobilization regimen is initiated. However, once the deformity is fixed, then the prognosis for a good outcome is poor. These patients should be monitored weekly while they are in the orthosis to check the skin as well as to assess for any changes in swelling.

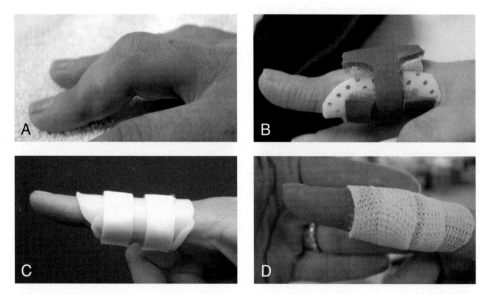

FIGURE 18–29 A, Closed boutonniere deformity sustained after a fall. **B,** Volar PIP immobilization orthosis with dorsal padding to secure extension position. **C,** Circumferential 'clamshell' design using thermoplastic material. **D,** QuickCast 2 used offering maximal pressure distribution, making this a comfortable option (Patterson Medical).

If swelling decreases, the orthosis may become too loose, requiring adjustment. After the 6-week period, PIP flexion is gradually introduced with extension immobilization continued between exercise sessions for another 2 to 4 weeks. The immobilized tendon is fragile and lacks the normal tissue properties (tensile strength, hydration, and collagen cross-linking); therefore, care must be taken to not be overly aggressive when initiating flexion. Most importantly, watch for increases in swelling and any developing extension lag. Because of the unique anatomy in zones III and IV, there is a high risk for scarring and adhesions to occur. In zone IV, there is a high ratio of tendon to bone and this fact, combined with poor tendon excursion in this zone, leads to a large area for the tendon to adhere to the bone. When the tendon is immobilized for 6 weeks, it is relying on extrinsic healing to occur (i.e., healing via scar tissue). As PIP joint motion is initiated, if the tendon is adhered in zone IV, attenuation can occur over the PIP joint, which leads to an active extension lag. This is why progression of motion must begin slowly.

Functional impairments for the untreated boutonniere can include lack of ability to extend the finger when reaching into a small space (pockets, gloves, etc.) as well as difficulty with fine motor coordination because of lack of DIP flexion. Often, patients are more bothered by the appearance of the finger when the PIP joint is enlarged.

Open Injuries

Open injuries are less common. Depending on the amount of soft tissue loss, the patient can begin a **short arc of motion (SAM) protocol** after surgical repair, as outlined by Evans (2011). For this protocol, the patient is immobilized in full extension, and two exercise orthoses are fabricated for the patient (Fig. 18–30A–D). The first exercise orthosis is for PIP flexion and it allows the PIP to flex to 30°. The patient actively flexes to the orthosis block then actively extends the PIP fully. The second exercise orthosis is for DIP flexion. If the lateral bands are not repaired, then the DIP is allowed to flex fully during exercise sessions while the PIP is held at zero. If the lateral bands are repaired as well as the central slip, the template is fabricated with the PIP held at zero and the DIP allowed to flex to 30°. During exercise sessions, the patient positions the wrist in slight flexion, which decreases the viscoelastic tension on the tendons. After the second postoperative week, if no extensor tendon lag has developed, then the patient is allowed to flex to 40°. Approximately 10° of flexion are added each week as long as no active lag has developed. Full composite flexion is allowed by week 5 and gentle strengthening exercises by week 6 (at which point the extension orthosis is discontinued). The rationale for this protocol, as outlined by Evans (2011), is to allow for slight tendon excursion and promote tendon healing (applied from the principles gleaned from flexor tendon research). Evans (2011) also advocates treating closed boutonniere injuries with SAM protocol; however, the results are unpublished at the time of this publication, and it is recommended that this is discussed with the referring physician prior to initiating this protocol.

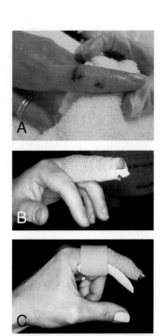

FIGURE 18–30 A, Open extensor tendon zone II injury over the PIP joint. Three splints used for the SAM protocol. **B,** A volar PIP/DIP immobilization splint is used between exercise sessions. **C,** The first exercise splint allows 30° of flexion at the PIP joint and 20 to 25° of flexion at the DIP joint. **D,** The second exercise splint blocks the PIP joint so that the lateral bands can glide distal to the repair site.

Zones V and VI

Zone V lies over the MCP joint and contains the sagittal bands and the EDC tendon. Zone VI spans the length of the metacarpals and involves the EDC tendons just distal to the wrist joint.

Closed Injuries

Rupture of the sagittal bands can lead to subluxation of the extensor tendon off of the MCP joint. Usually, it is rupture of the radial bands, which are weaker than the ulnar bands. The long finger is the most commonly involved finger with this type of injury (Young & Rayan, 2000). Treatment of the closed injury can be done conservatively with immobilization (Slater & Bynum, 1997) (Fig. 18–31A–D). Operative treatment may be indicated in cases of complete radial sagittal band disruption or in instances of failed conservative treatment.

Open Injuries

Tendons in zones V and VI that are repaired can also be treated with immobilization. This may be appropriate if the patient cannot be compliant with a more complicated early mobilization protocol or if there are other structures that

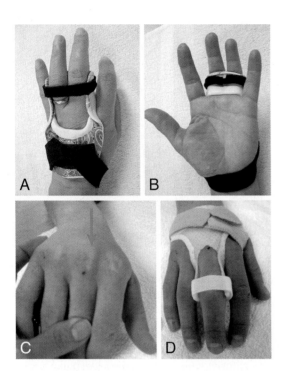

FIGURE 18–31 **Closed extensor tendon zone V injury. A and B,** Two digits involved and **(C and D)** middle finger only included in this volar/dorsal MCP joint immobilization orthosis. Note the radial orientation of the extensor tendon over the 3rd MCP indicated by the arrow.

need to be immobilized. It is important to keep in mind that the more traumatic the injury, the greater the likelihood of scar tissue and adhesion formation.

If only the EIP or EDM is lacerated, then only the involved digit needs to be immobilized. However, if the EDC is lacerated, then all digits need to be included in the orthosis because of the action of the juncturae (Fig. 18–32A,B). The orthosis positions the wrist in 30° of extension and the MCP

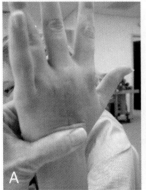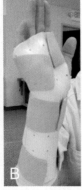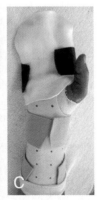

FIGURE 18–32 **Laceration and repair of extensor tendon zone VI injury. A,** Note adherence over scar. **B,** Wrist and MCP immobilization orthosis allowing IP ROM to prevent distal stiffness and promote edema reduction. **C,** If PIP joint flexion contractures are a concern, provide patient with a removable hand-based orthosis that can be worn over the longer orthosis. This may be worn at night or intermittently during the day as needed.

joints in full extension for 4 to 6 weeks, with buddy taping to provide protection for another 2 weeks (Griffin, et al., 2012). The IP joints are left free in the orthosis, but there must be enough thermoplastic volarly on the proximal phalanx to support the MCP joint, not so long as to prevent IP flexion. It is important to monitor the patient and make sure that he or she is not developing PIP flexion contractures. If there seems to be a potential for this, the patient can wear a night orthosis that positions the entire hand in full extension (Fig. 18–32C).

Gentle active motion is initiated at week 3, with the initial focus on isolated MCP joint motion. Using the principles of tenodesis decreases the tension from the surrounding soft tissue: MCP flexion with the wrist in slight extension and MCP extension with the wrist in slight flexion. Composite flexion is begun at postoperative week 4 or 5 if there is no extension lag, and the orthosis is discontinued at week 6.

Zones VII and VIII

Zone VII is over the wrist and contains the extensor reticulum—the broad fibrous structure divided into six compartments for the tendons to pass through. The retinaculum is synovial, which provides nutrition to the tendons, yet there is increased risk for scar formation in this region. Loss of extensor retinaculum may lead to bowstringing of the tendons and result in an extension lag at the MCP joint(s). Zone VIII is the area of the dorsal forearm just proximal to the extensor retinaculum and includes the musculotendinous junctions of the digit and wrist extensors. The immobilization and exercise regimen is essentially equal to the treatment for zones V and VI, with a slight modification: The wrist is placed within the orthosis at 40 to 45° of extension (Fig. 18–32).

Thumb Extensor Tendons

The extensor tendons in the thumb are divided into five zones (with odd numbers over the joints) (Fig. 18–27). The EPL inserts on the base of the distal phalanx of the thumb and is the only tendon that can *hyper*extend the IP joint. IP joint extension to neutral can occur through contributions to the dorsal hood from the intrinsic muscles, but not hyperextension. The EPL is also the only tendon that can perform retropulsion (the ability of the thumb to extend off of the table). Injury can occur either through laceration or rupture. Rupture can occur at the distal insertion or at the level of Lister's tubercle (such as after distal radius fracture). If this is the case, the patient will likely need a tendon transfer (e.g., EIP to EPL) because the ruptured tendon ends are often not in suitable condition for direct repair. After direct repair or tendon transfer, the thumb and wrist are positioned in extension to put slack on the repair. The EPB inserts on the base of the proximal phalanx and passes through the first dorsal compartment at the extensor retinaculum (along with the APL).

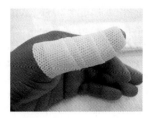

FIGURE 18–33 Thumb extensor tendon zone I injury with QuickCast 2 used to immobilize the IP joint (Patterson Medical).

Zone TI

This is a mallet type of injury to the EPL and is treated the same as zone I digit extensor tendon injuries. The IP joint of the thumb is held continuously in slight hyperextension for 6 to 8 weeks if there is no surgical repair. If the tendon was repaired, then active flexion can begin earlier, at week 5 or 6. In either situation, motion is initiated gradually, with the orthosis worn between exercises for an additional 2 weeks (Fig. 18–33)

Zone TII

Zone TII lies over the proximal phalanx and also involves the EPL tendon. The orthosis is hand based, with the MP and IP joints in extension and the thumb in radial abduction (Fig. 18–34). A short arc active mobilization protocol can be initiated at week 3 and gradually progressed weekly. The orthosis is discontinued by week 6 as long as there is no active extension lag.

Zones TIII and TIV

Zones TIII and TIV reside over the MCP joint and thumb metacarpal, respectively. The orthosis used is forearm based, with the wrist in 30° of extension and the thumb in radial abduction and MP/IP extended (Fig. 18–35A). There is little published information on rehabilitation in this zone. Injuries here can be treated with immobilization, early AROM, or with dynamic passive mobilization. As mentioned earlier, knowledge of flexor tendon healing and early mobilization can be applied to the thumb. Khandwala, Blairm, Harris, Foster, and Elliot (2004) and Elliot and Southgate (2005) found that EPL tendons treated with a dynamic passive mobilization orthosis had good to excellent results (Fig. 18–35B). However, both authors point out the promising results seen with early AROM in the

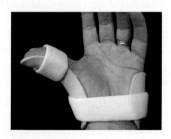

FIGURE 18–34 Hand-based thumb MP and IP immobilization orthosis for thumb extensor tendon zone II injury.

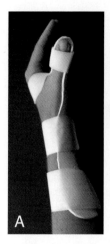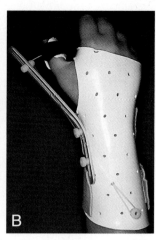

FIGURE 18–35 Options for managing thumb extensor tendon zones III to V repairs including **(A)** immobilization orthosis and **(B)** mobilization orthosis (Digitec Outrigger System shown, Patterson Medical).

finger extensors and advocate a move toward an early AROM protocol for the EPL (as opposed to passive mobilization via dynamic orthosis), which will require a less bulky orthosis.

Zone TV

Injuries in this zone involve the extensor retinaculum, which is synovial. This poses an increased threat to adhesion formation. If there is limited ability for the tendon to glide, changes in wrist position can affect the position of the thumb (Chinchalkar, Pipicelli, Laxamana, & von Dehn, 2010). Because of this increased risk, early AROM or PROM is recommended. It has been found that the EPL achieves the greatest amount of glide at the wrist when the wrist is positioned in 30° of extension when compared to other wrist positions (Chen, Tsubota, Aoki, Echigo, & Han, 2009).

The orthosis recommended places the wrist in 30° of extension, the MP at neutral, and the IP dynamically held in extension (allowing for up to 60° of active IP flexion) (Fig. 18–35B). In therapy, the orthosis is removed for passive tenodesis exercises (no more than 20° of wrist flexion) and place/hold exercises with the wrist in 20° of flexion and the thumb in radial abduction and MP/IP joints in extension. Graded increases in individual joint motion are initiated at weeks 3 to 4 and composite flexion is initiated at week 5. The orthosis is discontinued by week 6.

Extensor Tendon Protocols

Early Active Mobilization

There are multiple benefits to mobilizing a tendon early, such as decreased potential for joint contractures, tendon adhesion, decreased time in therapy, and earlier return to function. The rationale is that early stress to the tendons promotes healing both intrinsically and extrinsically. If feasible, this should be the protocol of choice for treatment of extensor tendon injuries in zones V to VII. There are also various early controlled active mobilization protocols that allow for active ROM within the limitations of the orthosis (Khandwala et al., 2000; Merritt, Howell, Tune, Saunders, & Hardy, 2000; Sylaidis et al., 1997). Early controlled AROM protocols require orthoses that are simpler and less expensive to fabricate than a mobilization orthosis; they are also less cumbersome for the patient to wear, which is likely to maximize compliance.

Immediate Controlled Active Motion

This protocol, also referred to as "relative motion splinting," was first described by Merritt et al. in 2000 and again by Howell et al. in 2005. This theory is based on the premise that positioning the injured tendon 15 to 20° proximally in relation to the uninvolved adjacent digits allows for the repaired tendon ends to approximate. Early motion can progress without placing stress on the repair as long as this relative motion is maintained. Biomechanical studies support this theory (Sharma, Liang, Owen, Wayne, & Isaacs, 2006), and 96% of patients in this study had excellent results (Howell et al., 2005). This regime can be used with both simple and complex repairs as long as there is one intact extensor tendon. Merritt et al. (2000) has also used this protocol with sagittal band ruptures.

This protocol requires two orthoses. A wrist immobilization orthosis is fabricated placing the wrist in 20° of extension. The distal palmar crease is cleared to allow for full MCP ROM. Then a separate **yoke orthosis** is fabricated that places the involved digit in 15 to 20° of extension relative to the adjacent digits (Fig. 18–36A,B) (Howell et al., 2005). If the index finger is lacerated, then the yoke also places the small finger in extension to create balance (and vice versa if it is the small finger that is lacerated). The following describes the phases of this protocol:

- **Phase 1 (days 0 to 21):** The patient is allowed full AROM within the confines of the orthoses (which are not to be removed by the patient).

- **Phase 2 (days 22 to 35):** The wrist orthosis is removed for wrist AROM and light activities, but the yoke stays on at all times.

- **Phase 3 (days 36 to 49):** The wrist orthosis is discontinued and the patient can remove the yoke for AROM exercises but continues to wear the yoke with ADLs.

The Norwich Regime

This protocol came out of the United Kingdom as a way to mobilize extensor tendons early without the bulk of a dynamic orthosis (Sylaidis et al., 1997). The orthosis includes the wrist placed in 45° of extension, the MCP joints flexed to 50°, and the IP joints in full extension.

During the first 4 weeks, the patient performs two exercises within the orthosis: full MCP/IP extension and full MCP extension with IP flexion. At 4 weeks, if there is no extension lag, the orthosis is discontinued and progressive flexion exercises are allowed. If there is a lag, then the orthosis is continued another 2 weeks. In this study, 92% of patients had good/excellent results (Sylaidis et al., 1997).

Khandwala et al. (2000) took the EAM premise of the Norwich regime and modified the orthosis to allow for synchronous motion at the MCP, PIP, and DIP joints. The orthosis includes the wrist in 30° of extension, the MCP joints at 45° of flexion, and the IP joints left free (Fig. 18–37A–C). During the first 3 weeks, the patient is allowed full AROM within the orthosis (extension to neutral only). At week 3, the MCP joints are flexed to 70° in the orthosis. The exercise regimen remains the same with full active extension, with the addition of a hook fist within the orthosis. The orthosis is discontinued by week 5. In this study, 93% of patients had good/excellent results, which was comparable to results experienced with patients in a dynamic orthosis group (Khandwala et al., 2000).

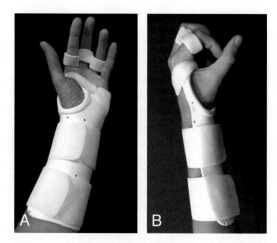

FIGURE 18–36 A and B, Yoke orthosis used in ICAM protocol. Two orthoses are fabricated: a yoke, which positions the injured finger in slight extension relative to the adjacent digits, and a wrist orthosis, which clears the distal palmar crease to allow for MCP flexion.

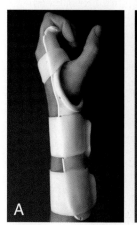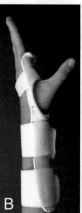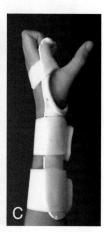

FIGURE 18–37 Early active motion, Khandwala protocol. A, MCP joints are placed in 45° of flexion; IPs are left free. **B,** Full AROM is allowed within the orthosis, and patient can actively extend MCP joints to neutral. **C,** At week 3, hook fist within the orthosis is added and the orthosis is modified to allow for 70° of MCP flexion.

Early Passive Mobilization

The use of dynamic orthoses for zone V and proximal is considered a passive mobilization protocol (although it is likely that there is some active extension occurring in the dynamic orthosis). The orthosis is molded dorsally with the wrist in 40° of extension. The outrigger (homemade or via commercially available kit) is attached dorsally, allowing for finger sling placement holding the MCP joints at neutral. The slings are attached to the outrigger with rubber bands or elastic thread (Fig. 18–38A). The MCP joints are allowed to flex to 30° (a mechanical block is placed on the outrigger to prevent further flexion). The elastic tension of the rubber bands then passively extends the MCP joints back to neutral. The IP joints can flex with the MCP joints held in neutral via the sling. After 3 weeks, progressively, more MCP flexion is allowed with full composite fist and orthosis discontinuation by week 6. The dynamic mobilization orthosis regimen works best with patients who can understand the precautions. The orthosis itself is time consuming and expensive to fabricate. It can also be bulky and cumbersome, making dressing and sleeping difficult. An extension immobilization orthosis for sleeping can be made, although insurance may not cover both orthoses (Fig. 18–38B). These are factors to consider when choosing a postoperative protocol.

Immediate Active Tension

The immediate active tension protocol as outlined by Evans (2011) includes a mobilization (dynamic) orthosis fabricated as described earlier (Fig. 18–38A). Gentle passive tenodesis exercises are performed (but not allowing more than 40° of MCP flexion with the wrist in full extension, and not allowing the wrist to flex more than 20°). This is followed by active place and hold exercises: performed with the wrist in 20° of flexion and MCP joints at

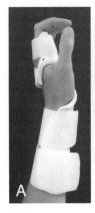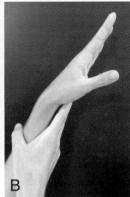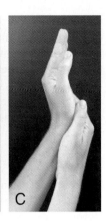

FIGURE 18–39 **A,** Immobilization orthosis used in zones V to VIII. Early phase exercise regimen performed with therapist: **B,** Active place/hold MCP extension with the wrist in 20° of flexion. Patient can also flex MCP joints to 30° and actively extend to neutral from this position. **C,** Wrist extension with MCP flexion to 40°.

neutral. Then, with the wrist still in 20° of flexion, the MCP joints are actively extended from 30° of flexion to neutral. These exercises are done under the supervision of the therapist in the clinic while the patient performs the PROM protocol (mentioned earlier) while at home. Progression of exercises is the same as in the dynamic protocol. Evans (2011) advocates using a dynamic orthosis with this protocol; however, this same tenodesis exercise progression can also be performed using a static orthosis between exercise sessions: The wrist is positioned in 30 to 45° of extension, MCP joints flexed to 20°, and the IP joints free. Active place and hold tenodesis exercises are performed in a protected range as mentioned earlier (Fig. 18–39A–C) (Gallagher, 2006a).

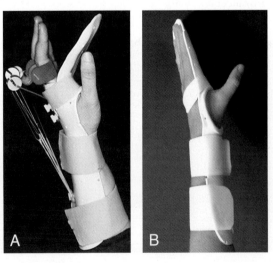

FIGURE 18–38 **A,** A dynamic MCP extension mobilization/flexion restriction orthosis used for an EPM program for zones V to VII extensor tendon repair (Phoenix Outrigger System shown, Patterson Medical). **B,** A wrist/hand extension immobilization orthosis is worn during rest to complement an EPM program for zones V to VII extensor tendon repair.

Conclusion

Rehabilitation to flexor and extensor tendon injuries has come a long way in the past 70 years. Research and experience have shown that early mobilization tends to result in better functional outcomes for the patient. However, tendon adhesions and joint stiffness continue to be issues faced by physicians and therapists. Further research in this area is recommended, particularly in concern to rehabilitation of the tendons of the thumb where research is scant. The general trend has been toward early ROM, either passive or active, and toward orthoses that are less bulky and less complicated, which not only saves time and money but also increases patient compliance with the postoperative protocol. Tendons can be interesting and exciting to treat; however, choosing an appropriate treatment protocol and accompanying orthosis requires good communication among the treating team and sound clinical judgment skills.

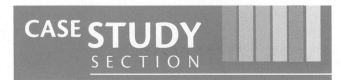

CASE STUDY 1: Flexor Digitorum Profundus Avulsion

JF is a 56-year-old lawyer who ruptured his left middle finger FDP tendon when his hand became caught in someone else's shirt while dancing at a wedding. He was seen preoperatively for orthosis fabrication and instruction on what to expect postoperatively. He had a lot of anxiety about his injury and the surgeon wanted him placed in a protected position to prevent retraction of the tendon. A wrist and hand extension restriction orthosis was fabricated for him with his wrist in 10° of flexion, his MCP joints in 70° of flexion, and his IP joints straight (Fig. 18–7A). He wore this until surgery. Surgically, his FDP was reattached to the distal phalanx with a pull-through suture to a button on his nail (Fig. 18–14). He had also suffered a middle phalanx fracture that was treated with screw fixation. He brought his orthosis with him to his first postoperative visit at day 3, when his dressing was removed. The physician felt that the fracture was stable enough and the tendon repair strong enough to participate in an EAM program. He was started on an HEP of passive digital flexion and active extension to the roof of the orthosis (Fig. 18–9A,B). Gentle passive tenodesis was performed in the clinic, but because his finger was edematous and stiff combined with his anxiety level, it was decided to wait until his next visit before initiating place and hold tenodesis exercises.

At his next visit (postoperative day 5), his HEP was reviewed. He demonstrated almost full passive flexion, so it was decided to add gentle composite fist place and hold tenodesis to his home program (10 repetitions, five times per day) (Fig. 18–12A,B). He was followed three times per week for edema control, wound care/scar management, and upgrade of home program. At 2 weeks postoperatively, place/hold hook fist was initiated to increase glide of the FDP tendon and place/hold straight fist to maximize FDS glide (Fig. 18–12C, D). He also was developing a PIP flexion contracture, so at 2.5 weeks, a finger immobilization orthosis was fabricated for him to wear at night within his dorsal block orthosis.

JF continued to make nice progress and was able to maintain the place/hold composite, hook, and straight fists. It was decided to continue him on his current home program until 4 weeks postoperatively when active tendon glide exercises were introduced as well as active tenodesis. His PIP flexion at that point was 90° and DIP flexion was 3°. At 5 weeks, his DIP flexion remained the same, so gentle blocking exercises were introduced.

At 6 weeks, his button was removed and the dorsal block orthosis was discontinued except when in crowds (on the subway, while out jogging, etc.). Light functional tasks were introduced in the clinic. Because he still had a slight PIP flexion contracture, his finger immobilization orthosis was continued at night. It was felt that the PIP contracture was likely caused by soft tissue tightness around the PIP joint and not caused by extrinsic flexor tightness. He continued to make gains in PIP/DIP flexion, so resistive exercises were not begun until 8 weeks postoperatively. JF continued in therapy until 12 weeks postoperatively. Final ROM measurements taken are the following: PIP, 10/100; DIP, 0/50. At that point, he was discharged from therapy.

Additional case studies can be found on the companion web site on thePoint.

Chapter Review Questions

1. Name the two digit flexor tendons and describe their path from origin to insertion.

2. What is the most common orthosis used for flexor tendon rehabilitation and how can this be altered to address a developing PIP flexion contracture?

3. How can scar management be integrated into an orthosis used to protect a tendon repair?

4. What are the theories behind early passive mobilization (EPM) and early active mobilization (EAM) in flexor and extensor tendon repair management?

5. Describe the various orthoses that may be used to address a mallet finger or injury in zone I.

Peripheral Nerves Injuries

MaryLynn Jacobs, MS, OTR/L, CHT

Chapter Objectives

After study of this chapter, the reader should be able to:

- Appreciate the motor, sensory, and vasomotor pathways as well as the healing and regeneration principles of a peripheral nerve.
- Be able to identify the deficiencies of the three main peripheral nerves to the hand: **radial**, **ulnar**, and **median nerves**.
- Appreciate the various degrees of injury associated with traumatic and compressive nerve insults.
- Determine the appropriate therapeutic and orthotic intervention for each nerve injury.
- Understand the popular surgical techniques and the various types of peripheral nerve repairs.
- Appreciate the role of **nerve grafts**, conduits, and **nerve transfers** in this patient population.
- Describe the common tendon transfers and orthotic management to replace lost function for each of the peripheral nerves.

Key Terms

Anterior interosseous nerve syndrome	Froment's sign	Pronator syndrome
Ape hand deformity	Guyon's canal	Radial nerve
Axonotmesis	Jeanne's sign	Radial tunnel syndrome
Carpal tunnel syndrome	Median nerve	Resistant tennis elbow
Claw hand deformity	Multiple-crush syndrome	Saturday night palsy
Cubital tunnel syndrome	Nerve grafts	Second-degree injury
Double-crush syndrome	Nerve laceration	Sixth-degree injury
Elbow flexion test	Nerve transfers	Third-degree injuries
End-to-end repairs	Neurapraxia	Tinel's sign
End-to-side repairs	Neurotmesis	Ulnar nerve
Epineurial repair	Peace sign deformity	Wallerian degeneration
Fifth-degree injuries	Peripheral nerve injury	Wartenberg's sign
First-degree injury	Phalen's test	Wartenberg's syndrome
Fourth-degree injury	Posterior interosseous nerve syndrome	Wrist drop

The need for corrective splintage in peripheral nerve injuries has been recognized for a long time, but only recently has it been appreciated that a good splint should do more than merely prevent deformity, it should also encourage function.

—WYNN PARRY, 1981

Introduction

Orthotic intervention for **peripheral nerve injury (PNI)** is challenging, thought provoking, and always specific to the individual. This chapter describes orthotic management for deficiencies of the three main peripheral nerves: median, ulnar, and radial. **Nerve lacerations**, common mixed lesions, compression neuropathies, lesions associated with other injuries, and tendon transfers are addressed. A table is provided to aid the therapist in nerve injury identification and appropriate selection of orthoses.

Assessment of the nerve-injured hand requires sound knowledge of nerve healing, functional anatomy, physiology, and kinesiology as well as a thorough understanding of motor, sensory, and vasomotor pathways. With this information, the therapist can recognize abnormalities and determine the appropriate therapeutic and orthotic intervention. The therapist must appreciate (1) the type and degree of motor and sensory loss, (2) the importance of cortical reintegration, (3) protection of the healing nerve, (4) prevention of deformity, (5) education of adaptive techniques, (6) the role of exercise, and (7) continual reassessment of nerve return to achieve the best functional results for the patient (Fig. 19–1).

Advances in nerve repair have allowed surgeons to employ the peripheral nerve's regenerative capabilities and apply these to creative techniques for nerve reconstruction. This has opened the door for the therapist to participate in pioneering complimentary orthotic management and rehabilitation protocols.

Definition

PNIs commonly seen by a therapist are either traumatic in nature or as a result of an entrapment or a compression neuropathy. Most traumatic injuries occur in association with other injuries, such as fractures or tendon lacerations. Compression neuropathies usually occur in specific anatomic areas where the nerve is vulnerable as it passes through a soft tissue restraint, such as the median nerve as it traverses beneath the transverse carpal ligament in carpal tunnel syndrome (American Society for Surgery of the Hand [ASSH], 1995; Diao, 2011; R. G. Eaton, 1992; Mackinnon, 1992; Thomas, Yakin, Parry, & Lubahn, 2000). Compression neuropathies are typically chronic in nature because they are a result of prolonged compression to the nerve. Acute compression neuropathies are associated with traumatic events, such as in compartment syndrome or with a direct hit or blow to the nerve (Elfar et al., 2010). A nerve can also be entrapped at more than one site along the nerve's pathway, resulting in a **double-crush** or **multiple-crush syndrome** and/or phenomenon (Bindra & Johnson, 2011; Jacoby, Eichenbaum, & Osterman, 2011; Mackinnon, 1992). Nerves are vulnerable to injury as they slide, glide, pass, and/or rub over or between soft tissue structures and bony prominences (e.g., ulnar nerve at the cubital tunnel, radial nerve as it traverses through the soft tissue structures of the forearm) (Topp &

Boyd, 2012). Neuropathies can occur secondary to repetitive use/cumulative trauma, endocrine disorders (e.g., diabetes or hypothyroidism), renal failure, hormonal changes (e.g., pregnancy or menopause), electrical injury, traction, ischemia, rheumatoid arthritis, Guillain-Barré syndrome, myasthenia gravis, amyotrophic lateral sclerosis, sarcoidosis, or tumors/soft tissue masses (Cameron & Klein, 2010; Dellon, 1992; Diao, 2011; K. L. Smith, 1995, 2011).

A nerve injury produces changes within the nerve itself and in the tissues that it innervates. Symptoms of nerve injury include weakness or paralysis of the muscles innervated

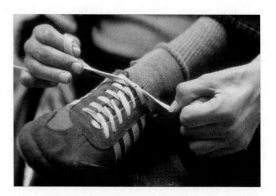

FIGURE 19–1 Although nerve injuries are devastating, many patients can learn adaptive methods for functioning independently. Note the ulnar nerve atrophy of the left thumb dorsal web space.

by the motor branches of that particular nerve and sensory loss to areas innervated by the sensory branches of the injured nerve. Early symptoms of compression neuropathy may be vague but usually include some combination of pain, tingling, numbness, and weakness. Pain may be sharp and burning with accompanying paresthesias over the corresponding dermatome or sensory distribution. These signs may occur proximal and/or distal to the site(s) of compression (Bell-Krotoski, 2004; Mackinnon, 1992; Slutsky, 2005a, 2011; K. L. Smith, 1995). Applying an orthosis that positions the limb in such a way that tension or compression stress is decreased on the nerve may relieve some, or all, of the nerve symptoms (Topp & Boyd, 2012; Walsh, 2012).

The reader should keep the following points in mind while progressing through this chapter:

- Atrophy begins immediately.
- The more proximal the diagnosis, the worse the prognosis.
- The more severe the injury, the worse the prognosis.
- A more favorable prognosis is associated with early repair.
- Sensation can return up to 3 years postinjury.
- Peripheral nerves have excellent regeneration potential.
- Complete functional recovery is rarely attained in an adult.
- Nerve transfer should be undertaken as soon as it is determined that spontaneous recovery, primary repair, or grafting will be of little benefit.

Nerve Anatomy

The nervous system is made up of two parts: the peripheral nervous system (PNS) and the central nervous system (CNS). The PNS consists of the spinal and cranial nerves, and the CNS incorporates the brain and spinal cord (Carpenter, 1978). The PNS serves as the mediator (or transporter) of neural impulses traveling between the sensory receptors, muscles, and CNS. A bundle of axons (nerve fibers) in the PNS is called a nerve, and a network of nerves is referred to as a nerve plexus. A collection of nerves outside the cell bodies is a ganglion. Peripheral nerve fibers are made of an axon, myelin sheath, and neurolemma or sheath of Schwann cells. After a nerve has been injured, the changes that happen to the nerve are collectively termed Wallerian degeneration (Bindra & Johnson, 2011; Boscheinen-Morrin, Davey, & Conolly, 1985; Carpenter, 1978; Elfar et al., 2010; Mackinnon, 1994; Parry, 1981; K. L. Smith, 1995, 2011; Walsh, 2012).

Figure 19–2 shows the anatomy of a nerve cell and its pathway to the target organ. A peripheral nerve is surrounded by three layers of connective tissue that offer strength and protection to the nerve itself (Elfar et al., 2010). The layers are the epineurium, a sheath that encompasses the entire nerve; the perineurium, which encloses a small bundle (fasciculus) of nerve fibers and forms a more fragile connective tissue sheath

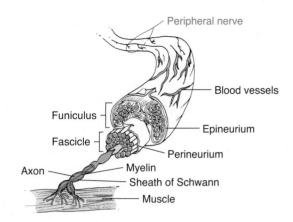

FIGURE 19–2 Anatomy of a nerve cell and its pathway to the target organ.

than the epineurium; and the endoneurium, a thin connective tissue sheath that surrounds the individual nerve fibers (Bindra & Johnson, 2011; Boscheinen-Morrin et al., 1985).

Figure 19–3 illustrates nerve injury and regeneration (Boscheinen-Morrin et al., 1985). After any significant neural insult, degeneration of the axon and myelin sheath occurs distal to the injury site. Degeneration also occurs proximal to the injury and to the previous node of Ranvier (constrictions of the myelin sheath). During this process of Wallerian degeneration, the axon atrophies, but the connective tissue sheath remains open to accept regenerating axonal fibers. In general, axons grow approximately 1 to 2 mm per day or, in an adult, 1 cm per month. If there is no axonal activity soon after injury or if axons never make contact with a motor end organ, muscle atrophy will occur with irreversible loss by 24 months (Slutsky, 2011). This may account for poor motor outcomes in above elbow injuries, especially in the adult (Slutsky, 2005a, 2011; Terzis, 1991). In contrast to motor end plates, the sensory end organs remain preserved after denervation (Elfar et al., 2010). The potential for reinnervation of a sensory nerve is therefore more optimistic by comparison, providing protective sensation even several years after insult (Elfar et al., 2010; Slutsky, 2011).

Different types of nerve lesions result in different prognoses; therefore, it is important to appreciate the effect and extent that each type of nerve injury may have on its

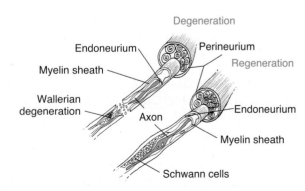

FIGURE 19–3 Nerve degeneration and regeneration.

respective nerve cell, axon, and target organ. This information is also important for assessing nerve regeneration, applying appropriate orthoses and therapy intervention, and timely orthotic modifications. The more proximal the injury, the worse the prognosis is, possibly because there is a greater distance from the site of insult to the target organ (Lundborg, 1988; Lundborg & Rosen, 2004; Moore & Agur, 1995). By the time the regenerated axon reaches the end organ, significant muscular atrophy may have occurred. Regenerated axons may not always find their end organs (Bathen & Gupta, 2011; K. L. Smith, 2011). For example, a sensory axon may reach a motor plate or vice versa. Age can be a significant factor in potential nerve recovery. In general, young children have a better functional result than adults. This may be due to the shorter distances axons have to grow (smaller, shorter limbs) to reach their target organ and for the great capacity young brains have to integrate centrally and reorganize incoming information (Bindra & Johnson, 2011; Elfar et al., 2010; Parry, 1981). Cortical plasticity and its importance to nerve recovery gained increased attention, particularly with sensory relearning techniques (Anastakis, Chen, Davis, & Mikulis, 2005, 2008; Duff, 2005; Novak, 2011; Walsh, 2012). Proximal injury in adults may require that functional or antideformity orthoses be worn for extended periods of time.

A crush or compression injury may cause damage to the axon but can leave the connective tissue layers of the nerve intact, maintaining a conduit to guide the growing axons to their ultimate destinations. However, when a nerve is severed, the part distal to the injury degenerates, and only careful surgical anastomosis will provide a chance of functional recovery (Elfar et al., 2010; Lundborg, 1988; Mackinnon, 1994, 1997; Moore & Agur, 1995). Some of these surgical options are reviewed later in this chapter.

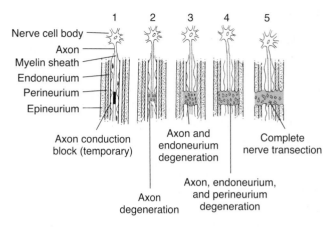

FIGURE 19–4 Sunderland's five degrees of nerve injury: (1) conduction block; (2) axonal degeneration; (3) axonal and endoneurial degeneration; (4) axonal, endoneurial, and perineurial degeneration; and (5) complete nerve transection.

Nerve Injury Classification

Seddon (1943) was the first to classify nerve injuries (K. L. Smith, 1995), using the terms **neurapraxia**, **axonotmesis**, and **neurotmesis**. In 1951, Sunderland (1952) expanded this classification to five more precise degrees of injury (Fig. 19–4) (Horn & Crumley, 1984; K. L. Smith, 1995). Mackinnon (1994) identified a sixth lesion, a mixed injury that includes normal fascicles with some or all of Sunderland's five degrees (Bathen & Gupta, 2011). Regardless which classification the reader chooses to reference, the most important part of these classifications is the prognosis. Table 19–1 summarizes and compares the Seddon and Sunderland classifications.

TABLE 19–1

Comparison of Sunderland and Seddon Classification of Nerve Injuries

Author	Descriptive Term	Nature of Injury/Neuropathology
Sunderland Seddon	First-degree injury Neurapraxia	Demyelinating injury with a temporary conduction block
Sunderland Seddon	Second-degree injury Axonotmesis	Distal degeneration of the injured axon but with almost always complete regeneration due to intact endoneurium
Sunderland Seddon	Third-degree injury Neurotmesis	Sunderlands third-degree injury is less severe than the neurotmesis category of Seddon since the perineurial layer is intact. Regeneration occurs but is incomplete due to endoneurial scarring and loss of end-organ specificity within the fascicle
Sunderland	Fourth-degree injury	Axon, endoneurium, perineurium are disrupted with extensive scarring that blocks axonal regeneration and often results in a neuroma in continuity.
Sunderland	Fifth-degree injury	Severed nerve trunk without possibility of spontaneous regeneration.

Doyle, J. R. (2006). *Hand and wrist.* Philadelphia, PA; Lippincott Williams & Wilkins.

First-Degree Injury (Neurapraxia)

First-degree injury involves a localized area of conduction block, which is reversible. Recovery is quick, usually complete motor and sensory function within 12 to 16 weeks. The mechanism of injury is commonly acute compression and local ischemia (Elfar et al., 2010). Wallerian degeneration does not occur in neurapraxic lesions because the perineurium is left intact.

Second-Degree Injury (Axonotmesis)

In the **second-degree injury**, damage to the axon occurs, and regeneration of the nerve proceeds at the standard rate of approximately 1 mm per day or 1″ per month. An advancing **Tinel's sign** is present. The Tinel's sign is a common technique used to assess nerve regeneration; a gentle tapping is performed along the nerve's pathway, distal to proximal (although many therapists perform this proximal to distal), which, when performed carefully, should elicit paresthesias into innervated tissue (Allan & Vanderhooft, 2005; Bell-Krotoski, 2004; Diao, 2011; Lundborg, 1988; Mackinnon, 1994; Parry, 1981). The recovery rate for second-degree injuries is slow; yet, complete return of function can be expected. If the injury occurs proximal to the distal target, the time required to reach the end organ makes the recovery pattern slower than normal (Lundborg, 1988).

Third-Degree Injury (Axonotmesis or Neurotmesis)

Third-degree injuries have the most unpredictable degree of recovery, which ranges from almost normal to no recovery at all. With this type of injury, there is some scarring within the endoneurium, making it difficult for the axon to reach the appropriate receptor. The lesion may be iatrogenic in nature, occurring when a patient sustains a nerve injury during a surgical procedure. These injuries recover slowly, and patients eventually achieve some, but usually not all, function.

Fourth-Degree Injury (Neurotmesis)

In a **fourth-degree injury**, a segment of the nerve is completely blocked by scar. The nerve is in continuity but only because of the fibrous bond. The internal structure of the nerve is severely damaged. There is no function or nerve conduction through the fibrous block of scar. Surgical repair or grafting is most often recommended.

Fifth-Degree Injury (Neurotmesis)

In **fifth-degree injuries**, the nerve is completely severed. The patient must undergo surgical intervention, which may include direct repair or a nerve graft, depending on the size of the deficit. Functional recovery depends on factors such as the time since injury and/or repair, wound status, patient's age, surgeon's skill, and the degree of tension on the repair.

Sixth-Degree Injury (Mixed Injury or Neuroma in Continuity)

The **sixth-degree injury** is a mixed lesion that includes some normal fascicles in combination with all or any of Sunderland's five degrees of injury (Bathen & Gupta, 2011; Mackinnon, 1994). This lesion includes several patterns of injury from fascicle to fascicle. The variation in injury can also be seen along the length of the nerve. Complicated upper extremity lesions are often the result of devastating injuries such as gunshot wounds, traumatic crushing, and traction injuries, or they can occur from a combination of the previously stated mechanisms. Surgical intervention may include a combination of procedures such as neurolysis, nerve graft, and/or direct repair. Mixed lesions are challenging injuries for the surgeon to treat and the therapist to rehabilitate, owing to the variability of injury, repair, and recovery.

Nerve Reconstruction

Prior to treating a nerve-repaired structure, the clinician must have knowledge of the exact reconstruction performed. Questions presented in Box 19–1 are only some of the questions that a clinician should consider when referred a patient with a postoperative nerve repair. Close communication with the surgeon is paramount.

Introduction of Nerve Reconstruction

It is not the intent of this chapter to discuss the vast options and advances in surgical procedures because there are many detailed resources available. Rather, this chapter is meant to provide the clinician with a basic foundation and familiarity with terms related to PNI and surgery in order to fully appreciate the selection and application of appropriate

BOX 19–1

Questions the Clinician Should Ask

1. What type of repair/reconstruction was done (epineurial, perineurial, end-to-end, end-to-side)?
2. Was there tension on the nerve repair?
3. How much of the nerve was injured and/or repaired?
4. Was the injury/repair to a motor, sensory, or combined nerve?
5. Was the repair primary or via nerve graft, conduit, or transfer?
6. If a donor nerve was used, what is the expected deficit from the donor site (sensory, motor)?
7. When orthotic protection/positioning is prescribed, what are the exact joint positions desired?
8. What are the parameters for immobilization, mobilization, and/or restriction of the repaired structure?

orthotic intervention. The clinician will find short descriptors of the most common procedures for quick reference and are encouraged to seek further study in this exploding area of nerve repair and reconstruction. The definitions listed in the following text highlight common definitions the therapist will encounter in the realm of peripheral nerve surgery.

Definitions Related to Peripheral Nerve Repair

- Primary repair is typically done within 48 hours (K. L. Smith, 2011) and does not involve the use of grafting or other supplemental techniques.
- Early secondary repairs are performed within the first 6 weeks.
- Late secondary repairs are done after 3 months (K. L. Smith, 2011).
- **Epineurial repair** is a quick, simple, and most common technique used to repair a completely transected nerve. The outer epineurium is debrided proximal and distal from the nerve stumps until all signs of damage are removed. The nerve stumps are then realigned, and sutures are placed in the epineurium to secure closure (K. L. Smith, 2011). The goal is to establish continuity of the nerve with minimal tension (Elfar et al., 2010) (Fig. 19–5).
- **Perineurial repair** (group fascicular repair) is the second most common peripheral nerve repair technique. In this repair, the outer and inner epineurium are dissected away from the nerve stumps. The fascicles are then matched and aligned using the least amount of suture to close. An advantage of this repair is the matching of similar fascicles (motor and sensory), but the disadvantage can be the risk of intraneural fibrosis secondary to the increased use of suture and the overall surgical handling (Elfar et al., 2010; K. L. Smith, 2011).
- **End-to-end repairs** are direct clean nerve ends sutured together.
- **End-to-side repairs** have been described mainly for sensory reconstruction. The proximal stump of a nerve is sutured into the side of a distal receptor. It is an alternative in cases that the distal nerve stump is not accessible or retrievable.
- **Fibrin glue** can be used with epineurial repairs in order to reduce suture materials and adequately seal the repair site. The role of fibrin glue in peripheral nerve repair is becoming more popular due to the ease of application versus microsuture (Sameem, Wood, & Bain, 2011).
- Neurotization is the implantation of a nerve into a paralyzed muscle.
- **Neurorrhaphy** is the suturing of a divided nerve.
- Nerve grafting is used to bridge a deficit in a nerve using a donor graft. A nerve graft can be nonvascularized (a conventional graft) or vascularized. A vascularized graft is either pedicled or free flaps (Slutsky, 2005a; Terzis & Kostopoulos, 2005).

- **Nerve conduits** are also used to bridge nerve gaps. The conduits can be of biologic or nonbiologic origin (Herman, 2005).
- **Neurosensory flaps** are innervated flaps that provide sensory feedback. These flaps can be either pedicled or free flaps (Slutsky, 2005b).

Nerve Healing

After insult, a peripheral nerve can regenerate spontaneously, but this requires both axon regrowth and remyelination by Schwann cells. Without surgical intervention, healing naturally may lead to poor results such as (1) a mismatch when the end organ is attempting to innervate a receptor, (2) the axon may lose its continuity, and (3) the end organ may have too long a distance to travel, therefore becoming degenerated by the time it reaches the end target (Bathen & Gupta, 2011). Other factors that influence healing are patient's age, the length of time since injury, level of injury, the quality of surrounding tissues, and the amount of scar formation about the injured area (K. L. Smith, 2011).

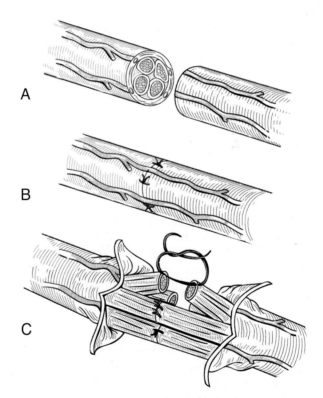

FIGURE 19–5 A, Schematic representation of a traumatic nerve laceration. **B,** A traditional epineurial repair done to establish proper alignment while minimizing tension. **C,** A group fascicular repair is often advantageous over epineurial repair if the sensory and motor group fascicles are in near alignment to their corresponding sensory and motor group fascicles in the distal stump. Borrowed with permission from Elfar, J., Petrungaro, J. M., Braun, R. M., et al. (2010). Nerve. In W. C. Hammert, R. P. Calfee, D. J. Bozentka, & M. I. Boyer (Eds.), *ASSH manual of hand surgery* (p. 332). Baltimore, MD: Lippincott Williams & Wilkins.

Nerve Grafting

A nerve graft provides a regenerating axon with a protective pathway to the distal stump (Slutsky, 2005b). The nonvascularized nerve graft is considered to be the treatment of choice in reconstructing nerve gaps. The grafting procedure normally takes place approximately 3 weeks after injury using a suitable, accessible donor (Elfar et al., 2010). Vascularized nerve grafts have been shown to work well in areas of a scarred recipient bed when there is poor or scant vascularization or when a traditional nerve graft has been unsuccessful (Elfar, 2010; Terzis & Kostopoulos, 2005). The patient should be accepting of the choice of donor nerve. Some of the more commonly used nerves are the anterior and posterior interosseous nerves (PINs), the medial and lateral cutaneous nerves, and the sural nerve from the lower extremity (Elfar et al., 2010; Slutsky, 2005a). The length of the donor nerve needs to be long enough to allow a tension-free repair. This is a critical question the clinician must ask when applying an orthosis to these patients.

Nerve Conduits

A nerve conduit can act as a guide, connecting the neural gap in order to contain, align, and direct the regenerating axons (Taras, Nanavati, & Steelman, 2005). A nerve conduit is made of either an autogenous material (i.e., vein) or a synthetic material (i.e., collagen) that is placed between the nerve ends, incorporating the end stumps into the conduit. Soon after the nerve ends are placed into the conduit, a serous fluid begins the process of creating a platform for regeneration (Elfar et al., 2010). Tension on the repair site is not a factor in regards to initiation of early rehabilitation; therefore, early active motion can commence soon after repair, incorporating appropriate orthotic management; protective, guarded motion; and motor and/sensory reeducation principles (Slutsky, 2011). Orthosis positioning should include a degree of flexion if the nerve repair is volar and extension if the repair is dorsal (Taras et al., 2005). Extension restriction and flexion restriction orthoses are excellent choices for this patient population. Restriction orthoses do not completely block motion; instead, they allow a protected arc of motion that will assist in prevention of adhesion formation and facilitate gentle nerve and tendon glide. A digital nerve repair that is tensionless will most often not require orthosis management (Taras et al., 2005). Most orthotic intervention is discontinued between 4 and 6 weeks.

Nerve Transfers

Recent developments in peripheral nerve reconstruction introduced nerve transfer to the upper extremity. In injuries where primary nerve reconstruction or grafting is not possible or where the outcome is expected to be poor, the surgeon may consider nerve transfer. Nerve transfers can restore at least some degree of motor or sensory function (Slutsky, 2011). A donor nerve is required; therefore, thoughtful discussion with the patient is important to consider how the loss of the donor would impact function. The patient must clearly understand the deficit left by the harvesting of the donor, the purpose of the transfer, and the intended outcome. The therapist is well versed in functional (motor and sensory) anatomy and can be of great help to the patient and family through this decision-making process.

A therapist may see such transfers in patients with a brachial plexus lesion, a high ulnar nerve injury or traumatic injury to several of the peripheral nerves of the same extremity such as seen in a gunshot wound (Elfar, 2010). Protective orthotic intervention, motor reeducation, sensory retraining, and ongoing patient education are a large part of postoperative management.

Motor Transfers

The best donor for a motor transfer is a pure motor nerve. This muscle should be of adequate strength (grade 4) being able to work against gravity, ideally with light resistance (Elfar, 2010). Orthotic management is based on close communication with the surgeon because the surgeon has firsthand knowledge of the quality of the tissue transferred and the amount of tension desired for that transfer. Orthotic management may consist of weekly adjustments as the tissue heals and motor innervation commences.

Examples of common motor donors that a clinician may see (Elfar, 2010) are as follows:

- Elbow flexion
  - Intercostal nerve or partial ulnar nerve transfer to biceps branch of musculocutaneous nerve
- Shoulder abduction/flexion
  - Spinal accessory nerve transfer to suprascapular nerve
  - Posterior triceps branch of radial nerve to axillary nerve
- Hand intrinsic function
  - Anterior interosseous nerve (AIN) to motor branch of ulnar nerve or recurrent branch of median nerve

Sensory Nerve Transfers

Most devastating to functional use of the hand, besides loss of motor innervation, is sensory loss. When there is sensory loss to the volar aspect of the hand, radial border of the index finger (IF), ulnar border of the thumb, and ulnar border of the hand, sensory nerve transfer should be considered (Elfar et al., 2010; Slutsky, 2011). These can restore, at best, protective sensation (Elfar et al., 2010). The sensory nerve end organs remain viable for longer periods of time than do those of a motor nerve, making sensory nerve transfer less common than a motor nerve transfer. In a patient that has sustained a severe nerve injury, the therapist may commonly see a sensory nerve transfer performed at the same time as a motor transfer. An example would be a patient with a high ulnar nerve injury losing intrinsic function and sensation to the ulnar innervated digits as seen in Figure 19–1. Orthotic management is similar to that described for a motor transfer.

Examples of common sensory nerve donors that a clinician may see (Elfar, 2010) are as follows:

- Radial sensory nerve transfer to ulnar aspect of the thumb and/or radial aspect of IF
- Ulnar digital nerve of IF to radial aspect of IF
- Ulnar digital nerve of long finger to ulnar aspect of small finger (SF)
- Palmar cutaneous branch of median nerve to ulnar sensory branch of ring and SF

Nerve Innervations and Pathology

The extent of functional loss from a nerve injury depends on where along the nerve's pathway it has been injured. In this chapter, the author will discuss injuries that affect the forearm, wrist, and hand.

Lesions and/or lacerations are generally referred to as high (injury proximal to the elbow) or low (injury near or distal to the elbow joint). Figures throughout this chapter detail the specific muscles an individual nerve innervates and at what level/order the innervation generally occurs. There can be variations in nerve innervations that can be functionally significant. Clinicians should be aware of these possible connections and how they may complicate the clinical presentation (Bas & Klienert, 1999). The two most common examples are the links between the median and ulnar nerves in the proximal forearm and the hand (Figs. 19–6 and 19–7).

- **Martin–Gruber Connection.** This association is seen when a portion of the median nerve communicates with the ulnar nerve in the proximal one-third of the forearm. There are many variants of Martin–Gruber connections that have been identified. Several are noted in Figures 19–6 and 19–7 (Elfar et al., 2010). These connections are generally proximal to the AIN branch or distal within the flexor digitorum profundus

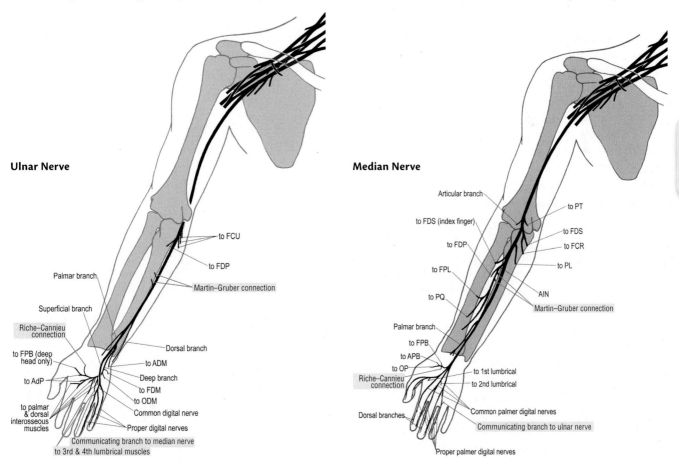

FIGURE 19–6 AND FIGURE 19–7 Schematic representation of the ulnar nerve and median nerves with their common connections to each other.
Of these variant connections, the most common are those between either the median and ulnar nerve or, the anterior interosseous nerve and ulnar nerve. When these variant connections are present, a complete lesion of the involved nerve (median or ulnar) may not cause full motor or sensory loss because of the "additional" communication from the neighboring nerve.

(FDP) muscle occurring in approximately 10% to 25% of the population (Gellman & Owens, 2011; Leversedge, Goldfarb, & Boyer, 2010; Toby & Ritter, 2011). This connection may contain a mix of fibers from the median nerve or AIN or just motor fibers or just sensory fibers. When this anastomosis is present, a complete lesion of the median nerve may not cause paralysis or sensory loss in all the median nerve–innervated muscles because some of the muscles may be receiving innervation from the ulnar nerve. This puzzling presentation, which can exist at various levels, may make the therapist question whether the nerve has been completely severed (Leversedge et al., 2010; Matloub & Yousif, 1992; Moore & Agur, 1995).

- **Riche–Cannieu Connection** (refer to Figs. 19–6 and 19–7). This is a connection between the recurrent branch of the median nerve and the deep branch of the ulnar nerve in the volar hand offering, ulnar nerve innervation to the intrinsic thenar muscles (Elfar et al., 2010). This occurs in approximately 50% to 77% of the population (Gellman & Owens, 2011; Leversedge et al., 2010). Variations in this anastomosis have been observed, but the most common effect seen by a clinician would be ulnar innervation to intrinsic thenar muscles such as the body of the flexor pollicis brevis (FPB). Other variations include the thenar common digital nerve connecting to the deep ulnar nerve and connections appearing deep within the abductor pollicis brevis or in the first lumbricals (Elfar et al., 2010). When this anomalous interconnection is present, clinicians will note that full or near full thumb motion will be preserved.

Peripheral Nerve Pathology

The following section will describe the pathology associated with each of these peripheral nerves, further divided into sections for high lacerations, low lacerations, and compressive neuropathies.

Median Nerve Injuries

Laceration to the Median Nerve

HIGH LACERATION

High median nerve injury is often associated with traumatic injury of the upper extremity, which may include several neurovascular structures (Fig. 19–8). Clinical signs of isolated high median nerve injury are a loss of the following:

- Forearm pronation
- Wrist radial flexion
- Independent proximal interphalangeal (PIP) joint flexion from the IF through the SF
- IF and middle finger (MF) distal interphalangeal (DIP) and metacarpophalangeal (MCP) joint flexion

BOX 19–2

Order of Innervation for Median Nerve

1. Pronator teres
2. Flexor carpi radialis
3. Palmaris longus
4. Flexor digitorum superficialis
5. Radial half of flexor digitorum profundus
6. Flexor pollicis longus
7. Pronator quadratus
8. First lumbrical
9. Second lumbrical
10. Abductor pollicis brevis
11. Flexor pollicis brevis
12. Opponens pollicis

- Thumb interphalangeal (IP) flexion, opposition, and palmar abduction
- Thumb MP flexion weakness caused by the partial innervation of the FPB radial head
- Sensation to the volar radial aspect of the hand

The hand will posture in a **peace sign deformity**–like position (Fig. 19–9). This devastating injury robs the hand of normal function. Rehabilitation should involve preservation of joint range of motion (ROM), education on sensory

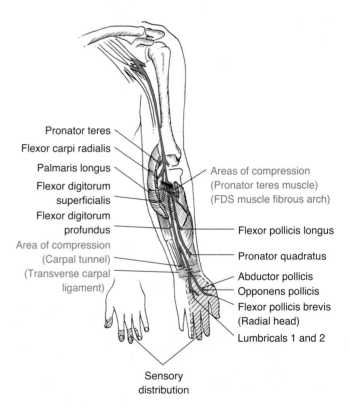

FIGURE 19–8 The motor portion of the median nerve innervates most of the wrist and digital flexors. The sensory distribution of the median nerve plays an integral role in providing sensation to the volar radial aspect of the hand.

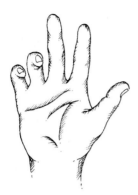

FIGURE 19–9 A high median nerve laceration causes a peace sign posturing of the hand, owing to the loss of the FDP, FDS, and intrinsics of the IF and MF.

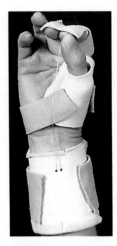

FIGURE 19–10 A wrist and IF/MF finger extension restriction orthosis. This tenodesis orthosis employs power from the radial nerve to allow light functional pinch of the IF and MF to the thumb.

precautions, and careful orthotic intervention to maximize function and prevent deformity (Fig. 19–10).

LOW LACERATION

Low median nerve injury, at the level of the wrist, may be associated with flexor tendon injury. Motor, sensory, and sometimes vascular innervation to all structures distal to the injury site may be affected. In this laceration, there may be loss of the following:

- IF and MF MCP flexion (lumbricals IF and MF)
- Thumb opposition and palmar abduction
- Thumb MP flexion (weakness caused by partial innervation of the FPB radial head)
- Sensation to the volar radial aspect of the hand

The sensory loss is extremely disabling because there is no sensory input to most of the volar surface of the radial digits. The clinical presentation of this injury is often referred to as **ape hand deformity** because of the loss of stabilizing thenar musculature to the volar radial aspect of the hand with inability to position the thumb out of the palm (Fig. 19–11A–C). Simple activities such as writing and

holding a utensil can be greatly impaired not only due to the motor loss but also to the inability to feel the object with the radial digits and thumb.

If wrist, thumb, or digital flexor tendons are involved, treatment includes a wrist/hand flexion immobilization or restriction orthosis (also referred to as a dorsal blocking orthosis) to decrease tension on the nerve repair and associated soft tissue structures (Fig. 19–12). If the median nerve was repaired in isolation, an orthosis that positions the radial aspect of the wrist and MCPs in flexion (allowing IP motion) with the thumb in opposition and palmar abduction is often acceptable (Fig. 19–13A,B). When healing allows (at 4 to 6 weeks), a small opposition strap can be used to enhance and facilitate functional pinch (Fig. 19–14). Orthotic fabrication is used in combination with the referring physician's postoperative protocol, which may include such techniques as wound care, edema reduction, and guarded active or passive ROM.

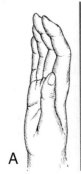
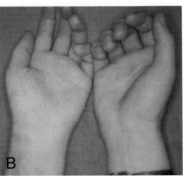
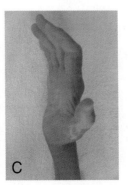

FIGURE 19–11 **A and B,** A low median nerve laceration leaves an apelike hand. Note left hand thumb adduction secondary to the loss of thumb abductor and opponens pollicis. Posture further influenced by the innervated thumb adductor and 1st dorsal interossei. **C,** In this radial view, the devastating loss of the hand's arches and muscular tone is appreciated.

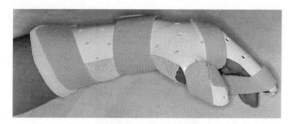

FIGURE 19–12 A wrist/hand flexion immobilization or restriction orthosis (dorsal blocking orthosis) is used to protect a repaired median nerve as well as repaired flexor tendons and other soft tissue structures.

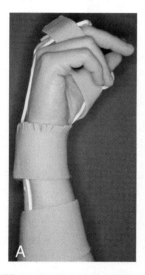 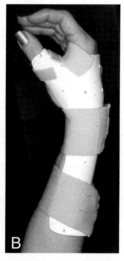

FIGURE 19–13 A, A wrist/IF-MF MCP flexion, thumb opposition/abduction immobilization orthosis to protect an isolated median nerve repair. **B,** Another option for orthosis management is incorporating gentle wrist flexion, thumb opposition/palmar abduction, with the MCPs free. If the thumb web is not supported in opposition and abduction, the unopposed ulnar-innervated intrinsics will pull the thumb web into adduction, eventually leading to contracture.

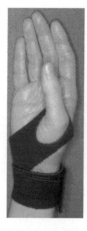

FIGURE 19–14 A simple strap can be used to allow functional opposition. This neoprene strap allowed an OB/GYN surgeon to resume limited work activities by giving assistance to weak re-innervating median nerve musculature.

Compression Neuropathies of the Median Nerve

PROXIMAL MEDIAN NERVE NEUROPATHY (PRONATOR SYNDROME)

Compression in the proximal forearm is commonly referred to as **pronator syndrome**; however, proximal median nerve compression is not localized solely to the pronator teres muscle. The most common site of proximal neuropathy is in the region of the fascial bands and muscular anomalies of the pronator teres muscle and the fibrous arcade of the flexor digitorum superficialis. Other less common potential sources of compression are the ligament of Struthers, lacertus fibrosis, an accessory bicipital aponeurosis, an anomalous muscle, a space-occupying lesion, or scarring from trauma (Eversmann, 1992; Hartz, Linscheild, Gramse, & Daube, 1981; Moore, Dalley, & Agur, 2010; Toby & Ritter, 2011). Symptoms may include intermittent or consistent pain and paresthesias in the volar forearm and hand, which increases with active use or provocative positioning. The thenar muscles may feel weak and fatigued with only an occasional loss of sensation in the median nerve distribution of the hand. There is often a positive Tinel's sign in the volar forearm, weak or negative **Phalen's** and reverse Phalen's tests (positioning in extreme wrist flexion/extension, creating paresthesias in the median nerve distribution), pain with resistive pronation, and pain in the forearm with resistance to the flexor digitorum superficialis (FDS) of the MF and ring finger (RF).

Proximal median nerve neuropathy or pronator syndrome is often seen in patients who do heavy manual labor; those whose jobs require resistive, repetitive forearm rotation; and quite often in musicians who maintain awkward postures or bear the weight of their instruments on their hands for long periods of time (Charness, 1992; Eversmann, 1992; Mackinnon & Novak, 1997). Care must be taken to examine and rule out carpal tunnel syndrome and cervical radiculopathy. Orthosis management is usually in combination with rest, activity modification, appropriate therapeutic modalities, gentle nerve-gliding exercises, and anti-inflammatory medication. Suggested orthosis positioning includes elbow flexion, forearm pronation, and wrist neutral.

ANTERIOR INTEROSSEOUS NERVE SYNDROME

The AIN is a motor branch of the median nerve, originating 5 to 8 cm distal to the level of the lateral epicondyle (Lundborg, 1988). **Anterior interosseous nerve syndrome** is purely a motor lesion and may occur secondary to trauma (fracture, puncture, and compression), vascular insult, or compression under tendinous bands. Symptoms can include weakness or paralysis of the flexor pollicis longus (FPL), FDP of the IF and MF, and pronator quadratus muscle. Injury to the AIN results in the inability to perform tip and three-point pinch properly (Eversmann, 1992). If the patient is unable to make the "OK" sign, it is likely there is AIN loss (Fig. 19–15A,B).

Orthosis intervention is not common but may be considered to prevent thumb IP (Fig. 19–15C), IF DIP, and

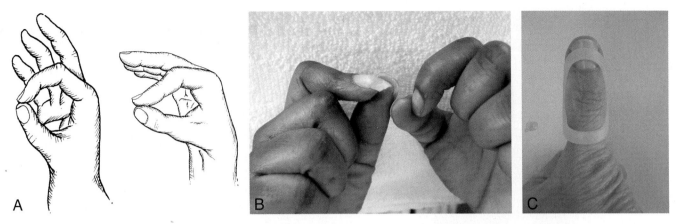

FIGURE 19-15 **A and B,** With an AIN injury, loss of thumb IP and IF DIP flexion results in the inability to perform the okay sign as seen in this patients right hand. **C,** This Oval-8® Finger Splint (3-Point Products, Stevensville, MD) applied to the thumb IP joint helps maintain a small degree of flexion for an improved pinch.

sometimes MF DIP extension contractures if applicable. The clinician must impart the importance of maintaining passive motion of these distal joints as the patient is awaiting nerve return. If nerve regeneration is not noted after a reasonable amount of time, other treatment options for complete loss of this branch may be considered, including surgical decompression, nerve, or tendon transfer.

CARPAL TUNNEL SYNDROME

Carpal tunnel syndrome (CTS) may be recognized as one of the most common compression neuropathies of the upper extremity. The carpal tunnel is a narrow space in which the median nerve and nine digital flexor tendons traverse. The tunnel is bordered on three sides by carpal bones and on the volar aspect by the thick, dense transverse carpal

ligament (Lundborg, 1988). This narrow space is just wide enough for the structures within it to pass (Fig. 19–16). Any additional pressure, inflammation, or obstacle—such as an osteophyte or scar tissue—within this space may cause compression of the nerve. Compression of the median nerve at this level may occur owing to a multitude of factors, including inflammatory conditions, metabolic disorders, status post fracture or dislocation of the distal radioulnar joint, and tenosynovitis of the digits and wrist flexors caused by arthritis or repetitive stress motions (Lundborg, 1988).

The median nerve is a mixed nerve with both motor and sensory fibers; and because of this, the symptoms can be varied. Some complain of only numbness, whereas others may complain of shooting volar forearm pain and weakness. Most commonly, however, the patient experiences nocturnal

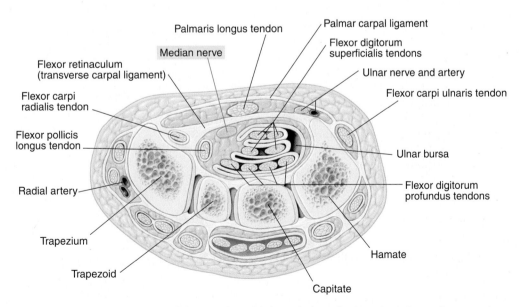

FIGURE 19-16 Cross section of the carpal tunnel through the wrist. Note how the median nerve is surrounded by nine tendons within a small space. Borrowed from Tank, P. W., & Gest, T. R. (2009). *Atlas of anatomy.* Philadelphia, PA: Lippincott Williams & Wilkins.

CHAPTER 19

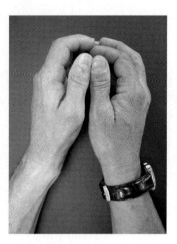

FIGURE 19–17 Note the thenar atrophy on the left thumb of this man as compared to his right.

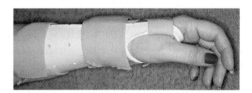

FIGURE 19–18 When the median nerve is compressed at the level of the wrist, an orthosis that positions the wrist in neutral can decrease symptoms since the nerve is in a relaxed, tension free position.

burning pain and paresthesias, clumsiness with routine tasks (e.g., drying hair, taking dishes out of the dishwasher), or radiating pain along the volar forearm. Continued compression and irritation to the nerve may result in weakness of thumb abduction, opposition, and the median nerve–innervated intrinsics (Fig. 19–17). The patient may have difficulty with fine motor manipulation because of the described weak musculature and the sensory disturbance to the volar thumb, IF, MF, and radial half of the RF (Boscheinen-Morrin et al., 1985). The patient may have a positive Tinel's sign with tapping over the carpal tunnel and a positive Phalen's test. Conservative treatment consists of rest; activity modification; a volar wrist immobilization orthosis, with the wrist in neutral for night use; nerve-gliding exercises; and anti-inflammatory medication and/or injection (Fig. 19–18) (Sailor, 1996). Surgical intervention is an option if symptoms persist.

Ulnar Nerve Injuries

Lacerations to the Ulnar Nerve

HIGH LACERATION
Lacerations of the ulnar nerve at or above the elbow result in loss of the following (Fig. 19–19):

- Ulnar wrist flexion
- DIP and MCP flexion of RF and SF
- Abduction and adduction of all digits
- Adduction of thumb

BOX 19–3
Order of Innervation for Ulnar Nerve

1. Flexor carpi ulnaris
2. Ulnar half of flexor digitorum profundus
3. Abductor digiti minimi
4. Flexor digiti minimi
5. Opponens digiti minimi
6. Fourth web space interossei
7. Third web space interossei
8. Second web space interossei
9. Fourth lumbrical
10. Third lumbrical
11. Adductor pollicis
12. First web space interossei

- Thumb MP flexion (weakness owing to partial innervation of the FPB ulnar head)
- Sensory loss of the dorsoulnar aspect of the hand, radiating along the ulnar side of the forearm
- Significant loss of grip and pinch strength

Clinical signs of chronic high-level ulnar nerve injury may include a mild **claw hand deformity** of the hand (hyperextension of the RF and SF MCP joints secondary to loss of the stabilizing intrinsics, weakened or stretched MCP joint volar plates, and overpull of the intact extensor tendons) with a loss of the hypothenar and interosseous muscles (Fig. 19–20). The patient may be unable to adduct the SF secondary to paralysis of the third volar interossei (**Wartenberg's sign**)

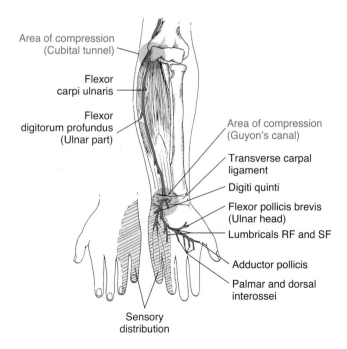

FIGURE 19–19 The ulnar nerve provides innervation to the ulnar aspect of the wrist and hand. The sensory branches innervate the dorsal ulnar and the volar aspect of the SF and the ulnar half of the RF.

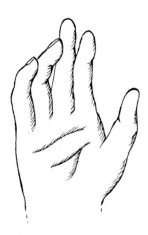

FIGURE 19–20 A high ulnar nerve laceration does not cause the pronounced RF and SF PIP/DIP flexion posturing that is seen with a lower ulnar nerve lesion secondary to the paralysis of the associated FDP tendons.

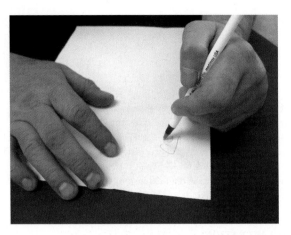

FIGURE 19–22 Froment's sign: with ulnar nerve injury, the patient loses the ability to contract the adductor pollicis; and when combined with the loss of the first dorsal interossei, attempted lateral pinch is significantly impaired. Lateral pinch is compensated for by the median nerve–innervated FPL, resulting in flexion of the thumb IP as shown here.

and abduct the IF owing to paralysis of the first dorsal interossei (Lundborg, 1988) (Fig. 19–21). The patient may also exhibit the inability to contract the adductor pollicis; and when combined with the loss of the first dorsal interossei, attempted lateral pinch is significantly impaired. Lateral pinch is compensated for by the median nerve–innervated FPL, causing extreme flexion of the thumb IP joint during attempted pinch (**Froment's sign**) (Fig. 19–22); and with chronic loss of innervation, this clinical picture may eventually include hyperextension of the thumb MP joint known as **Jeanne's sign** (Fig. 19–23A) (Doyle, 2006; Lundborg, 1988; Parry, 1981).

Treatment may consist of education regarding sensory precautions, preservation of ROM, and orthotic intervention to maximize functional use and prevent joint contractures while waiting for nerve regeneration (Fig. 19–23B).

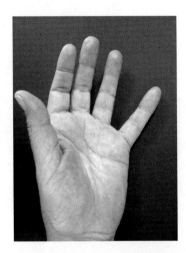

FIGURE 19–21 Wartenberg's sign: demonstrating the inability of the small digit to actively adduct secondary to intrinsic weakness.

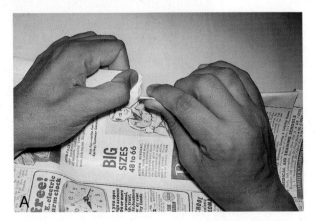
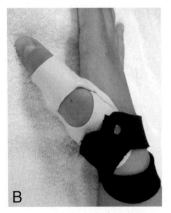

FIGURE 19–23 **A,** Jeanne's sign: with ongoing chronic loss of the ulnar nerve, the patient displays all that is described with the Froment's sign. In addition, over time, the volar structures of the thumb MP become lax, eventually causing pronounced thumb MP hyperextension (Borrowed from Doyle, Hand & Wrist 2006, LWW page 219). **B,** A thumb MP extension restriction orthosis can be used to position the thumb MP in slight flexion (better mechanical advantage), which supports a functional position for pinch and prevents further stretching of the volar MP structures.

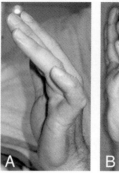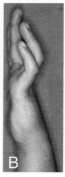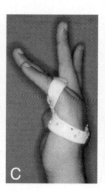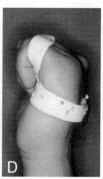

FIGURE 19–24 A low ulnar nerve laceration leads to partial claw deformity. **A,** Low lesion; note the DIP flexion here caused by the innervation of the FDP SF. **B,** High lesion; there is an increase in MCP volar laxity and a loss of distal innervation to the DIP. An RF/SF MCP extension restriction orthosis allows RF and SF digit extension **(C)** and flexion **(D).**

LOW LACERATION

Low ulnar nerve injury at the wrist is often seen in combination with flexor tendon, median nerve, and vascular injury. Injury of the ulnar nerve at this level results in loss of the following:

- MCP flexion of RF and SF
- Abduction and adduction of all digits
- Adduction of thumb
- Sensory loss of the ulnar aspect of the hand
- Thumb MP flexion (weakness caused by partial innervation of the FPB ulnar head)
- Significant loss of grip and pinch strength

A clawing deformity of the RF and SF is more prominent than with a high lesion secondary to the intact profundus tendon to these digits (Fig. 19–24A,B). In chronic conditions, the patient may progress to the point that the Wartenberg's, Froment's, and Jeanne's signs are present. The use of an orthosis that places the MCPs in flexion can prevent overstretching of the volar soft tissue supports and can facilitate functional use while waiting for nerve return (Fig. 19–24C,D).

Combined Ulnar and Median Nerve Injury

A combined median and ulnar nerve injury can result in a claw hand deformity. In a low lesion, clawing of all the digits occurs secondary to complete loss of intrinsic control and a functioning profundus tendons (Fig. 19–25A,B). If the injury is high, clawing still occurs but is significantly less pronounced.

Intervention (for high and low combined lesions) includes patient education regarding sensory precautions as well as fabrication of a daytime functional orthosis that includes all the MCPs in flexion (and thumb abduction/opposition if necessary) to prevent MCP joint extension/PIP flexion contractures while providing a position for functional use. Furthermore, a nighttime wrist/hand immobilization orthosis is used to place the structures in an antideformity position while waiting for nerve return (Fig. 19–25C–E). The elbow joint is incorporated into the orthosis (positioned at 90° flexion) if at least one of the involved muscle–tendon unit's origin is at or above the humeral condyles (Fig. 19–25F) (Doyle, 2006).

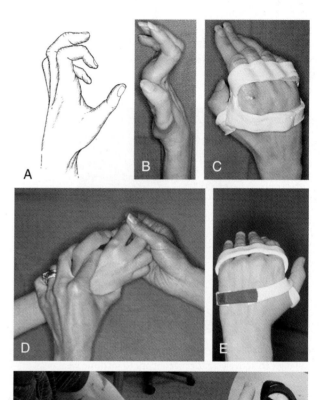

FIGURE 19–25 A–E, Atrophy of the hypothenar and the first dorsal interossei muscles may cause muscle atrophy/indenting along the lateral borders of the hand, making application and removal of an orthosis quite difficult. A trap door (using hook loop closure) helps with orthosis application and removal. **F,** The elbow is incorporated after surgical repair of a high ulnar laceration and complex flexor tendon injury. Note the soft crossed neoprene strapping in the anterior elbow fossa.

Compression Neuropathies of the Ulnar Nerve

CUBITAL TUNNEL SYNDROME

The cubital tunnel is formed by a tendinous arch joining the ulnar and humeral attachments of the flexor carpi ulnaris (FCU) tendon. The boundaries of the cubital tunnel are the medial epicondyle, the ulnohumeral ligament, and the fibrous arch formed by the two heads of the FCU tendon (Rayan, 1992). Many factors can cause or contribute to **cubital tunnel syndrome**, a common compression neuropathy, including direct trauma; fracture or fracture and dislocation of the medial or lateral epicondyles; arthritis; a subluxing ulnar nerve; or postural stress caused by sleeping positions, vocational demands, or recreational activities.

The clinical symptoms of cubital tunnel syndrome are paresthesias and numbness in the ulnar portion of the hand and forearm; vague, ulnar-sided arm pain that is sometimes described as a sharp, radiating pain that may worsen with an increase in activity level; and reported weakness of grip and pinch strength. Novak, Lee, Mackinnon, and Lay (1994) found that the cubital tunnel can be quickly screened by performing an **elbow flexion test** (prolonged elbow flexion positioning resulting in paresthesias along the ulnar nerve distribution) combined with pressure on the ulnar nerve. A positive Tinel's sign over the ulnar nerve at the elbow, sensory changes in the ulnar nerve distribution, decreased grip and pinch strength, and atrophy of the intrinsic muscles of the hand are also common indicators (Novak et al., 1994). In some cases, chronic compression may lead to positive Wartenberg's, Froment's, and Jeanne's signs. The differential diagnosis should rule out thoracic outlet syndrome, C8/T1 nerve root compression, and compression of the ulnar nerve distally at the Guyon's canal.

Conservative management usually involves rest and avoidance of provocative activities (e.g., prolonged elbow flexion, repetitive elbow flexion/extension, and weight bearing on the medial elbow), gentle nerve-gliding exercises, anti-inflammatory medication if appropriate, and some type of night elbow immobilization orthosis (slight elbow flexion, neutral forearm to slight pronation, and wrist neutral with slight ulnar deviation) (Fig. 19–26) (Harper, 1990; Sailor, 1996; Tetro & Pichora, 1996; Warwick & Seradge, 1995).

If the patient cannot tolerate a thermoplastic orthosis for nighttime use (or insurance will not cover it), other

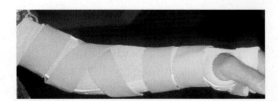

FIGURE 19–26 A night resting elbow immobilization orthosis minimizes compression on the nerve as it passes through the cubital tunnel. Restriction of elbow flexion during sleep may decrease irritation in this area.

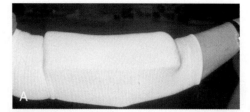
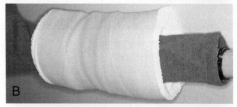
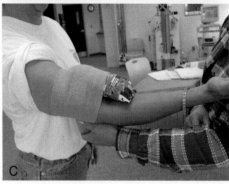

FIGURE 19–27 **A,** A foam pad applied to the anterior aspect of the elbow can provide some light resistance to full elbow flexion. **B,** A towel wrapped about the elbow can also prevent full elbow flexion while sleeping, allowing a less restraining option to rigid immobilization. **C,** A small pillow or rolled up towel can be secured with an elasticized bandage as yet another option.

options can be considered. A piece of foam or a small pillow can be placed on the anterior aspect of the elbow crease to prevent elbow flexion. The foam should extend proximally to the middle upper arm and distally to the midforearm; it can be held in place with a stockinette or a light circumferential wrap. Another option is to wind a towel around the elbow, securing it with a circumferential wrap (Fig. 19–27A–C). These methods are intended to restrict full elbow flexion and may be tolerated better than a rigid orthosis. During the day, soft padding (foam or silicone) about the posterior and medial elbow (cubital tunnel region) may protect the nerve from further trauma and provide a sense of security for the patient (Fig. 19–28A,B). If symptoms continue, surgical decompression or transposition of the nerve may be warranted.

ULNAR TUNNEL (GUYON'S CANAL) SYNDROME

The ulnar tunnel, also referred to as **Guyon's canal**, is formed by the volar carpal ligament, hook of the hamate, and the pisiform bones. This space is small and somewhat superficial, making the nerve vulnerable to injury. Just proximal to the wrist, the nerve divides into a dorsal superficial sensory branch and a volar deep motor branch. Compression of the sensory branch, motor branch, or both branches may occur

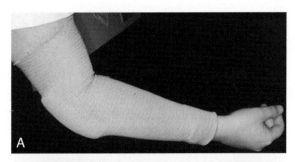

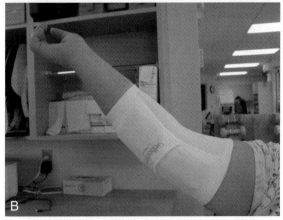

FIGURE 19–28 **A and B,** Soft padding or use of silicone gel sheets (or similar products) over the cubital tunnel area may help protect and absorb vibration/forces to a hypersensitive or regenerating ulnar nerve.

depending on the level of impingement. If only the motor branch is involved, the intrinsic muscles are affected, but sensation is left intact. An isolated lesion to the deep motor branch may be seen in people who use tools intensively, such as a screwdriver or pruning shears. They do not usually complain of pain, just weakness and atrophy (Boscheinen-Morrin et al., 1985; Matloub & Yousif, 1992).

The compression of the ulnar nerve at this level can be caused by repetitive trauma (cycling, hammering, use of vibrating tools), fracture of the hook of the hamate or pisiform bones, arthritis in the pisohamate joint, ganglion, anomalous muscle or ligament, or possibly an ulnar artery aneurysm or thrombosis (Lundborg, 1988; Moore & Dalley, 1999; Moore et al., 2010). Symptoms include vague pain, paresthesias or numbness of the SF and ulnar half of the RF, and weakness of the intrinsic muscles. In some cases, the patient may demonstrate positive Wartenberg's, Froment's, and Jeanne's signs owing to the weakness of the ulnar innervated muscles. When the sensory branch is involved, examination may reveal a positive Phalen's test and Tinel's sign over the ulnar tunnel.

Treatment of these low lesions focuses on rest, immobilization, avoidance of symptomatic activities, and anti-inflammatory medication. If symptoms persist, surgical intervention may be necessary. Orthoses may be used initially to immobilize the wrist and ulnar aspect of the hand for symptom relief. Once symptoms subside, orthoses can be fabricated to protect the ulnar tunnel during vocational or recreational activities. Padding the ulnar wrist over the ulnar tunnel area with gel or high-density foam may aid in absorbing vibration and compression stress to this vulnerable area. An orthosis can then be formed directly over this padded area (Fig. 19–29A–C).

Radial Nerve Injuries

Lacerations of the Radial Nerve

The radial nerve innervates the triceps muscle, which provides elbow extension, and innervates all of the wrist,

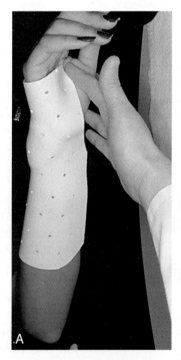

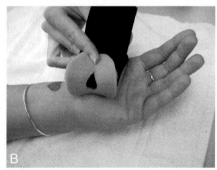

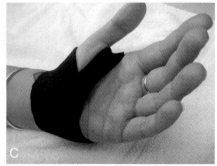

FIGURE 19–29 **A,** An ulnar wrist immobilization orthosis can be fabricated by incorporating silicone gel or high-density foam over the volar ulnar aspect of the wrist to protect the ulnar nerve in this region. **B and C,** A donut of foam rests over Guyon's canal and is incorporated into this small custom fabricated neoprene orthosis.

BOX 19–4
Order of Innervation for Radial Nerve

1. Brachioradialis
2. Extensor carpi radialis longus
3. Supinator
4. Extensor carpi radialis brevis
5. Extensor digitorum communis
6. Extensor carpi ulnaris
7. Extensor digiti minimi
8. Abductor pollicis longus
9. Extensor pollicis longus
10. Extensor pollicis brevis
11. Extensor indicis proprius

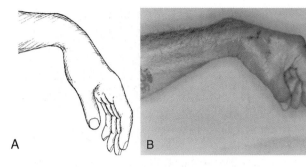

FIGURE 19–31 A and B, High radial nerve injury with wrist drop.

digit, and thumb extensors as well as the supinator muscle (Fig. 19–30). Sensory loss of the radial nerve is much less functionally significant than that of the ulnar or median nerve.

HIGH LACERATION
Laceration to the radial nerve in the upper arm is often associated with a midshaft humerus fracture or traumatic injury to the nerve from a gunshot or stabbing injury. The radial nerve travels in close proximity to the humerus and is extremely vulnerable to injury if the humerus is involved. If lacerated at this level, the patient experiences loss of the following:

- Wrist extension
- Forearm supinator (weak)
- Thumb and digital extension
- Independent IF and SF digital extension
- Sensation over the dorsal radial aspect of the forearm and hand

This clinical presentation is often referred to as **wrist drop** (Fig. 19–31). The radial nerve cannot innervate its distal musculature, making wrist and digital extension impossible. Orthosis intervention can be used to place the wrist and digits in a more neutral/functional position to prevent overstretching of the involved extensor muscle–tendon units, prevent joint contractures, and provide a mechanical advantage for the flexor tendons while waiting return of radial nerve function (Fig. 19–32A,B) (Colditz,

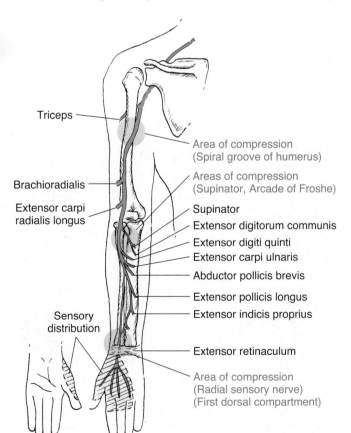

FIGURE 19–30 Injury to the motor portion of the radial nerve is functionally disabling.

Triceps

Brachioradialis

Extensor carpi radialis longus

Sensory distribution

Area of compression (Spiral groove of humerus)

Areas of compression (Supinator, Arcade of Froshe)

Supinator
Extensor digitorum communis
Extensor digiti quinti
Extensor carpi ulnaris
Abductor pollicis brevis
Extensor pollicis longus
Extensor indicis proprius
Extensor retinaculum
Area of compression (Radial sensory nerve) (First dorsal compartment)

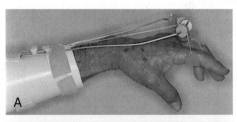

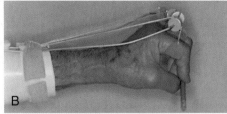

FIGURE 19–32 A, A wrist/MCP/thumb extension mobilization orthosis (for radial nerve palsy) is used to enhance hand function for a patient waiting for radial nerve reinnervation. The wrist is passively extended as the digits actively flex through this mobilization device; **(B)** and when the wrist actively flexes (through the functioning flexor tendons), the digits passively extend. The proximal dorsal orthosis was fabricated out of ³/₃₂″ material; the mobilization component is a Phoenix Extended Outrigger Kit. Design of this orthosis modified from Colditz, J. C. (1995). Splinting the hand with a peripheral nerve injury. In J. M. Hunter, E. J. Mackin, & A. D. Callahan (Eds.), *Rehabilitation of the hand* (4th ed., pp. 679–692). St. Louis, MO: Mosby Year Book.

CHAPTER 19

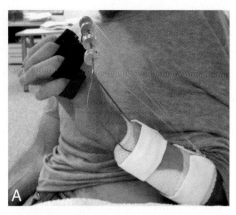

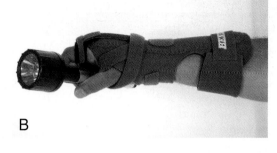

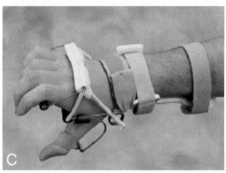

FIGURE 19–33 **A,** Custom bent aluminum wire and soft neoprene slings can be an alternative when not all kit components are available, affordable or appropriate for the patient. Note the dorsal orthosis 'cuff' with elasticized strap closures. **B,** The Tunnel Forearm Splint. *Photo courtesy of Benik Corp (Silverdale, WA).* **C,** LMB™ Radial Nerve Splint Wrist Extension with MCP Extension Assist and Adjustable Thumb Extension Assist. *Photo courtesy of DeRoyal Industries (Powell, TN).*

1987; Duff, 2005). There are several options of orthoses available to the therapist, including both custom and prefabricated designs (Fig. 19–33A–C). These are mentioned in Table 19–2.

A wrist extension immobilization orthosis can also be used for day functional use; however, the therapist should caution the patient on potential MCP flexion and IP extension contractures due to loss of active extension. Nighttime immobilization may consist of a simple wrist/hand/thumb immobilization orthosis. Figure 19–34 shows a simple wrist extension immobilization orthosis that is worn for day use; then for night, an extension attachment was added to prevent flexion contractures of the digits and of the first web space. The use of elastic therapeutic tape such as Balance Tex™ or Kinesio® tapes can be used in conjunction with an orthosis to assist the digits and thumb into extension (Fig. 19–35A,B).

When surgical tendon transfer or repair is warranted, similar orthosis intervention is appropriate after the initial postoperative phase. Postoperative orthoses can be used to facilitate muscle reeducation and functional use, maintain balance of muscle–tendon unit length(s), and prevent joint contractures.

LOW LACERATION

Distal and anterior to the lateral epicondyle (at 8 to 10 cm), the radial nerve divides into a sensory and a motor branches. The sensory branch provides innervation to the dorsoradial forearm while the motor branch (PIN) continues distally to innervate the digit and thumb extensors. The radial

wrist extensors—the extensor carpi radialis longus (ECRL) and extensor carpi radialis brevis (ECRB)—are innervated proximal to this bifurcation. Therefore, with low injury to the PIN, wrist extension is normal with only the loss of digit and thumb extension. The intrinsics attempt to extend the PIP and DIP joints, but the MCPs cannot be extended by the

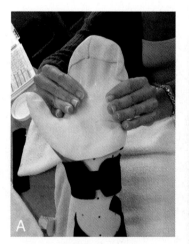

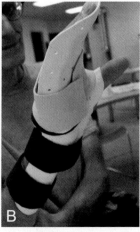

FIGURE 19–34 **A,** A night digit/thumb extension piece is being fabricated over the day wrist extension orthosis to prevent IP flexion contractures and shortening of the flexor tendons; which can occur as a consequence of this injury. **B,** A simple volar piece was added to this day orthosis in order to keep digits extended, the thumb MP & IP are free yet the orthosis incorporated the first web to provide for a wide first web space minimizing contracture.

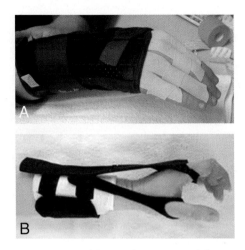

FIGURE 19–35 **A,** A prefabricated wrist immobilization orthosis supports the wrist into neutral, whereas the elastic therapeutic tape is applied to assist the digits into extension. **B,** A low-profile wrist/MCP extension orthosis can be an alternative design for a radial nerve palsy orthosis as described in Figures 19–32 and 19–33 (refer to Chapter 14).

inactive extrinsic extensor tendons. Orthosis management is essentially the same as for a high lesion. The inclusion of the wrist is optional and not recommended if there is adequate wrist extension strength (Fig. 19–36A–E).

Compression Neuropathies of the Radial Nerve

HIGH COMPRESSION

The radial nerve courses about the humerus at the level of the spiral groove. Injury may occur owing to local compression of the radial nerve against the humerus for an extended period of time, also known as **Saturday night palsy** (i.e., falling asleep with arm against a hard object,

a forceful squeeze). There may be tenderness directly over the compression site with little other pain noted. This area of compression block may cause a neurapraxia, resulting in impairment of the muscles innervated below this level. With time, this weakness or paralysis may resolve with little or no functional deficit (C. J. Eaton & Lister, 1992; Lundborg, 1988; Moore & Dalley, 1999; Moore et al., 2010; Parry, 1981). The goals of orthosis intervention consist of prevention of joint contractures, protection against overstretching of the involved extensor muscle–tendon units, and maximizing functional use of the hand and wrist while waiting for nerve return.

RADIAL TUNNEL SYNDROME

The PIN passes deep to the origin of the ECRB and the arcade of Frohse (proximal margin of the supinator) and then passes between the two heads of the supinator to supply the supinator (Lundborg, 1988; Moore & Dalley, 1999; Moore et al., 2010). Compression can occur at any one of the sites through which the nerve passes; however, the arcade of Frohse is by far the most likely anatomic structure to compress the PIN (Lundborg, 1988; Moore & Dalley, 1999; Moore et al., 2010). **Radial tunnel syndrome**, also known as **resistant tennis elbow**, is often characterized by pain with repetitive rotational movement of the forearm (Roles & Manudsley, 1972; Simmons & Wyman, 1992). Pain is described as aching and radiating toward the dorsal part of the wrist. There is profound tenderness on palpation directly over the extensor muscle group and supinator, 3 to 4 cm distal (over the arcade of Frohse) to the lateral epicondyle (Lundborg, 1988; Rayan, 1992). Resistance to supination, wrist extension, and MF extension usually reproduces the pain. Pain can occur during the day with forearm rotation activities; however, it is usually most evident at night. Radial tunnel can be misdiagnosed as lateral epicondylitis (tennis elbow). A careful differential

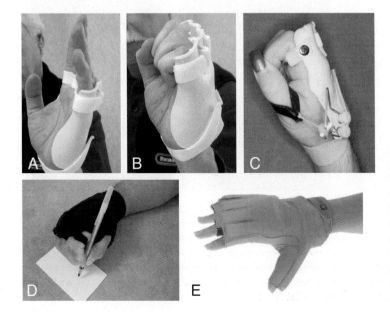

FIGURE 19–36 **A and B,** PIN injury can be managed with a hand-based MCP/Thumb MP extension mobilization orthosis. This orthosis maintains passive MCP/Thumb MP extension **(A)** while allowing **(B)** active digital flexion. A lightweight material is used to contour about the dorsum of the hand. **C,** A thumb extension outrigger is not always necessary and may be cumbersome to some patients; however, here it helped the patient carry out work responsibilities. Prepadding the dorsal MCPs may assist in decreasing migration, shear stress, and increasing comfort. **D,** The Hand-Based Tunnel Splint® and **(E)** The Robinson Hand-Based Nerve Splint. *Photo courtesy of Alimed, Dedham MA.*

diagnosis should be done. In lateral epicondylitis, pain is directly over the lateral epicondyle, wrist extension may be weak and painful, and pain is most often during and/or after work or recreational activity (C. J. Eaton & Lister, 1992; Lundborg, 1988; Newcomer, Martinez-Silvestrini, Schaefer, Gay, & Arendt, 2005).

Management should include rest, avoidance of provocative positions, activity modification, anti-inflammatory medication or modalities, nerve-gliding exercises, and orthosis application with the elbow gently flexed (optional) and forearm supinated with wrist extension.

POSTERIOR INTEROSSEOUS NERVE SYNDROME

The same pathology and therapeutic intervention as described for the low radial nerve laceration applies to **posterior interosseous nerve syndrome**. Although not common, the PIN can be damaged, compressed, or lacerated at this level (Thomas et al., 2000). Injury may occur from a mass pressing on the nerve (e.g., ganglion, lipoma, or fibroma), from a traumatic incident (e.g., an injection, plate or pin fixation while repairing a proximal radius or ulna fracture), rheumatoid arthritis of the elbow, or a forearm compression injury (Dell & Guzewicz, 1992). Symptoms usually include some degree of pain and weakness. Physical examination reveals no sensory deficit and a temporary partial or complete paralysis of the extrinsic digit and thumb extensors.

SUPERFICIAL RADIAL SENSORY NERVE SYNDROME (WARTENBERG'S SYNDROME)

The sensory branch of the radial nerve is vulnerable to injury as it approaches the radial styloid of the wrist. Therapists and surgeons often see injury and/or irritation at this level. In superficial radial sensory nerve syndrome or **Wartenberg's syndrome**, the nerve can become entrapped in scar from a laceration or from a surgical incision, as occasionally seen with a deQuervain's release. Irritation to this branch can also be caused by friction from pin placement, jagged orthosis edges, sharp or compressive orthosis straps, or excessive edema (Colditz, 1995). Sensory alterations (paresthesias and numbness) occur in the dorsoradial aspect of the hand (Lundborg, 1988). Intervention focuses on orthosis management, with a silicone gel cushion or pad placed directly over the radial styloid (Fig. 19–37). For an acute, painful injury, a doughnut may be used over this area to avoid direct contact. An orthosis can offer protection and decreased tension on the nerve. Other therapeutic modalities may be used as warranted. Surgical decompression is considered when all conservative management fails.

Digital Nerve Lacerations

Digital nerves can be lacerated in isolation but most often are seen in combination with tendon injury in zones II to IV. If seen in isolation, the involved digit is placed into a hand-based immobilization or restriction orthosis (depending on the physician's protocol). The

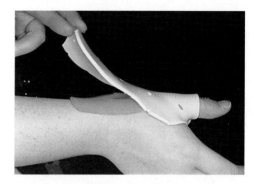

FIGURE 19–37 Place a silicone gel cushion or pad directly over or around the radial styloid process and under the orthosis for protection of the nerve absorption of vibration and distribution of pressure.

position of the digit is in a gently flexed posture to minimize stress on the surgical anastomosis. Protective orthotic management is used for 4 to 6 weeks; the patient is put into progressively greater extension per physician's orders (Fig. 19–38A–D).

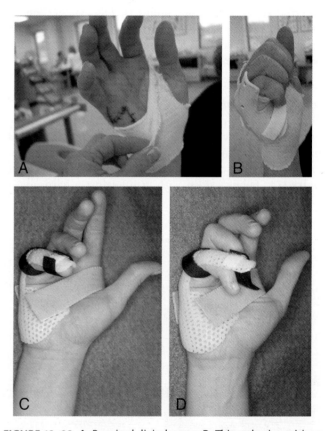

FIGURE 19–38 A, Repaired digital nerve. **B,** This orthosis positions the repaired digital nerve in a shortened position while allowing gliding of the flexor tendons through the incision area, minimizing the risk of adhesion formation. **C,** This design further protects the length of the nerve when increased precaution is necessary. **D,** Removal of the straps allows periodic gentle ROM within the orthosis confines.

During the initial weeks, a guarded ROM program is begun, which usually involves unrestricted flexion and some degree of restricted extension. If tendons are involved, the wrist and/or thumb must be incorporated into the orthosis, following the physician's preferred tendon protocol. Patient education regarding sensory precautions, wound care, edema control, and protected ROM must be reviewed.

Brachial Plexus Injury

Injuries to the brachial plexus are extremely varied, ranging from simple compression and irritation injuries to complex traumatic avulsions. The brachial plexus supplies the principal motor and sensory innervations to every muscle of the upper extremity with the exception of the levator scapulae and trapezius muscle (Leversedge et al., 2010; Moore et al., 2010). Trauma (i.e., gunshot wounds, avulsions), disease, stretching, and compression (Erb's palsy, Saturday night palsy) in the axilla or lateral cervical triangle of the neck may produce a brachial plexus injury (Moore et al., 2010). The type of distal pathology the clinician will see depends where the plexus was injured. The location of injury and the anticipated pathology can be appreciated in Figure 19–39A. Although a review of this nerve complex is beyond the scope of this chapter, it is important to value the complex path (root → trunk → division → cord → branch) the peripheral nerve takes to end in its terminal branch. It is also relevant to mention that orthotic intervention is based on the predicted distal pathology and potential deformity (Hunter & Whitenack, 1995; Jacobs, 2003; Lowe & O'Toole, 1995) (Fig. 19–39A). Pain is often a consequence of these injuries and can play a major role in the therapist's ability to manage the patient. The therapist should recognize that the peripheral nerves, nerve plexuses, spinal nerves, and nerve roots may all become a source of pain and thus may limit the plan of care (Barbis & Wallace, 1995; Elvey, 1997).

The same general orthosis management principles, considerations, and precautions discussed in this chapter apply to brachial plexus injuries as well. Orthosis intervention to preserve functional motion and minimize overstretching of the denervated muscles is most important especially with an extended recovery (Colditz, 1987).

The level at which the brachial plexus is injured determines the most appropriate orthotic intervention for preventing deformity and maximizing function (Hunter & Whitenack, 1995; Lowe & O'Toole, 1995). Often, there is not a clear-cut pattern of deformity, especially with untreated lacerations and long-standing compression injuries. In addition, the patient may have developed joint contractures

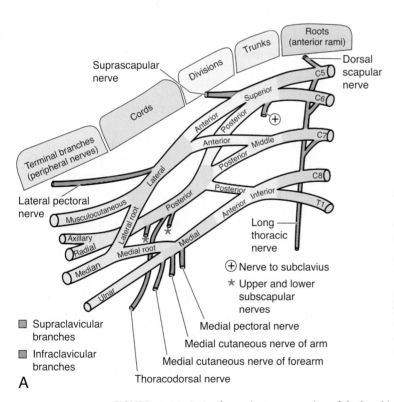

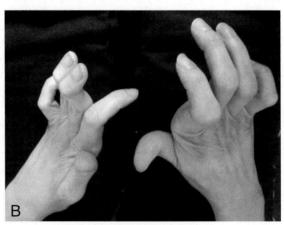

FIGURE 19–39 A, A schematic representation of the brachial plexus. The clinician can appreciate the complex origin of each terminal branch. From Moore pg 722 6.44B. **B,** This patient has a long-standing brachial plexus injury sustained during a bilateral first cervical rib resection. In Moore, K. L., Dalley, A. F., & Agur, A. M. (2010). *Clinically oriented anatomy* (6th ed.). Philadelphia, PA: Lippincott Williams & Wilkins

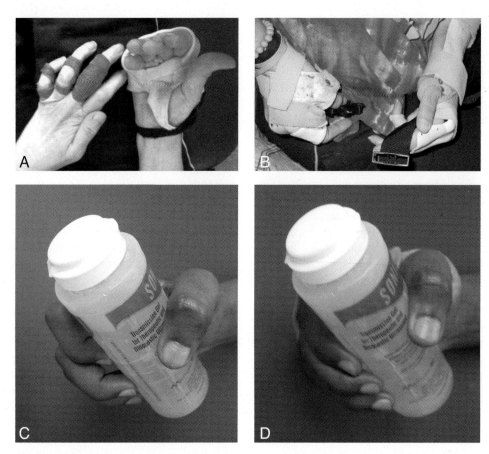

FIGURE 19–40 A, Various bilateral orthoses provide this patient with the ability to function somewhat independently. **B,** Bilateral orthoses are used to attach the seat belt and proceed to drive a car with a modified steering wheel. **C,** Note the gross grasp this patient displays without an orthosis and **(D)** the position of digits and thumb while wearing an MCP extension restriction orthosis with the thumb included. The orthosis placed the MCPs in flexion and the thumb in opposition allowing a better mechanical advantage for the work of the flexor tendons.

and/or compensatory patterns, which may lead to deforming forces acting on the distal hand (Fig. 19–39B).

For example, a patient with an injured **medial cord** of the brachial plexus has involvement of the ulnar nerve as well the contributions to the median nerve. This type of injury results in remarkable loss of the ulnarly innervated intrinsic hand muscles and causes some median nerve deficits as well. The patient essentially presents with a claw hand deformity as noted in Figure 19–39. Applying an IF through SF MCP flexion restriction orthosis may preserve function while the patient waits for nerve return. For those patients who will not fully regain normal function, these orthoses become a crucial component of everyday existence. The patient may need to depend on these orthoses in order to perform even the simplest of tasks (Fig. 19–40A–D).

Injury to the **posterior cord** of the brachial plexus results in damage to all of the extensors of the forearm, wrist, thumb, and fingers and to the deltoid, which abducts the shoulder at the glenohumeral joint. The patient presents with a wrist drop deformity that can be managed with an immobilization

orthosis, a mobilization orthosis, or a combination of both as shown in Figures 19–32 and 19–33. The mobilization orthosis allows for a light functional grasp using the natural tenodesis of the hand. The therapist should teach the patient sensory precautions, passive ROM exercises, carefully guided nerve-gliding exercises, the use of adaptive techniques, and postural awareness (Barbis & Wallace, 1995; Lowe & O'Toole, 1995; Topp & Boyd, 2012; Walsh, 2012).

General Principles of Orthotic Intervention for Peripheral Nerve Injuries

Table 19–2 summarizes PNI management focusing on orthosis considerations. This table is not intended to include all the options of therapeutic procedures or orthotic interventions available to treat the nerve-injured hand.

Goals in Managing the Upper Extremity Peripheral Nerve Injury

When caring for a patient with a PNI, the therapist should have the following goals in mind:

- Reduce pain and edema.
- Provide a balance among the innervated and denervated muscle–tendon structures while waiting for motor return.
- Keep denervated muscles from remaining in a lengthened position.
- Appreciate cortical plasticity while applying sensory relearning techniques.
- Promoting sensorimotor/sensory reeducation strategies.
- Prevent joint stiffness and joint/soft tissue contractures.
- Prevent development of abnormal substitution patterns.
- Position the hand and wrist in the best biomechanically prudent position to maximize functional use and substitute for loss of motor function.
- Decrease pain and paresthesias associated with nerve compression injuries.
- Protect the surgically repaired or injured nerve and associated injuries.
- Protect and teach the patient/caregiver how to protect insensate areas.
- Keep abreast on current findings on neural regeneration and cortical reorganization.

Considerations and Precautions for Orthotic Intervention

The therapist should keep the following considerations and precautions in mind when fabricating an orthosis for this patient population:

- Sensory and motor return should be monitored and orthoses modified accordingly.
- Watch for deformities that may not initially be clinically or functionally evident. As reinnervation occurs, the deformity may become increasingly more apparent; therefore, corrective orthotic intervention is mandatory (e.g., in a returning high ulnar nerve lesion, the FDP eventually becomes innervated and the distal claw deformity becomes more prominent) (Dell & Guzewicz, 1992).
- If patients with nerve injuries must wear an orthosis for function, keep the design simple and low profile. An orthosis that is cumbersome and bulky may interfere with the function of uninvolved joints. Patients are less likely to comply with an orthosis-wearing schedule when the orthosis is big and cumbersome.
- Be aware of the most common distributions of the sensory branches of the three major peripheral nerves in order to appreciate strap placement and orthoses borders and avoid compression of these structures.
- Educate patients regarding their sensory deficits, teaching careful skin examination after fabrication. This will prevent the possibility of excess pressure/friction caused by extended wear of the orthosis (Blackmore & Hotchkiss, 1995; Jacobs, 2003). Meticulous skin inspection after wear is crucial, especially with sensory loss.

Material Selection

Lightweight, contouring, and highly drapable materials may be the most appropriate choice for management of the nerve-injured hand. Many of these injuries have accompanying sensory loss, which limits the patient's ability to detect shear or compressive stress. Great care should be taken to ensure proper length, width, and weight distribution. Corners and borders should be rounded and flared to prevent skin irritation and maximize the orthosis strength, comfort, and cosmesis. The perforated nature of some materials, although lighter in weight, can be problematic. The holes in the material may cause shear/friction stress against the skin as the patient attempts to move. If a perforated material is chosen, patient education regarding diligent and meticulous skin inspection is paramount (Austin, 2003).

Materials that tend to retain heat (during the molding process) may be uncomfortable and even painful for some patients with nerve involvement. Select a material that has a lower heating temperature but can still provide an intimate fit with minimal handling (refer to Chapters 5 and 6) (Austin, 2003). As mentioned throughout this chapter and detailed in Chapter 14, neoprene materials, either alone or in combination with thermoplastics, can provide an alternative for some patients.

Component Selection

The use of components, such as outriggers, slings, and line guides, should be minimized. Every additional component makes the orthosis more complicated to apply and wear. Finger and hand slings should be cautiously applied to the insensate hand. Close attention should be given to avoid creation of shear and/or compression stress under these slings (Austin, 2003). If components are necessary to maintain active function, the therapist must educate the patient, family, and/or caregiver in the correct application and wearing schedule as well as stress the precautions of orthosis wear. The selection of the components should be as low profile as possible. Carefully read instructions for applications and precautions. Commonly, mobilization orthoses are worn for functional day use, complemented by a night immobilization orthosis to prevent joint contractures.

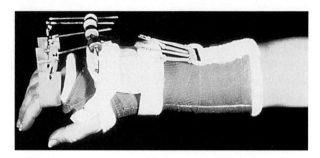

FIGURE 19–41 Extension mobilization orthosis can be fabricated over a cast to maximize functional hand use while waiting for nerve return. For this orthosis, a drapable ⅛″ plastic material was used to contour to the ridges of the fiberglass. Rolyan® adjustable outrigger kit is shown here.

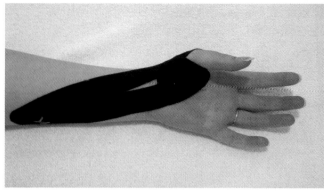

FIGURE 19–42 For a returning median nerve, elastic therapeutic tape is used to position the thumb gently in palmar abduction and opposition. As the wrist is extended, the thumb is carried farther into opposition and abduction, providing the capacity for light tip pinch. This taping technique can be used in conjunction with other orthosis interventions.

Strapping Selection

Straps should be conforming and soft. They should be strategically placed to minimize migration and increase comfort. Neoprene and soft straps conform nicely around joints and through web spaces, minimizing skin irritation (Austin, 2003).

Other Management Options

Other options to manage PNIs may include simple taping techniques (see Chapter 13) or the creative use of neoprene (see Chapter 14). These other options can be performed either alone or in combination with thermoplastic material, casting material, or an orthosis that is either prefabricated or custom made as shown in Figures 19–35A,B, and 19–41. A simple "off-the-shelf" orthosis such as a wrist orthosis (sold by many manufacturers) can be a complement to a custom-fabricated program (worn only for certain events/activities), or in some cases can be used alone. For example, a patient may not be able to afford therapy sessions due to copayments/coinsurance/deductibles costs or the patient may object to wearing a custom orthosis; in this case, a cost-effective option to consider is a prefabricated device.

The Robinson InRigger soft leather glove (AliMed Corporation, Inc., Dedham, MA) or the Tunnel Splint® (Benik Corporation, Silverdale, WA) are just a few additional options for management of such nerve injuries. These are both prefabricated, low-profile, glove-like designs (they come with or without the wrist and/or with or without the thumb) that provide some degree of wrist and/or thumb and/or digit extension after active flexion. A few examples of such orthoses are shown in Figures 19–33B,C. These types of gloves can be used to manage PIN injury, radial nerve injury, combined PNIs, distal pathology from a brachial plexus lesion, and distal nerve degeneration from a chronic neuromuscular disease. Reference to Chapter 11 is encouraged for a more thorough description of the avail-

able prefabricated options. Chapter 14 reviews the use of neoprene for the creative modification of prefabricated orthoses as well as using neoprene (and a combination of other materials) to fabricate "soft" low-profile options for this population.

Elastic therapeutic taping (such as Kinesio® Tape, Balance Tex™ tape, SpiderTech™ Tape) can be used to help position and increase the function of the hand. For example, the thumb can be taped in abduction and opposition after a median nerve injury. A Figure-8 design around the proximal phalanx can enhance tip pinch during wrist extension (Figs. 19–42 and 19–43). Chapter 13 provides additional information and techniques for the use of elastic therapeutic taping.

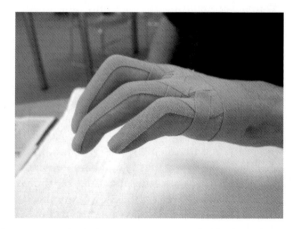

FIGURE 19–43 Elastic therapeutic taping used to facilitate digit extension in this patient who lacerated his median and ulnar nerve. He was a late referral to therapy and had developed PIP flexion contractures. Note the hypothenar atrophy.

TABLE 19–2

Peripheral Nerve Injury: Orthosis Management and Considerations

The guidelines and recommendations outlined in this chart are not meant to be inclusive of every possible product or management technique; rather, the guidelines are to stimulate thought and provide a foundation to build a treatment plan.

Diagnosis	Therapy Goals	Orthosis Guidelines and Recommendations	Considerations
Median nerve			
High and low lacerations	• Prevent adduction contractures of the thumb • Prevent overstretching of the thenar muscles • Prevent IF MCP joint contractures • Prevent tension on the surgical repair	• Week 1 (postsurgery): elbow flexed (high lesion only), wrist flexed, thumb midpalmar/radial abduction immobilization orthosis • Week 3: increase wrist extension of orthosis to tolerance • Weeks 4–5: discontinue elbow for high lesions • Weeks 5–6: discontinue wrist, continue protective orthosis for night and at-risk situations only; children and tenuous repairs 1 week longer; thumb abduction/opposition mobilization strap for day; maintain thumb abduction at night • Week 8: begin gentle mobilization orthosis, if necessary	• Maintain IF passive ROM: extend distal borders of thumb abduction portion of the orthosis (for comfort) • Apply soft material under web portion of orthosis to provide intimate fit (elastomer or silicone gel) • Weeks 5–6: attempt thumb opposition to MF with day orthosis to allow functional pinch through the common origin of the FDP
Pronator syndrome	• Relieve pain and paresthesias • Rest inflamed structures • Prevent provocative motions of the wrist and forearm	• Day: forearm pronation, wrist neutral to slight flexion, immobilization orthosis • Night: for severe symptoms, include elbow in slight flexion	• Fabricate with patient in supine for gravity assist • Careful placement of straps to prevent direct pressure over tender area • The orthosis should be worn until symptoms have subsided and should be only part of a comprehensive rehabilitation program.
Anterior interosseous nerve syndrome	• Simulate pinch while waiting for nerve return • Prevent thumb IP and IF DIP extension contracture	• IF DIP/thumb IP flexion immobilization orthosis (or casts); optional	• Consider orthosis in this position if thumb IP and IF DIP function is required for vocational functional tasks • Thin thermoplastic materials or thin casting materials such as QuickCast or Orficast™ can be used, leaving volar pads free for sensory input
Carpal Tunnel Sydrome	• Decrease pain and paresthesias • Avoid repetitive and/or provocative motions • Rest inflamed structures	• Mild symptoms: day use is optional or depends on physician's preference; wrist immobilized in neutral • Severe symptoms: consider night wrist/hand orthosis to immobilize entire muscle–tendon length	• Allow unimpeded MCP flexion and thumb mobility • The orthosis should be worn until symptoms have subsided and should be only part of a comprehensive rehabilitation program.

CHAPTER 19

(continued)

TABLE 19–2

Peripheral Nerve Injury: Orthosis Management and Considerations (Continued)

Diagnosis	Therapy Goals	Orthosis Guidelines and Recommendations	Considerations
Ulnar nerve			
High and low lacerations	• Prevent RF/SF MCP extension, PIP flexion contractures • Prevent overstretching of intrinsic muscles • Prevent RF/SF MCP collateral ligament shortening • Protect and decrease the tension on surgical repair	• Week 1 (postsurgery): elbow flexed (high lesion only), wrist flexed, immobilization orthosis • Week 3: increase wrist extension in orthosis to tolerance • Weeks 4–5: discontinue elbow for high lesions • Weeks 5–6: discontinue wrist; continue MCP flexion protective orthosis for night and at-risk situations only; children and tenuous repairs 1 week longer; use RF/SF MCP extension restriction orthosis for day • Week 8: begin gentle mobilization orthosis, if necessary	• Allow for full RF/SF MCP flexion • The dorsal component should be well molded to distribute pressure. • Prevent RF/SF collateral ligament shortening • Atrophy of the hypothenar muscles may make the day orthosis difficult to don and doff; incorporate an opening (on dorsal aspect) to ease application.
Cubital tunnel syndrome	• Prevent repetitive and prolonged elbow flexion • Decrease shearing stress on the nerve as it travels through the cubital tunnel • Position the nerve in a resting state	• Day: posterior medial elbow pad; buddy tape SF to RF (if needed) • Night: elbow at 30–40°; wrist neutral with slight ulnar deviation immobilization orthosis • Alternative: elbow flexion restriction orthosis to allow a protected, limited ROM, avoiding full elbow flexion • Alternative: foam on anterior elbow or towel wrap around elbow to prevent elbow flexion at night	• Severe symptoms may require orthosis use during day. • Avoid pressure over epicondyles • Posterior orthosis designs should be well padded over cubital tunnel. • Restriction orthosis may be used for intermittent symptoms and does not allow elbow flexion beyond 90°.[b] • Avoid straps directly over tender or inflamed areas • The orthosis should be worn until symptoms have subsided and should be only part of a comprehensive rehabilitation program.
Ulnar tunnel/ Guyon's canal syndrome	• Decrease stress on the ulnar nerve as it passes through the ulnar tunnel • Protect from direct forces over the pisiform • Avoid provocative activities	• Day and night: immobilization orthosis with wrist 0° to slight flexion; consider padding ulnar/volar wrist area • Alternative: soft neoprene orthosis for work and leisure activities	• Consider applying a silicone gel patch directly over the sensitive area before orthosis fabrication, or use a foam doughnut • The orthosis should be worn until symptoms have subsided and should be only part of a comprehensive rehabilitation program.

TABLE 19–2

Peripheral Nerve Injury: Orthosis Management and Considerations (Continued)

Diagnosis	Therapy Goals	Orthosis Guidelines and Recommendations	Considerations
Combined median and ulnar nerves			
High and low lacerations	• Same goals as listed for each nerve • Maintain three-point pinch	• Week 1 (postsurgery): elbow flexed (high lesion only), wrist flexed, thumb midpalmar and radial abduction immobilization orthosis • Week 3: increase wrist extension in orthosis to tolerance • Weeks 4–5: discontinue elbow for high lesions • Weeks 5–6: discontinue wrist, continue with IF-SF MCP flexion/thumb abduction orthosis for night and at-risk situations only; children and tenuous repairs 1 week longer; use IF-SF MCP extension restriction orthosis for day, with or without thumb • Week 8: begin gentle mobilization orthosis, if necessary	• Orthosis may be difficult; some patients may benefit from an orthosis that recruits power from the radial nerve. • These injuries most often occur in combination with tendon and vascular injury; check with physician for specific protocol. • Paramount to maintain PROM of all involved joints
Radial nerve			
High laceration or compression injury	• Recreate tenodesis action while waiting for nerve return • Prevent overstretching of the wrist, thumb, and digital extensors • Prevent joint contractures (wrist, MCP, and PIP flexion)	• Week 1 (postsurgery): if repair is proximal to the elbow, consider orthosis or casting as follows—elbow flexion/wrist extension/digit and thumb extension immobilization • Weeks 2–3: nonsurgical or compressive injury; use wrist/MCP/thumb extension immobilization orthosis (IPs are free) for day; use wrist extension/MCP flexion/IPs and thumb extension immobilization for night • Alternative: tenodesis orthosis (wrist flex/MCP extension; MCP flex/wrist extension) • Alternative: consider fabricating a wrist immobilization orthosis for work if the tenodesis orthosis is too cumbersome or not appropriate • Alternative: Robinson forearm-based radial nerve glove with wrist (AliMed®) • Alternative: Forearm-based Tunnel Splint® (Benik Corporation) • Alternative: Neoprene custom made (see Chapter 14) • Alternative: LMB™ radial nerve Splint with MCP extension	• Avoid pressure over ulnar styloid; consider prepadding • Take care when fitting all the proximal phalanx slings • Check for appropriate tension when fabricating tenodesis orthosis • The orthosis should be worn until symptoms have subsided and should be only part of a comprehensive rehabilitation program. • Prolonged orthosis use may contribute to weakened extensors.

CHAPTER 19

(continued)

TABLE 19–2

Peripheral Nerve Injury: Orthosis Management and Considerations (Continued)

Diagnosis	Therapy Goals	Orthosis Guidelines and Recommendations	Considerations
Low laceration and posterior interosseous nerve injury	• Recreate tenodesis action while waiting for nerve return • Prevent overstretching of the wrist, thumb, and digital extensors • Prevent joint contractures	• Day: wrist flexion/MCP extension; MCP flexion/wrist extension mobilization orthosis (tenodesis orthosis) • Night: wrist/thumb/digit extension immobilization orthosis • Alternative: hand-based MCP extension mobilization orthosis, with or without thumb extension outrigger • Alternative: Robinson radial nerve glove (AliMed®) • Alternative: Hand-based Tunnel Splint® (Benik Corporation) • Alternative: use of elastic therapeutic taping to assist in digit/thumb extension; can be worn alone or under an orthosis • Alternative: neoprene custom made (see Chapter 14)	• Take care when fitting all the slings • Avoid pressure over the ulnar styloid; consider prepadding • Check for appropriate tension when fabricating tenodesis orthosis • For hand-based orthosis, avoid MCP irritation • Correct thumb position
Radial tunnel syndrome	• Prevent repetitive resisted supination • Avoid provocative positions • Position the nerve in a resting state	• Day and night: wrist extension (30–40°), forearm neutral rotation immobilization orthosis	• When in combination with lateral epicondylitis, orthosis the elbow in 60–90° flexion and the forearm in supination • Avoid strap compression over tender area • The orthosis should be worn until symptoms have subsided and should be only part of a comprehensive rehabilitation program.
Superficial radial nerve syndrome, Wartenberg's syndrome	• Eliminate irritation of the cutaneous branch of the radial nerve about the radial styloid • Protect the area from direct trauma while healing	• Day and night: radial wrist immobilization orthosis that positions the wrist and thumb column to minimize tension on the radial sensory nerve	• Take care when molding; avoid direct pressure over the radial styloid • For severe irritation, consider lifting the material up by making a doughnut to relieve pressure on the entrapped nerve • Alternative: apply silicone gel or padding over this area before applying the orthosis

TABLE 19–2

Peripheral Nerve Injury: Orthosis Management and Considerations (Continued)

Diagnosis	Therapy Goals	Orthosis Guidelines and Recommendations	Considerations
Digital nerves			
Lacerations	• Protect and decrease tension on the surgical repair • Prevent joint MCP, PIP, or DIP contractures • Sensory precautions	• Day and night: hand-based MCP/PIP/DIP extension restriction orthosis (MCP: 45°, PIP: 30°; DIP slight flexion)	• Orthosis position depends greatly on level of digital nerve injury and involvement of other structures (e.g., neurovascular, tendon, ligament). • When orthosis, pay extra attention to the orthosis' borders, making sure they do not dig into insensate areas.

[a]This table is meant as only a guideline for injury management. Keep in mind that other nerve innervations may be present, and the pattern of nerve return is never predictable. This table does not include all possible mixed lesions. Remember that orthosis modifications occur frequently to accommodate motor return. Evaluate for sensory loss, and teach patients careful skin inspection.

[b]Data from Colditz, J. C. (1995). Splinting the hand with a peripheral nerve injury. In J. M. Hunter, E. J. Mackin, & A. D. Callahan (Eds.), *Rehabilitation of the hand* (4th ed., pp. 679–692). St. Louis, MO: Mosby Year Book.

[c]Data from Matloub, H. S., & Yousif, N. J. (1992). Peripheral nerve anatomy and innervation patterns. *Hand Clinics, 8,* 203–214; Bindra, R. R., & Brininger, T. L. (Eds.). (2010). *Advanced concepts in hand pathology and surgery: Application to hand therapy practice* (pp. 145–179). Rosemount, IL: ASSH; and Elfar, J., Petrungaro, J. M., Braun, R. M., Cheng, C. J., Gupta, R., LaBore, A., & Wong, J. E. (2010). Nerve. In W. C. Hammert, R. P. Calfee, D. J. Bozentka, & M. I. Boyer (Eds.), *ASSH manual of hand surgery* (pp. 294–342). Philadelphia, PA: Lippincott Williams & Wilkins.

Tendon Transfers

Tendon transfers are surgical procedures that reestablish balance and active motion to a nerve-injured hand or one that has experienced a complex tendon avulsion or rupture. A tendon transfer procedure uses the tendon of a functioning muscle; it is detached, mobilized, rerouted, and resutured to the tendon of a muscle that has lost innervation or into a bony insertion (Bednar, Judson, & von der Hyde, 2010; Brand, 1995; Hammert et al., 2010; Jones, 1994). Described in this chapter are only common tendon transfers related to specific PNI of the median, ulnar, and radial nerves will. Tendon transfers can be performed for related injuries such as spinal cord injury, stroke, traumatic brain injury, cerebral palsy, and brachial plexus lesions, in which the therapeutic and orthotic intervention may have a similar postoperative course. The reader is referred to the Suggested Reading list for a more in-depth review of the transfers outside the scope of this chapter and detailed discussion of orthotic intervention.

Patients may undergo tendon transfers to substitute for motion of a paralyzed muscle in which peripheral nerve function has not been restored within a reasonable period of time (Bednar et al., 2010; Jones, 1994). The best functional results seem to occur when (1) all involved joints are supple and have full passive motion, (2) edema has subsided and scars have matured, and (3) ulnar and median nerve sensation is at least partially present, although some patients seem to do quite well despite a sensory loss. In most cases, the patient cannot maximize use of the hand without adequate sensory feedback; therefore, the results of the surgical reconstruction will be marginal at best.

Tendons are transferred and repaired with a distinct degree of tension, and the postoperative orthosis program should adequately protect the surgical reconstruction during the healing period (Barbis & Wallace, 1995; Blackmore & Hotchkiss, 1995; Brand, 1995; Chan, Jaglowski, & Kaplan, 1994; Colditz, 1995; Elvey, 1997; Hunter & Whitenack, 1995; Jones, 1994; Lowe & O'Toole, 1995; R. J. Smith, 1987). The postoperative orthosis should relax tension on the surgically transferred muscle(s) by placing the joint that the transferred muscle–tendon unit crosses in a shortened position to allow rest (Bednar et al., 2010). It is also important that the orthosis positions the joint(s) in a manner that protects the proper direction of the transferred tendon's pull. For example, when an opponensplasty has been performed using a slip of the RF FDS tendon guided through an FCU pulley, the orthosis should hold the thumb in a palmar abduction/opposition with the wrist in neutral to slight flexion and ulnar deviation.

The therapist should review with the surgeon the exact reconstruction that was performed before seeing the patient. With good surgeon–therapist communication, a clear picture can be established regarding which muscle–tendon unit was used, what function has been restored, and what the appropriate orthosis design should be (e.g., dorsal vs. volar design). This information can guide the therapist in thorough patient education, proper orthosis fabrication, and optimal therapeutic intervention.

This section reviews functional deficits relative to specific levels of nerve injury. A general discussion is presented; the reader must fully research the specific tendon transfer performed for each patient. The orthosis recommendations given here are meant as only guidelines. Each patient must be evaluated and immobilized or mobilized according to his or her needs and in accordance with the surgeon's protocol. Table 19–3 summarizes orthosis management for common tendon transfers.

Selection of Tendon Transfers

In an ideal situation, the therapist, patient, and surgeon decide on what function is to be restored and what is available to use as a possible donor. The selection process includes the analysis of the anticipated strength of a donor muscle after the transfer, its potential excursion, how many joints it must cross, the direction it must pull in to be effective, and the overall effect the transfer has on the balance of other muscle–tendon units in the extremity (Bednar et al., 2010; Brand, 1995; Colditz, 1995; Jones, 1994; Mackinnon, 1994; R. J. Smith, 1987). Before surgical intervention, the following therapy considerations should have been met:

- Prevent or correct substitution patterns from developing or progressing while awaiting transfer by providing preoperative therapy and orthosis fabrication to encourage the natural use of the hand.
- Achieve and maintain full passive ROM of all involved joints.
- Elongate the involved skin and soft tissue adhesions and joint contractures (Brand, 1995; Colditz, 1995; Jones, 1994; Walsh, 2012).
- Strive to achieve maximal strength (4+) of the donor muscle(s) considered for transfer (Bednar et al., 2010; Brand, 1995; Elfar et al., 2010).
- Patient education regarding postoperative course of the therapy and the importance of orthosis compliance.

Postoperative Therapy Considerations

If a tendon transfer is performed on a *young child*, placing an orthosis on the hand postoperatively may not be appropriate. Children do quite well with the use of a cast for the required healing time (4 to 8 weeks) and then progress directly into the rehabilitation phase. Applying an orthosis that is potentially removable on a young person may tempt him or her to take it off, possibly jeopardizing the surgical reconstruction. The stiffness encountered while wearing the cast is a small price to pay for the security the cast provides to the parents and physician. Joint and musculotendinous tightness can be addressed readily in the young patient.

The application of an orthosis should protect and position the joints properly to avoid too much or too little tension at the transfer site. Too much tension can cause attenuation, rupture, or gap on the anastomosis. Too little tension can cause excessive tightness and tissue contracture.

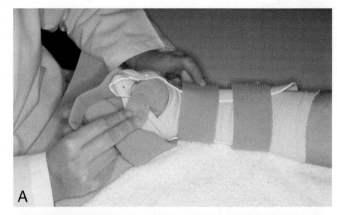
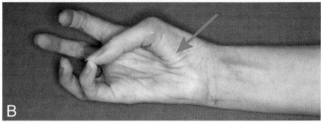

FIGURE 19–44 A, Dorsal wrist and thumb flexion immobilization orthosis, allowing distal strap removal to perform passive exercise as shown here. **B,** During active ROM, the transfer is prominently visible during opposition.

All fabricated orthoses should be carefully inspected for possible areas of compression. Depending on the nerve deficit, sensation can be greatly impaired. It is the therapist's responsibility to teach the patient vigilant skin inspection under the confines of the orthosis and its straps.

Orthoses can be used to initiate limited, guarded active exercise under supervision of a therapist. As shown in Figure 19–44A, the therapist is performing passive and active assistive ROM within the confines of the orthosis. The postoperative exercise regime is dependent on the surgeon's preference, strength of transfer, and any other factors that may influence early motion. Orthoses are generally worn for 3 to 4 weeks then active motion is begun (Fig. 19–44B). The use of a protective orthosis continues for an additional 3 to 6 weeks during at-risk activities and while sleeping.

As the patient progresses, exercise orthoses can be helpful in strengthening a transferred muscle. For example, when approved by the surgeon, exercising with a thumb IP immobilization orthosis after an opponensplasty can (1) block the strong extrinsic FPL tendon from overpowering the weak, newly transferred tendon; (2) retrain the transferred muscle–tendon unit (cortical reorganization) to do its new job; (3) minimize adhesion formation; and (4) increase blood flow and nutrition to the repair site (Fig. 19–45).

Excluding problems from the tension of the transfer, daytime orthoses are generally discontinued at 6 weeks for flexor tendons and approximately 8 weeks for extensor tendons. Extensor tendons are generally weaker than flexor tendons; and therefore, greater caution (held in a shorter resting state)

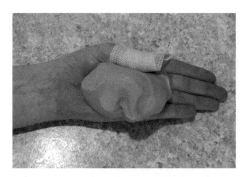

FIGURE 19–45 A small thumb IP immobilization orthosis used to isolate palmar abduction and opposition after an opponensplasty.

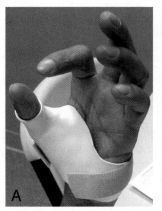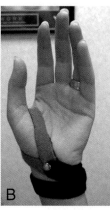

FIGURE 19–46 **A,** A hand-based orthosis can be used after the initial period of rest to free the wrist and position the thumb in opposition and abduction; this decreases the stress on the repair while allowing for light functional use. **B,** At approximately 6 to 8 weeks postsurgery, an opposition strap made from neoprene may be worn intermittently to support and augment the tendon transfer.

and longer protection (8 weeks) should be implemented (Bednar et al., 2010; R. J. Smith, 1987; Stanley-Goodwyn, 1995). The therapist should explain this time frame to the patient/family and consider this when designing the orthosis. Night orthotic management continues as long as necessary to address potential contractures and/or tension-related complications (Bednar et al., 2010).

Mobilization orthoses can be initiated after the initial phase of immobilization (8 to 12 weeks) to gently stretch tight structures, such as tight intrinsic muscles after an extensor tendon transfer. Orthoses used to encourage motion can be fabricated out of lightweight material and used for a home program. For example, immobilizing the IP joint of the thumb can prevent the FPL from overpowering a weak opponensplasty. Various taping and strapping techniques can also be used to facilitate appropriate movement such as thumb palmar abduction and opposition (Walsh, 2012) (Figs. 19–42 and 19–46A,B).

TABLE 19–3
Tendon Transfers

Nerve Involved	Functional Loss	Common Tendon Transfer Options	Orthosis
Median nerve			
High	• Flexion of the thumb IP joint • Flexion of the IF and possibly MF PIP and DIP joints • Thumb opposition and palmar abduction • Wrist radial flexion (FCR)	• BR to FPL to restore IP joint flexion of the thumb • IF and MF FDP side-to-side suture to RF and SF FDP to restore FDP flexion • ECRL to FPL • ECRL to FDP • See also low median nerve tendon transfers	• The elbow is held in 90° of flexion if BR used. The wrist, digits, and thumb are immobilized in some degree of flexion (wrist: 20–30°; MCP: 40–60°; PIP/DIP: neutral to slight flexion; thumb MP and IP: 30°; CMC: midabduction). • Maintain for approximately 4 weeks, with an additional 1–2 weeks for protection only • Consideration should be given to providing a comfortable balance between wrist, digit, and thumb position when this procedure is done in combination with an opponensplasty. • Transfers restore opposition and palmar abduction.

(continued)

TABLE 19–3

Tendon Transfers (Continued)

Nerve Involved	Functional Loss	Common Tendon Transfer Options	Orthosis
Low	• Thumb opposition and palmar abduction • Thumb MCP joint flexion may or may not be noticed secondary to the dual innervation from the ulnar nerve	• EIP to APB or proximal phalanx • FDS RF to FCU pulley to base of thumb proximal phalanx or into APB • PL to APB • EDM to APB	• The wrist from neutral to approximately 30° of flexion; exact position depends on whether a flexor or extensor tendon was used as the donor, and if the approach was via a dorsal or volar route. • EIP: wrist approximately 30° flexion, thumb full abduction, slight palmar flexion, and opposition to approximately MF tip for 4–5 weeks; use as additional protection for 2 weeks. • FDS: wrist neutral, thumb full abduction, slight palmar flexion, and opposition to approximately MF tip for 3–4 weeks; use as additional protection for 1–2 weeks.
Ulnar nerve			
High	• Ulnar wrist flexion (FCU) • DIP joint flexion of RF and SF • See also low lesion	• High ulnar nerve injury can be functionally devastating, grip strength is severely affected; transfers restore grip capabilities and balanced wrist function. • FDS MF or IF to FDP RF and SF to restore digit flexion • FCR to FCU to restore ulnar deviation and wrist flexion	• The wrist is immobilized in neutral to slight extension (15–20°), the MCPs are flexed, and the PIP/DIPs are extended. Thumb CMC in 30° palmar abduction (P Abd). Immobilization is mandatory for 3 weeks with an additional 3 weeks for protection.
Low	• Digital abduction or adduction • MCP joint flexion of RF and SF • PIP and DIP joint extension of RF and SF • Thumb adduction	• Transfers provide MCP flexion and PIP extension (prevent clawing). • FDS MF to radial lateral bands of RF and SF • FDS MF or IF to pulleys of RF and SF (Zancolli lasso operation) • FDS MF to ADP • ECRL or ECRB (with tendon graft) to lateral bands of RF and SF (Brand transfer)[c] • ECRB to ADP with APL accessory to first dorsal interosseous to restore thumb adduction	• See high lesion

TABLE 19–3

Tendon Transfers (Continued)

Nerve Involved	Functional Loss	Common Tendon Transfer Options	Orthosis
Combined median and ulnar nerves			
Low and high	• Thumb abduction and adduction (lateral pinch and opposition) • Thumb IP and IF/MF DIP flexion (tip and three-point pinch) • SF adduction • MCP IF through SF flexion and PIP and DIP extension (claw hand) • Wrist flexion • Volar hand sensory loss	• Transfers provide balance and at least partial function. • Low: (1) ECRB to APB for lateral pinch, (2) EIP to APB/EPL for thumb opposition, (3) APL to first dorsal interossei (possible arthrodesis of MP joint) to restore tip pinch, (4) ECRL or BR to IF through SF A2 pulley area for MCP flexion • High: (1) see low injury, (2) BR to FPL for thumb IP joint flexion, (3) ECU to FCU for wrist flexion	• The wrist is positioned in neutral; the MCPs are flexed; the PIP/DIPs are extended; and the thumb is held in slight flexion, abduction, and opposition. • Check with surgeon for specific positioning measurements
Radial nerve			
High	• Wrist extension • Digit extension and thumb extension • Radial thumb abduction	• The inability to actively control or position the wrist makes grasp and release activities nearly impossible. • Common transfers restore wrist, digit, and thumb extension. • PT to ECRB, FCU to EDC, PL to EPL • PT to ECRB, FCR to EDC, PL to EPL • PT to ECRL plus ECRB, FDS MF to EDC MF/SF, FDS RF to EIP and EPL, FCR to APL and EPB	• Postoperative cast position includes elbow flexion to 90°, maximum pronation, wrist extension to 30–40°, MCPs at 0°, CMC in extension and abduction, and PIP/DIP joints free. • Maintain in a cast for 3–4 weeks, unless the protocol differs • After 4 weeks, orthosis for 3–4 weeks in the same position with gradual weaning for supervised exercise and hygiene
Low	• Digit extension • Thumb extension	• Transfers restore digit and thumb extension. • FCU to EDC, PL to EPL • FDS MF to EDC MF/SF, FDS RF to EIP and EPL, FCR to APL and EPB • FCR to EDC, PL to EPL	• Same position and time frame as for high lesion with exclusion of the elbow

[a]This table is meant as only a guideline for injury management. It provides the basic background information needed for challenging cases. Remember that the exact design and position of joints within the orthosis must be determined by close communication with the surgeon. This table does not include all possible tendon transfers and does not list all available orthotic interventions.

[b]Data from American Society for Surgery of the Hand. (1995). *Regional review courses in hand surgery* (Vols. 4 & 21). Englewood, CO: Author; Jones, N. F. (1994). Tendon transfers. In M. Cohen (Ed.), *Mastery of plastic and reconstructive surgery* (pp. 1579–1597). Boston, MA: Little, Brown; and Smith, R. J. (1987). *Tendon transfers of the hand and forearm*. Boston, MA: Little, Brown.

[c]Data from Jones, N. F. (1994). Tendon transfers. In M. Cohen (Ed.), *Mastery of plastic and reconstructive surgery* (pp. 1579–1597). Boston, MA: Little, Brown; and Brand. P. W. (1995). Mechanics of tendon transfers. In J. M. Hunter, E. J. Mackin, & A. D. Callahan (Eds.), *Rehabilitation of the hand* (4th ed., pp. 715–727). St. Louis, MO: Mosby Year Book.

[d]Data from Blackmore, S. M., & Hotchkiss, R. N. (1995). Therapist's management of ulnar neuropathy at the elbow. In J. M. Hunter, E. J. Mackin, & A. D. Callahan (Eds.), *Rehabilitation of the hand* (4th ed., pp. 665–677). St. Louis, MO: Mosby Year Book.

Data from Bednar, M., Judson, E., & von der Hyde, R. (2010). Tendon transfers to restore upper limb function. In R. R. Bindra & T. L. Brininger (Eds.), *Advanced concepts in hand pathology and surgery: Application to hand therapy practice* (pp. 165–179). Rosemount, IL: ASSH.

ADP, adductor pollicis; *APB*, abductor pollicis brevis; *APL*, abductor pollicis longus; *BR*, brachioradialis; *CMC*, carpometacarpal; *ECU*, extensor carpi ulnaris; *EDC*, extensor digitorum communis; *EDM*, extensor digiti minimi; *EIP*, extensor indices proprius; *EPL*, extensor pollicis longus; *FCR*, flexor carpi radialis; *PL*, palmaris longus; *PT*, pronator teres.

Conclusion

This chapter has focused on the role of the orthosis in various conditions of nerve injury and/or repair. With the information in this chapter, the reader should appreciate the importance of orthotic intervention in this patient population. Not only is the orthosis used to protect the body part after injury and/or surgical repair but it also can play a critical role in granting functional independence. The future for the surgeon and clinician managing the nerve-injured hand is exciting. Early referral to a "nerve" specialist combined with developments in surgical techniques and procedures, innovative motor and sensory nerve grafting and transfers, and the skilled intervention of a hand therapist foster improved functional outcomes for this challenging patient population.

CASE STUDY SECTION

The case studies presented here are meant as a teaching guideline only. Treatment and orthosis protocols vary greatly from surgeon to surgeon and from therapist to therapist. The therapist should check with the referring physicians and colleagues to define the preferred treatment and appropriate orthotic intervention.

CASE STUDY 1: High-Level Radial Nerve Injury

GH is a 39-year-old, right-dominant female who sustained a right midhumeral fracture, right distal radius fracture, and radial nerve injury during a hit-and-run accident. In the emergency room, she was placed in a long arm cast with her elbow at 90°, forearm pronated, wrist in slight flexion, and digits left free. Because of the edema in her hand and digits and her inability to extend her digits, she was referred to hand therapy with a question of radial nerve injury.

Upon clinical examination, it was noted that she did indeed have symptoms consistent with radial nerve compression or injury. GH was unable to extend her digits or thumb actively within the cast. Therefore, an MCP extension mobilization orthosis was fabricated to fit directly over the cast similar to Figure 19-41. This allowed the patient to use her digits purposefully and prevent overstretching of the digit and thumb extensors (Fig. 19–41).

The cast was removed 6 weeks later. Upon examination, GH demonstrated weak triceps function and no active wrist, digit, or thumb extension. She had impaired sensibility over the dorsoradial aspect of her forearm. She required continued orthosis intervention to substitute for loss of muscle function. A wrist flexion/MCP extension, wrist extension/MCP flexion orthosis was chosen (radial nerve orthosis). This design allowed the patient to take advantage of the natural tenodesis effect of the digits with wrist movement. When the wrist extends, the digits flex; when the wrist flexes, the digits extend (Fig. 19–33A). This orthosis design allows full use of the palmar surface of the hand and is light in weight. GH continued with the orthosis for approximately 6 weeks. At night, she wore a simple wrist/hand/thumb immobilization orthosis (Fig. 19–34), which she found did not disrupt her sleep. In therapy, the patient worked on regaining wrist motion and strength.

When her wrist extensors were strong enough to support themselves against gravity, she was placed in a hand-based MCP/thumb extension mobilization orthosis (Fig. 19–36C) while waiting for the return of the distal motor branch of the PIN. GH wore the orthosis for activities of daily living (ADLs) and work-related tasks. Compliance with wearing the orthosis was not an issue because of its low-profile design. She was able to take it off with increased frequency while waiting return of nerve function, which took an additional 5 weeks. Eventually, she discarded all orthoses and worked on a general strengthening program.

Additional case studies can be found on the companion web site on thePoint.

Chapter Review Questions

1. Name the three main peripheral nerves of the upper extremity, describing the motor and sensory function of each.

2. What are the general principles in managing a peripheral nerve injury? What are the unique roles of immobilization, mobilization and restriction orthoses in this patient population?

3. Describe the conservative management for a compression injury of the median nerve.

4. Describe the injury associated with a high radial nerve laceration and what distal orthotic intervention(s) a therapist can provide to allow for some functional use.

5. Not initially prominent, in a high ulnar nerve injury, what must a therapist be concerned with? What interventions should a therapist consider?

The Athlete

Kimberly Goldie Staines, OTR, CHT
Evan D. Collins, MD*

Chapter Objectives

After study of this chapter, the reader should be able to:

- Describe common sport-specific diagnoses of the upper extremity.
- Understand the clinical reasoning process for selecting the most appropriate orthosis for an athlete.
- Explain how management of the athlete differs from other patient populations when managing upper extremity diagnoses.

- Appreciate the unique sport-specific factors related to orthotic intervention.
- Identify various materials and application techniques used in the management of this unique population.

Key Terms

Bennett's fracture
Biceps tendon rupture
Boutonniere deformity
Bowler's thumb
Carpal tunnel syndrome
Cubital tunnel syndrome
Cyclist's palsy
DeQuervain's tenosynovitis
Distal radius fractures

Distal ulna instability
Flexor digitorum profundus avulsion
Handlebar palsy
Intersection syndrome
Lateral epicondylitis
Mallet finger
Medial epicondylitis
Metacarpal fractures
Olecranon bursitis

Phalangeal fractures
PIP joint dislocation
Playing orthosis
Pronator syndrome
Radial tunnel syndrome
Scaphoid fracture
Thumb MP joint sprain
Triangular fibrocartilage complex

Introduction

Hand and wrist injuries are common among athletes, equaling approximately half of all sporting injuries sustained by the general population (Simpson & McQueen, 2006). Although the hand does not often bear weight and these injuries do not always sideline an athlete, careful attention must be made when treating injuries of the hand and wrist (Alexy & De Carlo, 1998). Fabricating orthoses for upper extremity injuries poses unique challenges for the clinician. These challenges do not arise primarily from the injuries seen but are often related to the unique demands of the athlete. Approximately one in four

---

*This chapter is based on the first edition chapter written by Lisa Schulz Slowman, MS, OTR/L, CHT.

injuries sustained in sports involves the hand and wrist (Barton, 1997). The injured athlete, whether high school, collegiate, professional, or recreational, is generally eager to return to activity and competition as soon as possible. Often, the therapist is asked to provide an orthosis that offers adequate protection to facilitate the early return to sports without simultaneously limiting or interfering with the athlete's performance nor posing a risk of injury to other athletes in the game.

The purpose of this chapter is to highlight common sport-specific injuries and review options in orthotic management. Common upper extremity injuries include bony and ligamentous injuries to the elbow, forearm, wrist, hand, thumb, and digits in addition to a variety of other soft tissue injuries.

Implications for Orthotic Fabrication

As with any condition, the orthotic requirements for upper extremity injuries in athletes change as the athlete progresses through the phases of rehabilitation, from acute injury to return to sport (Schulz, Busconi, & Pappas, 1995). Several factors need to be considered when fabricating an orthosis, which include a prior history of similar injuries, the athlete's age and level of competition, the sport-specific demands of the athlete, and the rules established by the governing bodies relating to the use of protective devices during competition (Bertini et al., 2011).

General Orthotic Considerations

Athletes with upper extremity injuries progress through the phases of rehabilitation. These phases include acute injury management, initial rehabilitation, progressive rehabilitation, integrated functions, and return to sport (Skerker & Schulz, 1995). In the early phases of rehabilitation, orthotic goals are generally to provide rest and protection to the injured structure(s) while allowing easy removal of the orthosis for initiation of a range of motion (ROM) program and management of soft tissue trauma. Other rehabilitation goals during this initial period are to decrease edema and pain.

As the athlete progresses, orthotic goals begin to focus on providing protection to the injured structure(s) while minimally interfering with the upper extremity function of the athlete. For example, a hockey player who sustains a metacarpal fracture initially requires a wrist and metacarpophalangeal (MCP) joint immobilization orthosis to protect the fracture; the player removes the orthosis to do protected ROM exercises. As the athlete advances to return to competition, he or she may be

fitted with a similarly positioned hand-based orthosis that fits into the hockey glove; this facilitates early return to competition.

Any orthosis or protective device provided to an athlete should protect the injured structure(s) and prevent reinjury, allow safe and effective participation in the sport, should not pose an injury threat to an opposing athlete, and should meet the demands of the governing bodies for the sport and the local game officials (Bertini et al., 2011; DeCarlo, Malone, Darmelio, and Rettig, 1994). The specific rules regarding the use of orthoses, casts, and other types of protective equipment depend on the sport and the level of competition. Information regarding the rules and guidelines is readily available; some sources are listed in Table 20–1.

Close communication between the treating physicians, team athletic trainers, and/or coaches is crucial to provide safe return to play while limiting stress to the involved structures in order to limit the risk of reinjury (Singletary & Geissler, 2009). These team members provide valuable information regarding the injury and help the therapist gain an understanding of the sport-specific demands to help maximize the orthotic intervention. Specific demands include the level of competition, type of sport, and position played. It is also important to know the athlete's goals for continued participation in the sport. For example, a high school field hockey player with the prospect of a collegiate sports scholarship may have a stronger desire to return to competition compared to a high school freshman playing field hockey for the first time.

If the athlete uses gloves or other equipment (e.g., sticks, clubs, bats, braces, handlebars), it is important that the athlete has them when any orthosis is fabricated. This allows the therapist to make any necessary modifications to permit continued effective use of the equipment while protecting the injury without creating pressure areas or impingement from the orthosis (Fig. 20–1).

TABLE 20–1

Sports Rules and Regulations

National Collegiate Athletic Association (NCAA)

6201 College Blvd.

Overland Park, KS 66211-2422

913-339-1906

www.NCAA.org

College sports

National Federation of State High School Associations (NFHS)

P.O. Box 20626 (64195-0626)

11724 Northwest Plaza Circle

Kansas City, MO 64153

816-464-5400

www.NFHS.org

High school sports

American Alliance for Health, Physical Education, Recreation and Dance (AAHPERD)

1900 Association Dr.

Reston, VA 20191

703-476-3400

www.AAHPERD.org

High school sports

Finally, educating the athlete and team staff about the purpose of the orthosis is imperative. The athlete should understand why the orthosis is necessary, when and how it should be used and cared for, and the plan for duration of use and weaning from the orthosis. The better the athlete understands the purpose of the orthosis, the greater the chance for compliance and the lower the patient's risk for reinjury. It is also important that the athlete's coach, athletic trainer, team members, and family understand the purpose and importance of the orthosis to help reinforce its use.

Material Selection

There are various materials and strapping systems that may be good choices for athletes. The choice of material depends on the objective for the orthosis. In the initial phases of rehabilitation, the goal for the orthosis may be to provide protection during daily activities and to allow removal for hygiene and ROM exercises. For protective purposes, a ⅛″ material is typically appropriate for orthotic fabrication. As the athlete returns to practice and competition, a **playing orthosis** may be suitable. Thick external padding of a rigid orthosis works well as a transitional orthosis by providing impact absorption while continuing to rigidly protect healing structures. If only soft support is necessary, a neoprene orthosis with or without a rigid support may be appropriate (Fig. 20–2). Neoprene material is a synthetic, latex-free rubber that is available in various thickness, densities, elasticity, and perforations. It is able to provide flexible support and compression via prefabricated or custom-fabricated orthoses (see Chapter 14 on Neoprene for further information).

The body part being fitted also influences the material selection. A thinner material with memory, such as ¹⁄₁₆″ or ³⁄₃₂″ Aquaplast or Orfit thermoplastic, is an option to consider for digit-based immobilization orthoses used after a fracture (Fig. 20–3). This thinner material may not be appropriate for a wrist and thumb immobilization orthosis, for example, following a scaphoid fracture, which requires a ⅛″ thermoplastic for greater durability, rigidity, and protection (Fig. 20–4).

When determining the best material to use for a protective orthosis for an athlete returning to competition, the therapist should consider the hardness (rigidity) of the material (must be strong enough to protect and stabilize

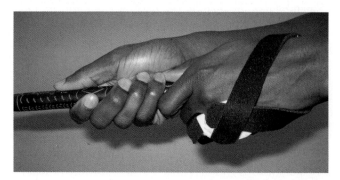

FIGURE 20–1 The therapist must consider the injured athlete's sports equipment when fabricating or fitting an orthosis. This RF and SF digit immobilization orthosis is protecting a healing SF PIP joint injury in this golfer.

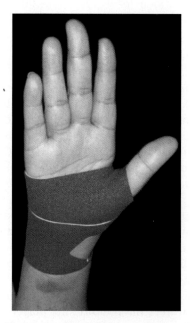

FIGURE 20–2 Neoprene offers support, warmth, and restriction of joint motion.

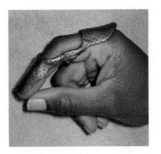

FIGURE 20–3 A PIP extension restriction orthosis for a volar plate avulsion fracture fabricated from ¹⁄₁₆″ material.

the injured structures), the ability of the material to absorb an impact (flexibility), and the rules of the sport's governing body and local officials regarding playing with orthoses and/or casts (DeCarlo et al., 1994). Consider that professional and collegiate athletes can usually return to competition with a hard cast or an orthosis provided that it is covered with soft padding, but this is generally not allowed in high school contact sports. The sport's governing body may dictate the thickness and type of padding material, but generally closed-cell foam at least ¾″ thick is appropriate to encompass the device. If the athlete requires padding only in competition, consider securing the padding in place with an elastic wrap so that it can be removed when the athlete is not competing (Fig. 20–5A,B).

Material options include low-temperature thermoplastics, room-temperature vulcanizing (RTV) silicone rubber, tape, fiberglass-based materials (Scotchcast™ and Plastazote®),

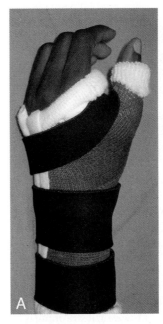 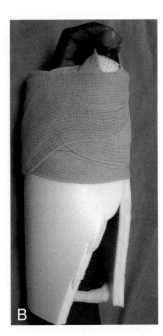

FIGURE 20–5 **A,** A Delta-Cast® conforming thumb and wrist orthosis for a scaphoid fracture; split and secured with elasticized loop to allow for edema and skin care. **B,** Cast covered with ½″ closed cell padding and secured with an elastic bandage for return to sport.

Delta-Cast® Conformable Casting Tape (BSN medical Inc., Charlotte, NC), and neoprene materials (Bouvette, Malanga, Cooney, Stuart, & Miller, 1994; Canelon, 1995; Colditz, 1999). Materials applied circumferentially, such as QuickCast 2 and Orficast™ that contain a combination of rubber and fiberglass, have simplified many orthotic applications. A circumferential digit orthosis fabricated from either of these materials eliminates the need for straps. If the orthosis is made without a liner, the athlete does not have to remove the cast for hygiene because of the material's mesh-like quality. In addition to the benefit of air exchange, these materials are extremely durable, allowing the athlete to sweat, bathe, or swim with limited risk of maceration. This works especially well for acute boutonniere and mallet injuries; the ability to get the hand wet is appreciated along with the slim custom fit (Fig. 20–6).

Additional considerations for orthotic material selection include the use of perforated materials to decrease perspiration and minimize skin irritation. The use of colored materials and strapping to coordinate with uniforms should also be considered, which may improve wear compliance. The therapist should be aware of the temperature and environment in which the athlete will be wearing the orthosis. A diver may require a perforated orthosis to limit skin irritation, whereas a rugby player in Texas may not tolerate thermoplastic material due to the heat exposure and humidity.

Strapping Selection

The strapping systems used for athletic orthoses are unique, especially for those used in conjunction with other equipment. For example, a thumb immobilization orthosis that is

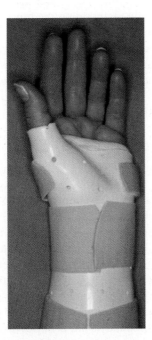

FIGURE 20–4 Wrist and thumb immobilization orthosis fabricated from ⅛″ material to provide a rigid support for a healing scaphoid fracture. Note full clearance of the IP joint.

CHAPTER 20

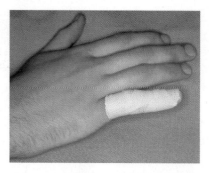

FIGURE 20–6 Circumferential digit immobilization orthosis fabricated from QuickCast 2 allows this patient with an acute central tendon injury to bathe with the orthosis on.

fabricated for a motorbike racer who is returning to competition may not require a strap. Rather, the orthosis may be held in place by the bike glove (Fig. 20–7). A strap in this case is unnecessary and could interfere with the cyclist's feel and grip of the handlebars in the palm. However, if strapping is to be used under equipment, consider soft strapping material or taping to minimize the risk of skin irritation from friction.

Sometimes, it is appropriate to use a circumferential elasticized wrap, such as an elastic bandage (Coban™ or Ace™ Wrap), to hold an orthosis in place. This secures the orthosis while distributing the pressure evenly on the body part. A padded wrist orthosis used during practice by a football blocker may best be secured with an elasticized bandage (Fig. 20–5B).

Another option for securing a return to sport orthoses is tape. There are a multitude of options that can be used to limit migration of the orthosis and bulk under equipment. You may use ½″ paper or silk tape for the application of a finger orthosis, whereas athletic tape or elastic therapeutic tape (Kinesio®) may be used to secure a hand- or forearm-based orthosis. Be sure that the tape selected has enough adhesion to secure the orthosis with sweat and friction from external sports equipment. When using high tack tapes,

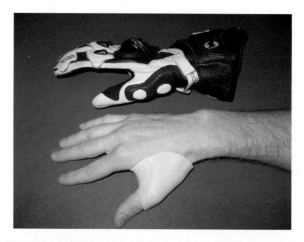

FIGURE 20–7 Thumb immobilization orthosis using thermoplastic material that can be secured inside a motocross glove without additional strapping.

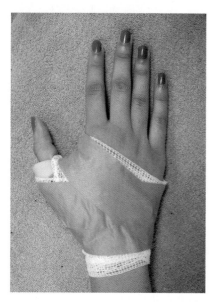

FIGURE 20–8 Wrapping the hand with gauze prior to taping on the orthosis will prevent skin irritation and ease removal/reuse.

such as athletic tape, be sure to use roll gauze (Kerlix) or prewrap to allow for easy removal and reuse of the orthosis (Fig. 20–8).

It is important that the strapping best suits the needs of the athlete. Whenever possible, the athlete should bring the sports equipment that will be used or worn while wearing the orthosis to the clinic. The athlete should practice using the orthosis with the equipment prior to leaving the clinic so the therapist can make any reasonable alterations to the orthosis. The therapist must work with the athlete to customize the strapping system and allow maximal upper extremity use while maintaining the function of the orthosis and protecting the injury. Athletes should be given additional sets of strapping, especially those involved in aquatic activities such as rowing, kayaking, swimming, water polo, and diving so that dry straps are always available for securing the orthosis. This is necessary for maintaining good skin integrity under the straps.

Orthosis Options

Orthotic fabrication includes articular and nonarticular, immobilization, and restriction orthoses involving the elbow (EO), wrist hand (WHO), hand (HO), hand finger (HFO), and finger (FO) that includes the thumb (Bash et al., 2011). Articular orthoses stabilize or restrict the motion across a joint. Examples of articular orthoses include a thumb MP immobilization orthosis (FO) used to protect a healing ulnar collateral ligament (UCL) on a cyclist (Fig. 20–7) and a proximal interphalangeal (PIP) joint extension restriction orthosis (FO) used to prevent reinjury of the volar plate in a soccer player (Fig. 20–3). Nonarticular orthoses do not cross a joint but provide stability to soft tissue or bony structures to treat or prevent injury. Examples of nonarticular orthoses are a proximal phalanx orthosis (FO), also known as a pulley ring,

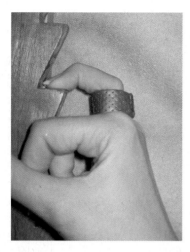

FIGURE 20–9 Nonarticular proximal phalanx orthosis (pulley ring) to limit bowstringing of flexors for return to sport after tendon injury.

for a rock climber to protect against flexor tendon sheath injury (Fig. 20–9) and a proximal forearm orthosis (EO), also known as an epicondylitis strap, used to absorb and disperse forces of the forearm muscles as they approach the medial and/or lateral epicondyle(s) (Fig. 20–10) (Warme & Brooks, 2000; Whaley & Baker, 2004; Wichmann & Martin, 1996).

Sport-Specific Injuries

Hand and wrist injuries are more common in adolescents than adults. Over a 10-year period, the Cleveland Clinic found that 14.8% of athletic participants younger than the age of 16 years sustained upper extremity injuries. Of these, 16% involved the hand, whereas 9% involved the wrist (A. C. Rettig, 1998). Management of specific common upper extremity injuries such as fractures, fracture/dislocations, ligamentous injury, muscle/tendon ruptures, and nerve injury are discussed in detail elsewhere in this book (see Chapters 16, 18, and 19). A brief description of common sport-related injuries are reviewed in the following text. Table 20–2 summarizes orthotic selection and fabrication for sport-specific injuries. Relying on basic science knowledge of connective tissue healing, protection, and immobilization is important

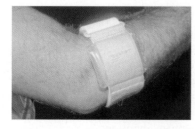

FIGURE 20–10 A proximal forearm orthosis (counterforce brace or epicondylitis strap) used to reduce stress at the proximal muscle insertion.

in the first phase of healing (Kannus, Parkhari, Jarvinen, Jarvinen, & Jarvinen, 2003).

Fractures

In sport, upper limb fractures are much more common than lower limb and axial skeletal fractures, accounting for 76.7% of sports fractures seen (Aitken & Court-Brown, 2008). When treating an athlete with an acute fracture, the therapist must consider the stability of the injury as well as the patient's age, level of competition, position played, and desire to return to sport. Fractures sustained by athletes during competition due to low impact forces can be stable injuries treated with immobilization followed by a transition into a playing orthosis for early return to competition (A. C. Rettig, 1991). Fabrication of an orthosis for an unstable fracture requires the stabilization of the joint proximal and distal to the fracture. Unstable fractures may require surgical intervention, resulting in a more variable course of treatment. Refer to Chapter 16 for more comprehensive information regarding orthotic management for fractures.

Distal Radius

Distal radius fractures are common in sporting activities; the usual mechanism of injury is a fall on an outstretched hand (FOOSH). These injuries tend to be high-energy fractures and involve the articular surfaces, causing disruption of the distal radioulnar and distal radiocarpal joints (M.E. Rettig & Raskin, 2000). After cast removal, a wrist immobilization orthosis with a circumferential design may offer the most protection for the athlete while he or she begins to progress through the later stages of rehabilitation. A custom bivalved or zipper-type orthosis may be used for initial return to practice and conditioning as well as transition to return to play with padding (Fig. 20–11A,B). Returning to full sport participation depends on the sport-specific requirements and the demands placed on the healing extremity. For example, a soccer player (except the goalie) may be able to return to play before a football player because of the individual upper extremity demands of the sports.

Scaphoid

A **scaphoid fracture** in sports can occur with a fall on an outstretched arm with maximum wrist extension (football, soccer, biking). Stable nondisplaced fractures are often immobilized in either a long arm or a short arm thumb cast (Fig. 20–12), followed by orthosis application during the initial return to play (Fig. 20–4) (M. E. Rettig & Raskin, 2000). If bone healing is slow and both the physician and the athlete agree that return to a guarded level of performance may be of benefit, then a protective playing cast made from conforming cast material and external padding may be appropriate (Canelon & Karus, 1995; A. C. Rettig, 1991). In the collegiate or professional athlete, percutaneous fixation of nondisplaced scaphoid fractures may be done to facilitate early return to competition in a playing cast. Whether or not the athlete may return to play with a scaphoid fracture is controversial and depends on the

TABLE 20–2

Orthoses for Sports Injuries

Diagnosis	Orthosis Options	Return to Sport	Considerations	Return to Play
Distal radius and/or ulna fracture	After surgery or cast removal: • Wrist immobilization orthosis	• Circumferential wrist orthosis (primarily with contact sports) • Neoprene wrist orthosis	• Adapt playing orthosis to athlete's upper extremity demands • Well padded on outside for contact sports	• With confirmed healing, protective orthosis worn for 2–4 weeks per physician recommendation and sports-specific position requirements
Scaphoid fracture	After surgery or cast removal: • Wrist and thumb MP immobilization orthosis	• Circumferentially padded wrist and thumb immobilization orthosis • Neoprene wrist/thumb orthosis • Wrist/thumb taping	• Adapt playing orthosis to athlete's upper extremity demands • Trim thumb portion of neoprene orthosis to allow necessary motion • Tape to limit full thumb motion, protecting against hyperextension and radial deviation forces	• Per physician recommendation and sports-specific position requirements • Use of playing orthosis depends on status of scaphoid healing and sport demands on the hand/wrist
Metacarpal fracture	After surgery or cast removal: • Wrist and MCP or hand-based MCP immobilization orthosis	Depends on fracture stability and sport-specific demands • Buddy taping • Wrist and MCP or hand-based MCP immobilization orthosis	• Make sure orthosis is adapted to equipment used by athlete (hockey stick and glove, bicycle handlebars, ski glove and pole) • Pad the exterior of return to play orthosis to prevent slipping on equipment	• Per physician recommendation and sports-specific position requirements • May return to play with sport orthosis depending on fracture healing and demands of sport
Phalangeal fracture	After surgery or cast removal: • Hand-based digit immobilization orthosis • Buddy taping	Depends on fracture stability and sport-specific demands • Digit or hand immobilization orthosis for injured digit(s) only • Digit or hand immobilization orthosis for injured and adjacent digits • Buddy taping to adjacent digits	• Orthosis should provide enough stability to protect fracture and be adapted to allow athlete to meet upper extremity demands • Adapt orthosis to equipment as necessary	• Per physician recommendation and sports-specific position requirements
PIP fracture and/or dislocation (volar plate injury)	Acute (nonoperative management): • Hand-based PIP extension restriction orthosis (extension allowed is increased weekly until full extension is attained)	• PIP extension restriction orthosis • Buddy taping to adjacent digit	• Orthosis should position PIP in appropriate degree of flexion determined by fracture reduction • Early motion program and edema management are important	• PIP extension restriction orthosis used for initial 2–4 weeks • Buddy taping continues for 4–6 months during competition

TABLE 20–2

Orthoses for Sports Injuries (Continued)

Diagnosis	Orthosis Options	Return to Sport	Considerations	Return to Play
Central tendon rupture (Acute boutonniere injury)	Acute (nonoperative management): • PIP or IP extension immobilization orthosis • Serial digital cast immobilizing PIP joint while allowing DIP flexion	• Digital cast with PIP and DIP extension to protect DIP from hyperextension injury • PIP or IP immobilization orthosis • Taping	• Watch for problems with skin maceration or breakdown at dorsal PIP joint • Changes in edema require frequent adjustments • Orthosis must maintain PIP in full extension when DIP is actively flexed with exercise	• Used 4–6 weeks (day and night) • Used 4–8 weeks between ROM exercises and at night • Used 8 or more weeks at night and as required during the day
Terminal tendon rupture (Mallet finger)	Acute (nonoperative management): • DIP extension immobilization orthosis • Digital cast immobilizing DIP joint while allowing PIP flexion	• DIP extension immobilization orthosis • Digital cast immobilizing DIP joint while allowing PIP flexion • Circumferential IP taping • Neoprene DIP orthosis	• Watch for problems with skin maceration or breakdown at dorsal DIP joint • Changes in edema require frequent adjustments • Watch for inadvertent removal of orthosis if used under glove	• Use 6 weeks (day and night) • Use 6–8 weeks ROM exercise and at night • Use 8 or more weeks at night and as needed during the day
FDP avulsion (jersey finger)	After surgical repair: • Wrist flexion/MCP flexion/IP extension immobilization orthosis	• Dorsal DIP immobilization orthosis with DIP slightly flexed • Circumferential DIP cast • Circumferential DIP taping	• With repaired tendon, follow protocol precautions • Generally, athlete will not return to competition for at least 12 weeks	• Use 4–6 weeks (day and night) • Use 6–8 weeks for additional protection only
Thumb UCL injury (skier's or gamekeeper's thumb)	After surgical repair (Stener lesion): • Wrist/thumb MP immobilization orthosis After cast immobilization: • Thumb immobilization orthosis Return to sport: • Hand-based orthosis during sport for 1–2 months Partial tear: • Hand-based thumb MP immobilization orthosis • Taping	• Hand-based thumb MP immobilization orthosis • Neoprene thumb orthosis • Thumb MP circumferential taping	• Adapt orthosis to equipment used by athlete	• After surgery: use for approximately 8 weeks • After casting: use 6–8 weeks • Partial tear: use 4–6 weeks

(continued)

TABLE 20–2

Orthoses for Sports Injuries (Continued)

Diagnosis	Orthosis Options	Return to Sport	Considerations	Return to Play
Medial epicondylitis (golfer's elbow)	• Proximal forearm orthoses (counter-force brace: Epitrain, Nirschl Count'R Force brace) or custom-made nonarticular forearm orthosis • Taping (Chapter 13)	• Proximal forearm orthosis • Taping (Chapter 13)	• In addition to bracing, patient education, anti-inflammatory treatment, massage, ice, activity modification, and equipment modification (wider handle) may help	• Depends on symptoms
Lateral epicondylitis (tennis elbow)	• Proximal forearm orthoses—prefabricated or custom (counterforce brace: Epitrain, Nirschl Count'R Force brace) • Taping	• Proximal forearm orthosis • Taping	• In addition to orthotic management, patient education, anti-inflammatory treatment, massage, ice, activity modification, and equipment modification (wider handle, string tension) may help	• Depends on symptoms
Guyon's canal syndrome (handlebar palsy)	Acute symptoms: • Wrist immobilization orthosis in neutral to slight flexion and ulnar deviation Return to sport: • Padded biking gloves	• Padded biking gloves • Custom strap with padding	• Padding may require modification (doughnut) to relieve pressure on the nerve	• Depends on symptoms
Dorsal impaction syndrome (gymnast's wrist)	Return to sport: • Wrist immobilization orthosis to decrease wrist hyperextension • Neoprene orthosis • Taping	• Neoprene orthosis	• Minimize palmar contact area in the hand with orthotic material and strapping • Patient education regarding changing hand position and periodic stretching • Consider prefabricated or neoprene orthosis to restrict hyperextension	• Continuous use for practice and competition • Not used for daily activities

IP, interphalangeal; *PROM*, passive range of motion.

sport, athlete, location of the fracture, stability of the fracture, and ability to safely participate in a cast/protective orthosis (Jaworski, Krause, & Brown, 2010).

Thumb Metacarpal

Fracture of the base of the first metacarpal, a **Bennett's fracture**, is often associated with a fall on a hyperextended thumb, as in a baseball player diving for a ball or sliding into a secured base. The fracture is accentuated by the strong pull of the abductor pollicis longus (APL) tendon as it inserts on the base of the first metacarpal. The athlete generally undergoes a period cast immobilization (Fig. 20–12), progressing to a return-to-sport wrist and thumb immobilization orthosis (Fig. 20–4). For unstable first metacarpal fractures in athletes, especially for the professional athlete, surgical fixation may be the treatment of choice because surgical fixation may facilitate an earlier return to play.

Digit Metacarpals

Fracture of the neck, shaft, or base of the metacarpal bone(s) can be sustained from blunt trauma (hit with a lacrosse stick, goalie block in soccer) and, more commonly, from

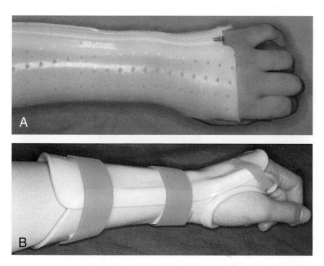

FIGURE 20–11 Circumferential wrist immobilization orthoses. **A,** Rolyan® AquaForm™ Zippered Wrist Splint and clamshell design (**B**) with interlocking volar and dorsal pieces.

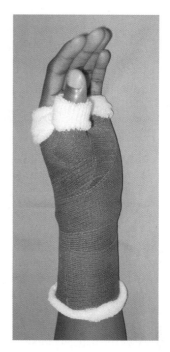

FIGURE 20–12 Wrist and thumb cast used after scaphoid fracture.

punching-type sports (boxing, karate, blocking sports). Initially, metacarpal shaft fractures may be immobilized in a cast or orthosis including the wrist and digits (Fig. 20–13A,B). In some instances, metacarpal shaft fractures may be adequately treated with a simple nonarticular metacarpal immobilization orthosis (Fig. 20–13C), which traverses the involved metacarpal and adjacent structures. Often, this orthosis is supplemented with finger buddy taping to limit lateral and rotational forces across the fracture. When

treating a young athlete, the therapist should consider adding the proximal phalanx within the orthosis (Fig. 20–13D). Including the MCP joint in the orthosis provides greater protection and stability against external forces across the proximal injury (Jaworski et al., 2010).

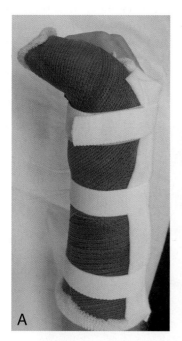
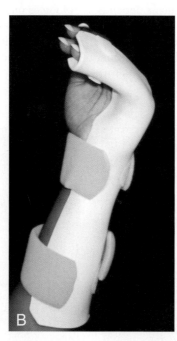
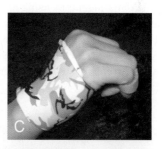
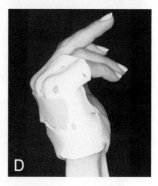

FIGURE 20–13 Various ways to immobilize a metacarpal fracture. **A,** Ulnar-based wrist and digit Delta-Cast® Conforming Cast. **B,** Forearm-based design in the antideformity position. **C,** Nonarticular metacarpal orthosis with buddy taping RF/SF. **D,** Hand-based design with MCP joint included to further protect distal metacarpal fractures.

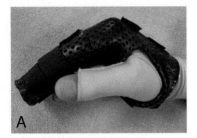
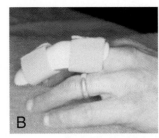
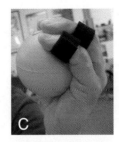

FIGURE 20–14 **A,** Hand-based index finger (IF) and MF orthosis for proximal phalanx fracture; notice edema glove used beneath. **B,** PIP joint extension restriction orthosis for a volar plate avulsion fracture. **C,** Buddy taping of RF and SF can be challenging because of the difference in the length of the digits. Custom straps to accommodate for this difference are necessary to allow unrestricted joint motion.

A metacarpal neck fracture of the ring finger (RF) or small finger (SF) can be managed after cast removal with an orthosis that immobilizes the ulnar two metacarpals along with the middle finger (MF) metacarpal, positioning the MCP joints in flexion (Fig. 20–13D). Anchoring the RF and SF to the MF decreases the natural mobility in the ulnar side of the hand. Metacarpal base fractures are treated in the same manner; however, the wrist is included in the orthosis to provide optimal fracture alignment with or without the digits (Fig. 20–13B).

Phalangeal

Fractures of the proximal or middle phalanges are common in the athlete (Jaworski et al., 2010). **Phalangeal fractures** can occur in various sports, including tumbling events in gymnastics, wrestling maneuvers, football, and lacrosse. Fracture management using an orthosis depends on the location (articular versus nonarticular), type of fracture, stability of the fracture, presence of dislocation/ligamentous injury, and need for surgical intervention. There are many options for orthotic intervention: fracture bracing (Fig. 20–14A), circumferential casting (Fig. 20–6), restrictive orthoses (Figs. 20–3 and 20–14B), and buddy taping (Fig. 20–14C).

Sprains, Ligamentous Injuries, Dislocations

Injury to ligamentous structures in the upper extremity is common in athletes. The degree of injury depends on the amount of force applied to the body part and the direction of that force on the joint. These two factors directly affect the recommended medical and orthotic intervention.

Elbow Ulnar Collateral Ligament Injuries

Medial-side elbow injuries are common in any sport requiring forceful overhead or side arm movements, for example, with baseball pitching (Fig. 20–15A). Owing to the combination of forces on the elbow during the final stages of cocking and initiation of the acceleration phase, the ulnar collateral ligament (UCL) and ulnar nerve can undergo significant microtrauma, resulting in both acute and chronic injuries, such as progressive degeneration of the UCL. Rest (immobilization in an orthosis

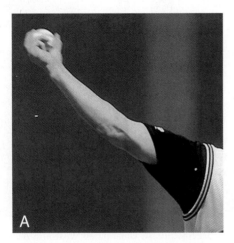
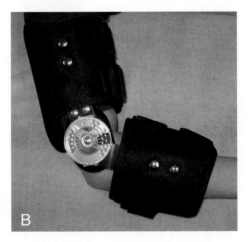

FIGURE 20–15 **A,** Pitching places tremendous stress on the medial structures about the elbow. Note the prominence of the ulnar nerve at the medial elbow. **B,** Hinged elbow restriction orthosis to allow for limited motion after soft tissue injury or fracture. The hinge also prevents lateral forces about the elbow.

to limit lateral stress to the elbow), followed by strengthening of the flexor pronator mass, stabilization of the proximal joints, and evaluation of throwing mechanics are the initial treatment recommendations. In chronic cases, reconstruction of the UCL may be indicated. Symptoms of ulnar neuropathy often occur simultaneously; therefore, an ulnar nerve release or transposition may be performed at the same time (Alley & Pappas, 1995). Postoperative management involves protection in a long arm orthosis immediately after surgery and initiation of gentle elbow flexion and extension 1 week later. Protection against lateral stresses is accomplished with an elbow restriction orthosis (hinged) that can allow for progressive increases in elbow mobility until the athlete achieves full ROM (Fig. 20–15B).

Triangular Fibrocartilage Complex Tears

As the primary stabilizer of the radioulnar joint, injuries to the **triangular fibrocartilage complex** (TFCC) can result in significant disability for the athlete. Injury is often a result of a FOOSH, resulting in compression of the TFCC between the head of the ulna and the carpus or torqueing of the forearm while loaded (Rettig, 2003). This injury is seen in athletes who break a fall with the hand (gymnasts) or who undergo excessive rotational force (e.g., racket and throwing sports) (Howse, 1994). A nonsurgical or surgical approach may be taken with this population, depending on the severity of the disruption. Orthoses can be an important component of the rehabilitation plan and return to competition. Initial injury may require a rigid cast for complete immobilization. As rehabilitation progresses, a wrist immobilization orthosis can be used and weaned to a less rigid support, such as taping or neoprene orthosis. Soft supports may be appropriate to allow initiation of guarded activity with continued protection (Fig. 20–16). Chapter 14 (PP. 12) reviews the fabrication of a neoprene orthosis for this patient population and those with wrist instability.

Wrist Instability

Carpal instability can often be associated with athletes that use equipment (baseball, lacrosse, golf, etc.) requiring wrist

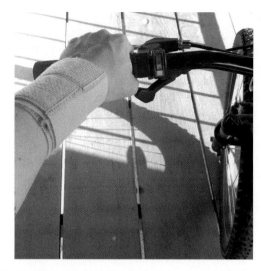

FIGURE 20–16 Prefabricated orthosis for stabilization of the TFCC while allowing wrist extension in this cyclist.

deviation along with rotation of the forearm. Midcarpal instability often presents with a trivial injury or no injury at all, clinically presenting with a painful wrist and spontaneous "clunk." The laxity of the extrinsic stabilizing ligament of the wrist can lead to a carpal instability (Lichtman & Wroten, 2006). Many orthotic designs to manage carpal instability have been reported (Chinchalkar & Young, 2004; Skirven & DeTullio, 2006; Staines, Konduris, & O'Brien, 2003; T. W. Wright & Michlovitz, 2002) (Fig. 20–17A–C). These orthoses are designed to stabilize the extrinsic ligaments of the carpus and are used in conjunction with activity modification and strengthening exercises (extensor carpi ulnaris [ECU] primarily) (Staines et al., 2003).

Thumb MP Joint Injury

Thumb MP joint sprain most often occurs from forceful thumb MP hyperextension, resulting in MP volar dislocation.

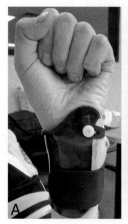
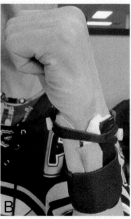
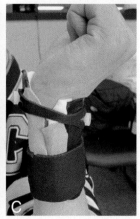

FIGURE 20–17 **A–C,** A "pisiform boost" orthosis for mid carpal instability will allow wrist extension while stabilizing the ulnar side of the carpus. In this orthosis note the use of neoprene as the counterforce, anchoring the volar to dorsal segments.

In addition, lateral forces at the MP joint can disrupt the collateral ligaments, resulting in joint instability. A UCL sprain, also known as gamekeeper's or skier's thumb, occurs commonly in sports after a fall onto the hand with the thumb in abduction, such as when gripping a ski pole or racquet (Melone, Beldner, & Basuk, 2000) (Fig. 20–18A). Orthoses are commonly used to place the ligament in a stress-free, shortened position while healing occurs (Fig. 20–18B). As with other ligamentous injuries, a range of damage can occur, from a midsubstance tear to an avulsion fracture where the ligament inserts on the thumb proximal phalanx. In a pure ligamentous injury, a Stenar lesion can occur (the adductor is interposed between the UCL and its insertion). A rotated fracture or a Stenar lesion is generally an indication for surgery (Badia & Khanchandani, 2011; Baskies & Lee, 2009; Melone at al., 2000). Patients who require surgery usually undergo a period of postoperative immobilization in a thumb cast progressing to an immobilization orthosis that can be used for protection during sport to prevent reinjury (Little & Jacoby, 2011). Radial collateral ligament (RCL)

disruptions can also occur, but those injuries are much less common. Injury to the RCL is also managed with a thumb immobilization orthosis with weaning to taping or a neoprene restriction orthosis for return to competition.

PIP Joint Dislocations

PIP joint dislocation can result from an axial load, lateral stress, or hyperextension force applied to the PIP joint in sports such as volleyball, basketball, soccer (primarily goalie), rock climbing, and gymnastics (Fig. 20–19A,B). The severity of this injury depends on the amount and direction of force applied as well as any concurrent injury such as fracture (Glickel & Barron, 2000; Little & Jacoby, 2011; Vitale, White, & Strauch, 2011). Injury can occur to a single collateral ligament, both collateral ligaments, and/or the volar plate. If the volar plate is disrupted, then at least one of the collateral ligaments is usually involved. This injury can include an avulsion fracture of the middle phalanx associated with the volar plate (fracture dislocation of the PIP joint).

Orthosis selection is affected by the degree of injury and stability of the joint. Collateral ligament injuries may be managed with buddy taping to an adjacent digit (Fig. 20–14C) or a restrictive orthosis, including hinge or Figure-8 type (Fig. 20–19C,D); whereas volar plate involvement usually requires a dorsal-based PIP extension restriction orthosis (Fig. 20–14B). Orthotic fabrication after surgical intervention may also be necessary and should be customized to the surgical procedure (Little & Jacoby, 2011; Najarian & Lawton, 2011).

DIP Joint Dislocations

A forceful blow to the distal finger is most often the cause of a distal interphalangeal (DIP) joint dislocation (Hritcko, 2006; Little & Jacoby, 2011). Sprain and/or dislocation of the DIP joint can occur in many sports, but these injuries are most often associated with ball-handling sports such as volleyball, basketball, and football. Thermoplastic materials, taping techniques, and silicone-lined products are a few options available for protecting an injured distal phalanx.

Tendon Injuries

Tendon injuries can occur in any sport in which the tendon is placed in a vulnerable position (e.g., excessive force loading, forceful hyperextension, or flexion). Refer to Chapter 18 for more comprehensive information regarding orthotic management for tendon injuries.

Distal Biceps Tendon Rupture

Distal **biceps tendon rupture** can occur after a fall on a hyperextended elbow or with a sudden eccentric load to the biceps brachii muscle during a sport such as snowboarding, rock climbing, wrestling, and bodybuilding (Bertini et al., 2011; Williams, Hang, & Bach, 1996). Athletes usually note a "pop" during the activity and present with a deformity of the upper arm (fullness in bicep area) with pain and difficulty supinating the forearm. Management of these patients can be surgical or nonsurgical. Surgical repair to preserve

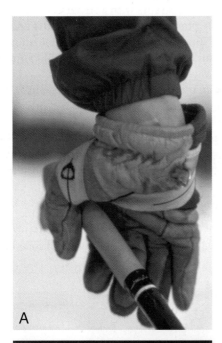

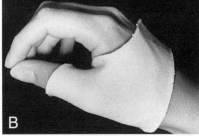

FIGURE 20–18 A, Note that holding a ski pole places the thumb MP joint at risk for injury. **B,** Hand-based thumb MP immobilization orthosis including the ulnar side of the hand to further prevent stress to UCL.

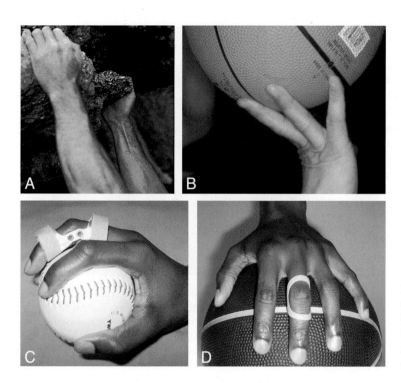

FIGURE 20–19 **A,** The interphalangeal (IP) joints are stressed during rock climbing, placing them at risk for injury. **B,** PIP hyperextension injuries are common in basketball and volleyball players. **C,** PIP restriction orthosis with hinges to prevent lateral stress to healing ligaments. **D,** PIP extension restriction orthosis prevents hyperextension stress while playing sports.

elbow flexion and supination strength is one option for the highly competitive athlete. Rehabilitation protocols after surgical repair of the ruptured biceps tendon depends on the method and stability of the repair. Newer protocols advocate early, restricted ROM in a hinged elbow restriction orthosis, whereas older protocols favor an extended period in an elbow immobilization orthosis. The elbow restriction orthosis allows for gradual increases in amount of allowed ROM (Fig. 20–15B). Returning to preinjury level of competition is dictated by the surgeon and may warrant several months of rehabilitation for regaining full strength for sports

participation (Cohen, 2008; Morrey, 1993). More recently, postoperative care may only involve a few weeks of immobilization beginning protective active motion as early as 10 days to 2 weeks (Blackmore, 2011; Ivy & Spencer, 2011).

Mallet Finger

Injury to the terminal extensor tendon, a **mallet finger**, can occur from hitting the fingertip against an oncoming ball (volleyball, baseball) or on an opponent's athletic equipment such as pads or helmet (Scott, 2000) (Fig. 20–20A). The injury can be managed with various orthosis designs,

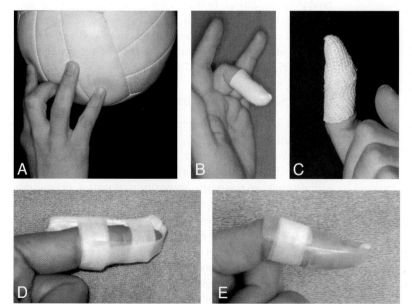

FIGURE 20–20 **A,** Force directed at the DIP joint into flexion can result in a mallet finger deformity. Various types of orthoses can be used for mallet finger management: thin thermoplastic material **(B)** or QuickCast 2 material **(C),** or a prefabricated orthosis such as Aluma-Foam® **(D)** and Stax **(E).**

prefabricated or custom, with the DIP positioned in neutral to slight (~15°) hyperextension. The orthosis is worn continuously for approximately 6 to 8 weeks to allow for adequate healing (Little & Jacoby, 2011; Wichmann & Martin, 1996). Orthoses can be custom fabricated from thin (1/16″) thermoplastic material or circumferential casting tape such as QuickCast 2 or Orficast™ (Fig. 20–20B,C). In some cases, a prefabricated orthosis such as an AlumaFoam® or Stax can be used (Fig. 20–20D,E). When applying an orthosis, dorsal or volar, consideration should be given to the specific sport demands, such as whether there is a need to preserve sensation in the fingertip to manipulate sports equipment. The orthosis can be secured with cloth tape, cohesive bandage, or traditional hook-and-loop straps. The skin under this orthosis should be evaluated regularly to check for maceration and possible skin disruption.

Flexor Digitorum Profundus Avulsion

Flexor digitorum profundus (FDP) avulsion (jersey finger) usually occurs when a player grabs the jersey of another player and gets the fingertip caught in the uniform while the opposing player continues forward momentum, most commonly seen in the RF FDP tendon (Allan, 2011; Stamos & Leddy, 2000) (Fig. 20–21). This is a severe injury requiring surgical intervention to restore FDP function and should be managed according to the treating physician's flexor tendon protocol (see Chapter 18 for details). For professional athletes and promising collegiate athletes, the option to not repair the ruptured tendon may be exercised. The athlete may require taping of the digits upon return to sport.

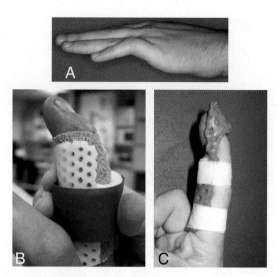

FIGURE 20–22 **A,** Posturing of digit with disruption of the central tendon overlying the PIP joint. **B,** PIP joint immobilization orthosis allowing DIP motion to mobilize the lateral bands. **C,** Digit immobilization orthosis ("drop out" design); note the DIP is in slight flexion while the PIP is held in extension for correction of deformity.

Postseason or at the end of the athlete's career, secondary tendon repair options or a DIP fusion may be considered.

Acute Boutonniere Injury

Rupture of the extensor mechanism at the PIP joint can result in flexion posturing of the PIP, a **boutonniere deformity**, owing to rupture of the insertion of the central tendon and volar migration of the lateral bands (Scott, 2000) (Fig. 20–22A). These injuries can occur from a fall or from striking the hand against another player or athletic equipment. Immobilization of the PIP joint in extension for 6 to 8 weeks is necessary for conservative management of these injuries. Various orthoses can be used to achieve this goal (Fig. 20–22B,C). In most cases, the DIP joint is left free for ROM to encourage and facilitate gliding of the lateral bands dorsally. Orthosis use may be continued throughout the rest of the sport season as a precautionary measure (H. H. Wright & Rettig, 1995).

Other Soft Tissue Injuries

Overuse injuries in athletes can result from repetitive microtrauma that leads to inflammation of the involved muscle–tendon units and local tissue irritation and/or damage. These injuries are most likely to occur when an athlete changes the mode, intensity, or duration of training. Soft tissue injuries can occur from a single traumatic event or from repetitive stress due to overtraining. Soft tissue injuries can be managed not only with orthotic intervention, but consideration should be given to other materials such as taping and neoprene. These alternative materials can play a significant role in allowing healing while even returning to light activity.

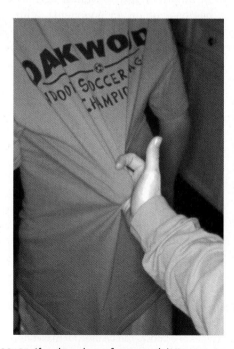

FIGURE 20–21 If a player has a finger stuck in an opponent's jersey, the DIP joint will be forced to flex strongly as the opponent continues to run, possibly resulting in an FDP rupture.

Bicep/Triceps Tendinosis

Tendon-specific inflammation in sports is generally characterized as acute (macrotrauma) or chronic (microtraumatic overuse, cumulative trauma, or overuse syndrome) (Bertini et al., 2011; Leadbetter, 1995). Clinically, sports-induced soft tissue inflammation may resolve spontaneously; however, often this may become chronic and a major problem for the athlete. Bicep tendinosis is seen primarily at the bicep proximal insertion and is often seen in a sport that requires repetitive overhead reaching (basketball, weight lifting) or in sports in which handheld equipment may come in contact with resistance (lacrosse, golf, etc.). Triceps tendinosis, also known as "jumper's knee" of the elbow, develops after the triceps tendon at the distal attachment to the olecranon gets irritated. This is specifically seen in sports requiring excessive forces to propel the body such as gymnastics, track and field, and snow sports (Vidal, Drakos, & Allen, 2004). The aging process contributes a tendency toward chronic soft tissue inflammation (Leadbetter, 1993). Medical management of these injuries often includes the use of nonsteroidal and steroidal anti-inflammatory treatments as well as altering the technique that causes inflammation of the specific structure. In addition, bicep and triceps counterforce strapping can off-load the inflamed area while allowing return to play, much as a Cho-Pat™ strap is used for patellar tendon inflammation (Fig. 20–23).

Olecranon Bursitis

The olecranon bursa is a fluid-filled sac at the posterior elbow that may become inflamed from pressure or a direct blow to the olecranon process, with resultant **olecranon bursitis**. This is sometimes seen in golfers with repeated grounding of the club or during athletic competition from direct blows sustained to this region from a piece of playing

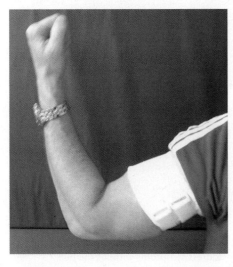

FIGURE 20–23 Nonarticular arm orthosis (large version of counterforce brace) used to off-load the bicep for management of tendinosis.

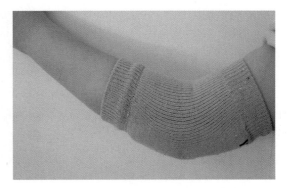

FIGURE 20–24 Soft elbow pad can be placed over posteriorly to prevent contact stress to the olecranon bursa.

equipment (hockey stick, baseball bat, tennis racket). Treatment options include aspiration, cortisone injection, edema control techniques, and the use of a soft compressive orthosis such as a soft elbow protective pad (Heelbo®) (Fig. 20–24). Return to sport is recommended when the athlete can use the piece of sporting equipment with adequate force and no pain. Weight bearing should be performed painlessly before returning to any sport requiring such maneuvers (e.g., gymnastics).

Epicondylitis

Injury to the muscles and tendon origins at both the medial and lateral elbow are seen in a variety of athletes. Repetitive microtrauma to either the wrist extensor mass (**lateral epicondylitis**) or the flexor pronator mass (**medial epicondylitis**) can result in injury, ranging from acute inflammation to chronic degeneration and fibroblastic changes (Ciccotti, Schwartz, & Ciccotti, 2004; Fedorczyk, 2011; Whaley & Baker, 2004) (Fig. 20–25A). Management of these injuries focuses on rest (refraining from the sport), nonsteroidal anti-inflammatory drugs (NSAIDs), and/or injection (corticosteroid, platelet-rich plasma or prolotherapy) (Sanchez, Anitua, Orive, Mujika, & Andia, 2009). Orthosis use or therapeutic taping (Fig. 20–25B) to decrease activity of the involved muscle–tendon units may be beneficial, including the use of a nonarticular forearm orthosis (counterforce strap) (Borkholder, Hill, & Fess, 2004; Meyer, Pennington, Haines, & Daley, 2002; Struijs et al., 2001) (Fig. 20–10). It is important for the athlete and therapist to determine the factors that may be contributing to the development of the condition (grip size, racquet stringing, and technique) (Alley & Pappas, 1995). Although the orthosis may decrease the advancement of the microtrauma and allow for tissue healing, appropriate activity changes should be made to deter recurrence.

DeQuervain's Tenosynovitis

DeQuervain's tenosynovitis involves the tendon and synovial sheath of two thumb muscles: the extensor pollicis brevis (EPB) and the APL. These tendons share a common

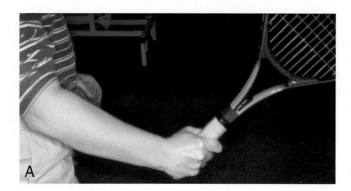

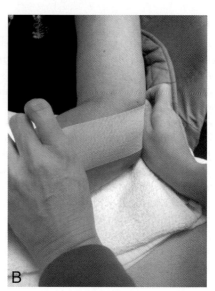

FIGURE 20–25 A, When treating a tennis player with lateral epicondylitis, the therapist should critique technique as well as equipment. **B,** Therapeutic taping is one technique that can improve muscular symptoms.

tendon sheath (first dorsal compartment) and can become inflamed when there is too much friction within the sheath as a result of activities requiring grip with wrist deviation such as improperly using a golf club or racquetball racket (Fig. 20–26A,B). A direct blow to this area can also result in an acute onset of deQuervain's tenosynovitis. Pain occurs with ulnar deviation of the wrist with thumb flexion (Finkelstein test) and most often radiates proximally along the thumb column into the forearm. Management is similar to other tendinopathies, including rest (orthoses and activity modification), NSAIDs, anti-inflammatory injection, and activity/equipment modification. The appropriate orthosis for this condition is one that immobilizes the wrist and thumb such as a wrist and thumb immobilization orthosis (Fig. 20–4). Taping and soft orthosis use can also be considered (Fig. 20–26C,D).

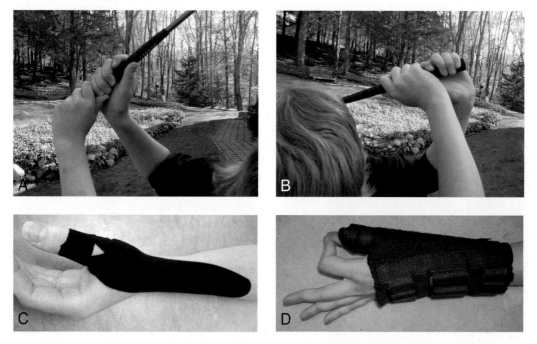

FIGURE 20–26 A and B, When treating golfers, evaluation of their swing with attention to wrist deviation is essential. **C,** Therapeutic taping is a low-profile way to address symptoms without the bulk of an orthosis. **D,** Prefabricated thumb orthoses can also be used for a more restrictive support early on in management of radial sided wrist pain.

Intersection Syndrome

Intersection syndrome is inflammation or tenosynovitis at the junction of the first and second dorsal compartments of the wrist (Servi, 1997). Intersection syndrome most often occurs from overuse of the radial wrist extensors, for example, in skiing when the pole is pulled from deep snow. It may also be seen in weightlifters, rowers, and indoor racket sport players (Servi, 1997). Signs and symptoms include tenderness, crepitus, and swelling over the dorsal radial aspect of the forearm. Crepitation, or squeaking, may be noted with active wrist extension or passive motion. Treatment is similar to that for deQuervain's tenosynovitis: orthoses, NSAIDs, and activity/equipment modification. Orthosis use should incorporate the wrist positioned in extension, usually with the thumb left free to move (Fig. 20–27). Care should be taken not to irritate the median nerve by positioning the wrist in extreme extension (>30°).

Extensor Carpi Ulnaris Tenosynovitis

The ECU tendon is a prime muscle providing wrist extension and ulnar deviation. ECU tenosynovitis can occur in athletes who participate in racket, stick, and rowing sports because of the repetitive ulnar deviation involved in these activities. Management consists of rest, evaluation of equipment, and technique modification. The wrist should be positioned in extension and slight ulnar deviation in order to off-load the ECU tendon (Fig. 20–27). The athlete should be transitioned from immobilization to a conditioning program once the inflammation and pain have been controlled.

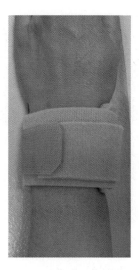

FIGURE 20–28 Custom nonarticular distal forearm orthosis (using hook, loop, and padding) to stabilize the distal radioulnar joint (DRUJ) for impact activities such as biking, cheerleading and gymnastics.

Distal Ulna Instability

Distal ulna instability can be acute or chronic in nature. Acute instability is often associated with a fracture of the ulna styloid and disruption of the TFCC. Treatment of this type of injury may be surgical or may require 6 weeks of cast immobilization (Morgan, 1995). Chronic instability often results from a late diagnosis after a "wrist sprain" (common with gymnasts and snowboarders). Treatment of these injuries is generally surgical and involves a period of immobilization after surgery. After using a wrist immobilization orthosis (Fig. 20–27), a soft support such as therapeutic taping, neoprene, or custom nonarticular orthosis may be recommended to aid in the transition from practice to competition (Fig. 20–28).

Pisotriquetral Joint Synovitis

Pisotriquetral joint synovitis, or degeneration between the pisiform and triquetrum, can cause pain with activities that require gripping or pressure along the volar ulnar aspect of the palm, such as batting, gymnastics, and field sports. Arthritic changes in this joint can be an indication for pisiform excision. A gel-lined or cushioned orthosis may be helpful to protect this area from direct trauma during competition (Fig. 20–29).

Hypothenar Hammer Syndrome

Athletes exposed to blunt trauma to the hands, for example, catchers in baseball, are at risk for injury to the ulnar artery called hypothenar hammer syndrome. This can result in ischemia to one or more digits depending on the athlete's palmar arch configuration. Use of custom padding (donut shaped) in the glove to minimize trauma and vibration may be necessary to alleviate symptoms (Mueller, Mueller, Degreif, & Rommens, 2000) (Fig. 20–30). For the cyclist, handlebar and positional alterations may be necessary to complement the device dispensed.

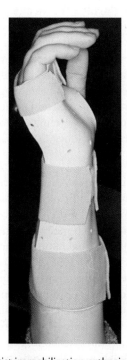

FIGURE 20–27 A wrist immobilization orthosis is commonly used to treat tendonitis about the wrist, forearm, and elbow regions. Note the position can be modified for the specific wrist condition.

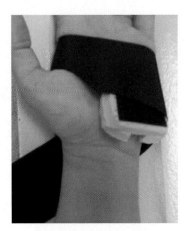

FIGURE 20–29 Soft padding secured to hand via hook and loop to protect the inflamed region and reduce pressure on the pisiform.

Nerve Injuries

Sports-related nerve injuries are not as common as the bony and soft tissue injuries described previously. Many sports activities lead to compression and direct trauma to the nerves of the upper extremity. Refer to Chapter 19 for more comprehensive information regarding orthotic management for nerve injuries.

Ulnar Nerve

Injury to the ulnar nerve in athletes most commonly occurs either at the elbow (**cubital tunnel syndrome**) or in the hand at Guyon's canal (**handlebar** or **cyclist's palsy**) (Kennedy, 2008; Wichmann & Martin, 1996). Ulnar neuropathy at the elbow is often seen in throwing athletes secondary to the significant valgus stretch placed on the elbow and its surrounding soft tissue structures during the late cocking and acceleration phases of the pitch (Fig. 20–15A). In professional and collegiate athletes, ulnar nerve release or transposition surgery is often the treatment of choice. Orthosis use after surgery depends on the type of procedure and involvement of other structures (UCL reconstruction). Often, an elbow

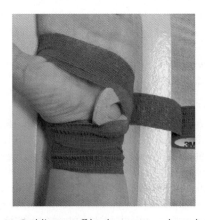

FIGURE 20–30 Padding to off-load pressure on hypothenar area applied with adhesive elasticized wrap; low profile to fit inside a glove. Custom fabricating an insert using neoprene and padding would provide a more permanent solution.

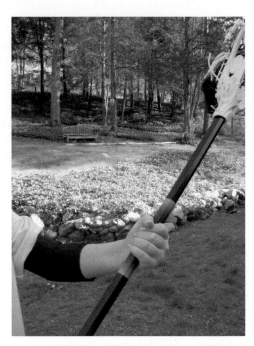

FIGURE 20–31 Custom restrictive elbow orthosis fabricated from neoprene for this lacrosse player to limit elbow extension and medial stress at elbow with cradling and throwing.

immobilization orthosis with the wrist included is fabricated for use during the early phases of rehabilitation. Transition to a soft elbow pad (Fig. 20–24), a neoprene restrictive orthosis, or taping can be used for return to competition in order to limit extension and valgus extremes (Fig. 20–31).

Compression of the ulnar nerve at Guyon's canal is seen most commonly in cycling but can be seen in other sports in which the ulnar wrist is exposed to excessive pressure or sustained extreme wrist extension. Positioning and pressure of the hands on the handlebars in cycling is usually the biomechanical cause of injury. Clinical management consists of making adjustments to the type and position of the handlebars as well as use of padded cycling gloves or custom orthoses (Slane, Timmerman, & Ploeg, 2011) (Fig. 20–32A–C).

Median Nerve

Neuropathy of the median nerve at the wrist (**carpal tunnel syndrome**) can have a significant effect on the athlete's performance. Nighttime use of a wrist immobilization orthoses, with the wrist positioned in neutral, is the initial conservative management for carpal tunnel syndrome (Lawrence, Mobbs, Fortems, & Stanley, 1995) (Fig. 20–27). Again, modification to the activity and equipment should be evaluated.

Pronator syndrome, or entrapment of the median nerve proximally, can occur at several sites, including the pronator teres, lacertus fibrosis, and proximal portion of the flexor digitorum superficialis (Servi, 1997). An arm- or forearm-based orthosis as well as activity modification may be helpful to place the structures at rest (Fig. 20–27). Techniques such as taping and soft orthoses offer an alternative

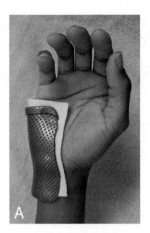
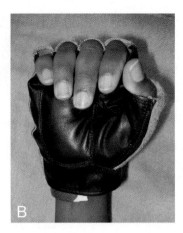
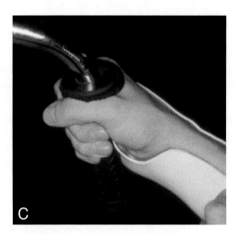

FIGURE 20–32 **A and B,** Custom thermoplastic insert for use under padded cycling gloves. **C,** Gel-lined options for thermoplastic material molded on the wrist of a weight lifter to reduce stress on the ulnar palm region.

to more restrictive orthoses and often can be used to transition back to play.

Radial Nerve

Acute trauma to the radial nerve can occur at multiple locations along its course, commonly at the spiral groove of the humerus or in the proximal forearm. Compression of the radial nerve, **radial tunnel syndrome**, can occur where the nerve enters the intermuscular septum or at the radial tunnel. These injuries are uncommon in sports but may be seen in athletes who perform repetitive pronation and supination (Jebsib & Engber, 1997; Long, 1995; Stanley, 2006) such as racquet sports, gymnastics, and field sports. An arm- or forearm-based orthosis that limits rotation may be helpful to place the structures at rest (Fig. 20–27).

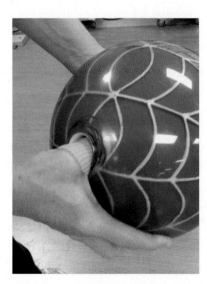

FIGURE 20–33 Note the lateral stress to the MP joint of the thumb while grasping the bowling ball. Gel-lined digit sleeves can pad the area and decrease pressure on the digital nerves.

Digital Nerves

One of the most common sites of neuropathy in the digital nerves is the thumb of bowlers (Sweet, Kroonen, & Weiss, 2011; H. H. Wright & Rettig, 1995). **Bowler's thumb** is a painful neuroma that can develop at the point where the thumb grips and releases the ball. Widening the size of the thumbhole in the bowling ball may be necessary to decrease pressure on the nerve. The use of padding, taping, or a gel sleeve at the base of the thumb may be useful for management of this condition (Fig. 20–33).

Treatment and Return to Sport

Stretching, strengthening, and conditioning exercises are critical to the successful return to sport; they include eccentric and concentric loading as well as sport-specific drills. The clinician or athletic trainer should review proper technique, provide information for equipment modification, teach adequate warm-up and cool-down exercises specific to the injury, and, if appropriate, provide orthoses or taping for use during and/or after exercise. The athlete should initially monitor the intensity and duration of exercise and report any signs and symptoms of reoccurring symptoms.

Communication with the physician, athlete, coaching staff, and trainers ensures that the most appropriate orthosis options are being considered. Appropriate prefabricated orthoses or sport-specific equipment that may not be commonly used (skiing gloves with thumb MP support) may be available to meet the performance demands of the athlete (refer to Chapter 11 on prefabricated orthoses for further information). The athlete, coaches, or trainers may be familiar with such equipment, and it is important for the therapist to investigate these options. If other management options are explored, the therapist must make sure that the equipment meets the medical needs of the athlete.

In some cases, taping may be an option for protection of the injured structures (Dievert, 1994; Little & Jacoby, 2011). For example, after acute management of volar plate injuries, buddy taping adjacent fingers helps prevent undue stress to healing structures. Some of the goals that can be met with taping are restriction of ROM, managing edema, providing anatomical support, and protecting against reinjury (Birrer & Poole, 1996). Taping of the wrist, thumb, and digits is common after injuries to these areas and can be used with or without custom thermoplastic supports (refer to Chapter 13 on taping for further information) (Jebsib & Engber, 1997).

Also, the therapist should stay abreast of any changes in the sport and make necessary modifications as the sport evolves. For example, the potential for decreased impact attenuation properties of artificial turf compared to natural turf may require increased padding and/or rigid support for hand and wrist injuries (Williams, Hume, & Kara, 2011).

Conclusion

All school-aged children participate in sports, whether in gym class or as a member of the school's football team. In addition to the recreational and professional athletes, this makes for a large population at risk for an upper extremity injury. There are numerous benefits of physical activity well documented that include improved cardio-pulmonary function (Braith & Stewart, 2006), glycemic control (Limke, Erbs, & Hambreacht, 2006), and psychological well-being (Lawlor & Hopker, 2001). Weight-bearing structures directly affect an athlete's ability to move, overshadowing injuries to the upper extremity (Strickland, 1995). The athlete moves well but may not be able to perform his or her sports. If neglected, upper extremity injuries can cause permanent damage and hinder daily activities as well as athletic performance (Plancher & Minnich, 1996). As such, upper extremity injuries in athletes confront therapists with often challenging situations. Although therapists are not expected to be experts on every sport, knowledge of the demands of the sport and a thorough understanding of the athlete's injury guide the therapist to appropriate orthosis selection. This chapter reviewed some of the common injuries therapists see in clinical practice and provided general guidelines for orthotic intervention. For information about other injuries, see other chapters in the book and the suggested reading list.

CASE STUDY SECTION

The case studies presented here are meant as a teaching guideline only. Treatment and orthosis protocols vary greatly from surgeon to surgeon and from therapist to therapist. The therapist should check with the referring physicians and colleagues to define the preferred treatment and appropriate orthotic intervention.

CASE STUDY 1: **Fifth Metacarpal Fracture**

RP is a 25-year-old right-handed professional hockey player. He sustained a fifth-metacarpal base fracture to his right SF during a fight. The fracture was managed by cast immobilization. The patient was referred to hand therapy at 3 weeks postinjury. RP presented with evidence of early fracture healing.

RP was placed in an ulnar wrist extension/RF-SF MCP flexion immobilization orthosis (wrist: 20° extension; MCP: 60° flexion; PIP/DIP: free) (Fig. 20–24). He was instructed in orthosis removal for active ROM (AROM) exercises of the wrist and digits. At 4 weeks after injury, his orthosis was modified to include only the hand (fifth MCP joint). The orthosis was small enough to fit into the hockey glove (Fig. 20–10) and was used for protection during practice and, eventually, for safe return to competition.

Additional case studies can be found on the companion web site on thePoint.

Chapter Review Questions

1. Describe the most appropriate material options for use with an athlete and explain how these options differ with other patient populations.

2. What is a playing orthosis? What must a therapist consider when fabricating one of these?

3. Describe a "jersey finger"? Can the athlete return to sport after this injury? If so, when?

4. Name two common types of tendonitis in the hand and forearm. How are these typically managed in the athlete?

5. What is a mallet finger? What is one option to manage this so that the athlete may return to sport as quickly as possible?

Adult Neurologic Dysfunction

Salvador Bondoc, OTD, OTR/L, BCPR, CHT, FAOTA*

Chapter Objectives

After study of this chapter, the reader should be able to:

- Define terms that describe and influence the muscle and tissue response that a neurologically impaired patient may possess.
- Understand and describe the clinical reasoning for selecting the most appropriate orthosis for a neurologically impaired patient.

- Explain the rationale for material choices in this patient population.
- Recognize the role orthoses can play in improving functional independence for the neurologically impaired.
- Identify the precautions for the use of casts, immobilization, or mobilization orthoses for this patient population.

Key Terms

Cerebrovascular accident
Decerebrate
Decorticate
Dependent distal edema
Dyssynergia
Elastic therapeutic tape
Flaccid upper extremity
Flaccidity

Hyporeflexia
Hyperreflexia
Low-load, prolonged stretch
McConnell technique
Multiple sclerosis
Neuromuscular electrical stimulation
Paresis
Postural control

Primitive reflexes
Spasticity
Spinal cord injury
Subluxed shoulder
Traumatic brain injury
Tremors
Weakness

Introduction

This chapter addresses orthotic intervention for adults with central nervous system (CNS) disorders (Chapter 22 addresses the pediatric population). This chapter discusses the common manifestations of neurologic dysfunction and offers the clinician guidance in clinical reasoning and problem solving when it comes to the application of an orthosis. Attempts have been made to ensure that the most current evidence is incorporated into this chapter. However, as literature on the use of orthotic devices for the neurologically impaired populations continues to emerge, the clinician is advised to keep current on this information and engage in critical reflection. Key to the success of integrating orthoses in practice is sound clinical reasoning based on evidence, theory, and assessment findings.

*This chapter is based on the first edition chapter written by Sue Ann Ordinetz, MS, CAS, OTR/L.

Common Adult Neurologic Conditions

Cerebrovascular accident (CVA), **traumatic brain injury (TBI)**, **spinal cord injury (SCI)**, and **multiple sclerosis (MS)** represent four common adult neurologic conditions seen in physical rehabilitation. Each condition has its own unique set of clinical considerations. Depending on the lesion site and the primary and secondary effects, an orthosis may be indicated. The orthosis can aid in addressing the presence of impairments in the upper extremity structures and functions. *Primary* effects or signs following an insult to the CNS are the direct manifestation of a neurologic lesion such as those that affect muscle tone (i.e., **flaccidity**, **spasticity**), stretch/deep tendon reflex (i.e., **hyporeflexia**, **hyperreflexia**), muscle strength and activation (i.e., **paresis** or **weakness**), and coordination (i.e., **tremors, dyssynergia**). On the other hand, *secondary* effects are manifestations that emerge because of the primary effects. Spasticity or flaccidity and weakness contribute to lack of mobility and functional use, which lead to complications including soft tissue contractures, atrophy, edema, and pain. Furthermore, disuse along with the lack of normal muscle activation patterns around a joint and the loss of soft tissue support may lead to joint deformation or instability over time.

In developing an intervention plan that involves orthoses for the upper extremity, it is crucial for the therapist to take into consideration the onset of the condition, the current neurofunctional status of the upper extremity, and its progression. For instance, in the early stages of recovery where tone is likely to change, the need for an orthosis may also change. There is no one single most effective orthosis for each diagnostic condition. Therefore, the therapist must apply clinical reasoning based on knowledge of the condition, upper extremity biomechanics, evidence, and patient/client contexts and preferences during the design, fabrication, and training process.

Considerations for Orthotic Intervention

Depending on the goals of orthotic intervention, there may be instances when a specific orthosis may be applicable across conditions. For instance, the management of contracture by the use of a mobilization orthosis (such as serial static and static progressive designs) may follow the same treatment principle of low-load, prolonged stretch (Glasgow, Tooth, & Fleming, 2010). However, there are also typical patterns of impairment that may be specific to the condition and thus warrant special consideration when it comes to the use of orthoses. These will be described in the following text.

Cerebrovascular Accident

Following an insult caused by ischemia or hemorrhage, the brain of a stroke survivor undergoes a series of physiologic events, which are considered part of spontaneous recovery. According to Dombovy (as cited in Teasell, Bayona, & Bitensky, 2012), this period of recovery, which occurs around 4 to 6 weeks postinsult, constitutes resolution of cerebral edema and a return of circulation around the area of the ischemia. Although the spontaneous recovery period may continue for more weeks, another period of recovery marked by CNS reorganization ensues, lasting for several months (Duncan & Lai, 1997; Teasell et al., 2012). These two periods of recovery are apparent in the patient's clinical presentation. During the acute recovery period, cortical functions immediately surrounding the area of ischemia are depressed. Consequently, muscle tone is marked by flaccidity, stretch reflexes are absent or decreased, and muscle activation is also absent or decreased. As the brain continues recovery, muscle tone and stretch reflexes increase, and voluntary muscle activation may then be possible. The extent of voluntary motor control and the evolution of spasticity and its severity varies from patient to patient. This makes early prediction, and thereby early intervention, of severely disabling spasticity challenging for clinicians (Wissel et al., 2010).

During the flaccid period, the hand and arm may rest in a dependent position. With the emergence of proximal control without return of extensor activity of the hand and wrist, the resulting posture may be a wrist-drop configuration (Fig. 21–1). When the hand is unsupported, the finger extensors are placed in passive tension, causing the metacarpophalangeal joint to be pulled into extension or hyperextension. From a flaccid state, spasticity may emerge in the upper extremity (Brunnstrom, 1970; Gowland, 1982; Wissel et al., 2010). The onset of spasticity varies in severity, timing, and location. However, there are muscle groups where spasticity becomes more pronounced and may lead to stereotypical posturing of the upper extremity. This posture includes the humeral adductors, humeral internal rotators and elbow flexors proximally, and digit/wrist flexors distally

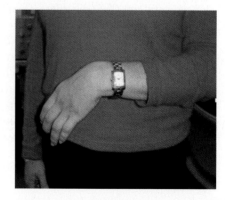

FIGURE 21–1 Patient presenting with wrist drop during the flaccid period following a CVA. Courtesy of Salvador Bondoc, Associate Professor of Occupational Therapy, Quinnipiac University.

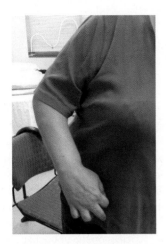

FIGURE 21-2 Spasticity becomes more pronounced, leading to a stereotypical posturing of the upper extremity

(Teasell, Foley, & Bhogal, 2011) (Fig. 21–2). Such a stereotypical pattern is implicated in abnormality of reach, grasp, and manipulation, and, with disuse or nonuse of the arm and hand, the formation of contracture deformity becomes an inevitable sequel (Shumway-Cook & Woollacott, 2010).

During the flaccid stage, the glenohumeral joint is at risk for subluxation because of loss of contractile tension from the deltoid and supraspinatus muscles (Fig. 21–3). In addition, with the humeral head slipping in inferior-lateral or inferior-anterior directions, the superior capsular structures become overstretched. During the spastic stage, shoulder subluxation may remain. The deformation is further complicated by the onset of increased spasticity in the subscapularis and pectoralis major muscles (Teasell et al., 2011). Hecht (1995) noted that spasticity in these muscles is the primary contributory factor in causing shoulder pain because of its tendency to restrict external rotation during humeral elevation (Teasell et al., 2011). During humeral elevation (e.g., abduction), external rotation clears the greater

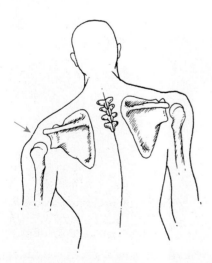

FIGURE 21-3 Note the flaccid left shoulder and the indentation just proximal to the humeral head.

tubercle of the humerus from coming in close contact with the acromion and thus preventing impingement.

Sling and Shoulder Support

Various sling and shoulder support designs have been commercially fabricated and studied to address shoulder subluxation. A simple *biomechanical design* comparison table is provided in Table 21–1. Regardless of the design, sling use has its own share of controversies, in large part because of some of the risks associated with its use. The therapist must carefully monitor patients who are using slings to ensure that they are removing the sling, monitoring joint and soft tissue integrity, and providing exercise as recommended to prevent complications of stiffness and **dependent distal edema**. In a Cochrane systematic review, Ada, Foongchomcheay, and Canning (2005) found insufficient evidence that slings and positioning devices (i.e., shoulder supports) prevent or reduce shoulder subluxation. In addition, sling use has been criticized for its impact on a patient's **postural control** and body image. However, slings and shoulder supports are still clinically useful to the **subluxed shoulder** and the **flaccid upper extremity**. They can assist in prevention of further injury especially during transfers and ambulation by keeping the arm secure against the patient's torso and lessening its tendency to flail around (Fig. 21–4A). As neuromuscular function improves, therapists may exercise judgment on the need for these devices. Several versions of slings used to support a subluxed shoulder are commercially available; however, the GivMohr® Sling (GivMohr® Corporation, Albuquerque, NM) is an option with emerging evidence support (Fig. 21–4B). In a comparative study, the GivMohr® Sling resulted in improvements in the vertical alignment of the glenohumeral joint based on x-ray studies (Dieruf, Poole, Gregory, Rodriguez, & Spizman, 2005). This device can be adjusted to hold the shoulder in near neutral rotation and the arm in a functional position.

As a rule of thumb, sling use and shoulder supports should be diminished as the therapist notes evidence of muscle contraction of shoulder stabilizers. Persistent use of a sling may only encourage disuse, pain, and contracture. It must be noted that many sling designs place the upper extremity in humeral adduction and internal rotation with elbow flexion (Fig. 21–5). These positions reinforce the synergy pattern described earlier and can be deleterious to upper extremity recovery. Instead, therapists should consider the use of other evidence-based interventions for shoulder subluxation such as **neuromuscular electrical stimulation** (NMES), task-oriented practice, and exercise. Information about these evidence-based interventions is beyond the scope of this text.

Taping

Another alternative to sling use is strategically applied tape. Tape application affords the clinician to directly influence at least partial alignment of the joint by constraining the joint and the movement of supportive bony structures. The

TABLE 21–1

Comparison of Shoulder Slings

Characteristic	Standard Sling	Arm Cuff	Holster Design
Commercial examples	North Coast Hemi Sling (North Coast Medical, Morgan Hill, CA)	AliMed® Hemi Sling (AliMed, Dedham, MA)	GivMohr® Sling (Patterson Medical, Warrenville, IL)
Mechanism of support	Sling support is applied at the elbow, forearm, and wrist; a strap is attached to the sling and loops around the upper back to produce a superiorly directed pull on the arm and forearm.	Cuff support is applied at the mid–proximal arm; two to three straps are attached to the cuff and are anchored over the opposite shoulder. The straps are intended to apply a superior-posterior pull on the humerus.	The hand and forearm are supported by a wide semielastic Figure-8 strap that loops around the hand through a plastic cylinder and crosses at the dorsal wrist. The straps continue proximally to the shoulder anteriorly and posteriorly that cross on the upper back and continue as a loop on the opposite shoulder. The flaccid extremity is supported from the palmar surface of the hand, providing compressive force through bones and joints of the arm, resulting in reduction of shoulder subluxation.
Effect on shoulder mobility	Immobilizes the glenohumeral joint in internal rotation and adduction but shoulder flexion is possible	Affords shoulder abduction but restricts some movement in the sagittal (flexion-extension) and transverse planes (internal-external rotation)	Affords maximal shoulder abduction and extension and moderate flexion and external rotation
Effect on elbow, wrist, and hand	Elbow is immobilized in flexion; wrist may rest in flexion. Hand may not be used.	Affords full movement of the elbow and distal joints. Hand may be used.	Affords movement in the elbow; hand/wrist is saddled on a semiflexible plastic tube. Hand use is limited.
Effect on postural control and mobility	Shifts the center of gravity superiorly and anteriorly	Allows arm swing during gait	Facilitates thoracic extension; affords/facilitates arm swing during gait
Potential sensory effects	Forearm and hand are not exposed.	Forearm and hand are fully exposed.	Moderate hand and forearm exposure to external environment; strapping configuration provides gentle joint compression; provides sensory input through dynamic compression

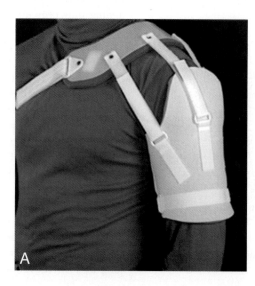 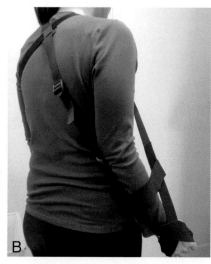

FIGURE 21–4 A, The AliMed® Hemi Shoulder Sling with a humeral cuff to support the weight of the affected extremity in a functional position. Photo courtesy of AliMed (Dedham, MA). **B,** The Giv-Mohr® Sling is designed after the Figure-8 harness, facilitating thoracic extension and providing better positioning of the scapula and glenoid fossa.

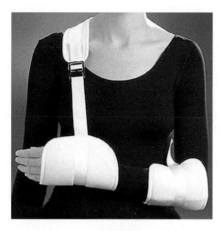

FIGURE 21–5 A Rolyan® CVA Sling promotes a pattern of shoulder adduction and internal rotation as well as elbow flexion. Photo courtesy of Patterson Medical (Warrenville, IL).

application of tape to treat shoulder subluxation has its own share of controversies. Several approaches to taping or strapping have been proposed (Ancliffe, 1992; Hanger et al., 2000; Morin & Bravo, 1997). However, recent studies (Appel, Mayston, & Perry, 2011; Griffin & Bernhardt, 2006) point to the benefits of taping or strapping to manage pain, but evidence remains limited whether taping or strapping improves shoulder subluxation.

Two common taping options for shoulder subluxation are the **McConnell technique** and **elastic therapeutic tape** (see Chapter 13 on "Taping Techniques" for more detail).

MCCONNELL TAPE

McConnell tape is a rigid/nonelastic tape applied over a thin layer of protective undertape (Fig. 21–6). The undertape is extremely important because it protects the skin

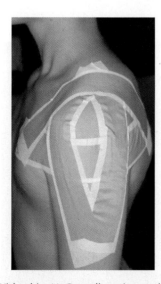

FIGURE 21–6 With this McConnell taping technique, the tape should be applied distal to proximal to provide proper support when correcting an anterior-inferior shoulder subluxation.

from shearing forces from the strong holding adhesive of the brown (overtape) tape. In general, McConnell taping is employed to reduce pain and improve muscle function and biomechanics. Proper analysis of the underlying pathology is essential to maximize the effectiveness of the method, which focuses on reestablishing a proper length/tension relationship and motor control.

McConnell taping for the shoulder may occasionally cause skin irritation, depending on the condition of the muscle carrying the weight of the arm. The vertical strip serves to support the weight of the arm and provide upward lift of the humerus, and the transverse strip supports the humeral head in the glenoid, serving as a reinforcement of the anterior ligaments. When taping a patient who has suffered a CVA or who has weakened deltoids, the use of two vertical, parallel, and overlapping strips may assist in reducing the load on the skin. This taping may stay in place for 3 to 4 days depending on the patient's age, overall medical condition, diagnosis, and skin condition. McConnell taping for shoulder subluxation also works well for anterior instability because the tape strips create a perpendicular capsular support. In this case, a shorter vertical strip may be used to avoid upward compressive forces that may result in subacromial impingement.

ELASTIC THERAPEUTIC TAPE

Elastic therapeutic tapes are tapes made from cotton, which have varying degrees of stretch depending on the tape chosen (e.g., Kinesio® Tape, Balance Tex™ Tape, SpiderTech™ Tape; Patterson Medical, Warrenville, IL). Elastic therapeutic tape has become a popular option in part because of the ease of application and friendliness of wear. The elastic recoil of the tape combined with proper application affects the superficial fascia, creating a light skin "lift" on the tissue it rests on. Not only do these reactions cause a reduction in subcutaneous interstitial pressure and improve lymphatic drainage, but as movement occurs, there is also constant tactile stimulus to the low-threshold cutaneous mechanoreceptors of the skin (Fig. 21–7A,B). This stimulates muscle, decreases pain, and enhances proprioception for neuromuscular reeducation. The high elastic recoil of the tape also provides support to weak muscles, reducing fatigue and overstretching. The thickness and weight of the tape is approximately the same as skin so the patient does not normally perceive the tape.

Both the McConnell technique and the use of elastic therapeutic taping should be combined with a comprehensive strengthening program for the muscles affecting the joint to provide extrinsic stability and prevent further damage or stretching of supporting ligaments and joint structures. Whether the choice is taping or a sling/shoulder supportive device, the clinician must also consider preventive positioning. Typical positioning recommendations for the affected upper extremity are elbow/wrist extension and shoulder abduction and external rotation. Positioning options that may be used to prevent contractures and promote proper alignment include adjustable tables, lap trays, and arm troughs.

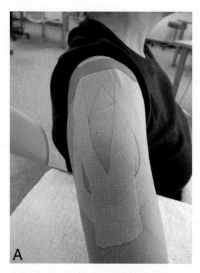

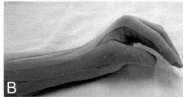

FIGURE 21–7 **A,** Elastic therapeutic taping to the shoulder using Kinesio® Tape. **B,** Elastic therapeutic tape applied to a post-CVA patient whose hand underwent surgical releases for digital flexion contractures. The tape assists in facilitating digit and thumb extension after a therapy session.

Traumatic Brain Injury

TBI, also known as acquired brain injury or head injury, happens because of a sudden traumatic event that results in damage to the brain. There are different types of TBI based on the mechanism of injury—from a simple concussion to one that involves fracture or penetration into the skull. In addition to the initial trauma, damage to the brain is worsened by the shearing forces that the brain undergoes, heavy bleeding, development of hematoma, and a decrease or absence of oxygen supply (National Institute of Neurological Disorders and Stroke, 2002).

Patients with TBI may be seen for individualized rehabilitation from the early stages of recovery in the intensive care unit. The path of recovery may be progressive, starting from low levels of arousal, consciousness, and limited neuromotor activity to emerging levels of consciousness and the onset of spasticity and **primitive reflexes**. Early in the recovery process, the use of orthoses may be indicated to assist with appropriate positioning and prevention of contractures. More involved patients may exhibit exaggerated whole body stereotypical responses known as **decorticate** and **decerebrate** posturing or rigidity. In the upper extremity, decorticate rigidity consists of shoulder extension and internal rotation, elbow flexion and forearm pronation, and finger and wrist flexion. In contrast, decerebrate rigidity presents itself as shoulder adduction and internal rotation with elbow flexed, forearm pronated, and fingers and wrist flexed (Fig. 21–8). When muscle tone is rigid, the resistance to passive movement is strong and constant throughout the range. Such condition places the patient at risk for contractures. Thus, the aim of therapy and the provision of an orthosis is to maintain and/or increase available range of motion (ROM) (Fig. 21–9).

To reduce contracture, prolonged stretch over an extended period of time may be favored. As detailed in Chapter 13, the use of serial casting is a preferred treatment option for this issue. One study suggested that in severe tone-induced contractures, the preferred approach is to apply a cast for short durations of 1 to 4 days to maximize ROM and minimize complications (Pohl et al., 2002) (Fig. 21–10).

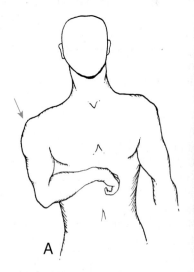

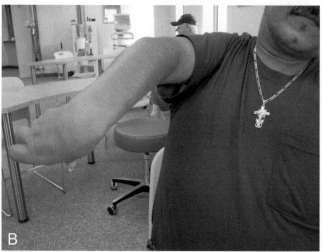

FIGURE 21–8 **A and B,** Decerebrate posturing including shoulder adduction and internal rotation, elbow flexion, and pronation with fingers and wrist flexed.

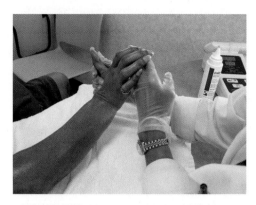

FIGURE 21–9 Passive stretching of the digital flexors being performed prior to reapplication of an orthosis.

Complications such as pain, swelling, tissue breakdown, and contractures may arise. Therefore, the therapist must exercise extra caution when applying and removing a cast on a patient with severe tone. As a patient's level of consciousness improves, serial casting may continue with lesser risk for complications (Pohl, Mehrholz, & Rückriem, 2003) (Fig. 21–11). The advantages of serial casting are in the evenness of circumferential pressure or force application and its neutral warm inhibitory effect on muscle tone (Colditz, 2000, 2002, 2011; Radomski & Trombley Latham, 2008).

Spinal Cord Injury

Some neuromotor signs such as spasticity and hyperreflexia found in SCI may share similarities with brain-based lesions (i.e., CVA, TBI), but the pattern of clinical manifestations and the course of recovery are unique. In SCI, the functional prognosis is directly linked to the level of injury. This is clearly illustrated by a series of practice guidelines published by the Consortium for Spinal Cord Medicine (2000). The goal of rehabilitation is to optimize the patient's function that corresponds to neurologic level. There is potential for improvement in the presence of partial innervation below

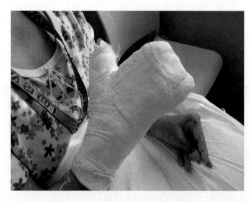

FIGURE 21–10 Initial cast application for dense digital flexion contractures. The cast provides a prolonged duration of gentle continual stress to these tight tissues. Note the posturing of the left hand.

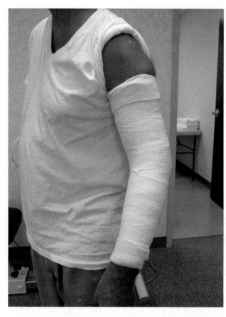

FIGURE 21–11 Serial static elbow extension mobilization cast using plaster of paris.

the neurologic lesion known as the zone of partial preservation (McKinley, Jennings, & Pai, 2011). For instance, a patient with a neurologic level of C6 may have fair power in the long finger flexors, which corresponds with C8 functional level. Therefore, the therapist must regularly examine the patient's neuromuscular functions for any indication of functional return that exceeds the expected prognosis (Fig. 21–12). Depending on available motor function and

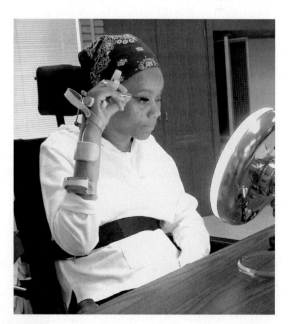

FIGURE 21–12 C6 complete tetraplegia using a wrist-driven, wrist hand orthosis. Reprinted with permission from Radomski, M. V., & Trombley Latham, C. A. (2008). *Occupational therapy for physical dysfunction* (6th ed.). Baltimore, MD: Lippincott Williams & Wilkins.

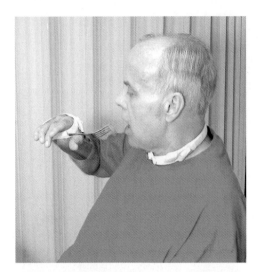

FIGURE 21–13 C5 tetraplegia using a universal cuff as part of a wrist immobilization orthosis. Reprinted with permission from Radomski, M. V., & Trombley Latham, C. A. (2008). *Occupational therapy for physical dysfunction* (6th ed.). Baltimore, MD: Lippincott Williams & Wilkins.

expected functional prognosis, orthoses may be used as adjunct to functional training by providing support to joints and substituting for denervated muscles. The following provides examples of orthotic intervention for the various levels:

- C5 tetraplegia without the functional ability to use the hand for manipulation—a wrist immobilization orthosis could be used with an attachment for a universal cuff (Fig. 21–13). This adaptation provides support to the wrist in the absence of wrist extension and would enable the patient to self-feed through the universal cuff because shoulder elevation and elbow flexion power may be adequate.
- C6 and C7 tetraplegia—the presence of innervated radial wrist extensors would enable them to use tenodesis action to achieve grasp (Fig. 21–14A,B). Harvey (1996) advocated for the use of progressive orthotic intervention to promote the development of tenodesis grasp. Wrist-driven wrist–hand orthoses based on the original design of the Rehabilitation Institute of Chicago (RIC) tenodesis orthosis (Michela, Sabine,

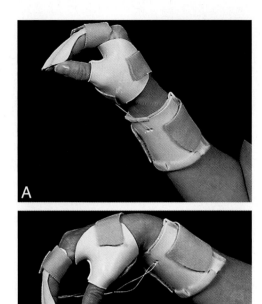

FIGURE 21–15 **A and B,** Reciprocal tenodesis orthosis harnesses the power from the radial nerve for light functional pinch/use. Wrist extension provides digit flexion and wrist flexion allows digit extension.

& Sammons, 1959) may also be provided, especially when prehension is desired (Fig. 21–15A,B).
- C8 tetraplegia present with hand function based on the availability of innervated extrinsic finger and thumb flexors and extensors. Intrinsic function may be absent, and therefore, hand dexterity is limited. Without intrinsic power during grasp, the hand is subject to muscle forces that position the MCP joints in hyperextension and the IP joints in flexion. This claw hand or intrinsic-minus configuration is not functional especially when the task requires a cylindrical prehension pattern (e.g., grasping a cup). An MCP flexion immobilization orthosis with an opponens component may be one orthotic consideration used to augment the lack of muscle innervation of the intrinsics (Fig. 21–16A,B).

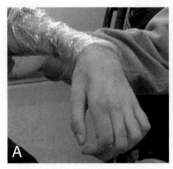
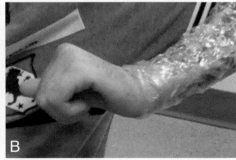

FIGURE 21–14 Tenodesis: **(A)** Wrist flexion, digit MCP joints extended; **(B)** Wrist extension, MCP joints flexed. Courtesy of Salvador Bondoc, Associate Professor of Occupational Therapy, Quinnipiac University.

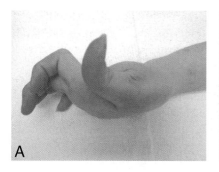
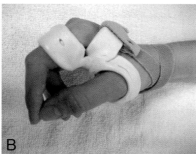

FIGURE 21–16 A, Severe claw hand deformity caused by long-standing brachioplexopathy. **B,** MCP and thumb MP extension restriction orthosis. Note how the orthosis places the digits in a better position for attempts at functional use.

Multiple Sclerosis

MS is an unpredictable CNS condition that affects the orchestration of movement, sensory perception, and cognition. In the upper extremity, two of the most common complaints are tremors and loss of proprioception (PubMed Health). Because of the unpredictable nature of MS, the functional presentation of the hand and upper extremity will vary from patient to patient. In a small study involving six participants with MS, a commercial wrist orthosis was used as one of many strategies to limit tremors and enhance hand function (Hawes, Billups, & Forwell, 2010). Both the participants and the investigators of the study had a mixed reaction to the intervention effects.

The presence of contractures or functional hand deformities varies and may sometimes mimic a peripheral nerve injury. To date, there is no single "most effective" orthosis that may circumvent hand impairments. It is the therapist's clinical reasoning based on knowledge of hand biomechanics, motor control, and task analysis that are most critical in determining the most effective intervention tool (orthosis) for that patient. For instance, one common issue in patients with MS is lost of grip strength caused by weakness in extrinsic flexors and wrist extensors that minimize their ability to engage in self-care activities such as holding on a toothbrush or utensils; a therapist may try using a wrist immobilization orthosis that positions the wrist in 20° of extension to optimize grip control (Fig. 21–17A). Another common issue is wasting of the intrinsic muscles of the hand resulting in flattening of the hand and loss of thumb opposition. Consequently, a patient with such problem may have difficulty with fine motor prehension (e.g., tripod or tip pinch). A simple solution is to provide a patient with a hand-based carpometacarpal (CMC) immobilization orthosis that enables the approximation of the distal segments of the thumb and the index finger while maintaining the first web space for correct hand aperture (Fig. 21–17B).

Clinical Reasoning on the Use of Orthoses in Adult Neurologic Conditions

There are three general purposes for the use of orthoses in adult neurologic conditions:

1. To prevent or manage an existing contracture/deformity
2. To provide joint support because of muscle weakness
3. To assist with neuromuscular reeducation

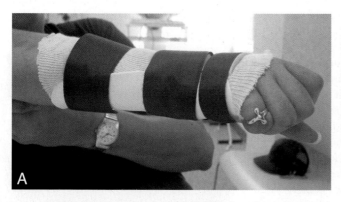
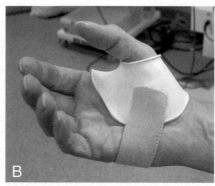

FIGURE 21–17 A, Wrist immobilization orthosis prevents excessive wrist flexion, allowing for functional grasp. **B,** Thumb CMC immobilization orthosis to maintain first web space and position thumb optimally for function.

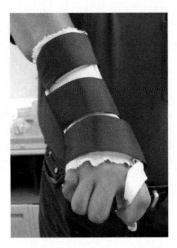

FIGURE 21–18 Custom-fabricated postoperative orthosis to support wrist. Additional index finger/middle finger web space thermoplastic "strut" was added to align index finger in opposition for pinch in order to assist with light functional use.

These purposes are not mutually exclusive. One type of orthosis may be used to satisfy more than one purpose. Furthermore, a patient may require the use of multiple orthoses to achieve various goals/objectives such as

- Support for the wrist while retraining manipulation (Fig. 21–17A)
- Protect and support postoperative procedures while providing some functional use (Fig. 21–18)
- Prevent spasticity-induced contractures through separate orthoses on the elbow and the wrist and hand (Figs. 21–10 and 21–11)

Managing Contractures Caused by Spasticity

Contractures may be defined as loss of extensibility of tissues leading to a loss of tissue and joint mobility. In patients with upper motor neuron lesions, contractures are proposed to be caused by degenerative changes in the elastic and contractile properties of muscle (Wissel et al., 2010). Because spasticity significantly limits the coordinated control of movement, the onset of contractures or deformities in patients with neurologic conditions is largely caused by spasticity-induced movement restrictions. This is not to suggest that the presence of spasticity determines the onset of contractures; contractures are preventable depending on their nature. Contracture may occur in either or both the contractile (e.g., sarcomeres) or/and the connective tissue elements of a muscle. When muscle is immobilized and unused, the contractile elements atrophy because of the reduction of sarcomeres in either length or cross-section (Farmer & James, 2001). Meanwhile, the connective tissue that lies within immobilized and disused muscles is lost at a

slower rate and tends to thicken because of abnormal cross-linking between fibers (MacDougall, 1986). Spasticity leads to a loss of productive motion and joint/tissue contracture if muscle is not stretched and activated.

The loss of motion is confounded by the presence of spasticity because it may limit muscle excursion during active movement. In the absence of active movement or relative immobility, spasticity may further lead to muscle imbalance, which then leads to stereotypical positioning of the limb, causing further muscle disuse and shortening over time. Typically in antagonistic muscle groups, the degree of spasticity is greater or more pronounced in one of the muscle groups. For example, although spasticity and hyperreflexia may be clinically assessed in both elbow flexors and extensors, elbow flexor spasticity may be more pronounced than in the elbow extensors, resulting in a stereotypical elbow flexion posture.

Spasticity may be defined as a pathologic increase in muscle tone and is marked by a resistance to stretch (Radomski & Trombley Latham, 2008). Resistance may be felt or observed when a muscle is stretched passively or when joint movement accelerates, causing the antagonistic (spastic) muscle to trigger the stretch reflex. For instance, in patients with active elbow extension, rapid reaching will cause the hyperactive stretch reflex in the elbow flexors to limit elbow extension toward the end range. Thus, spasticity is also velocity dependent. There are several theories proposed on the nature of spasticity; common to all of them is the lack of supraspinal or cortical inhibition at the spinal reflex arc (Gutman, 2007).

The use of orthoses to inhibit tone or address contracture formation in the neurologic population is wrought with controversy and confusion over proper nomenclature regarding these devices (Fig. 21–19). A systematic review consisting of 21 studies of varying quantitative methodologies and study quality indicate a mixture of positive and insignificant outcomes (Lannin et. al., 2003). The heterogeneity of the orthosis design, intervention regimen, and the study population limits the generalizability of this systematic review's recommendations. From an evidence-based practice perspective, the ability of the clinician to *critically appraise* the literature without bias is of crucial importance in judging the usability of evidence in everyday practice.

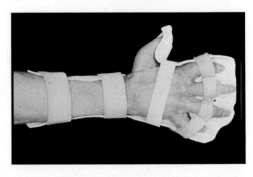

FIGURE 21–19 Several names have been used to describe this orthosis: finger spreader, hand abduction orthosis, or antispasticity orthosis.

Designs of Orthoses

The decision making to fabricate an orthosis on a spastic upper extremity may fall under two general frames of reference:

1. Neurophysiologic tradition of tone inhibition
2. Biomechanical tradition of tissue lengthening or contracture prevention

Tone Reduction

Designs that aim to reduce tone include the following (Jamison & Dayoff, 1980; Langlois, Pederson, & Mackinnon, 1991; Mathiowetz, Bolding, & Trombly, 1983):

- Cone orthoses (Fig. 21–20A,B)
- Resting/immobilization orthoses (Fig. 21–21A–E)
- Finger/forearm abduction orthoses (Figs. 21–19 and 21–22A,B)

Most often, the resting hand position is characterized by positioning the wrist between 10° and 30° extension, metacarpophalangeal joints in 40 to 45° flexion, interphalangeal (IP) joints in neutral extension to 20° flexion, and the thumb in midpalmar and radial abduction in order to maintain the first web space. Several variations of these orthoses designs exist through commercial and scientific literature.

The mechanisms for how these orthoses exactly inhibit tone are theoretically based. The original work of pioneers in neuromuscular rehabilitation including Rood (1954, 1956)

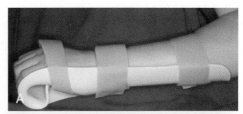
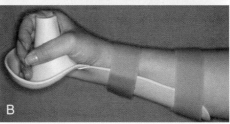

FIGURE 21–20 Rolling the finger platform on a wrist/hand immobilization orthosis (**A**) or forming a cone (**B**) in the hand portion of the orthosis may provide an LLPS to spastic digital flexors without overstretching them. Shown in **B** is a Preformed Spasticity Splint by DeRoyal, Powell, TN.

and Brunnstrom (1961, 1970) should be consulted for further details. The practice theories that emerged from these pioneers have spurned various designs over the years. To illustrate, Rood (1954) believes that pressure on tendon insertion has inhibitory effect. This theoretical influence may be

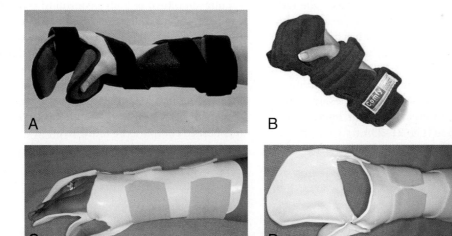
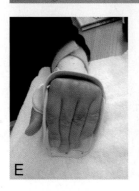
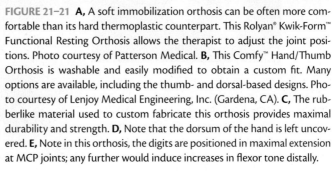

FIGURE 21–21 **A,** A soft immobilization orthosis can be often more comfortable than its hard thermoplastic counterpart. This Rolyan® Kwik-Form™ Functional Resting Orthosis allows the therapist to adjust the joint positions. Photo courtesy of Patterson Medical. **B,** This Comfy™ Hand/Thumb Orthosis is washable and easily modified to obtain a custom fit. Many options are available, including the thumb- and dorsal-based designs. Photo courtesy of Lenjoy Medical Engineering, Inc. (Gardena, CA). **C,** The rubberlike material used to custom fabricate this orthosis provides maximal durability and strength. **D,** Note that the dorsum of the hand is left uncovered. **E,** Note in this orthosis, the digits are positioned in maximal extension at MCP joints; any further would induce increases in flexor tone distally.

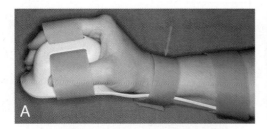
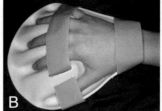
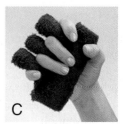

FIGURE 21–22 A, A dorsal wrist strap placed just proximal to the thumb CMC joint can help prevent orthosis migration. Shown here is a Preformed Neutral Position Hand orthosis by DeRoyal, Powell, TN. **B,** Hand-based Antispasticity Ball Orthosis by DeRoyal, Powell, TN. **C,** The Rolyan® Cone with Finger Separator prevents fingertips from digging into the palm and can prevent maceration in the palm and between the digits. Photo courtesy of Patterson Medical.

seen in the volar orthosis or cone orthosis designs in which the purported pressure application on the tendon insertions of spastic flexors may trigger an inhibitory response (Fig. 21–20). The Bobaths, on the other hand, believed that maintaining abducted fingers and thumb has a "reflex inhibitory" effect; a resting hand orthotic design with the thumb positioned in abduction and/or a volar-based finger abduction orthosis design are aimed to meet the intention of their approach (Figs. 21–19 and 21–22). Both cone and finger abduction orthotic designs and their modifications remain popular as indicated by their commercial presence in vendor catalogs.

The debate on the use of resting orthoses is further complicated by clinician preferences between volar and dorsal application of the resting hand orthosis. The rationalization for the choice of volar and/or dorsal application requires further study. Research studies are dated and do not indicate a clear advantage of one approach over the other (McPherson, Kreimeyer, Aalderks, & Gallagher, 1982; Rose & Shah, 1987; Takami, Fukui, Saitou, Sugiyama, & Terayama, 1992; Woodson, 1988). Design modifications that have emerged involve a volar hand support with a dorsal forearm base (Fig. 21–23A,B). One practical advantage of this design is class I leverage at the wrist. The deforming forces that originate from the flexors are balanced by an opposing lever applied on the forearm while maintaining a highly stable wrist. In purely volar or purely dorsal orthosis, the counterforces are based on how secure the straps are. In cases of severe spasticity, despite the best fit, the wrist has a tendency to buckle into flexion in the volar design; whereas in the dorsal design, the fingers tend to buckle into flexion, causing a distal migration of the orthosis (Fig. 21–24).

In the biomechanical tradition, the purpose of orthotic management is to preserve as much as possible the relative muscle balance between flexors and extensors and the intrinsic and extrinsic muscles of the hand (Bondoc, 2005). An uneven return of motor control to antagonistic muscles results in muscle imbalance; however, the onset of contractures caused by muscle shortening on one muscle group and the passive elongation of its opposing muscle group can become a vicious cycle and thus requires immediate intervention. Clinicians should constantly evaluate the muscle length to determine the onset of contracture and use diagnostic reasoning to differentiate contracture from tone. It is best to compare the more involved with the uninvolved

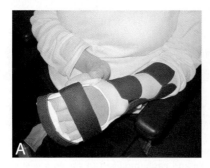
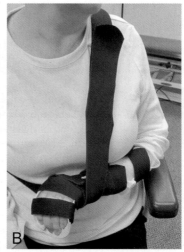

FIGURE 21–23 A, Dorsal/volar design using soft neoprene straps for closure. **B,** A custom neoprene shoulder support was made to assist the patient in holding up the weight of the orthosis because she had little control of the extremity.

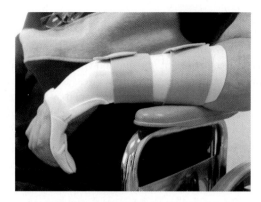

FIGURE 21–24 **Dorsal/volar design.** Note the counterforce generated through the orthosis and flexion posturing of digits because of tight flexor tendons. Over time, the orthosis can be serially positioned into more extension to lengthen the tendons.

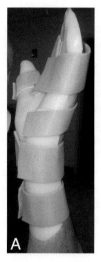
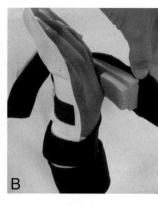

FIGURE 21–25 **A,** A wrist/hand extension immobilization orthosis used to preserve muscle tendon length shortly after neurologic insult. **B,** Wide widths of foam can be placed over the dorsum of the digits to impart a gentle stretch to the flexor tendons. The patient can assist in the amount of tension delivered by adjusting the straps.

or less involved side to further determine the presence of impairment.

- *Tone* is sensitive to rapid passive stretch; therefore, resistance may be felt at any point within the joint ROM.
- *Contractures* are usually felt as resistance to passive stretch at end range. If one is dealing with contractures of the ligamentous structures, the clinician must also consider when joints are in loose- and close-packed positions. When joints are in loose-packed positions, there is greater accessory motion (e.g., mediolateral gliding) that may be produced. Joints with contractures will have a decrease in the accessory motions.

The clinician should also apply conditional reasoning by attending to the typical recovery pattern or progression of the upper extremity following a CNS lesion. For instance, a patient with a CVA who may begin with flaccid tone may progress into a spastic flexor tone along with stereotypical posturing of the limbs. In such case, the anticipation of arm and hand posturing should guide the choice for an orthotic design. During the flaccid stage, the recommended orthosis position is wrist extension of 20 to 30° with composite extension of the fingers and the thumb (Fig. 21–25A,B). This position will prevent overstretching of the wrist and finger extensors, which could lead to a decrease in their mechanical advantage when the patient begins to regain more motor control of the hand. As the person continues to experience recovery, the clinician must provide ongoing monitoring and, if necessary, make adaptations to the orthosis design and intervention plan.

Contracture Prevention

Using an orthosis to treat or prevent contractures is based on the concept of **low-load, prolonged stretch** (LLPS). Although the original basis for LLPS came from animal studies, Tardieu and colleagues (1988) demonstrated in human spastic muscle that a minimum of 6 hours of sustained stretch is needed to preserve its normal physiologic length.

However, the treatment or prevention of contracture caused by spasticity cannot be simply addressed using orthoses. Lannin and colleagues (2007), who conducted a randomized controlled study on the effect of an orthosis on wrist extensibility following a stroke, found that fabricating an orthosis in either neutral or extended wrist position provided no benefit. They further concluded that the practice of orthotic intervention following a stroke should be abandoned. However, one significant deficiency in their study that may have deviated from best practice and may have contributed to unfavorable outcomes was that "stretches" of the extrinsic flexor muscle groups were not performed during the 6-week study period (Lannin et al., 2007). Therefore, a regimen of stretching and pain-controlling physical modalities (e.g., heat) should also be considered along with orthosis use to manage contracture.

The use of orthoses must take into consideration the severity of the limitation. Traditional intervention as indicated earlier may not be sufficient. Special consideration should also be given when dealing with severe spasticity because it is difficult to delineate tone from contracture-based limitations. A referral to a specialist (e.g., physiatrist, neurologist) is appropriate to determine if a patient is a candidate for pharmacologic intervention including OnabotulinumtoxinA or botulinum toxin A (Botox) injection, or oral medications such as dantrolene and baclofen that target spasticity (Kheder & Nair, 2012). The reader is advised to consult reliable sources and physician specialists before discussing these matters with the patient. Even when the patient receives pharmacologic management, the use of an orthosis may continue to achieve maximum effect on contracture management. In some cases, the use of serial casting provides a complement or alternative to orthotic and/or pharmacologic intervention.

SERIAL CASTING

The use of casts is commonplace to manage fractures and dislocations and is based on sound biomechanical principles to restrict movement and afford healing. The use of casts to manage contractures and manage spasticity has gained significant attention over the past decades (Mayer, Esquenazi, & Keenan, 1996; O'Dwyer, Ada, & Neilson, 1996; Pohl et al., 2002). Serial casting to manage a flexion contracture caused by spasticity requires passively stretching the flexed joint and applying the cast material circumferentially on the limb at maximum tolerable extension until the cast sets. In patients with impaired somatosensory functions, extra precaution must be undertaken to determine the adequacy of stretch by examining skin color and palpating muscle tension. Slightly less extension may be indicated if the clinician finds that the flexor resistance is steadily increasing. This is an indicator of stretch reflex activation, which may further continue and cause some complications after the cast application.

It is recommended to apply minimal padding to achieve maximum surface contact and minimize shear. Gel padding may be strategically applied on bony prominences as an additional precautionary measure. The cast is left on for several days (e.g., 4 to 7 days), removed, and then reapplied with greater joint extension. Serial casting is discontinued when the patient has plateaued in terms of ROM gains or when there is no more clinically meaningful change that can be derived. A cast may still be an appropriate way to maintain gains. A bivalved cast configuration is recommended so that the patient or a caregiver may be able to remove and reapply the cast for skin inspection, ROM exercises if appropriate, and hygiene purposes (Fig. 21–26A,B).

Between cast applications, ROM exercises and functional training (whenever appropriate) is recommended. The cast should also be monitored during and after cast application and before reapplication for presence of pain, swelling, pressure ulcers, or skin breakdown caused by stretch. The presence of these complications may require cast repositioning and/or an adjustment of the duration of wear (or even discontinuation of the cast). In one study (Pohl et al., 2003), complication rates ranged from 8% to 25% of the cases reviewed. The clinician should exercise judgment and caution with the use of casts as an intervention modality for contractures. The patient and/or appropriate parties should be well informed on the aforementioned complications in order to participate accurately in monitoring tissue responses to cast wear (see Chapter 12 on "Casting Techniques" for detailed information on fabrication of casts).

Providing Joint Support

A loss of motor control, especially when associated with weakness and hypotonia or flaccidity, renders the joint unstable. The goal for orthosis use is to provide support and achieve joint stability. When motor return is anticipated, such as in mild CVA or TBI, the clinician should consider the least restrictive orthosis to immobilize the targeted segment. For example, when a patient has poor control of the wrist but has the ability to partially grasp and release, a wrist immobilization orthosis may be sufficient (Fig. 21–17). But when motor return is not anticipated, the goal may be both protective and preventive. The hand and arm should be placed in a resting position that maintains musculotendinous balance and/or promotes optimal musculoskeletal function (Fig. 21–23).

Prefabricated or preformed immobilization orthoses are occasionally issued as a cost-saving measure and used for those patients who are too challenging to fabricate a custom orthosis. Chapter 11 on "Prefabricated Orthoses" reviews many of these orthoses in greater detail.

- **Preformed** (thermoplastic) orthoses with memory characteristics are preferable because the overall orthosis shape remains intact and through heating, the clinician can then adjust the fit directly onto the patient (Figs. 21–20B, 21–22A,B, and 21–27).

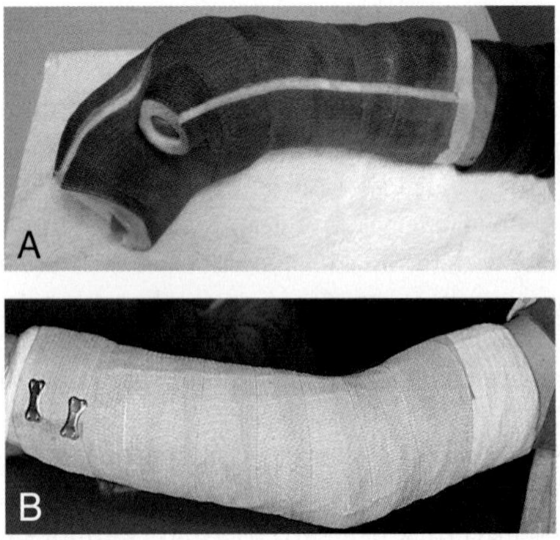

FIGURE 21–26 A, A bivalve cast to allow for donning and doffing. **B,** Note the use of an elasticized wrap to allow for removal of this bivalve elbow cast.

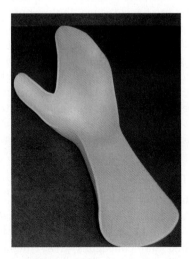

FIGURE 21–27 Preformed orthosis that can be reheated and *custom fit* to the patient.

- *Prefabricated* orthoses are generally soft and comfortable with a more forgiving and adjustable fit. Some have removable pieces or wire foam inserts that allow adjustment (Fig. 21–21A,B). Others contain air bladders that can be inflated to provide gentle stretch to the wrist and/or fingers. Prefabricated orthoses may be appropriate for patients with sensitive or fragile skin, such as the geriatric population. Softer orthoses, however, may be unable to provide adequate support for a large or heavy patient.

Whether a preformed or prefabricated orthosis is chosen for a patient, careful attention needs to be paid when evaluating for proper fit. Proper fit ensures against orthosis migration/slippage during wear. The importance of proper placement of the wrist strap cannot be overstated. This strap, when strategically placed, plays an important role in the orthosis's overall effectiveness that helps prevent migration (Fig. 21–22A).

Promoting Neuromuscular Reeducation

Orthoses for the neurological population were historically designed to influence muscle tone, prevent contractures, and provide joint support. With more recent evidence from the basic and behavioral neuroscience literature of motor learning, attention is steadily increasing toward the design and use of orthoses that may promote *active* use of the hand and arm and thus facilitate neuroplasticity with potentially long-lasting changes in motor behaviors (Hoffman & Blakey, 2011). Examples of such devices include SaeboFlex® (Saebo, Inc., Charlotte, NC), SaeboReach® (Saebo, Inc., Charlotte, NC),

and SaeboStretch® (Saebo, Inc., Charlotte, NC). For additional information regarding this treatment approach and products, contact Saebo, Inc. at www.saebo.com.

SaeboFlex® (Saebo, Inc.)

The SaeboFlex® is a dynamic orthosis that statically positions the wrist in optimal extension and dynamically extends the digits with spring-loaded traction in preparation for functional activities (Fig. 21–28A,B). The user is able to grasp an object by voluntarily flexing his or her fingers. The extension spring system assists in reopening the hand to release the object. The amount of tension may be adjustable to accommodate varying degrees of flexor spasticity. This orthosis allows patients suffering from neurologic impairments such as stroke the ability to incorporate their hand functionally in therapy and at home by supporting the weakened wrist, hand, and fingers.

SaeboReach® (Saebo, Inc.)

If a patient has a strong flexor synergy influenced during reach and requires an extension assist to the elbow, the clinician can fabricate a custom elbow extension orthosis or consider the SaeboReach®, which may provide an alternative option (Fig. 21–29). The SaeboReach® is a SaeboFlex® device fitted with a dynamic elbow extension component. It must be noted, however, that either the SaeboFlex® or SaeboReach® orthosis is not designed as a device to substitute for a loss of function but rather as a training device to *prepare* a patient to perform functional tasks without or with minimal support. The training program for the patient involves highly repetitive practice of arm and hand tasks using the orthosis (Hoffman & Blakey, 2011). When a patient has gained substantial flexor tone inhibition from active use and some semblance of release, the patient is encouraged to

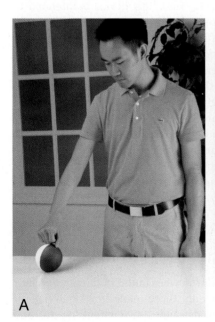
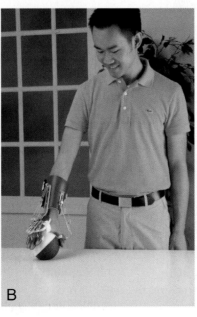

FIGURE 21–28 A, Grasping without and **(B)** with SaeboFlex®, which dynamically extends the fingers, allowing for grasp and release activities. For a patient who has synergistic mass grasp ability but poor or no ability to release, this device affords hand use by providing assistance to release. Photos courtesy of Saebo, Inc.

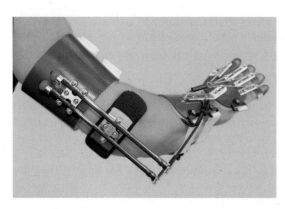

FIGURE 21–29 SaeboReach® addresses both elbow and hand involvement. Training in this device is part of both the clinic and home program; training includes repetitive task-oriented activities. Photo courtesy of Saebo, Inc.

use the arm and hand without the device. Pilot demonstration studies have shown promising results for stroke patients (Butler, Blanton, Rowe, & Wolfe, 2006; Farrell, Hoffman, Snyder, Giuliani, & Bohannon, 2007).

SaeboStretch® (Saebo, Inc.)

The SaeboStretch® uses a "stretch technology," which allows the fingers to flex within the device when tone in the hand increases protecting the finger joints from excessive force (Fig. 21–30A,B). It uses a low-load, long duration of stretch to return the fingers into extension. The SaeboStretch® addresses

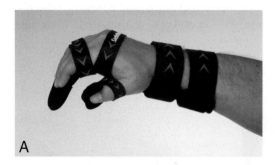

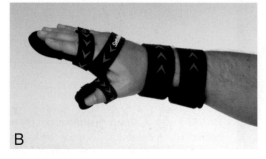

FIGURE 21–30 **A and B,** The SaeboStretch® liner is easily removable for routine cleaning. The straps are made of a nonskid material, which assists in preventing migration. Photo courtesy of Saebo, Inc.

issues such as deformity, joint damage, hypermobility, and contractures. This orthosis includes three hand pieces with various resistances to allow the therapist the ability to customize orthosis fit.

Neuro-Integrative Functional Rehabilitation and Habilitation (Neuro-IFRAH®) (Approach by Waleed Al-Oboudi MOT, OTR/L)

Another family of commercially available orthoses and therapy equipment is known as Neuro-IFRAH® Products (San Diego, CA). The Neuro-IFRAH® orthoses and therapy equipment are designed to serve as adjuncts to the Neuro-IFRAH® Approach. These devices purport to aid motor recovery by integrating its own unique Neuro-IFRAH® Approach concepts and applications with self-evident rehabilitation principles. These products include, but are not limited to, custom and prefabricated orthoses designed to prevent and address secondary effects of abnormal muscle activity in patients affected by lesions at the level of the brain stem and above. For example, the Prefabricated EWHO (elbow-wrist-hand hinged orthosis) and WHO (wrist–hand orthosis) may be adjusted to provide composite wrist-hand (digits) and elbow-wrist-hand extension and counteract abnormal involuntary activity in the flexors (Fig. 21–31A). The unique flat hand paddle designs are alternated with curved designs following specific protocols and strategies. The company also offers shoulder orthoses such as the Shoulder Support and the Humeral External Rotator. The Shoulder Support consists of a forearm cuff that may be clipped or hooked to a belt worn by the patient. The forearm support can be adjusted at various angles providing many options for alignment and support. The target effect is to support the weight of the arm to protect the patient's shoulder. Meanwhile, the Humeral External Rotator consists of a forearm trough supported by an L-bar that extends to a semicylindrical plate secured to the client's waist (Fig. 21–31B). This device is intended to prevent abnormal increased activity in the humeral internal rotators in patients affected by a stroke or brain injury by positioning the forearm lateral to the trunk and the humerus externally rotated lateral to the humeral sagittal plane. All the devices found on their Web site are said to be proprietary in nature. The originator of the Neuro-IFRAH® Approach maintains that all Neuro-IFRAH® Products are adjuncts and are part of a highly individualized whole person approach, and thus all products are not to be used, studied, or included in other protocols or approaches. For additional information regarding this treatment approach and products, contact the Neuro-IFRAH® organization at to www.neuro-ifrah.org. At this time, there are no published studies that directly evaluate the efficacy of these products.

Alternative Orthotic Devices

Other options for similar devices found both commercially and in research studies are those made from materials or combination of materials such as Neoprene, Lycra, and

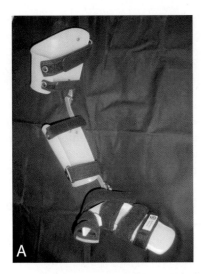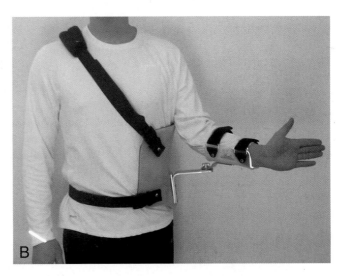

FIGURE 21–31 **A,** The Prefabricated EWHO (elbow-wrist-hand hinged orthosis) designed to decrease hypertonicity in flexors and increase passive mobility into extension. **B,** The Humeral External Rotator allows for adjusting of height, angle, and waist circumference. Photos courtesy of Neuro-IFRAH® Organization.

elastic. These types of garments are most often made from heavy-duty stretch materials that contour well on the body and offer substantial *support* to joints or *restriction* to certain movements and/or positioning (Fig. 21–32). They can be hand based, with the option of supporting the thumb in abduction and extension, or forearm based, including a spiral wrap that provides a dynamic assist into thumb abduction and extension and forearm supination or pronation (Fig. 21–33). Wilton (1997) also describes the use of Lycra orthoses to achieve more normalized active movement patterns of the upper extremity, including a sleeve-length (axilla to wrist) dynamic assist (elbow extension forearm supination or elbow flexion forearm pronation) model, a gauntlet style with a thumb abduction sleeve, and a full glove style. Recent studies on the use of Lycra or neoprene-based orthoses for increased tone/spasticity have been geared toward children with cerebral palsy (Elliott, Reid, Alderson, & Elliott, 2011). Commercially available resting orthoses are also available and can provide an LLPS to the fingers. The stretch can be adjusted by the progressive inflation of an air bladder placed in a palmar roll (Fig. 21–34).

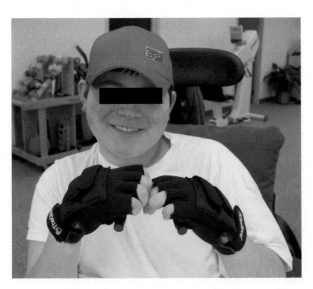

FIGURE 21–32 Thick neoprene and Lycra gloves support the MCP joints and position the thumb in this 16-year-old SCI patient.

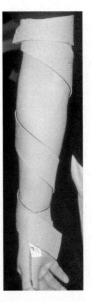

FIGURE 21–33 Neoprene's flexibility allows voluntary movement, whereas its elastic properties facilitate movement away from a spastic pattern. Shown is the Rolyan® Tone and Positioning (TAP™) orthosis by Patterson Medical.

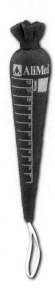

FIGURE 21–34 A Freedom® Finger Contracture Orthosis is recommended for a quick solution or when a more conventional orthosis is not indicated. Photo courtesy of Alimed (Dedham, MA).

Conclusion

The decision to use orthoses for the neurologically impaired adult is complex. The clinician must consider various factors including the patient's diagnosis and course of recovery, current and anticipated functional abilities, patient's goals and motivation, the purpose of the orthosis, and the patient's or caregiver's ability to follow through with the intervention. The clinician must also exercise judgment based on the available updated theoretical body of knowledge and current evidence.

The lack of convincing evidence to support or refute the use of orthoses for addressing neurologic dysfunction continues to be a source of controversy among clinicians and researchers alike. Many large studies and systematic reviews have cast scientific doubt on the use of orthoses for the neurologic population. However, it may be argued that neurorehabilitation is a highly individualized practice, and that one regimen of intervention may not always work for two similar patients. The therapeutic efficacy of orthotic intervention is no exemption. Like many other adjunctive treatment methods, orthoses should not be used as a stand-alone treatment. The clinician is encouraged to use sound reasoning that translates into skillful documentation that justifies and clearly elucidates the rationale for orthosis use. As evidence for the rehabilitation of upper extremity motor control continues to emerge, clinicians are advised to keep abreast of scientific developments in order to provide the best service for their patients.

CASE **STUDY**
S E C T I O N

The case studies presented here are meant as a teaching guideline only. Treatment and orthosis protocols vary greatly from surgeon to surgeon and from therapist to therapist. The therapist should check with the referring physicians and colleagues to define the preferred treatment and appropriate orthotic intervention.

CASE STUDY 1: **Part 1: Acute Cerebrovascular Accident—Inpatient Rehabilitation**

Thomas is a 63-year-old male who sustained a left middle cerebral artery (MCA) infarct resulting in right hemiparesis and expressive aphasia. Past medical history is remarkable for hypertension. He worked for the fire department and was quite physically active prior to the stroke. After days of acute hospitalization, he was discharged to an inpatient rehabilitation facility for intensive occupational, physical, and speech therapy. At initial evaluation, Thomas presented with maximal assistance in self-care and functional mobility. He is capable of sitting on the edge of the bed/mat with supervision, transitioning from sit to stand, and maintaining standing for at most 90 seconds given moderate assistance on the right side.

In terms of his upper extremity, Thomas has scapular elevation and emerging flexor activity to the elbow and hand. Extensor activity of the wrist and the hand is absent. The hand and wrist rest in partial flexion while seated or standing because of emerging spasticity. Mild clonus is felt upon quick stretch of the wrist flexors. Because of lack of movement, the hand has dependent edema. Thomas reports dull pain with passive composite extension of the wrist and fingers past the neutral position. When constrained to perform active use of the right arm and hand, the upper extremity goes in stereotypical flexor synergy pattern of scapular and humeral elevation, elbow flexion and forearm supination, and finger/wrist flexion.

As part of the occupational therapy intervention plan, a program of flexor stretching and inhibitory weight bearing on the palm while seated is initiated as a preparatory intervention for repetitive task training with massed push–pull movements of the right upper extremity. NMES of the elbow, wrist, finger, and thumb extensors was also added into the treatment as a complement to task-oriented training. After 1 week of NMES, trace muscle contraction was possible along with emerging stretch reflex response to the extensors. However, flexor spasticity of the wrist and fingers increased significantly. To sustain gains in extensor activity, the occupational therapist added orthotic intervention into the therapy plan of care. To maintain a balance of flexors and extensors of the wrist and hand, a dorsal forearm and hand-based immobilization orthosis was fabricated for use when Thomas was not active and for sleep (Fig. 21–35).

Initially, Thomas needed minimal assistance to apply the orthosis. The occupational therapist collaborated with the nursing staff to ensure carryover of wearing schedule and to provide

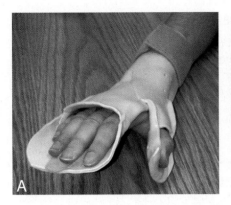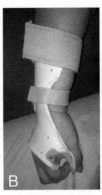

FIGURE 21–35 A, Note the additional finger-restraining straps added to prevent the tendency of the PIP joints to buckle into flexion that could eventually result in Boutonniere positioning. **B,** Dorsal-based wrist immobilization orthosis including thumb positioning. Courtesy of Salvador Bondoc, Associate Professor of Occupational Therapy, Quinnipiac University.

initial assistance to Thomas. Eventually, Thomas was able to independently wear the orthosis and report consistent compliance with wear and stretching schedule.

At the end of 4 weeks of intensive rehabilitation, Thomas was discharged to home with a plan for outpatient therapy services. At discharge, Thomas was able to dress and toilet with modified independence. He continued to need minimal assistance with heavy clothing and bathing. He ambulated at least 300 ft with a quad cane and contact guard assistance for safety. He formulated two to three word statements. He had greater upper extremity voluntary control as demonstrated by ~25% active shoulder elevation, ~75% active flexion of the elbow, massed flexion of the hand, and <25% extension during partial release.

During the last week of inpatient rehabilitation stay, Thomas was trained to use his massed flexion with greater functionality, such as grasping on a small ball or cylinder and carrying a small bag or weight using a hook grasp. But because of poor wrist extensor power, a dorsal wrist extension orthosis was fabricated to prevent passive wrist flexor posturing and to provide stability for active grip during task practice by maintaining functional wrist extension (Fig. 21–35B). Thomas continued the use of the immobilization orthosis for nighttime to prevent flexor contracture development. As tone increased in the digital flexors, modifications were made by gradually increasing the wrist extension and thumb abduction angle.

CASE STUDY 1: Part 2: Acute Cerebrovascular Accident—Outpatient Rehabilitation

Thomas was a highly motivated individual continuing his recovery through the course of his outpatient therapy. Outpatient occupational therapy was geared toward restoring Thomas's upper extremity function through intensive task training. After his initial evaluation, he met the minimum criteria for the SaeboFlex® training program (Fig. 21–28). In addition to having substantial arm elevation and elbow flexion and extension, he also demonstrated mass grasp and emerging active release. He displayed

tolerance of the immobilization orthosis that maintained his wrist and fingers in composite extension. Most importantly, Thomas demonstrated the motivation and capacity to carry out his home program.

Thomas had no known cardiac history prior to the stroke. But upon the occupational therapist's recommendation and with concurrence from his primary care provider, he underwent a stress test. The results of the stress test were highly favorable for him to begin a physical fitness program after 4 weeks of outpatient physical therapy. Upon discharge from physical therapy, he was walking with a small base quad cane and ankle–foot orthosis on even surfaces and close supervision on curbs and uneven surfaces. He was able to tolerate 30 minutes of cardio exercise using a combination of recumbent cycle and an ergometer with a hand-strap attachment.

Thomas received authorization for a total of 20 outpatient occupational therapy visits by his insurance. The plan of care was established so that Thomas would receive treatment twice a week for 10 weeks. He began the SaeboFlex® program 2½ weeks into the course. The main objective of participating into the program was for Thomas to complete most of the requisite number of repetitions doing reach-to-grasp and transport-and-release drills at home. The role of the therapist was to facilitate transfer of training. At the clinic, the SaeboFlex® exercises were also used as a precursor to active practice with the hand without extensor assistance. The repetitive grasp against resistance and release mimicked the proprioceptive neuromuscular facilitation (PNF) inhibitory technique of contract-hold-relax. With the SaeboFlex® orthosis off, Thomas was able to grasp and release tennis balls with the ulnar side of the hand. He developed improved control of mass grasp and release and was able to reach and transport objects away from the body with lesser compensatory movement. The biggest gain that Thomas made was his ability to move his arm in ipsilateral sideward, forward, and backward reach.

Thomas's next biggest barrier was the ability to use the radial side of the hand more functionally. Because most of the training with the SaeboFlex® orthosis was on gross grasp and release functions, the individual function of the fingers and thumb needed further training. In most MCA strokes, thumb adduction and flexion tone along with index finger flexor tone remain to be the most significant barriers to increased functional hand repertoire—especially one that involves precision grip and cylindrical grasp. The aperture of the hand required for pregrasp and the ability to assume precision finger patterns is grossly affected by the thumb–index hypertonic phenomenon. The flexor and adductor tone of the thumb and the index finger may be restrained using functional orthoses to directly address the fine motor control functions of the hand. Hence, the occupational therapist fabricated two orthoses: (1) proximal interphalangeal (PIP) flexion restriction orthoses and (2) first web space midpalmar/radial abduction orthosis (Fig. 21–36). These custom orthoses serve as adjunct to forced use interventions such as modified constraint-induced therapy or repetitive task training. More specifically, these orthoses allowed Thomas to expand on the repertoire of tasks that he could perform.

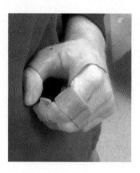

FIGURE 21–36 Functional orthoses used to promote improved use of left hand in completing daily tasks. Courtesy of Salvador Bondoc, Associate Professor of Occupational Therapy, Quinnipiac University.

Thomas would transition to only wearing the thumb abduction orthosis to practice more precision grasp activities beginning with cubes and then progressing to smaller objects. At the end of the 10-week period, Thomas had achieved a more advanced lateral grasp that mimics a basic tip and tripod pinch. With ongoing practice, Thomas will make more functional gains.

Additional case studies can be found on the companion web site on thePoint.

ACKNOWLEDGEMENT FROM SECOND EDITION

Sincere thanks to the following for providing input regarding their products/approaches included in this chapter: Paul Mohr, PT (GivMohr® Corporation), and Waleed Al-Oboudi, MOT, OTR/L (Neuro IFRAH® Organization).

Chapter Review Questions

1. What are common purposes for the use of orthoses in the adult with neurologic dysfunction?

2. What role can taping play in treating this population?

3. What is the theory behind the use of the Saebo products?

4. List a few prefabricated orthoses that may be indicated for use in joint contracture management.

5. What precautions must a therapist be mindful of when dispensing these devices?

22 The Pediatric Patient

Jill Peck-Murray, MOT, OTR/L, CHT*

Chapter Objectives

After study of this chapter, the reader should be able to:

- Appreciate the special developmental and environmental considerations in fabricating an orthosis for a pediatric patient.
- Describe the rationale for orthotic intervention in the pediatric population.
- List the most common diagnoses and appropriate orthotic intervention for the pediatric patient.
- Give examples of design considerations for custom and prefabricated orthoses for the small child.

Key Terms

Asymmetrical tonic neck reflex
Constraint-induced movement treatment
    protocol
Deformity
Gross and fine motor skills
Hypertonicity

Hypotonicity
Low-load, prolonged stretch
Muscle imbalances
Normal physiologic flexion
Pediatric upper extremity gross and fine
    motor development

Primitive reflexes
Spasticity
Stiffness
Tone
Weakness

Introduction

The pediatric patient is not just a "small adult." Therapy and orthosis provision need to be tailored for each child with special consideration for factors that are unique to pediatrics. Children lead an active lifestyle. They are growing and developing **gross and fine motor skills**. It is important for the therapist to remember normal hand skill development when assessing the need for intervention. The purpose and types of orthoses are similar to adult orthoses, but there are often differences in design, material selection, strapping, and padding application. Certain methods need to be used to enhance orthosis use and compliance, prevent self-removal, address primitive reflexes or abnormal tone, and protect the fragile infant. This chapter will describe a typical session for fabrication of an orthosis with suggestions for dealing with the challenges of fabrication and application of an orthosis on a wiggling infant or young child. The final

*This chapter is based on the first edition chapter written by Elaine Charest, MA, MBA, OTR/L

part of this chapter presents case studies of common pediatric conditions and diagnoses with recommendations for possible options for orthoses. It is beyond the scope of this chapter to describe all the orthoses that can possibly be made to treat the hands of children. The author of this chapter and the editors of this book provide the tools to critically assess a pediatric hand and teach the application of clinical reasoning skills to formulate an individual orthotic intervention plan for each unique child.

Normal Hand Skill Development

Assessing the child from a developmental perspective rather than from an anatomical perspective will allow the therapist to determine the most appropriate intervention that may include an orthosis (Ho, 2010). Table 22–1 is a brief summary of **pediatric upper extremity (UE) gross and fine motor development** with focus on grasp and hand skill development in the first 6 years of life. The therapist should do an assessment of the child's grasp and developmental skills because it is vital for therapeutic planning and goal setting. It is important for the therapist to remember details of **normal physiologic flexion** and **primitive reflexes** that predominate in the first few months of life. Parents may be concerned that the infant keeps his or her fingers and/or thumb flexed into the palm, but the therapist can explain that this is considered normal until age 4 months. If there are major delays beyond that age, an orthosis may be indicated. If an 8-month-old infant is still using a raking grasp or using the dorsal surface of the thumb for grasping, a soft neoprene thumb orthosis may help position the thumb to allow for more normal use (Fig. 22–1A–D). If that child is not yet crawling, the therapist may consider an orthosis to open the hand (Fig. 22–2). A weight-bearing orthosis positions the hand in the most effective position for weight-bearing activities (Kinghorn & Roberts 1996; Lindholm, 1986). Refer to Box 22–1 for fabrication instructions.

Purposes of Orthoses for the Pediatric Patient

The primary purposes of pediatric orthoses are to provide protection and support, proper positioning to enhance function, and to improve passive motion (Hogan & Uditsky, 1998).

Provide Protection and Support

After a child has undergone surgery or sustained an injury, the physician may request an orthosis to protect the healing tissue, skin, tendons, nerves, joints, and muscles. The body part may need to be protected or immobilized, whereas other parts are allowed to move for a certain period of time.

When there is **spasticity** or **weakness**, the maintenance of normal anatomical relationships is important to prevent permanent contracture and subsequent loss of function. An orthosis can provide proper positioning to align joints and prevent the shortening of soft tissues causing a deformity or the progression of deformity (Fig. 22–3A–C) (Schoen & Anderson, 1999). Refer to Box 22–2 for fabrication instructions. If the extremity is held tightly flexed by significant **tone** or severe **deformity**, an orthosis may be necessary to help maintain hygiene and skin integrity. To prevent skin breakdown, the areas that are held closed with minimal air circulation, such as a tightly fisted hand, adducted shoulder, or strongly flexed elbow, may need an orthosis to provide positioning (Fig. 22–4A,B).

Provide Positioning to Enhance Function

The pediatric patient may be born with a condition or sustain an injury to the ligaments, tendons, joints, or neurovascular structures that can affect joint stability. An unstable joint significantly alters the biomechanics of the hand or arm and thus affects function. Thumb hypoplasia (Table 22–2) or mild spasticity can cause a thumb to be unstable at the metacarpal joint so the child may not be able to hold finger foods. An orthosis can provide proximal stabilization to aid positioning that allows for function. The use of soft materials such as neoprene may provide enough support to allow for grasp and release tasks (Fig. 22–1A,B). If this does not provide enough support, thermoplastic material can be formed in the web space to place the thumb tip in opposition to the fingers for function (Figs. 22–1C and 22–5).

When there is weakness due to significant loss of muscle strength, an orthosis can provide the external support to a proximal joint to allow for distal use. The child with radial nerve palsy, brachial plexus palsy, arthrogryposis, or hemiplegia (Table 22–2) may lack active wrist extension so the hand is not held in an optimal position for use. A wrist orthosis that supports the wrist can provide the proper positioning to permit finger to thumb prehension and object manipulation (Fig. 22–6A–C).

TABLE 22–1

Pediatric Upper Extremity Gross and Fine Motor Skills

Age	Grasp and Skill Development	Age	Grasp and Skill Development
0–2 months	**Reflexive grasp** • Hand closes on objects placed in palm • Normal physiologic flexion (hands fisted), except with startle or stretching	10 months	**Pincer grasp** • Holds small object held with pads of index and thumb • Stands and cruises • Pokes with index finger • Beginning tool use (spoon)
2–3 months	**Ulnar palmar grasp** • Holds toy or block placed in hand on ulnar side of hand • In supine, moves arms overhead and brings hands together on chest	12 months	**Neat pincer grasp** • Holds small object with tip of index and thumb tip flexed • Walking independently, so more hand use • Uses hands in a coordinated manner (one hand stabilizes and other manipulates)
4 months	**Crude palmar grasp** • Contacts toy with palmar surface of hand • In prone, bears weight on ulnar side of forearms with good head control • Grasp reflex diminishing so thumb is no longer flexed in palm	15 months	**Forearm neutral palmar grasp** • Holds marker in palm with forearm neutral • Releases object with wrist extension into container • Stacks two blocks • Holds ball in two hands
5 months	**Palmar grasp** • Holds toy in palm enclosed by fingers with thumb adducted • In prone, pushes up on extended arms • In supine, can hold bottle with partial forearm supination	2–3 years	**Digital pronated grasp** • Holds marker with fingers and thumb with forearm pronated • Places small object into a hole with precision • Stacks 3–6 blocks into a tower
6 months	**Raking grasp** • Uses all fingers to rake small objects into palm • In prone, weight shifts on extended arms • In independent sitting, hands are now free for use • Grasp and release in purposeful manner	3.1–4 years	**Static tripod grasp** • Holds marker static with thumb, index, and long fingers • Stacks 7–9 blocks into a tower • Able to draw shapes • Beginning to cut with scissors
7 months	**Radial palmar grasp** • Holds toy or block in radial side of hand • In prone, pivots and combat crawls • In sitting, transfers objects from one hand to another	4.5–6 years	**Dynamic tripod grasp** • Holds marker with moving tips of thumb, index, and long fingers • Stacks 10–12 blocks into a tower • Able to write letters
8 months	**Developmental scissors grasp** • Holds small object with thumb and radial side of index • Crawling with weight bearing through shoulder, elbow, and wrist		
9 months	**Inferior pincer grasp** • Holds small object with thumb along distal radial side of extended index • Active forearm supination when reaching • Grasps toy or block using thumb and fingertips		

Modified from Charest, E. (2003). The pediatric patient. In N. Austin & M. Jacobs (Eds.), *Splinting the hand and upper extremity: Principles and process.* Baltimore, MD: Lippincott Williams & Wilkins; Ho, E. S. (2010). Measuring hand function in the young child. *Journal of Hand Therapy, 23*(3), 323–328; Erhardt, R., & Lindley, S. (2000). Functional development of the hand. In A. Gupta, S. Kay, & L. Scheker (Eds.), *The growing hand: Diagnosis and management of the upper extremity in children.* London, United Kingdom: Mosby.

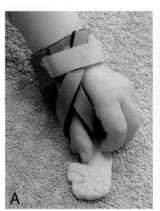 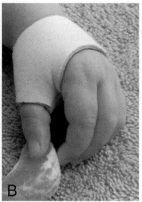 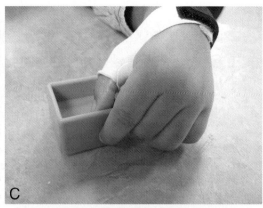

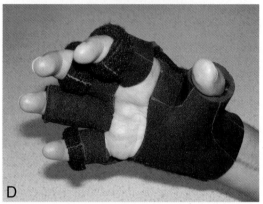

FIGURE 22–1 **A,** This prefabricated Thumb Abduction Splint (The Joe Cool Company, South Jordan, UT) can provide a subtle support and proper positioning of the thumb to allow for use. **B,** This custom-made neoprene thumb abduction orthosis can provide more support needed to mobilize the thumb for grasp. **C,** Thin thermoplastic can be substituted for neoprene if a more rigid support is necessary. **D,** This prefabricated thumb orthosis (BD-88, The Benik Corporation, Silverdale, WA) provides thumb support, and additional neoprene tubes have been added to it to position the fingers.

BOX 22–1

Weight-Bearing Orthosis

- Use a piece of ³⁄₃₂″ thermoplastic material 2″ wider and longer than the child's hand.
- Place a ball of Theraputty onto a nonadherent surface.
- Heat thermoplastic and mold onto supinated palm to form the palmar piece.
- While abducting the fingers and thumb, allow material to drape between web spaces to form finger separators.
- As material is partially set, carefully pronate hand into a weight-bearing position and press into the ball of Theraputty.
- As material sets, direct attention to the ulnar and radial edges forming borders to improve fit.
- After removal, use hole punch to make the following four slits in orthosis:
  - First web space
  - Index finger MCP joint
  - Base of thumb CMC
  - Small finger MCP joint
- Use a length of material (such as a ribbon or felt) and weave it through the slits and tie in a Figure-8 around the wrist as shown in Figure 22–2.
- Another option includes using traditional hook-and-loop closure.

CMC, carpometacarpal.

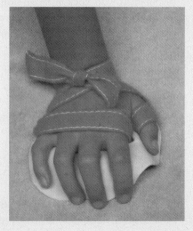

FIGURE 22–2 **Weight-Bearing Orthosis.** Thermoplastic material molded between the web spaces on the volar surface of the hand can help position the hand for weight bearing. Soft felt ribbon tied over the fingers and thumb and then around the wrist in a Figure-8 fashion secures the orthosis for crawling.

BOX 22–2

Volar/Dorsal Wrist and Hand Immobilization Orthosis

1. First heat the smaller hand segment.
2. Position child's hand by extending fingers with wrist in flexion.
3. Place material onto hand with base conforming into palmar arch.
4. While holding the thumb in abduction and extension, form thumb piece with gentle pressure, molding a trough for the thumb to rest.
5. Position the fingers into extension at IP joints and slight flexion at MCP joints while allowing the wrist to remain slightly flexed (except with significant extrinsic tightness, wrist should be moved into extension and fingers allowed to flex as needed).
6. Remove hand segment and prepare to heat and mold larger dorsal forearm-based segment.
7. Position child's arm by placing wrist into extension and allowing fingers to flex.
8. Place material onto dorsal forearm, gently smoothing down the sides. Distal edge should end at midmetacarpal region.
9. Allow the distal lateral pieces (wings), positioned ulnarly at the base of small finger and radially over web space, to "hang" while material sets.
10. Remove forearm segment.
11. Place hand segment on child and position wrist in maximal extension.
12. Reheat the "wings" on the forearm segment only in water to soften slightly.
13. Place dorsal forearm segment on child and gently mold "wings" around the ulnar and radial sides of the volar hand segment to attach in palm. Mark points where pieces overlap.
14. Remove both segments and permanently attach together. (Either use solvent or scratch off coating, followed by heating areas to bond with heat gun.)
15. Apply hook-and-loop straps as shown in Figure 22–3A–C.
16. Please note to wrist strap tension is key to help prevent slippage.
17. Be sure to choose a material with a protective coating to prevent inadvertent adherence during the molding process.

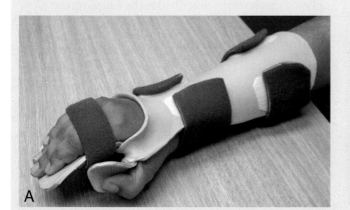

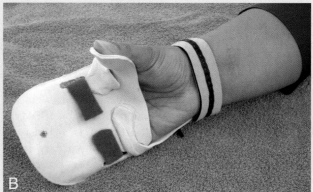

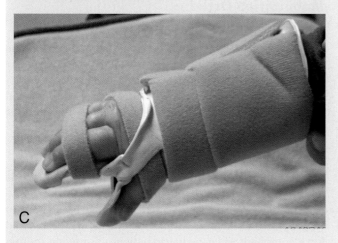

FIGURE 22–3 Volar/Dorsal Wrist and Hand Immobilization Orthosis. A and B, This immobilization orthosis with a dorsal forearm and volar hand piece can provide proper positioning to align joints and prevent contractures. **C,** This is an infant-size custom orthosis with a dorsal forearm and volar hand piece.

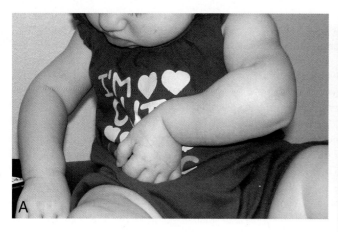
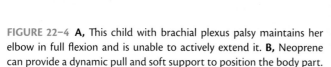
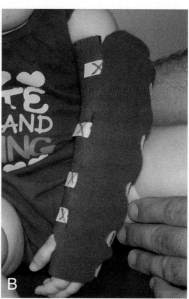

FIGURE 22–4 **A,** This child with brachial plexus palsy maintains her elbow in full flexion and is unable to actively extend it. **B,** Neoprene can provide a dynamic pull and soft support to position the body part.

Muscle imbalances can affect the position of an arm and ultimately interfere with normal developmental skills, such as crawling. The dynamic component of a stretchy material, such as neoprene or Fabrifoam®, can assist a weak muscle group to place the hand/arm in the position for function. For example, mobilization orthoses (Fig. 22–7A,B) can encourage supination and/or shoulder external rotation to position the arm appropriately for hand use or weight bearing and crawling.

Provide Stretch to Improve Passive Motion

When a cast is removed, **stiffness** typically resolves quickly in children. But if the passive range of motion (ROM) is limited, therapy may include the use of an orthosis to help gain motion and maximize tissue length. **Low-load, prolonged stretch** (LLPS) by the use of a cast or orthosis is the best, conservative way of increasing passive ROM (Fig. 22–8) (Duff & Charles, 2004). The orthosis can help maintain motion that was gained in therapy or help gain motion by placing the body part in a submaximal range (Exner, 2005).

Types of Orthoses for the Pediatric Patient

The types of orthoses chosen for the pediatric patient are similar to adult options, but there are often differences in design and material selection as well as strapping and padding applications. The following section will review the three categories of orthoses and the specific application to the pediatric patient. These are immobilization orthoses

(see Chapter 7), mobilization orthoses (see Chapter 8), and restriction orthoses (see Chapter 9). Orthoses in these categories can be custom fabricated, or a clinician may choose to use a prefabricated option (see Chapter 11). Within each of these categories, there are many design and material options, which will be described in the following text.

Immobilization Orthoses

Static Type

A static-type orthosis provides a firm base and immobilizes the joints it crosses. There are no movable parts. These supportive orthoses can protect joints or wounds, prevent deformity, or block motion in one joint while encouraging motion in another. Most pediatric orthoses are the static type. These can be custom made, or there are prefabricated options available.

Mobilization Orthoses

Serial Static Type

A serial static type is a mobilization orthosis that holds tissue at maximal length with periodic remolding to change the position. This type is effective to gain motion if a contracture has developed after injury or stiffness from a congenital anomaly, such as camptodactyly (Fig. 22–9) or arthrogryposis (Fig. 22–8).

Static Progressive Type

A static progressive type is another mobilization orthosis option using nonelastic components to provide an LLPS to gain mobility. Because the patient controls the amount of force applied to increase the motion, this type is best suited for a compliant older pediatric patient. Improving motion

TABLE 22–2

Orthotic Intervention for Common Pediatric Diagnoses

Diagnosis	Description	Therapeutic Intervention	Suggested Orthoses
Arthrogryposis	Congenital condition characterized by joint contractures and weakness Amyoplasia: shoulders internally rotated, elbow extended, wrist flexed, thumbs adducted Distal type: thumbs/fingers flexed, webbed, MCPs ulnarly deviated	Aggressive stretching to gain passive elbow flexion, wrist/hand extension, and thumb abduction	**Custom:** Serial casting, serial static, or static progressive mobilization orthoses (Figs. 22–3A and 22–8) **Prefabs:** LYNX WHFO™ (Alimed, Dedham, MA) (Fig. 22–14C); Comfy™ Pediatric Hand Thumb Orthosis and Comfyprene™ Pediatric Hand Orthosis (Lenjoy Medical Engineering Inc., Gardena, CA)
		Provide proper wrist position for hand use	**Custom:** Dorsal wrist immobilization orthosis (Fig. 22–6A) **Prefabs:** Liberty™ Wrist Brace (North Coast Medical, Morgan Hill, CA) (Fig. 22–6C); RCAI® Carpal Tunnel Splint (Restorative Care of America, St Petersburg, FL)
Brachial plexus palsy	Stretch injury to the brachial plexus resulting in varying degrees of weakness in the involved arm	Provide proper positioning for the wrist or elbow	**Custom:** Volar or dorsal wrist immobilization orthosis; elbow extension orthosis (Fig. 22–4B) **Prefabs:** Benik Neoprene Wrist Splints (Series 300)
		Correct elbow flexion <40° contracture	**Custom:** Serial static elbow extension orthosis (Fig. 22–8)
		>40° contracture	**Custom:** Serial casting
Camptodactyly	Congenital PIP contracture, usually of small finger	Reduce PIP flexion <30° contracture	**Custom:** Hand-based, finger extension mobilization, serial static orthosis (Fig. 22–9)
		>30° contracture	**Custom:** Serial casting
Cerebral palsy	Nonprogressive motor impairment caused by injury to the developing brain that causes irreversible upper motor neuron disorder characterized by abnormal tone, weakness, and progressive joint contractures	Maintain maximal soft tissue length to prevent elbow deformity or stabilize postoperatively	**Prefabs:** Comfy™ Pediatric elbow brace; Posey® soft-bead elbow splint (Posey, Arcadia CA); IMAK Pil-O-Splint® (IMAK®, Spirit Lake, IA), DynaPro™ Flex Elbow, Ultraflex Elbow Orthosis
		Maintain maximal soft tissue length to prevent wrist/hand deformity or stabilize postoperatively	**Custom:** Volar or volar/dorsal immobilization orthosis **Prefabs:** LYNX WHFO™ (Fig. 22–14C); Comfy™ Pediatric Hand Thumb Orthosis; Comfyprene™ Pediatric Hand Orthosis; TheraPlus® TA Hand Contracture Brace (Orthotic Rehab Products, Tampa, FL); Neuroflex™ Pediatric Thumb Ease (Fig. 22–21) (North Coast Medical); Pucci inflatable splint (DeRoyal Industries®, Powell, TN)
		Provide proper position to forearm to enhance distal function	**Custom:** Serpentine style forearm strap made of neoprene (Fig. 22–7A) or Fabrifoam® (Fig. 22–7B) **Prefabs:** McKie (McKie Splints, LLC Duluth, MN) or Benik supinator strap
		Provide proper position to wrist to enhance distal function	**Custom:** Dorsal wrist orthosis **Prefabs:** North Coast Liberty™ Wrist Brace (Fig. 22–6C); Benik Neoprene Wrist Splints (Fig. 22–14A); RCAI® Carpal Tunnel Splint
		Provide proper position to thumb or fingers to enhance distal function	**Custom:** Web space orthosis (Fig. 22–5); neoprene thumb abduction orthosis (Fig. 22–1B) **Prefabs:** Joe Cool Thumb Splints (Fig. 22–1A); Benik Thumb Splints (Fig. 22–1C); RCAI® Thumb Abduction Support

(continued)

TABLE 22–2

Orthotic Intervention for Common Pediatric Diagnoses (Continued)

Diagnosis	Description	Therapeutic Intervention	Suggested Orthoses
Charcot-Marie-Tooth disease	Hereditary sensorimotor polyneuropathy characterized by progressive weakness primarily in intrinsic weakness in feet and hands	Substitute for intrinsic finger weakness	**Custom:** Figure-8 orthosis **Prefab:** Oval-8® Finger Splint (3-Point Products, Stevensville, MD)
		Position thumb or fingers for use	**Custom:** Neoprene thumb abduction orthoses (Fig. 22–1B) **Prefabs:** Joe Cool Thumb Splints (Fig. 22–1A); McKie Thumb Splint; Benik Thumb Splints (Fig. 22–1C); RCAI® Thumb Abduction Support
Duchenne muscular dystrophy	Slowly progressive proximal to distal muscle weakness and wasting, eventually involves all voluntary muscles including respiratory muscles, which makes survival beyond age 20 years rare	Provide positioning to prevent contracture of the elbow	**Custom:** Elbow extension orthosis (Fig. 22–4B) **Prefabs:** Comfy™ elbow brace; Posey® soft-bead elbow splint; IMAK elbow support; IMAK Pil-O-Splint®
		Provide positioning to prevent contractures of wrist and hand	**Custom:** Volar or volar/dorsal immobilization orthoses (Fig. 22–3) **Prefabs:** LYNX WHFO™ (Fig. 22–14C); Comfy™ Pediatric Hand Thumb Orthosis; Comfyprene™ Pediatric Hand Orthosis; TheraPlus® TA Hand Contracture Brace
		Provide positioning of wrists for use	**Custom:** Dorsal wrist immobilization orthosis (Fig. 22–6B) **Prefabs:** North Coast Liberty™ Wrist Brace (Fig. 22–6C); Benik Neoprene Wrist Splints (Fig. 22–14A); Carpal Tunnel Brace from RCAI®
Fractures	Elbow fractures Distal ulna/radius fractures Finger fractures	Reduce postsurgical or cast removal stiffness	**Custom:** Serial static (Fig. 22–8) or static progressive (turnbuckle) mobilization orthoses **Prefabs:** Dynasplint® (Severna Park, MD), Ultraflex (Pottstown, PA), or JAS® (Effingham, IL) Braces for forearm, finger, or elbow (Fig. 22–10); LMB Finger Extension Splint (DeRoyal)
Hemiplegia due to stroke or other neurologic insult	Involvement of upper and lower extremity on same side; typically includes shoulder internal rotation, forearm pronation, wrist and finger/thumb flexion	Compensate for muscle imbalances in shoulder, elbow, and forearm	**Custom:** Serpentine style strap which is made of neoprene (Fig. 22–7A) or Fabrifoam® (Fig. 22–7B)
		Provide proper wrist/thumb position for hand use	**Custom:** Static dorsal wrist immobilization orthosis (Fig. 22–6B); weight-bearing orthosis (Fig. 22–2) **Prefabs:** North Coast Liberty™ Wrist Brace (Fig. 22–6C); Benik Neoprene Wrist Splints (Fig. 22–14A); Carpal Tunnel Brace from RCAI®
		Provide proper thumb positioning for use	**Custom:** Web space orthosis (Fig. 22–5) **Prefabs:** Joe Cool Thumb Splints (Fig. 22–1A); McKie Thumb Splints; Benik Thumb Splints (Fig. 22–1C)
		Constraint for noninvolved extremity to encourage use of involved extremity	**Custom:** Univalved cast made of polyester casting tapes (Fig. 22–8) **Prefabs:** PediWrap™ Pediatric Arm Immobilizers (The Med-Kid Co., Hemet, CA) (Fig. 22–23); Crandall (Bird and Cronin, Inc., Eagen, MN) Elbow Splint
Juvenile arthritis	Persistent swelling of joints with onset before age 16 years; may range from oligoarthritis (few joint involvement) to polyarthritis (many joint involvement)	Reduce pain and provide proper night positioning	**Custom:** Wrist/hand immobilization orthoses (Fig. 22–2A)
		Position wrist in extension to prevent loss of motion and reduce pain	**Custom:** Wrist immobilization orthoses (Fig. 22–6B) **Prefabs:** North Coast Liberty™ Wrist Brace (Fig. 22–6C); Benik Neoprene Wrist Splints (Fig. 22–14A); Carpal Tunnel Brace from RCAI®

TABLE 22–2

Orthotic Intervention for Common Pediatric Diagnoses (Continued)

Diagnosis	Description	Therapeutic Intervention	Suggested Orthoses
Nerve injuries	Radial nerve injuries common with humeral fractures	Positioning to prevent contractures	**Custom:** Wrist immobilization orthoses **Prefabs:** Benik Radial Nerve Tunnel® Splint; Liberty™ Wrist Splint (Fig. 22–6C)
	Ulnar nerve injuries	Positioning to prevent contractures	**Custom:** MCP blocking orthoses (Figs. 22–11 and 22–24)
Osteogenesis imperfecta	Hereditary connective tissue disorder characterized by defect in bone matrix calcification, resulting in some degree of bone fragility and deformity	Fracture management Protection Support	**Custom:** Immobilization orthoses supporting fracture sites or protecting vulnerable sites **Prefabs:** RCAI® Humeral Fracture Brace; RCAI® Wrist Fracture Orthosis
Radial ray deficiency	Congenital malformation of radial side of arm: radius, carpal bones, and/or thumb; clinically often severe radial deviation at wrist	Minimize soft tissue tightness due to radial wrist deviation posturing	**Custom:** Circumferential soft wrap (Fig. 22–25), ulnar-based wrist immobilization orthosis (Fig. 22–13B)
Rett syndrome	Progressive encephalopathy with loss of purposeful hand use with characteristic hand wringing and ataxia	Provide positioning to prevent excessive hand wringing or hand-to-mouth behavior	**Custom:** Elbow static orthosis **Prefabs:** PediWrap™ Pediatric Arm Immobilizer (Fig. 22–23); Benik Neoprene Elbow Sleeve
Syndactyly	Lack of differentiation of fingers, skin, and/or bones	Postoperative scar extension management and maintain extension of fingers	**Custom:** Finger extension orthosis lined with moldable silicone putty (Fig. 22–3B)
Sports injuries/ tendonitis	Overuse issues with pain, swelling, and limited use	Support to decrease pain and swelling	**Custom or Prefabs:** Immobilization orthoses as indicated by injury
Thumb hypoplasia	Underdevelopment of thumb clinically presents with various types from mild weakness to absent thumb	Preserve first web space and provide support for use	**Custom:** Web space opening orthosis (Fig. 22–5) **Prefabs:** Joe Cool Thumb Splints (Fig. 22–1A); McKie Thumb Splints; Benik Thumb Splints (Fig. 22–1C)
		Postsurgical protection after pollicization or opponensplasty	**Custom:** Thumb spica static-type immobilization orthosis
Thumb-in-palm deformities	Flexion posturing of thumb due to lack of thumb extension musculature	Position in full extension at night	**Custom:** Thumb extension immobilization orthosis (Fig. 22–20)
		Support thumb to allow for use	**Custom:** Opponens thumb orthosis; web space orthosis (Fig. 22–5); custom neoprene orthosis (Fig. 22–1B) **Prefabs:** Joe Cool Thumb Ssplints (Fig. 22–1A); McKie Thumb Splints; Benik Thumb Splints (Fig. 22–1C)
Ulnar deficiency	Congenital malformation of ulnar side of arm; clinically presents with wrist ulnar deviation	Maximize soft tissue length prior to surgery	**Custom:** Radially based wrist immobilization orthosis

RCAI, Restorative Care of America, Inc.

Modified from Charest, E. (2003). The pediatric patient. In N. Austin & M. Jacobs (Eds.), *Splinting the hand and upper extremity: Principles and process.* Baltimore, MD: Lippincott Williams & Wilkins; Ho, E., Roy, T., Stephens, D., & Clarke, H. M. (2010). Serial casting and splinting of elbow contractures in children with obstetric brachial plexus palsy. *Journal of Hand Surgery,* 35A, 84–91; Fuller, M. (1999). Treatment of congenital differences of the upper extremity: Therapist's commentary. *Journal of Hand Therapy,* 12(2), 174–177; Moran, S. L., & Tomhave, W. (2011). Management of congenital hand anomalies. In T. Skiven, L. Osterman, J. Fedorczyk, & P. Amadio (Eds.), *Rehabilitation of the hand and upper extremity* (6th ed., pp. 1631–1646). Philadelphia, PA: Mosby.

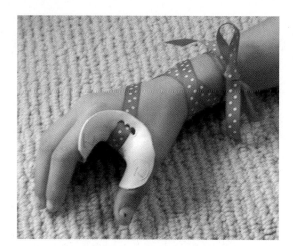

FIGURE 22–5 An orthosis formed in the web space can provide a more rigid support to position the thumb and index finger for use.

after an injury, such as an elbow fracture, can often be effectively managed with this type of orthosis (Fig. 22–10).

Dynamic Type

Dynamic types of orthoses use elastic components to exert a force to make gains in passive motion or to act as an assist for weak muscles. With adults, the orthosis often involves high-profile outriggers, but this orthosis would not be appropriate for a young child due to risk of injury from attachments and complex application. A low-profile design is preferred with the pediatric population. Soft materials with a stretchy

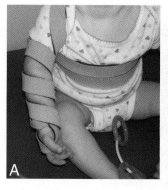
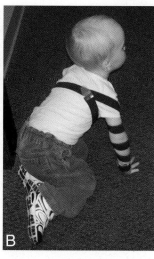

FIGURE 22–7 **A,** A mobilization orthosis made of neoprene assists forearm supination and shoulder external rotation to position the hand for use. **B,** A long strip of Fabrifoam® can be used to position the entire arm for crawling or weight bearing.

component such as neoprene can be a good choice for a dynamic orthosis (Figs. 22–1, 22–4, and 22–7).

Restriction Orthoses

Drop-out Type

A drop-out–type orthosis is a restriction/torque transmission–type orthosis that blocks motion in one direction

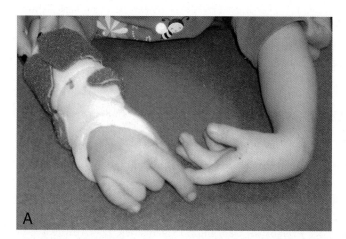

FIGURE 22–6 **A,** This child with arthrogryposis was unable to actively extend her wrist. This dorsal-based wrist orthosis provided better position for distal use. **B,** This child with hemiplegia was unable to actively extend her wrist. This dorsal-based orthosis provided position to prevent shortening of her flexor tendons with a compensatory tenodesis release pattern. Soft straps attached with finger rivets or a ribbon attached to the strap can prevent self-removal. **C,** This child with radial nerve laceration was unable to actively extend his wrist. This prefabricated Liberty™ Wrist Brace (North Coast Medical) provided wrist support. The MCP joints are free for motion because this orthosis does not cross the distal palmar crease.

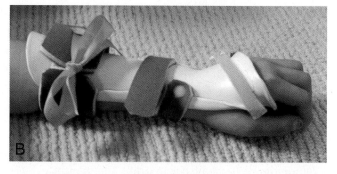
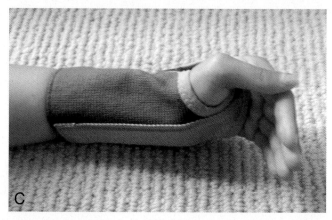

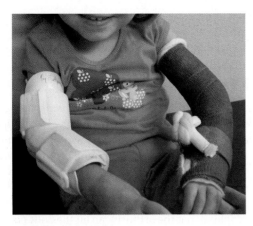

FIGURE 22–8 For this child with arthrogryposis, a cast was used to gain more passive elbow flexion, and custom thermoplastic immobilization orthosis was used to maintain gains. Note writing on orthosis to aid parents in proper application.

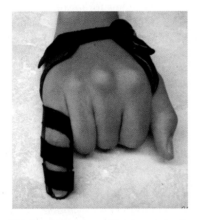

FIGURE 22–9 This hand-based mobilization orthosis can be used to improve PIP joint extension in a serial static manner.

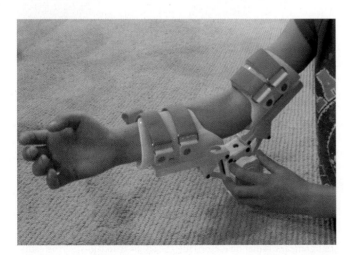

FIGURE 22–10 This elbow mobilization orthosis (JAS®) can provide static progressive stretch that is controlled by the patient to increase the tension with a turn of the knob.

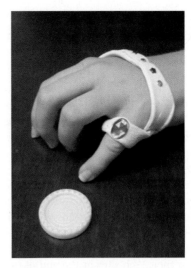

FIGURE 22–11 This orthosis can prevent hyperextension of the MP joint while encouraging PIP joint extension during exercise (pushing disc across table). Note decorations on the orthosis, which helped in maximizing acceptance and compliance.

while encouraging motion in the other direction. For example, an exercise orthosis to prevent hyperextension of the metacarpophalangeal (MCP) joint can be used to promote active proximal interphalangeal (PIP) joint extension (Fig. 22–11).

Articulated Type

Articulated types are mobilization/restriction orthoses that use a hinged joint to provide supportive motion in one plane. Prefabricated hinges are often too large for children, and custom hinges can be fabricated using speedy rivets or screw posts that are placed through holes in ends of thermoplastic strips attached to two circumferential cuffs (Fig. 22–12).

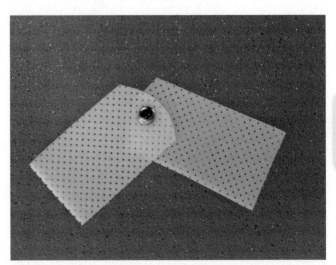

FIGURE 22–12 Homemade hinge fabricated from scrap thermoplastic material and a speedy rivet.

Orthotic Intervention for Specific Pediatric Diagnosis

The therapist must have a basic understanding of the various diagnoses that are specific to the pediatric population in order to design the most appropriate therapeutic intervention. The therapy program may involve the use of orthoses to enhance functional use and to provide proper positioning or protection before or after necessary surgical intervention. The therapist needs to select the most appropriate type of orthoses for each individual condition. The orthosis may be custom made out of thermoplastics or other materials. There are various types of prefabricated (prefabs) orthoses that also may be an option but should be selected carefully. Refer to the comprehensive listing of vendors and their Web sites at the end of this chapter for more information about prefabs. Table 22–2 provides description of common diagnoses, therapeutic intervention, and possible orthoses (custom or prefabricated) as indicated by the goals of therapy. However, the therapist should not decide on an orthosis based on the specific diagnosis. The final decision regarding orthotic intervention is made based on the limitations in specific movements, the type and severity of abnormal muscle tone, the extent of soft tissue and bony involvement, the child's functional level, the child's environment, and the frame of reference guiding therapy (Gabriel, 2008).

Proper Selection/Design for Pediatric Patients

Assessment and Treatment Planning

The therapist needs to base orthosis selection and design on multiple factors. It is essential to understand the diagnosis as well as the affected structures and systems. A complete evaluation will help reveal if there are issues related to the following:

- Motion
- Strength
- Joint stability
- Pain
- Wound healing
- Tonal abnormalities
- Scar formation
- Skin integrity
- Sensation
- Developmental delays

Then, the therapist needs to determine if an orthosis can address any of these issues. For example, an infant with type IV radial ray deficiency (Table 22–2) will exhibit significant wrist radial deviation (Fig. 22–13A). Surgical intervention is not an option until the infant is at least 1 year of age. So the goal of therapy is to maintain the soft tissue length of the involved structures. The parents are advised to perform

a stretching program with every diaper change and use a forearm–hand orthosis at all other times (Fig. 22–13B) (Moran & Tomhave, 2011).

Design Principles

Proper design should be based on good problem solving that is grounded in proper biomechanical principles (see Chapter 4). Appropriate decisions about location, width, and length are critical in design plans. In designing the orthosis, the therapist should use three points of pressure (one at each end in one direction and one in the middle in the other direction). If possible, the design should take advantage of this first class lever principle so that the orthosis can lift the body part rather than the straps forcing the body part into place. An example is a dorsal-based wrist orthosis (Fig. 22–6A,B) or ulnar-based orthosis (Fig. 22–13B). The design also needs to address the appropriate width and length of the orthosis (Fig. 22–6B). The width of the orthosis should be at least half the circumference of the body part, whether it is the upper arm, forearm, wrist, or finger/thumb. This will allow for maximal purchase from the straps when applied. The length should be as long as necessary to distribute the pressure appropriately, using joint creases as a guide to provide maximal length of levers. If the orthosis is a forearm based, then it should be designed to two-thirds of the length of the arm (Fig. 22–6B). The orthosis should be designed to support all necessary joints while allowing freedom of unaffected joints (Fig. 22–6B,C).

Selection of Prefabricated Orthoses for the Pediatric Patient

Fortunately, more options for prefabricated orthoses in pediatric sizes have recently become available. There are multiple

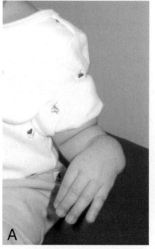
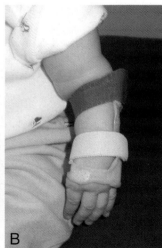

FIGURE 22–13 A, This child with type 4 radial ray deficiency exhibits significant radial deviation due to lack of structures on the radial side of the arm. **B,** The ulnar-based orthosis can provide the leverage needed to position the wrist in neutral. Small vertical snips have been added to the proximal strap to improve comfort.

resources for prefabricated orthoses (refer to listing at the end of this chapter including Web sites). The therapist needs to make a critical assessment of the orthosis before provision or ordering for a patient (see Chapter 11). The following issues need to be addressed:

- Is there an appropriate design needed for the patient to enhance function, provide support, or improve motion?
- Can the orthosis be ordered in the proper size? Having some sample sizes to try on the patient will help to determine if it provides proper positioning to aid function.
- Is it easy to apply for the family or patient? An orthosis that has multiple components may be too complicated for proper application.
- Do the straps allow for good purchase and positioning? A close examination of the strap placement is necessary to ensure that the appropriate forces are applied in the needed direction with necessary distribution of the pressure.
- Can the orthosis be adjusted for growth or change in position? Some of the newer styles are adjustable because they have thin thermoplastic (Fig. 22–14A), plastic, or malleable metal embedded within (Fig. 22–14B,C). There are other types that provide a dynamic stretch or serial progressive stretch to improve motion (Fig. 22–10).
- Is it washable? The materials should be washable and durable, especially if it is for long-term use.
- Who will be responsible for payment? The therapist needs to determine if the cost is affordable for the family if the insurance will not pay for it.

Fabrication of Custom Orthoses for the Pediatric Patient

Material Selection

- Functional limitations

There are many materials options to use for orthoses as described in Chapter 5. In pediatrics, it is important to start with the softest/thinnest/lightest material possible and choose thicker options as needed. Softer materials can include neoprene, soft foam strapping, Fabrifoam®, Plastazote®, and silicone-based putty. At the other end of the spectrum, the hardest materials include casting materials, such as plaster or the newer polyester casting tapes. Casting materials are very durable and conforming. They can be used for serially improving ROM in infants with arthrogryposis (Fig. 22–8) or teenagers with PIP joint flexion contractures. Some materials have the advantage of allowing the child to get them wet to swim or bathe. Casting materials are often used for fabrication of a constraint used in a **constraint-induced movement treatment protocol (CIMT)**. See Chapter 12 for more details on casting techniques.

Thermoplastics are the most common materials used for pediatric orthoses. The selection of the material type, thickness, and color may depend on multiple factors, including the required size and the function of the orthosis. The weight of the orthosis can be significant for infants and patients with weak muscles. Most materials come in various thicknesses: $\frac{1}{16}''$, $\frac{3}{32}''$, and $\frac{1}{8}''$. If the orthosis is required to be rigid to help manage spasticity, the material may need to be $\frac{1}{8}''$ thick or thinner with extra layers for reinforcement. An orthosis for a neonate is commonly made of $\frac{1}{16}''$ material to keep it thin and lightweight.

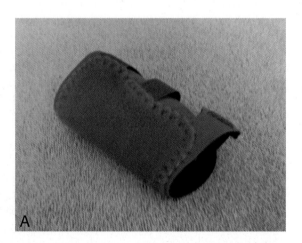

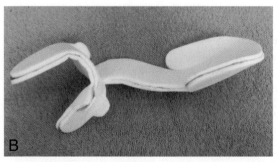

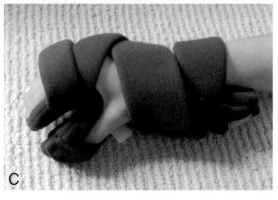

FIGURE 22–14 **A,** This prefabricated orthosis (Benik) with thin thermoplastic embedded inside the neoprene can add more support to position the body part. **B,** This is an example of the malleable metal with padding that is inside of several types of prefabricated orthoses. **C,** This orthosis (LYNX WFHO™) can be easily bent into correct position for fingers, thumb, and wrist.

This same thickness can be used to make a circumferential wrist orthosis that is supportive and easy to apply for an older child or teenager. Choosing a circumferential design allows for a thinner material because of how rigid an orthosis is when a body part is fully encompassed. Most pediatric orthoses are made of the thinner (¹⁄₁₆″ or ³⁄₃₂″) materials.

Each type of thermoplastic material has different properties, and selection should be based on what is necessary to correctly form the orthosis. The four major types of thermoplastics are plastic based, elastic based, rubber based, and combined plastic/rubber based (Armstrong, 2005). The plastic-based thermoplastics have a great deal of conformability but can be easily overstretched so they are best suited for small orthoses on the thumb or web space. Elastic-based thermoplastics have good conformability and resistance to stretch with a high degree of memory. This memory allows the entire orthosis to be remolded but can make it difficult to reform sections and smooth edges. The temporary bonding ability in an antigravity position is helpful when fabricating orthoses on children. The long working and setup time make this type of material difficult to use on squirming children, and the fact that these materials must be fully cooled on the patient to prevent shrinkage is also problematic at times. The rubber-based thermoplastics have a high resistance to stretch and minimal conformability. Due to the longer time for setup, the materials may need to be wrapped on with ace wraps for children with spasticity or limited cooperation. The combined rubber/plastic-based thermoplastics are durable with balanced control and conformability. These have mild to moderate resistance to stretch and are easy to remold and edge. There is a relatively short working and setup time that makes them a good choice for pediatric patients.

The color of the material for the orthosis may contribute to better compliance. The infant will not care about color, but the parent may not wish to have a blue orthosis or blue straps put on a baby girl. This parent may be pleased if a pink bow can be securely attached to the orthosis or strap. The young child may be more motivated to wear an orthosis made of colorful or patterned material, especially if they were allowed to choose it from a selection of materials. The teenager is often more compliant with a black orthosis or a neutral color with black straps (Fig. 22–9). The therapist should be cautioned that a thermoplastic material with a color or pattern will often not have the same properties as the original material, so it may act differently during formation (most often increased or decreased conformability).

Padding Selection

The practice of padding an orthosis has changed through the years. In the past, some therapists felt a need to make the inside of an orthosis soft for the child or infant, so they would line them with moleskin or soft padding material. Unfortunately, the bacteria, dirt, and moisture absorbed by open-cell padding can pose a challenge to clean. If the orthosis is formed correctly, the material should be left unpadded. This will allow the orthosis to be wiped clean daily. If a softer internal feel is desired, a sleeve of stockinette or a thin sock of an appropriate length may be applied to the arm under the orthosis.

Padding may be required over bony prominences to provide some pressure relief. The therapist needs to be aware that padding takes up space, so they need to take that into consideration prior to molding the orthosis. Closed-cell padding would be advisable, especially with an infant who might suck on the orthosis. If a perforated material is chosen, then the clinician may need to consider a soft, Moleskin type lining because the perforations may irritate thin, fragile, young skin.

Strapping Selection and Placement

Paying special attention to the straps with the pediatric patient is extremely important. The therapist should consider the strength, durability, elasticity, and texture of the strap (Gabriel, 2008). The straps need to hold the orthosis securely in place but not cause irritation to sensitive skin. They should be as soft as possible yet durable. The sharp edges of the straps may need to be softened with some small vertical snips (Fig. 22–13B). Because the straps are often the third point of control that will exert a force, the width of the straps should be appropriate to the size of the body part to help maximally distribute the pressure. On a child or teenager, the appropriate widths may be narrower than those for adults. Fingers are often secured with ½″ straps, wrists with 1″ straps, and forearms or upper arms with 2″ or wider straps. The infants and neonates require even narrower straps.

Maintaining the proper alignment of the orthosis is critical for a pediatric patient. On the volar surface, the strap should be placed along the wrist crease secured proximal to the bones of the hand to prevent migration distally (Fig. 22–6B). Providing the correct force from the strap can be a challenge. Placement of the strap in a slight diagonal may be helpful, and often two overlapping diagonals in an "X" pattern can facilitate a good hold on the dorsal surface. When attempting to gain finger positioning, it may be advisable to consider a finger strap in a spiral wrap. This can be used in a hand-based PIP joint extension orthosis for correction of a flexion contracture due to camptodactyly (Table 22–2) or for patients with limited PIP extension after fracture (Fig. 22–9).

The use of D-ring style straps to provide a "cinch" effect to hold the orthosis in place is often beneficial, especially for two-piece or circumferential orthoses (Fig. 22–8). The same effect can be accomplished by making a hole or slit into the material for the strap to run through. This may position the strap closer to the body part needing control (Fig. 22–15A,B). These holes or slits can be made with a hole punch or handheld electric drill and then the edges smoothed with dry heat.

Colorful straps may help increase the willingness of the child to accept the orthosis. Standard loop material comes in various colors. In addition, various types of soft strapping materials are now available, which can enhance comfort, compliance, and reduce issues of skin sensitivity (Figs. 22–3, 22–13B, and 22–15). Ribbon or shoelaces can also be used in place of strapping materials (Figs. 22–2 and 22–5).

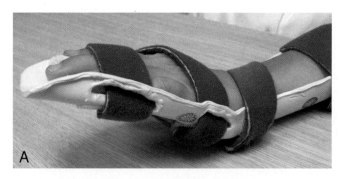
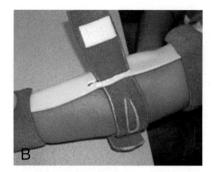

FIGURE 22–15 **A,** The use of a slit or hole for the strap to pass through can help position the strap closer to the body part needing control. **B,** This slit provides "cinch" effect to maintain the body part into the orthosis.

Enhancing Orthosis Use and Compliance

Therapists must take a multifaceted approach when encouraging compliance for a pediatric patient. First and foremost, it is important that the child accept the orthosis. Whenever possible, the therapist and parents must explain why the orthosis is necessary in terms that the child understands.

Understanding the rationale is not always enough for a child. Making the orthosis unique is essential to improve compliance and acceptance of the orthosis. For example, the therapist can offer a choice of colors for the thermoplastic, strapping, and decorating options. The material can be decorated using a permanent marker, fabric paints, adhesive-backed foam shapes, stickers, jewels, beads, etc. (Fig. 22–16A,B). All decorations should be securely attached, especially for any child who may try to place the orthosis in his or her mouth. Decorative accents can be added using bows, buttons, and lace that are sewn directly onto the straps (Fig. 22–17A,B). Naming the orthosis with appropriate child-friendly names may also help with compliance. For instance, an elbow orthosis decorated with an astronaut inside his "rocket ship" may help motivate the child to wear his orthosis (Fig. 22–16B).

Compliance goes beyond the child. Sometimes, the orthosis will be applied by the child, but most often, it will be applied by parents, nurses, school personnel, grandparents, or caregivers. These caregivers must understand proper application in order to comply with the use of the orthosis. To

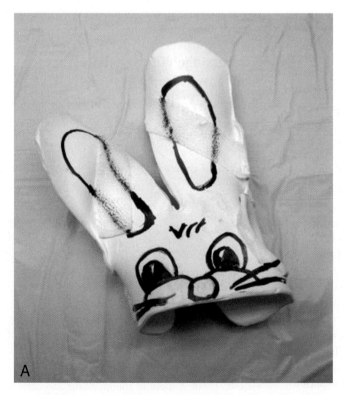
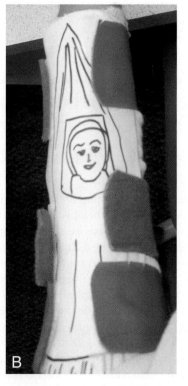

FIGURE 22–16 **A,** This orthosis became a "bunny" by decorating with permanent marker. **B,** This astronaut and his "rocket ship" motivated a young boy to wear his orthosis.

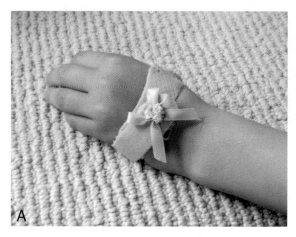
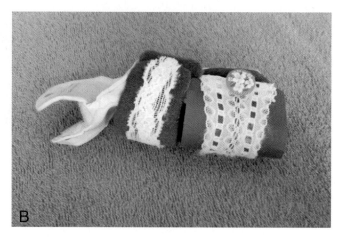

FIGURE 22–17 **A,** This pink bow was sewn onto the strap to help motivate a young girl to wear her orthosis. **B,** Lace and buttons were used to decorate this orthosis to maximize wearing compliance.

ensure proper application of the orthosis, it is often helpful to label the location of the orthosis (i.e., back of right wrist). A permanent marker can be used to label/number the corresponding hook-and-loop locations to aid in the ease of application. Providing the caregivers with a photo of the orthosis on the child or requesting that they take one with their cell phone camera is advisable. The caregivers and the patient should be provided with verbal and written instructions for application and a wearing schedule as well. As a reminder to apply the orthosis before bedtime, the orthosis can be stored in an obvious place, such as the nightstand or inside the patient's pillowcase. Using a compliance grid to keep track of the wearing time can allow the therapist to reward or praise the child for participation in the home program, including the use of the orthosis.

Challenges of Orthosis Provision for a Pediatric Patient

Preventing Self-Removal (Anti-Houdini Suggestions)

Many children act like Houdini and can wiggle out of any orthosis, even a cast. The therapist needs to use different techniques to keep an orthosis on a child. Simple hook and loop can easily be undone by a child of any age. Due to the small size of the straps, this can pose a choking hazard for the infant or young child. It is important to secure one end of the strap onto the thermoplastic material with a rivet (Fig. 22–6B) or an additional covering of thermoplastic material (Fig. 22–18). This option also reduces the chance that the strap will be misplaced. To help prevent self-removal, the other end of the strap can be attached using the "double locking" method. This is used when there is enough space for a long piece of adhesive backed hook that is attached to itself in the middle (Fig. 22–19).

If these methods are not successful, the therapist can apply tape or self-adhesive bandage over the outside of the strap to secure it in place. Placing a sock or stockinette tube over the entire orthosis may deter the persistent child. The therapist should use special care to prevent self-removal for a small orthosis on an infant or toddler due to risks of choking. Changing the strapping material to a shoestring or ribbon can allow for a more secured closure by tying a bow (Fig. 22–6B), a knot (Fig. 22–2), or using a cord lock (Fig. 22–20). The use of a friendship bracelet or a dog collar with a plastic clasp is another suggestion (Armstrong, 2005) for the older child (Fig. 22–18). In desperation, the therapist may even consider a small luggage lock placed through holes on each end of the strap.

Addressing Primitive Reflexes and Abnormal Tone

The presence of **primitive reflexes** can influence the application of the orthosis. For instance, the **asymmetrical tonic neck reflex (ATNR)** can be used to help extend the elbow and open the hand as the head is moved toward that arm. Tonal issues (**hypotonicity** or **hypertonicity**) may be

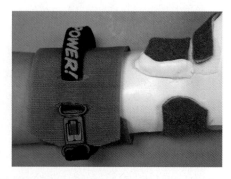

FIGURE 22–18 A piece of thermoplastic can cover the end of the strap to hold it in place. The friendship bracelet attached onto the strap can help prevent self-removal of the orthosis.

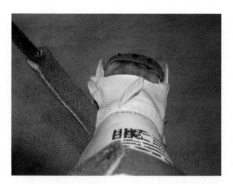

FIGURE 22–19 A piece of adhesive-backed hook attached to itself in the middle placed onto the orthosis may help prevent self-removal of the loop strap.

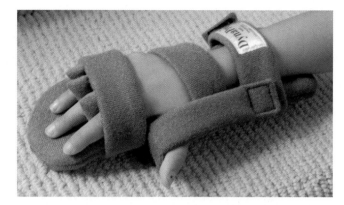

FIGURE 22–21 This prefabricated orthosis (Neuroflex® Pediatric Thumb Ease™) can provide position and adjust for changes with spasticity.

present in conditions such as cerebral palsy or hemiplegia (Table 22–2). It is important to keep in mind that the orthoses do not treat the source of the abnormal tone but attempt to manage the symptoms by preventing contractures (Fig. 22–3) or positioning the UE to enhance function (Fig. 22–1C). The dynamic and inconsistent nature of spasticity will present a challenge even for the most experienced therapist (Fess, Gettle, Philips, & Janson, 2005). Relaxation techniques prior to the fabrication or application of the orthosis may allow for best positioning. A custom orthosis for a child with fluctuating spasticity may require rigid material with extra reinforcement and proper fabrication to allow for the optimal positioning without stress to the joints (Fig. 22–3). Certain types of prefabricated orthoses (Fig. 22–21) have an insert that is flexible, providing a spring-back effect delivering an LLPS.

Special Considerations for the Fragile Infant

The therapist who works in the neonatal intensive care unit (NICU) or similar setting needs to use careful selection of the type and design of orthosis. They also need to be mindful when selecting the material and strapping due to the fragile

state of the infant, environmental issues, and nursing as primary caregivers (Tecklin, 2007). In addition, the therapist needs to use special care in fabrication and application. The infant may not tolerate handling or traction on nerves/joints/skin. There is a greater risk of fracture, dislocation, and skin breakdown (Anderson & Anderson, 1988). Other concerns that affect the treating therapists include time constraints, fear of harming the child, lack of family participation, and nursing compliance issues.

The material used for the orthosis should be soft and supportive. In the NICU at Rady Children's Hospital in San Diego, soft arm supports are made of 3″ wide Velfoam® wrapped circumferentially. Soft hand supports for neonates can be made of a tube of cylindrical foam with ½″ soft strapping in a Figure-8 pattern to hold around the wrist (Fig. 22–22A,B). If needed, more rigid support can be made from ¹⁄₁₆″ thermoplastic materials with closed-cell padding to line the entire device.

Simple instructions for orthosis application should be posted at bedside with a photo. Coordinating the wearing schedule with feeding times may make it easier for nurses to comply with the wearing schedule.

Tackling a Typical Session for Orthosis Provision for a Pediatric Patient

An adult hand therapist recently hired in a pediatric setting described her first session fabricating an orthosis on a child as "trying to change a tire on a moving vehicle." The fabrication can often be quite a challenge, especially if the child is a wiggling, crying infant. To streamline the process, the therapist should make a few changes to the environment and fabrication process.

Taking time to ensure that the area is safe and friendly to the child is essential. Putting away any sharp objects until needed will make the child feel less threatened upon entering the room. Placing out a few toys or a puzzle will make the room more friendly and inviting. Having a sample orthosis will allow the child and parent to understand the process. Allowing the child some opportunity to play with the

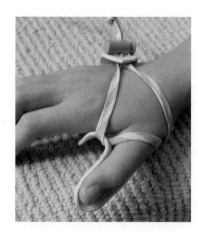

FIGURE 22–20 A cord lock has a spring closure that can securely hold a shoestring strap in place.

CHAPTER 22

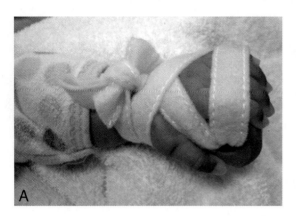 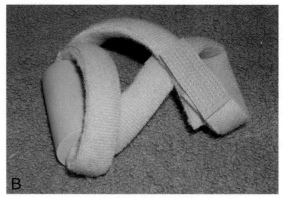

FIGURE 22–22 A, An orthosis made of cylindrical foam placed in the hand can be attached with soft ribbon and can provide a soft supportive position for the neonate. **B,** The orthosis can be made with smaller diameter cylindrical foam and thin soft strap to secure it around the hand and wrist.

softened material prior to fabrication may make the child less apprehensive when the warm material is later pulled out of the water to be placed on his or her arm.

If possible, place the child's hand onto a piece of paper towel or a more durable shop towel and draw the pattern. Cut out the pattern on the towel and then place it on the child, making all the necessary adjustments before using it to cut out the material. This minimizes the number of times that the warm material is placed onto the child for readjustments.

The therapist should then select a material for the orthosis of the correct thickness and properties for the child. If possible, allow the child to pick the color. The material should be placed into water of the correct temperature (150° for most plastic- and rubber-based materials and 160° for elastic-based material). After the material is soft, it can be removed from the water and placed on a towel to cool. Before placing the material on a child's extremity, the therapist should make sure it is not too hot. This is especially important when spot heating with a heat gun because this method tends to result in higher surface temperature (Gabriel, 2008). A piece of 1″ or 2″ stockinette can be placed onto the arm prior to applying the warm material. The child can be placed on the parent's lap or in a chair with the parent holding the proximal part of the arm to prevent the child from pulling away during fabrication.

When forming the orthosis, the therapist should place the material onto the arm or hand using gravity to assist if possible. Working quickly, the orthosis needs to be allowed to harden enough to maintain the form but removed to finish off the child's arm. The elastic-based materials will need to be left on longer to allow them to completely cool to prevent shrinkage. It may be advisable to quicken the process by applying something cold, such as a washcloth that has been soaking in ice water or applying a baggie of ice. After it has hardened, the edges can be smoothed with a heat gun. Finally, the straps should be added with special attention to strap placement to make sure there is proper purchase and control of the position. If possible, let the child pick the color of the straps or shoe strings.

After the final adjustments, the therapist should allow time to make the orthosis fun to wear by decorating and easy to apply by labeling the straps and parts. The family or caregiver should be instructed in the application and strap orientation. They should be observed donning/doffing the orthosis and have any questions clarified. The therapist should provide a wearing schedule beginning with short intervals to watch for skin irritation. Requesting the family to note any pressure problems from the orthosis and reminding them to bring the orthosis back at each visit for adjustments is advisable. The therapist should provide a reminder to the family that the orthosis will melt in a hot car and that pets can consider them as chew toys.

Conclusion

Orthosis provision for the pediatric patient can pose multiple hurdles. The therapist can rise to these challenges by using problem-solving ability that is grounded in good biomechanical principles to help design the most appropriate custom or prefabricated orthosis for each child. Additionally, there should be special consideration for factors that are unique to pediatrics, including methods to enhance orthosis use and compliance, prevent self-removal, address primitive reflexes or abnormal tone, and protect the fragile infant. The therapist should have a basic understanding of the various diagnoses that are specific to the pediatric population in order to design the proper therapeutic intervention. This therapy program may involve the use of orthoses to enhance functional use, provide proper positioning, or provide protection before or after necessary surgical intervention.

CASE STUDY
SECTION

The case studies presented here are meant as a teaching guideline only. Treatment and orthosis protocols vary greatly from surgeon to surgeon and from therapist to therapist. The therapist should check with the referring physicians and colleagues to define the preferred treatment and appropriate orthotic intervention.

CASE STUDY 1: **Camptodactyly**

Jamie is an 11-year-old who noticed increasing flexion contractures of her small fingers on both hands in the last several years. She had no previous injuries that would have caused these PIP contractures. She was recently seen by the orthopedist who felt that these are contractures due to the adolescent form of camptodactyly. The etiology is unknown but may have to do with anomalous insertion of the lumbricals or shortening of the flexor tendon. He explained that surgical release is unpredictable and associated with complications, such as the loss of flexion.

She presented for the first visit with both her small fingers held in flexion at rest. She admitted some concern about the appearance of her hands and frequently hides them under the sleeves of her sweatshirt. Her evaluation revealed that her ROM in both hands were within normal limits except in her bilateral small fingers, which lacked full PIP joint extension by 45° actively and 28° passively. Her grip strength was right: 20 lbs and left: 18 lbs. Manual muscle testing to lumbricals of both small fingers showed she exhibited a grade 3 strength. She denied any difficulty with use of hands in normal daily tasks, except she reported difficulty putting her hands in her pockets and placing her hands completely flat onto a table. She plays basketball and feels her ability to palm the ball has been diminished in the last few years.

Because her PIP joints could be reduced to less than 30° passively, she was a candidate for a serial static type mobilization orthosis (Fig. 22–9). She wore them nightly for at least 10 hours. She also participated in a home program, which involved heated stretching, active extension exercises, and activities such as playing "penny soccer" while wearing an MCP joint blocking orthosis (Fig. 22–11). She received weekly therapy that included paraffin, fluidotherapy, intrinsic strengthening activities, and finger extension strengthening with putty. Her orthosis was adjusted for more extension at each visit. After 3 months, her motion had improved to 8° from full extension. She was discharged from weekly therapy but advised to continue her home program. Because it is advisable to wear her orthosis until she reaches skeletal maturity, she returned every several months for modification to accommodate for growth.

Additional case studies can be found on the companion web site on thePoint.

PEDIATRIC PREFABRICATED ORTHOSES SUPPLIERS

3-Point Products	(888) 378-7763	www.3pointproducts.com
Benik Corporation	(800) 442-8910	www.benik.com
Bird & Cronin, Inc.	(800) 328-1095	www.birdcronin.com
Comfy Splints	(310) 353-2481	www.comfysplints.com
Dynasplint	(800) 262-8828	www.dynasplint.com
Joe Cool Company	(800) 233-3556	www.joecoolco.com
Joint Active Systems	(800) 879-0117	www.jointactivesystems.com
McKie Splints	(888) 477-5468	www.mckiesplints.com
North Coast Medical	(800) 821-9319	www.ncmedical.com
Ongoing Care Solutions, Inc. (OCSI)	(800) 375-0207	www.ongoingcare.com
Ottobock	(800) 328-4058	www.ottobockus.com
Patterson Medical	(800) 323-5547	www.pattersonmedical.com
Restorative Care of America, Inc.	(800) 354-9321	www.rcai.com
Restorative Medical	(800) 793-5544	www.restorativemedical.com
Silver Ring Splint	(800) 311-7028	www.silverringsplint.com
Ultraflex Systems	(800) 220-6670	www.ultraflexsystems.com

Chapter Review Questions

1. Describe three materials that were reviewed in this chapter that are appropriate for the pediatric patient. Provide rationale for these material choices.

2. Name three of the special developmental and environmental considerations when applying an orthosis on a pediatric patient.

3. Give two examples of creative, difficult to remove strapping applications for the pediatric orthosis.

4. Provide an example of an orthosis that enhances function for a pediatric patient.

5. Give two examples on how a clinician may encourage (patient and family) compliance and use of an orthosis to be worn on a pediatric patient.

Burns

Reg Richard, MS, PT
Jonathan Niszczak, MS, OTR/L

Chapter Objectives

After study of this chapter, the reader should be able to:

- Gain an understanding for burn injuries: severity, surface area, depth of wound, phases of healing, and long-term sequelae.
- Describe the considerations unique to orthotic intervention with the patient with burn injury.
- Identify the most common contractures seen in burn extremities.
- Understand the importance of material selection when addressing burn injuries and positioning.

Key Terms

Antideformity orthoses
Compressive stress
Contracture
Cutaneous functional units
Depth of injury

Epidermal
Full thickness
Inflammatory stage
Neuropathies
Partial thickness

Position of function orthoses
Proliferative phase
Shear stress
Skin grafts
Wound maturation phase

Introduction

The use of orthoses to treat patients with burn injuries is one approach in a cornucopia of treatment interventions that may be used in the rehabilitation of these patients (Richard et al., 2008). Construction of burn orthoses employs the basic orthotic principles described in Section I. Because the focus of this text is on how to correctly fabricate orthoses for patients and not on the treatment of patients overall, this chapter addresses the nuances of fabrication of orthoses that are unique to patients with burn injuries and highlights particular principles that can contribute to successful patient outcome. The most significant characteristic of orthoses fabricated for patients with burn injuries is that the orthosis is individualized to the specific needs of each patient based on assessment of the burn. However, before focusing on aspects of orthosis construction and implementation that apply to burns, some fundamental information about when and why patients need an orthosis is presented.

Burn Injury Considerations

The objectives when fabricating an orthosis for a patient with burns are as follows:

- Prevent burn scar contracture deformity
- Preserve range of motion (ROM) achieved in exercise sessions or through surgical release of a contracture
- Correct a scar contracture
- Protect tenuous joints and other delicate structures such as tendons, vessels, nerves, skin grafts, and flaps
- Decrease pain (Richard & Ward, 2005)

The decision to create an orthosis for a patient with a burn injury is based on the patient's age, level of cooperation, and the three aspects particular to the burn injury itself. Those aspects are the following:

1. The severity of the patient's injury
2. The patient's point of recovery regarding the phases of wound healing
3. The different biomechanical principles that are associated with the rehabilitation strategy of orthosis application (Richard, Hedmann, et al., 2009; Richard & Ward, 2005).

Because severe burn survival rates have exponentially improved, the ability of the burn therapist to accurately and precisely identify the correct plan for orthoses, particularly for injuries involving the hand and upper extremity, is a critical rehabilitation goal to support optimal functional return and improved quality of life (Esselman, Thombs, Magyr-Russell, & Fauerbauch, 2006; Richard, Hedmann, et al., 2009).

Burn Wound Severity

The severity of a patient's injury is judged by the extent, depth, and location of the burn wounds. Extent of injury involves the surface area of the body burned. A direct relationship exists between how much surface area of the body was burned and the number of scar tissue contractures a patient may develop (Esselman et al., 2006; Kraemer, Jones,

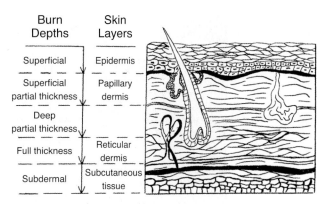

FIGURE 23–1 Layers of the skin and depth of tissue damage from different burn injuries.

& Deitch, 1988; Leblebici et al., 2006). The depth of the burn injury is classified into one of four categories relative to the level of skin damage (Richard, 2000). From a rehabilitation perspective, the location of the burn injury is of concern when it involves skin creases overlying or adjacent to joint areas (Richard, Lester, et al., 2009; Whitehead & Serghiou, 2009). In particular, skin recruitment (identified as **cutaneous functional units** [CFUs]) contributes to the motion of specific joints prone to burn scar contracture formation. A CFU involves a field of skin that extends well beyond the near proximity of the joint itself and uses up to 80% on average of available skin to produce specific ROM (Richard, Lester, et al., 2009).

The depth of burn is classified as **epidermal**, **partial thickness**, **full thickness**, and subdermal (Fig. 23–1). Partial-thickness burns can be subdivided into superficial and deep. The **depth of injury** is important from a wound-healing perspective because it relates to the formation of scar tissue and the potential for subsequent contracture development. Epidermal and superficial partial-thickness burns are of little consequence from an orthotic intervention perspective because minimal scar tissue is formed during the healing of these types of injuries (Fig. 23–2A,B).

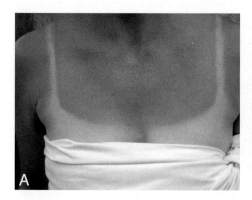

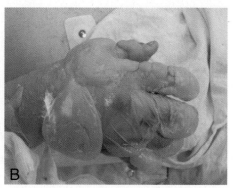

FIGURE 23–2 A, Example of a common epidermal burn (commonly seen in extreme sunburn exposures). **B,** Example of a superficial partial-thickness burn. Note the erythema, blisters, and moist appearance of this hand.

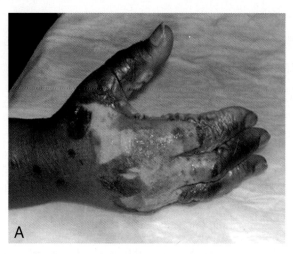
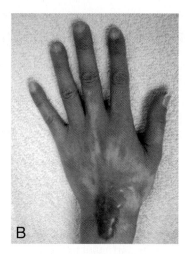

FIGURE 23–3 **A,** Example of a superficial deep partial-thickness burn. Note a more pale appearance of the skin and less erythema; scarring tissues are likely. **B,** Example of a superficial deep partial-thickness injury that healed by secondary intention. Note the thick appearance of the scar with tension in the surrounding dorsal skin that impacts wrist flexion.

Deep partial-thickness burns that heal by secondary intention (i.e., from the base upward without surgical closure) do so by production of dense scar tissue (Fig. 23–3A,B). Full-thickness burns, which typically require a skin graft to heal, have a far greater predilection for contracture formation than partial-thickness injuries (Fig. 23–4A,B) (Dobbs & Curreri, 1972; Kraemer et al., 1988). Finally, subdermal burns, commonly caused by electrical injury and followed by extensive tissue damage underlying the skin, likewise can cause functional deficits that require an orthosis (Fig. 23–5).

A consideration over the early application of orthoses centers on a decrease in blood perfusion to areas of deep partial-thickness burns. These burns have been noted to possess questionable blood flow (Rutan, 1998). In this event, orthoses applied with too much pressure can obliterate an already compromised blood flow and cause the initial burn area to convert to a full-thickness injury. Conversion of a partial-thickness burn to a full-thickness burn can be caused by termination of blood flow with subsequent tissue necrosis. Therefore, until a burn wound has fully demarcated itself within the first few days after injury, orthoses should be judiciously applied (Holavanahalli, Helm, Parry, Dolezal, & Greenhalgh, 2011; Richard et al., 2009).

The depth of injury is directly related to the potential for involvement of other structures in addition to the skin layers. Approaches for applying orthoses must take into account any involvement of tendon, joint capsule and ligaments, and neurovascular structures. In general, the structures should be positioned to prevent any excess stress that may disrupt their integrity and maintain a functional position if the structures have been disrupted. For example, when

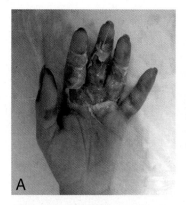
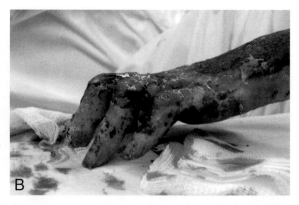

FIGURE 23–4 **A,** Example of a full-thickness burn. Note the depth on the volar aspect of the digits contributing to the likelihood of significant contracture and loss of function. **B,** Example of hypergranulation and delayed healing on a full-thickness burn to dorsal hand and PIP joints. Note the complete loss of MCP joint flexion, flattening of the palmar arch, PIP joint flexion contractures, and flexed wrist posture.

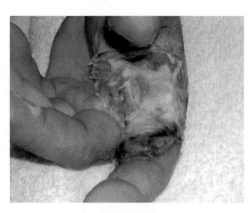

FIGURE 23-5 Example of a subdermal burn. Note the appearance of exposed bone as well as herniated muscle and tendons present. Definitive functional deficits and significant scar contraction will result.

deciding on the optimal joint positions when designing an orthosis for a dorsal hand burn with questionable extensor tendon integrity, there are many issues to consider. Ideally, the wrist and metacarpophalangeal (MCP) joints should be positioned to place the tendons in a slack position (wrist and joint extension); however, this position encourages the development of wrist and MP joint extension contractures. Therapists must use their clinical judgment and constantly reevaluate their patient's needs, which change as tissue healing evolves.

Another aspect to consider with orthosis use on patients with burns is the development of **neuropathies**. A frequent site for development of an upper extremity neuropathy as a result of an orthosis is at the brachial plexus with the use of a shoulder abduction immobilization, or an airplane orthosis. Brachial plexus injury may result from the patient being positioned in pure shoulder abduction over an extended period of time. The usual recommended position of the shoulder is 90°, but pressure on the brachial plexus can be relieved by horizontally adducting the upper extremity 10 to 15°. However, children have been positioned higher than this angle without any reported detrimental effects (Fig. 23–6).

A final factor that applies to the use of orthoses for patients with burn injuries is the variability of wound location. Burn orthoses can have a wide dispersion of designs and configurations, depending on the burn wound site. Table 23–1 outlines orthosis designs that have been suggested for use with upper extremity burns. In general, orthoses are applied on the surface of a burn to oppose the direction of the anticipated deformity. For example, a burn to the elbow antecubital surface requires an elbow extension immobilization orthosis placed on the anterior surface of the extremity to prevent an elbow flexion **contracture** from occurring. Circumferential burns involving joints may require alternating flexion/extension immobilization orthoses to oppose the direction of the anticipated deformity.

The most common contractures associated with upper extremity burns are the following:

- Shoulder adduction/extension
- Shoulder internal rotation
- Elbow flexion
- Forearm pronation
- Wrist flexion
- MCP joint extension
- Digit interphalangeal (IP) joint flexion
- Thumb adduction

Basic Burn Orthoses

An extensive review of designs for basic burn orthoses is available (Richard, Staley, Daugherty, Miller, & Warden, 1994). Although hand orthoses are considered standard therapy practice, no consensus was found for a specific design (Richard et al., 2008). Moreover, selecting, implementing, and designing the appropriate burn hand orthosis is of critical importance to the burn therapist providing therapy (Richard, Hedman, et al., 2009). Orthoses in this category are referred to by various names, but they essentially sort out into two groups: **position of function orthoses** and **antideformity orthoses**. Several suggested positions for the thumb were noted, which probably coincided with burn location based on clinical experience. Both types of orthoses position the wrist in some degree of extension. In general, position of function orthoses allow for some degree of flexion at the proximal interphalangeal (PIP) and distal interphalangeal (DIP) joints, whereas antideformity orthoses hold those joints in extension. The discriminating factor between the

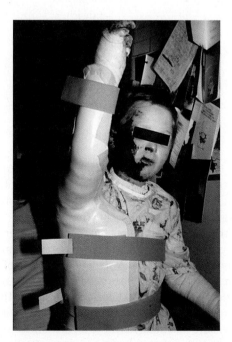

FIGURE 23-6 Example of a pediatric axillary, or airplane, orthosis (shoulder abduction/elbow extension immobilization orthosis) fabricated for more than 90° of shoulder flexion and abduction.

TABLE 23–1

Common Upper Extremity Burn Orthoses

Burn Wound Location	Common Orthosis Name	Reference
Axilla or shoulder	• Airplane	• Chown, 2006; Malick & Carr, 1982; Manigandan et al., 2005; Richard, Chapman, Dougherty, Franzen, & Serghiou, 2005; Richard & Staley, 1994b; Walters, 1987
	• Conformer/Figure-8	• Malick & Carr, 1982; Obaidullah et al., 2005; Richard et al., 2005; Richard & Staley, 1994b; Walters, 1987
	• Abduction	• Malick & Carr, 1982; Richard et al., 2005; Richard & Staley, 1994b
	• Clavicular strap	• Malick & Carr, 1982; Richard et al., 2005; Richard & Staley, 1994b; Walters, 1987
Elbow	• Dynamic	• Richard et al., 2005; Richard et al., 1995
	• Gutter or trough	• Richard et al., 2005; Richard, Schall, et al., 1994
	• Conformer	• Malick & Carr, 1982; Richard et al., 2005; Richard, Schall, et al., 1994; Walters, 1987
	• Three point	• Malick & Carr, 1982; Richard et al., 2005; Richard & Staley, 1994a; Wallace et al., 2009
	• Spiral	• Richard et al., 2005; Richard, Schall, et al., 1994
Wrist and hand	• Palmar pan	• Agrawal & Bhattacharya, 2011; Malick & Carr, 1982; Richard et al., 2005; Richard, Schall, et al., 1994; Walters, 1987
	• Position of function	• Kaine et al., 2008; Richard, Schall, et al, 1994; Richard & Staley, 1994a; Richard et al., 2005; Van Straten & Sagi, 2000
	• Antideformity	• Kaine et al., 2008; Richard, Schall, et al, 1994; Richard et al., 2005; Van Straten & Sagi, 2000
	• Thumb spica	• Daugherty & Carr-Collins, 1994; Richard, Schall, et al., 1994; Richard et al., 2005
	• C-bar thumb web spacer	• Richard et al., 1994; Richard et al., 2005; Walters, 1987
	• Palmar or dorsal extension	• Malick & Carr, 1982; Richard, Schall, et al., 1994; Richard et al., 2005; Schwanholt et al., 1992; Yotsuyanagi, Yokoi, & Omizo, 1994
	• Traction or banjo	• Malick & Carr, 1982; Richard et al., 2005; Richard & Staley, 1994b
	• Halo	• Richard et al., 2005; Richard & Staley, 1994a; Walters, 1987
	• Flexion glove	• Richard et al., 2005; Richard, Schall, et al., 1994
	• Sandwich	• Gilliam et al., 1993; Richard et al., 2005; Richard, Schall, et al., 1994; Walters, 1987
	• Bivalve	• Richard et al., 2005; Richard, Schall, et al., 1994
	• Gutter	• Richard et al., 2005; Rivers, Collin, Fisher, Solem, & Ahrenholz, 1984

orthoses is the amount of flexion allowed at the MP joints. Position of function orthoses place the joints at 60° or less of flexion, whereas antideformity orthoses position the MP joints in greater than 60° of flexion (Fig. 23–7).

A further consideration related to burn location is when the injury involves skin creases over multiple, consecutive joints. Previous work has shown that the position of an adjacent joint has an influence on skin excursion at the next joint in the series (Richard, Ford, Miller, & Staley, 1994). Therapists need to consider designs that incorporate all areas of involvement to ensure maximal benefit of an orthotic intervention by placement of an elongation stress over multiple, consecutive joint skin crease surface areas (discussed in the following text) (Cooney, 1984). In particular to the total hand burn,

special consideration must be paid to both the first and fifth digits because the dynamic pulling forces of developing scar tissue and the multiple planes of motion within each of these digits can create significant long-term complications if not continuously monitored with precise management of orthoses and carefully guided rehabilitation.

Wound Healing Phases

Wound healing can be divided into three phases that have some amount of overlap (see Chapter 3 for more specific details) (Greenhalgh & Staley, 1994). During the **inflammatory stage**, edema develops, which can be quite severe, especially in the hand (Fig. 23–8). During this initial stage

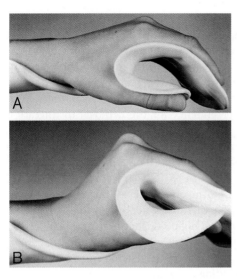

FIGURE 23–7 **A,** A position of function orthosis. **B,** An antideformity orthosis. Note the differences in degree of MCP and IP joint flexion.

of wound repair, which lasts 3 to 5 days under normal circumstances, orthoses should be avoided primarily for two reasons, unless needed to stabilize a joint. First, an orthosis fabricated and applied too early can cause vascular compromise when edema increases, making the orthosis too small. For the same reason, straps used to hold the orthosis in place can become constrictive, potentially impeding circulation. Second, an orthosis applied to the hand during the early stage of healing can limit active ROM, which in turn inhibits the muscle pump activity necessary to rid the area of edema. If orthoses are used during the acute phase of injury, they should be nonconforming to accommodate for fluctuations in edema.

The use of orthoses for patients who have moved beyond the emergent phase of treatment and into the **proliferative** and **wound maturation phases** depends on several factors (Richard, Staley, Miller, & Warden, 1996, 1997a, 1997b; Richard, Lester, et al., 2009). In the past, orthoses were applied routinely at the time of patient admission and after skin graft surgery, especially when the hand was involved. Currently,

therapists tend to delay the application of orthoses until a patient demonstrates a decrease in ROM (Holavanahalli et al., 2011; Richard, Schall, et al., 2009; Richard et al., 1996). Recently, an orthosis algorithm was proposed to help the therapist in the decision-making process for treatment of acute burn injuries (Heidenrich & Hansbrough, 1999). In general, immobilization orthoses are commonly used to prevent scar contractures, whereas mobilization orthoses are used to correct an existing scar contracture (Richard, Lester, et al., 2009; Richard, Shanesy, & Miller, 1995). Part of the reason for this difference is based on the biomechanical principles that underlie each type of orthosis.

Biomechanical Principles

Immobilization orthoses, which statically place a joint in a specific position, use the principle of stress relaxation on scar tissue (Richard & Staley, 1994a). Based on this principle, the amount of force required to maintain a given position of angularity decreases over time (Fig. 23–9). Essentially, tissues adapt to the stress placed on them. Burn wounds that remain open during the healing process are painful. Forceful stress on the tender tissues may increase the amount of pain experienced by the patient. When an immobilization orthosis is initially applied to a patient, there should be only slight discomfort, which lessens in a short period of time, owing to accommodation of the tissues. To avoid generating too much stress on delicate tissue, there is a tendency to use immobilization orthoses more than mobilization orthoses during this time.

After burn wound closure, as scar tissue continues to mature and contract, the ongoing biologic force needs to be counteracted by an equal or greater force. Once a burn wound is covered with new tissue, the primary source of pain is essentially removed and a greater demand can be placed on the tissue with less discomfort. If the patient has developed a scar tissue contracture during this phase of scar maturation, mobilization orthoses that operate under the principle

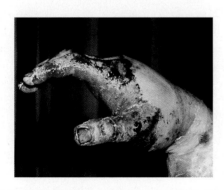

FIGURE 23–8 Massive edema as a result of a burn injury places the hand in a position that predisposes the development of claw hand deformity (MCP extension, IP flexion).

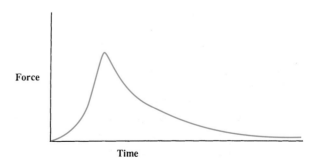

FIGURE 23–9 Soft tissue stress relaxation. After the peak stress is reached from the application of an immobilization orthosis, the amount of stress experienced by the tissue decreases. Reprinted with permission from Richard, R. L., & Staley, M. J. (1994). Biophysical aspects of normal skin and burn scar. In R. L. Richard & M. J. Staley (Eds.), *Burn care and rehabilitation—Principles and practice* (p. 65). Philadelphia, PA: Davis.

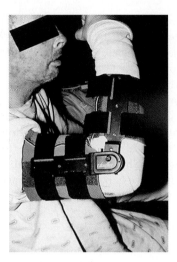

FIGURE 23–10 A commercial elbow mobilization orthosis.

of tissue creep are suggested (Fig. 23–10). Tissue creep is the process whereby the length of biologic tissue continues to elongate if tension is kept constant and maintained over a prolonged period of time (Fig. 23–11) (Richard & Staley, 1994b). The key to this principle is the constant application of force, which provides a stimulus for the tissue to lengthen by production and growth of additional tissue. (Refer to Chapter 15 on stiffness for additional information.)

Implications for Orthotic Intervention

General Considerations

Burn care literature commonly refers to orthoses as either nonconforming or conforming. Nonconforming orthoses are usually fabricated off the patient; conforming orthoses are molded directly to an area and result in a more intimate fit. Conforming orthoses have better pressure distribution than nonconforming orthoses and fewer tendencies to migrate on a limb. Caution should be used when applying nonconforming orthoses because their more generalized fit may lead to excessive pressure along the orthosis borders. Furthermore, there is a tendency for the orthosis to migrate along the extremity. Special attention also should be afforded when fabricating an orthosis over bony prominences to prevent skin breakdown. A positive side to prefabricated nonconforming orthoses is they can be made readily available to clinicians during emergencies. They may be useful at other times when therapists are not available, such as nights, weekends, and holidays. These orthoses can be applied relatively safely over bulky dressings by nursing personnel. Staff should, of course, be instructed in proper application, fit, and precautions with use.

A common concern regarding fabricating an orthosis is whether orthoses can be used over fresh **skin grafts** (Fig. 23–12). Generally, the area that has received a skin graft is heavily padded with dressings to absorb wound drainage and provide protection. Orthoses can be applied safely over skin grafts, particularly if the orthoses intent is to immobilize the area of injury until adherence of the graft to the wound bed is evident (Engrav, 1983; Friang, 1986). Caution should be used to avoid **shear** and/or **compressive stress** on any grafted site. Often, an orthosis may not be used because the bulkiness of the postoperative dressings alone can act as a block to prevent excessive joint motion.

A major consideration when fabricating an orthosis for the burned hand is the patient's age. With older patients who may have preexisting problems (e.g., arthritis), the degree to which fingers and other joints can be stressed and held immobile is less than for younger patients. Conversely, young children typically possess flexible joints. In these cases, positions of hyperextension of the MP joints can be made for palmar burns with minimal potential for causing MP joint extension contractures (Fig. 23–13) (Schwanholt, Daugherty, Gaboury, & Warden, 1992).

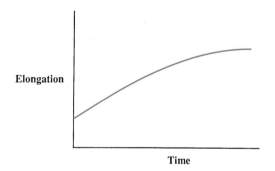

FIGURE 23–11 Continual tissue elongation, or creep, in response to a constant force applied to tissue over a prolonged period of time. Reprinted with permission from Richard, R. L., & Staley, M. J. (1994). Biophysical aspects of normal skin and burn scar. In R. L. Richard & M. J. Staley (Eds.), *Burn care and rehabilitation—Principles and practice* (p. 64). Philadelphia, PA: Davis.

The graph shows **Elongation** on the vertical axis and **Time** on the horizontal axis.

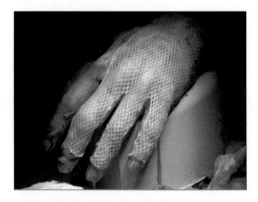

FIGURE 23–12 A fresh meshed, split-thickness skin graft that will require immediate postoperative immobilization in a volar orthosis to prevent graft loss.

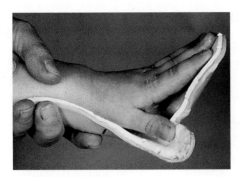

FIGURE 23–13 A pediatric volar orthosis for combined palmar expansion and finger/thumb hyperextension.

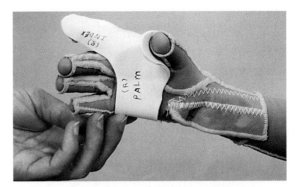

FIGURE 23–15 A pediatric CMC abduction immobilization orthosis (C-bar orthosis) for treating burns to the first web space.

A scar contracture problem that is unique to patients with hand burns is a web space syndactyly (Fig. 23–14). This condition can occur on the dorsum of the hand between any two fingers, but it is functionally most problematic at the first web space. A burn in this area may cause the thumb to contract into adduction or hyperextension. When applying an orthosis to the thumb, caution is needed to avoid damage to the collateral ligaments and subsequent instability of the thumb (Fig. 23–15).

The optimal amount of time that an orthosis should be worn has yet to be determined (Richard, Hedmann, et al., 2009). Each patient presents differently and should be approached individually. Initially, adults and children should wear orthoses at night and, for children, during naps. Depending on the area of the body involved and the depth of injury, uncooperative patients may need to use an orthosis continuously until they are able to actively participate in the therapy regime (Fig. 23–16).

Unconscious patients may or may not need orthoses. If the patient can be positioned properly, avoid orthosis use because the patient cannot communicate any problems with the device (Fig. 23–17). This situation is especially important

for skin grafts, which need close monitoring. These patients are at high risk for developing contractures and demand a therapist's attention regarding proper positioning, orthosis use, and exercise. A key burn therapist axiom is "the position of comfort is the position of contracture"; continuous and vigilant monitoring of the burn treatment intervention will help to achieve long-lasting functional recovery and outcomes.

Orthoses should be checked frequently for proper fit and adjustments made accordingly. During the day, mobility of alert patients should be encouraged until a decrease in ROM becomes apparent. (However, orthosis wear should be continuous except for dressing changes when exposed joints are present.) Clinically, a patient's ROM guides the wearing schedule of an orthosis. If ROM is decreasing, then the time spent in orthoses should be increased with all other treatment interventions and activity programs considered. Frequently, a 2-hour-on and 2-hour-off schedule is advocated, but no research exists to support this regimen. A review of the literature to find the origin of this approach reveals

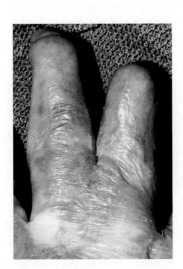

FIGURE 23–14 Dorsal hand scar tissue overgrowth of the web space between the middle and ring fingers.

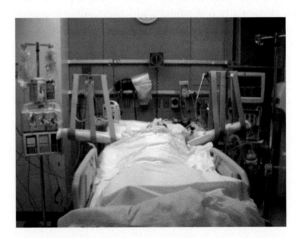

FIGURE 23–16 Modified bilateral shoulder abduction orthoses suspended with intravenous (IV) poles. These devices can be moved more easily than full airplane orthoses with a sedated patient and allow for easier positioning with a ventilator, multiple IV pumps, and nursing care.

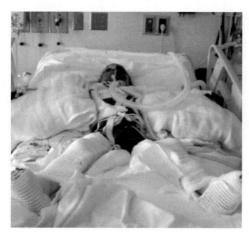

FIGURE 23–17 Positioning with pillows for upper extremities and knees. Ankle orthoses are used for foot positioning, and note no pillow to place the head in a neutral position.

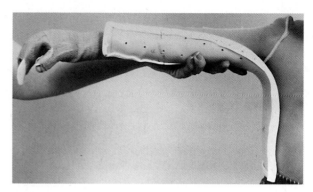

FIGURE 23–19 A combination of axillary and elbow extension orthoses.

only a recommendation that orthoses made of thermoplastic material should be removed every 2 hours for cleaning (Willis, 1969). Regarding the latter, disinfectant cleaning of orthoses was found more beneficial than air drying for burn orthoses (Richard & Staley, 1994a; Staley, Richard, Daugherty, & Warden, 1991).

If the patient is wearing pressure garments for scar control, pieces of loop strapping material can be sewn to the garment material to secure an orthosis. The hook portion of the strap is then attached to the orthosis material in a mirrored position (Fig. 23–18). This technique is especially useful to ensure that the orthosis is placed correctly each time it is worn. Oftentimes, when burns affect several areas, it is helpful to incorporate multiple orthoses into one design pattern. The more orthoses there are, the greater the chance of losing one. Furthermore, an all-inclusive orthosis design makes donning the orthosis easier for caregivers. For example, with small children particularly, a shoulder abduction and an elbow extension immobilization orthosis can be combined (Fig. 23–19) (Richard, Schall, Staley, & Miller, 1994). As another example,

the hand, wrist, and elbow can be incorporated into one orthosis (Richard, Schall, Staley, & Miller, 1994). A novel orthosis for treating bilateral axillary burns simultaneously is the T-shirt orthosis (Fig. 23–20) (Daugherty & Carr-Collins, 1994; Manigandan, 2003). The orthosis is worn on the anterior torso and secured with straps that crisscross over the back.

Material Selection

Commercially available orthoses can be used to treat patients with burn injuries if they fit properly. Acutely, prefabricated orthoses are often difficult to fit on the extremity, owing to the bulkiness of wound dressings and the frequent change in the amount of dressings that patients require. Additionally, dressing thickness must be accounted for because of the influence it can have on achieving an acceptable orthosis fit, especially when the hand is involved (Howell, 1994; Richard & Staley, 1994a).

Owing to the small anatomical structures of patients younger than 1 year of age, fabrication of orthoses is difficult and requires some fabrication experience to achieve a successful outcome. Therefore, it may be easier to position the extremity with the use of bulky dressings or insert material, such as Elastomer™ or foam, in lieu of an orthosis. Orthoses that do not fit correctly can place body segments in positions that encourage development of scar tissue contractures.

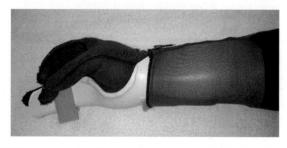

FIGURE 23–18 A modified hand fourth and fifth digit extension orthosis with a pressure garment glove and sleeve where the loop is attached directly to the hook on the volar aspect of the orthosis. Note the patient's upper extremity pressure garment is covering the forearm base of the orthosis.

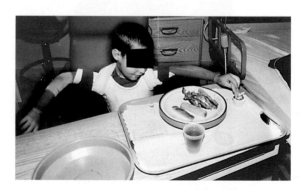

FIGURE 23–20 A T-shirt orthosis (bilateral shoulder abduction immobilization orthosis) used to position both extremities after a burn injury.

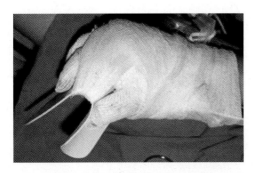

FIGURE 23–21 Poorly applied orthoses can further influence undesired positioning and contracture. Look closely at the position of the MCP and PIP joints relative to the orthosis platform, this position is supporting an intrinsic minus (claw hand) and not an intrinsic plus position.

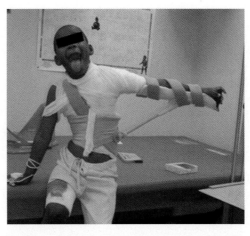

FIGURE 23–22 An airplane orthosis combination using colored thermoplastics helps to support compliance and ease pain in this pediatric patient postoperatively (note the donor site on the right thigh).

Therefore, the adage, "no orthosis is better than a poorly fitted orthosis," is one to heed in burn care (Fig. 23–21).

If therapists fabricate custom orthoses early during a patient's hospitalization, then a material that can be frequently remolded is recommended because of the number of modifications that may be needed to accommodate fluctuations in edema and bandage thickness. In 1969, the first use of a thermoplastic material to customize a burn orthosis was described (Willis, 1969). Since that time, a host of materials for orthoses have been advocated and used (Cox, Taddonio, & Thompson, 1991; Richard & Staley, 1994a; Willis, 1970). Generally, $\frac{1}{16}$″ material can be used with the pediatric population and in areas that do not bear much weight, such as the fingers. Thicker materials, $\frac{3}{32}$″ or $\frac{1}{8}$″, should be used for adult orthoses to ensure a rigid orthosis with adequate positioning. The material of choice for the burn therapist is largely dependent on the current stage of the wound healing process. Ideally, colored thermoplastics with moderate memory that have perforations but still maintain the rigidity to counteract positional forces are essential to support the modifications required from dressing and bandaging adaptations during the initial phases of healing and/or skin grafting. The inception of colored material and strapping has allowed patients to participate in creating the device, which may assist in compliance, especially for children, and also provides a device that is more readily identifiable among white wound bandages (Fig. 23–22). Fabrication of orthoses for the burned upper extremity can incorporate various types of materials (including aluminum, wood, high-temperature polycarbonates, and thermoformable foams), and the optimal selection is only limited to the imagination and resourcefulness of the treating clinician and the presenting wound/scar presentation (Agrawal & Bhattacharya, 2011; Forbes-Duchart & Niszczak, 2010).

Perforated or open-weave material is best used for patients who have a large amount of wound exudate or transudate and when topical antibiotic solutions are in use; the perforations allow the former to escape and the latter to penetrate through the dressings. Also, these plain thermoplastics (without combinations of foam, padding, or antibiotic properties) are more commonly used for ease of application and to create a well-fitting orthoses with bandaging or with pressure garments. Perforated material also allows for some air to reach the dressings, drying them and preventing wounds from becoming macerated. Thermoplastic materials are also available with antimicrobial built in to prevent bacterial growth on the surface and may protect against infection.

A major consideration with the use of thermoplastic material and its immediate fabrication at a patient's bedside is the anxiety evoked in patients with burns by the thought of having hot material placed on their wounds. This situation is especially heightened in children. To circumvent this issue, educate the patient and apply ample padding between the patient and material when fabricating the orthosis. A successful approach is to demonstrate the lack of heat conduction on a nonburn area using a piece of scrap material.

Traditional plaster cast material provides a cost-effective alternative to thermoplastics in some cases. Other casting type materials have been used (including 3M™ Scotchcast™ Plus fiberglass, Hexalite®, and Delta-Cast® Conformable polyester tape) in similar fashion to traditional casting to support optimal position and provide lightweight stability (Fig. 23–23A,B). These techniques and materials may not be the best choice during the acute phase of wound healing because frequent cast changes would be required. Cast material tends to absorb the wound exudate, which necessitates removal and application of a new cast. However, when patient compliance is an issue, serial casting can be a more effective medium than thermoplastic orthosis use. Also, consider thermoplastics when orthosis hygiene is an issue. These materials can be easily wiped clean, disinfected, and reapplied to the extremity. Casting may help in the later stages of wound healing to position joint(s) for a mobilization orthosis using serial static stress to improve

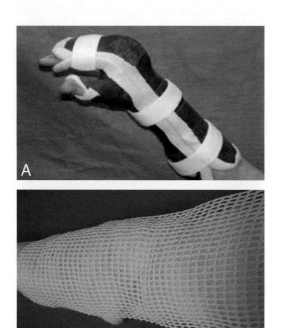

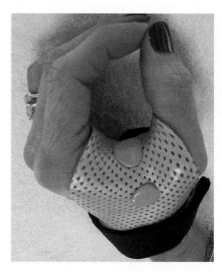

FIGURE 23–25 Technique of securing insert material to a perforated thermoplastic. The material protrudes through the holes and is flattened out, thus holding it in place on the orthosis.

FIGURE 23–23 **A,** Bivalve Delta-Cast® immobilization orthosis for a burn hand (BSN medical Inc., Charlotte, NC). **B,** This elbow extension orthosis is made of Hexalite®; note the open weave allowing for breathability and passage of heavy exudates.

and facilitate long-term ROM improvements (Daugherty & Carr-Collins, 1994).

Component Selection

Occasionally, dress hooks are glued to the fingernails so a traction force can be applied. The hooks act as terminal attachments for rubber bands that originate at the end of the pan portion of a hand or banjo orthosis (Fig. 23–24). This technique is useful when the finger joints are placed in extension. As an alternative, hook material can be glued to

the fingernails. A primary consideration before using any of these approaches is to ensure that the fingernails are viable and intact; otherwise, the traction force may disrupt the nail from its bed (Richard & Staley, 1994a; Wright, Taddonio, Prasad, & Thompson, 1989). This technique also should be avoided in very young children because of the instability of their fingernails.

For scar management, inserts made of putty (Elastomer™ or Otoform) can be incorporated into an orthosis nicely if perforated material is used (Richard & Staley, 1994a). Before the insert material hardens, it can be pushed through the interstices of the material (Fig. 23–25). The excess material that extrudes through the perforations is then flattened to form a rivet that secures the insert material in place (Costa, Nakamura, & Engrav, 1999; Ward, Schnebly, Kravitz, Warden, & Saffle, 1989). Additionally, thermoplastics bonded with silicone have been used to combine the use of both pressure and silicone in a single design (Fig. 23–26). The use of these

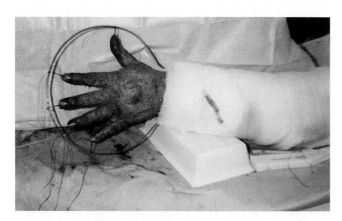

FIGURE 23–24 Dress hooks are applied to the fingernails to position the digits in extension for this digit extension/abduction immobilization orthosis—also known as a "banjo orthosis."

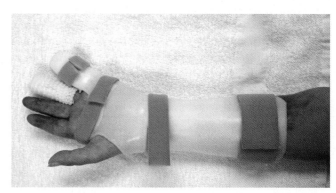

FIGURE 23–26 A volar-based fifth finger and wrist extension orthosis shown using Silon-LTS (thermoplastic material bonded with silicone) on the volar contact area of the entire orthosis. (Note that this silicone material is worn directly against the skin.)

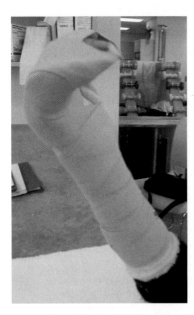

FIGURE 23–27 Circumferential elasticized bandage used to secure a volar wrist and hand immobilization orthosis.

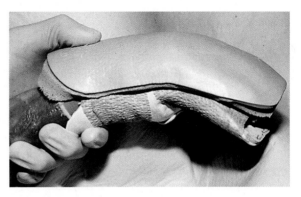

FIGURE 23–28 A sandwich orthosis (hand immobilization orthosis), also commonly known as a clamshell orthosis, includes two interlocking segments.

types of material has shown success for both pediatrics and adults to facilitate scar management in comparison to traditional thermoplastics (Serghiou & Niszczak, 2011). For children younger than the age of 3 years, therapists should avoid the use of small parts when making an orthoses (Richard, Schall, et al., 1994). If one of these pieces came loose, it would be a potential choking hazard.

Strapping Selection

The strapping methods used in adult and pediatric populations may differ. For compliant adults, a rolled gauze bandage, elastic wrap (e.g., Ace™ or Coban™), or foam straps (e.g., Velfoam®) offer an effective means to secure an orthosis (Fig. 23–27). Caution must be taken not to compress any superficial nerves or vascular structures; frequent monitoring is necessary.

A fabrication and design difficulty that often arises with children is getting the child to keep an orthosis on for extended periods of time. In burn care, orthoses are needed daily and for an extended period of time. The longer the child wears the orthosis, the greater the likelihood that he or she will find a way to remove it. Several methods can make the process of orthosis removal more difficult for the pediatric patient.

One method is to use a self-adherent elastic wrap, such as Coban™, to hold the orthosis in place instead of applying ordinary elastic wraps that fasten with clips or tape, as commonly used for adults (Richard, Schall, et al., 1994; Schwanholt et al., 1992). A second method is to use a sandwich orthosis (Fig. 23–28) (Gilliam, Hatler, Adams, & Helm, 1993; Ward et al., 1989). With this type of orthosis, recommended for use with the hand, a dorsal and volar piece is made that encases the hand. The use of self-adherent elasticized wrap is suggested for holding this orthosis together and in place. As an alternative, a bivalve hand cast can act as a type of sandwich orthosis.

Another technique for holding an orthosis in place and preventing distal slippage is to line the orthosis with Dycem or a similar nonskid material. This tacky material acts as a good interface between the orthosis and material in which it comes into contact, especially slick pressure garments commonly employed for burn management. Finally, simply increasing the angle of wrist extension in a hand orthosis, if appropriate, can prevent distal migration of the hand beyond the end of the orthosis.

Conclusion

The use of orthoses in the rehabilitation of patients with burn injuries is an integral part of a comprehensive treatment program. Specific considerations for orthosis use include burn wound extent, depth, and location as well as anatomical sites and phase of healing. Biomechanical principles should be taken into account based on the treatment objectives. Special considerations should be extended to pediatric and geriatric patients and the age-specific characteristics these populations possess.

Successful strategies demand a decision on whether to custom fabricate an orthosis or to use a prefabricated or commercially available orthosis. If an orthosis is custom made, attention should be paid to design and the type of material selected. The use of inserts, orthosis wear in conjunction with skin grafts, pressure garments, and the method used to secure orthoses can challenge a therapist's creativity. Treatment parameters, such as optimal duration of orthosis wear and ideal design, need further investigation and research.

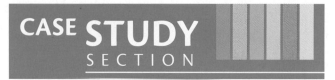

CASE STUDY
SECTION

The case studies presented here are meant as a teaching guideline only. Treatment and orthosis protocols vary greatly from surgeon to surgeon and from therapist to therapist. The therapist should check with the referring physicians and colleagues to define the preferred treatment and appropriate orthotic intervention.

CASE STUDY 1: Upper Extremity Burn Injury with Skin Grafting

MJS, a 41-year-old left-dominant female, was preparing supper and used an accelerant on smoldering briquettes in her outdoor barbecue grill when the charcoal suddenly erupted into flames.

The previously healthy patient was estimated to have experienced a 7% surface area burn of her dominant upper extremity. The palm of her hand was spared along with an area of skin on the medial aspect of her upper arm. She was diagnosed as having mixed deep-partial and full-thickness burns throughout (Fig. 23–29). When the therapist first evaluated the patient the morning after the injury, the patient's hand and remaining upper extremity were markedly edematous, and the hand and fingers were in a slightly flexed position. Joint motion was moderately restricted throughout, secondary to edema and pain. Surgery to apply skin grafts to the areas of full-thickness injury was scheduled for 2 days after injury. Owing to the swelling and impending surgery, the

therapist placed the upper extremity in an elevated position with external compression bandages and instructed MJS to perform limited active ROM to aid in edema reduction and maintenance of ROM.

By the time of surgery, the edema had subsided remarkably, and the areas of full-thickness burn had demarked themselves and were confined to the volar aspect of the arm and forearm, which involved the antecubital space. These areas were excised and covered with split-thickness sheet skin grafts harvested from a suprapubic donor site. The surgeon requested the therapist's attendance in the operating room, where a position of function hand orthosis was fabricated to immobilize the deep-partial thickness burns (Fig. 23–7A), and an elbow extension immobilization orthosis was formed and applied over the bulky dressings. MJS's elbow area was kept immobile for 3 days to allow for adherence of the skin graft.

After surgery and throughout the remainder of MJS's hospitalization, the hand orthosis was modified into more of an antideformity position (Fig. 23–7B). The patient's finger ROM increased through a program of progressive exercise. At 2 weeks after surgery, the patient wore the orthosis at night; the schedule progressed to an as-needed basis after the patient was discharged from the hospital.

When the elbow area was undressed for the first time after surgery and ROM was reinitiated, the patient lacked 25° of elbow extension with noticeable blanching of the skin graft when stress was applied. Apparently, her elbow had been slightly flexed when the bulky outer bandages were applied in the operating room, which was not apparent by visual inspection. MJS's existing postoperative elbow orthosis was remolded to form an elbow extension mobilization orthosis (Fig. 23–30).

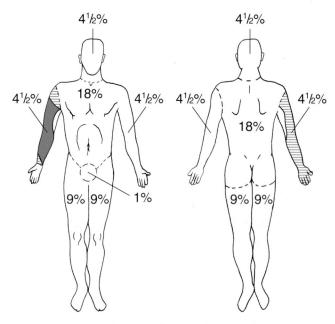

FIGURE 23–29 Distribution and depth of burns. The hatched areas represent partial-thickness burns, and the solid areas represent full-thickness burns.

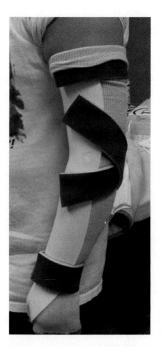

FIGURE 23–30 An elbow extension immobilization orthosis applied directly over healing skin grafts.

The patient received twice-daily therapy treatments. She showed minimal improvements in ROM, and the orthosis was modified as necessary. The nurses began having difficulty applying the orthosis at night owing to increasing elbow flexion tightness. A decision was made to change the intervention to a commercial elbow extension mobilization orthosis (Fig. 23–10). The rationale was that MJS could receive gentle stress applied intermittently throughout the day to the tight skin-grafted area while retaining functional use of the extremity. She continued to wear the serial static elbow mobilization orthosis at night.

The patient was compliant with the commercial orthotic program and, within 3 weeks, had regained full extension of her elbow. At that time, the orthosis was formally discontinued with instructions to continue the night orthosis regime for an additional month to maintain tissue length.

Additional case studies can be found on the companion web site on thePoint.

Chapter Review Questions

1. What important facts should the therapist consider when asked to apply an orthosis to a patient with burn injury? Discuss tissue considerations as well as material selections.

2. Describe the depths of burn injury and how this relates to orthotic intervention.

3. What is important about burn injuries that are over skin creases and what should the management involve in these situations?

4. How should a total hand burn be managed? Explain positions of each joint and list the precautions to look for.

5. What is web space syndactyly? Why is this significant and how can this condition be managed? What special considerations need to be taken when this occurs about the thumb?

The Musician

Colleen Lowe, MPH, OTR/L, CHT*

Chapter Objectives

After study of this chapter, the reader should be able to:

- Understand the unique evaluation and treatment approaches for the injured musician.
- Recognize the indications for use of orthoses and taping techniques for this patient population.

- Appreciate the diverse treatment approaches for the two main categories of injuries to the musician: traumatic injuries and repetitive injuries.
- Explain the fabrication of an orthosis for injuries related to handling instruments and playing orthoses for age-related problems.

Key Terms

FHRED oboe or English horn support
Functional movement analysis
Handling instruments

Musician's posture
Playing orthoses
Progressive ligament injuries
Repetitive use injuries

Soft tissue impact injuries
Training orthosis
Traumatic injuries

Introduction

Injured musicians are a client population that is interesting and challenging because of the artistic, physical, and psychological demands of playing an instrument. Instrumental musicians maintain static positions and repeat dynamic fine motor movements for hours, which are stressful on the tissues of their upper extremities, neck, and trunk (Lederman, 2003; Lederman & Calabrese, 1986; Lockwood, 1989). When musicians injure their upper extremities, it can be devastating. To treat musicians' injuries effectively, the therapist must have a thorough understanding of anatomy and kinesiology and a keen ability to observe and analyze dysfunctional movement patterns and muscle imbalances. Critical to the effectiveness of treatment is observing the musician playing his or her instrument and asking specific questions about the instrument, for example, how the musician has the instrument set up (i.e., weight and height of strings, action of keys, etc.), and questions about repertoire, practice schedule, warm-up, length of practice, and technique to understand what demands are being placed on the body. The therapist also needs to ask questions about any changes or concerns in the musician's artistry, work, leisure, and personal life because these aspects can contribute to the musician's physical well-being and recovery.

*This chapter is based on the first edition chapter written by Caryl Johnson, OTR/L, CHT.

Some instruments stand alone away from the musician's body, and the musician reaches and moves forward from a seated or standing position (piano, harp, drums), and others are held by the musician (violin, clarinet, guitar) to create sound. Some instruments require a combination of facial motor control and upper extremity action (French horn, trumpet, trombone), and others require elaborate fine motor control of the hand (flute, violin, cello, organ). Due to the variations in the way the instruments are played and how each musician has learned to play his or her instrument, a functional movement assessment and analysis of the musician's whole body adds specificity to understanding and treatment of his or her injuries.

Evaluation and Treatment Approach

When treating musicians' injuries, a thorough examination of posture, with and without the instrument; the upper quadrant; and a cervical screen combined with clinical problem solving is essential. Pain, muscle spasms, numbness, paresthesias, and tenderness are often treated initially with anti-inflammatory medication, immobilization with an orthosis, modalities, and soft tissue techniques, followed by graded remobilization and a timed practice schedule, building up to full performance at the instrument. After the acute stage of treatment, the therapist educates the musician in balanced and efficient body mechanics when performing and practicing and works with the musician to begin a realistic long-term strengthening and conditioning program to prevent further injury or reinjury.

Certain helpful parallels may be drawn between the treatment of musicians and the treatment of athletes. The fine motor control and elaborate coordination necessary to play an instrument requires regular physical conditioning and training, such as that required to achieve an elite skill in a sport. Musicians and athletes spend many hours each day training to improve their specific physical skills and enhance their innate talent-activating, efficient muscle synergies that are unique to the person and use dependent (Safavynia, Torres-Oviedo, & Ting, 2011; Ting & McKay, 2007). For both of these groups, external and internal demands for performance success may drive the person beyond his or her conditioning tolerance and/or abilities, resulting in injury. Gathering information about the correct playing position for the patient's instrument, the patient's level of skill, the demands of the repertoire, and the role music plays in his or her life assists the therapist in developing a plan of care. Treatment of the injury alone is not enough to enable the musician to resume performance; a total body-conditioning program should be implemented to improve overall strength and endurance along with thorough patient education about posture, body mechanics, and flexibility, and a balance of work and leisure are important to help the musician understand how to avoid reinjury.

Another important aspect for a successful recovery is a graded plan and schedule for return to the instrument. It is not simply enough to tell the musician to resume playing slowly. The amount of playing he or she can do should be progressive, based on the injury, stage of tissue healing, pre-injury practicing habits, and general physical status. From the student to the amateur to the professional performer, musicians frequently have strong emotional drives to play their instruments, which add intensity and anxiety to their responses to their injury, including fears about losing the ability to play and losing their artistic expression. Frequent reassurance, education about tissue healing and timing, guidance on how to resume full performance on their instrument, and support during the course of rehabilitation are important to the recovery of musicians.

Indications for Orthotic Intervention

Musicians of all levels, like the general population, are subject to traumatic upper extremity injuries. The most frequently seen are fractures, sprains, lacerations, crush injuries, and contusions. Although the initial phases of treatment are the same as those for a similar injury in any patient, a musician's urge to return to playing may put pressure on the therapist to speed up the steps of recovery; but assessment of healing and tissue response, determined by the treating physician and therapist, should be the deciding factor in planning for return to the instrument. However, return to the instrument should be as soon as physically and safely possible to allay any fears that the patient has and to maintain his or her motor control and sensorimotor organization of his or her upper extremity and digits at the instrument.

In addition to traumatic injuries, musicians frequently present with conditions resulting from playing their instruments, such as inflammation of muscle and tendon (usually related to insufficient conditioning or increased use or force), compression neuropathies (related to repetitive motion at extreme joint angles), and soft tissue injuries (related to repetitive impact to palm or finger and related to sustained static stretch of a muscle, e.g., scapular adductors, rotator cuff) when an instrument must be held or supported for long periods of time (Fig. 24-1). The most common repetitive use

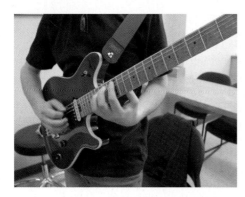

FIGURE 24–1 Notice the potential areas of concern on the guitarist's left side, including the compressive strap across the clavicle, sustained wrist flexed position, and soft tissue impact at the fingertips on the strings.

injuries, tendonitis/tendinosis and synovitis, are usually the result of misuse of the upper extremity or of insufficient conditioning for the physical demands placed on the player (e.g., increased playing time and intensity before an audition or performance). The challenging muscular coordination and specialized repetitive use of the musician's body and upper extremity require good posture and muscular balance at the instrument originating from a strong supportive framework, comprising strong trunk musculature, a stable pelvis and shoulder girdle, a flexible and relaxed forearm and hand, and overall strength and endurance to prevent injury.

Previously, the philosophy of care was to recommend that the musician return to playing when he or she could play without support or pain. The current practice is to assist the musician's return to playing as soon as possible because research shows that immobilization and lack of use for more than 12 hours reveals changes in motor performance, strength, and tactile discrimination (Huber et al., 2006; Weibull, Flondell, Rosen, & Björkman, 2011) and protective guarding or splinting impacts motor intent and motor planning (Mosley, 2004). Therefore, to keep motor and coordination skills at an elite level and maintain their competitive edge, musicians need to practice and perform. Not playing one's instrument for 2 weeks or longer is detrimental physically and psychologically for a musician.

Whether it is a traumatic or repetitive use injury, the resulting limits on playing time can represent a significant emotional and financial loss (Norris, 2002; Wilson, 1998). Orthoses that can be worn by the instrumentalist during recovery have been used successfully. This chapter describes the possibilities and practical considerations of creating **playing orthoses** for musicians, which are orthoses made to be worn and used while playing an instrument. Playing orthoses maximize extremity function by doing the following:

- Immobilizing and protecting areas of healing
- Stabilizing joints
- Rebalancing deforming forces

- Improving joint alignment
- Assisting and training muscle action

Playing orthoses are immobilizing, supportive, restricting, or assistive devices that serve a dynamic function. They can be constructed for the wrist, hand, fingers, or thumb. The upper extremity movements needed for playing the instrument together with the clinical purpose for the orthosis determine its design (Johnson, 1992a). The playing orthosis should do the following:

- Limit or assist only the joint motion needed.
- Conform closely to the body.
- Minimally interfere with the body motions of playing (Van Lede & Veldhoven, 1998).
- Not chafe the skin or rub against bony prominences.
- Be as lightweight as possible.
- Use minimal or no strapping.
- Not touch the instrument or interfere with its moving parts.

Orthotic Fabrication for Traumatic Injuries

Patients who have suffered **traumatic injuries**, including nondisplaced and/or stable upper extremity fractures, can be fitted with playing orthoses that brace the fracture against deforming forces. The orthosis can support and immobilize the healing bone to allow safe use when playing the instrument. Gutter playing orthoses (three-sided, U-shaped orthoses) can be used on long bones (distal radius and ulna), metacarpals, and on the phalanges.

For example, a recorder player with a fractured proximal phalanx may be immobilized in a volar hand-based orthosis that is removed only for exercise (Fig. 24–2A). In the later stages of healing, the patient may be able to safely return to the instrument by being fitted with a dorsal nonarticular proximal phalanx orthosis to support the fractured area (Fig. 24–2B). Evidence shows that longitudinal stress can hasten the formation of callus if alignment is not disturbed (Schenk, 1992). The nonarticular orthosis allows playing and provides additional longitudinal support to the fracture. An immobilization orthosis is worn when the patient is not playing to provide support and protection.

Many traumatic ligament injuries are amenable to the fabrication of an orthosis in a way that allows the performer to continue playing. The degree or nature of instability, alignment, and amount of swelling determine the choice of design of the orthosis (Fess, 2002; Mayer & McCue, 1990; Sadler & Koepfer, 1992) (Fig. 24–3). Orthoses used for acute injuries must be adjusted as swelling and contours change to ensure an appropriate fit. Although musicians who are able to make an earlier return to music will be more able to cope with the psychological feelings of loss caused by the injury, the use of playing orthoses should create no disruption to alignment, bony reduction, or healing, nor should playing orthoses create compensatory or substitution movements proximal or distal to the injury in the kinetic chain of the functional movement pattern. Lacerations or other skin lesions may need orthoses

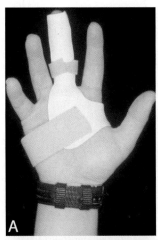

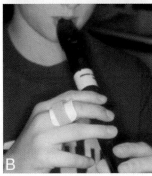

FIGURE 24–2 In this musician with a proximal phalanx fracture, a volar digit immobilization orthosis **(A)** and playing orthosis (for use with a recorder) **(B)** were used to protect the healing fracture.

fabricated to provide wound protection from contact, pressure, or percussion to avoid irritating the healing tissues.

Orthotic Fabrication for Repetitive Use Injuries

Repetitive use injuries, including tendonitis, synovitis, myositis, and compression neuropathies, are frequent presenting diagnoses for musicians (Johnson, 1992a, 1992b). A broad spectrum of therapeutic interventions can be used to treat these conditions, including heat/ice, soft tissue and

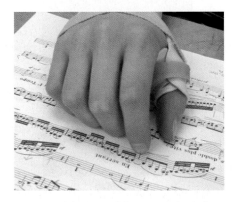

FIGURE 24–3 A thumb MP immobilization orthosis for UCL injury to prevent lateral stress on healing tissue fabricated out of rigid thermoplastic to allow early return to playing.

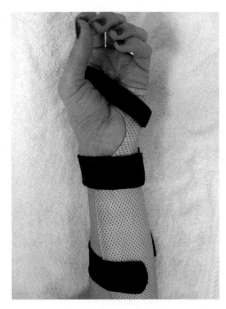

FIGURE 24–4 Because it is lightweight and has some flexibility, ¹⁄₁₆″ perforated material with memory was used to support the wrist in slight ulnar deviation in this wrist immobilization orthosis. Note full clearance of the MCP joints and thenar muscles.

joint mobilization, therapeutic exercise, and orthoses. Complete immobilization is used as an early intervention to rest inflamed tissues and inhibit provocative movements. After the acute phase, when pain and swelling have diminished, a playing orthosis can be used to block extreme or symptom-producing motions and allow the patient to return to his or her instrument. For example, a patient with extensor carpi ulnaris (ECU) tendonitis may be fitted with a playing orthosis to immobilize the wrist (Fig. 24–4). The wrist should be positioned in 20° of extension and the orthosis molded generously around the hypothenar eminence to restrict ulnar deviation. This orthosis supports the wrist in extension and prevents repetitive ulnar deviation placing the ECU on slack. The orthosis helps to educate the musician to avoid ulnar deviation when playing by providing tactile biofeedback. When indicated, Kinesio® tape can be also be used to support the ECU and restrict some wrist flexion and ulnar deviation while providing tactile biofeedback during use to educate the instrumentalist to play in safe positions, as seen with this violinist who has pain on the ulnar side of his right wrist when he uses his bow and on his left when he flexes his wrist and ulnarly deviates at acute angles (Fig. 24–5A,B).

Progressive ligament injuries that result from playing can be considered an overuse injury. Woodwind players who support the instrument on their right thumb are often found to have injured the ulnar collateral ligament (UCL) by repetitive stretching of the thumb at the metacarpophalangeal (MP) joint (Fig. 24–6A). A hand-based thumb immobilization playing orthosis can provide static alignment to the thumb MP joint and interphalangeal (IP) joint if needed (Fig. 24–6B). This orthosis can be used to decrease inflammation and decrease the external deforming force

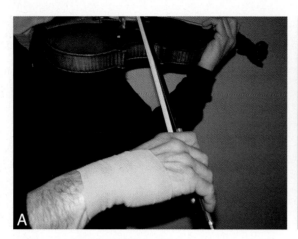
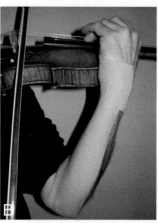

FIGURE 24–5 A, Elastic therapeutic tape (Kinesio® Tape shown here) applied to right wrist just ulnar to thenar crease and pulled tightly around dorsum of hand, supporting ulnar carpus and distal radio-ulnar joint (DRUJ). **B,** Kinesio® tape applied to left wrist and ulnar forearm to support ECU and ulnar side of wrist and forearm to provide tactile feedback to help musician recognize when he is flexing and ulnarly deviating his wrist too much.

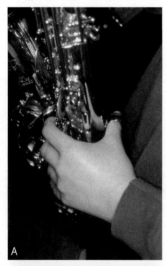

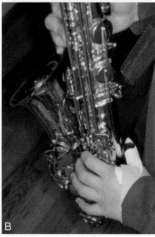

at the thumb MP joint in the same way that a wrist/thumb immobilization orthosis may be used to decrease inflammation and decrease the deforming external force at the thumb carpometacarpal (CMC) joint (Swigart, Eaton, Glickel, & Johnson, 1999). Many variations of a thumb MP immobilization playing orthosis can be used to treat musicians with overuse or cumulative trauma injuries. Playing orthoses can be constructed to stabilize any of the thumb joints laterally or longitudinally. The CMC joint can be blocked from excess adduction and/or dorsal subluxation, and the MP and IP joints can be stabilized laterally to prevent stress on the collateral ligaments (Bean, Tencer, & Trumble, 1999; Brandsma, Oudenaarde, & Oostendorp, 1996; Glickel, Malerich, Pearce, & Littler, 1993; Haelterman, 1996; Heyman, Gelberman, Duncan, & Hip, 1993) (Fig. 24–7).

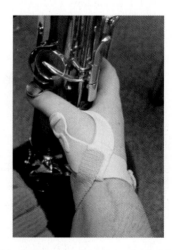

FIGURE 24–6 A, Note the lateral stress on thumb MP joint and UCL from holding a saxophone. **B,** A hand-based thumb immobilization orthosis that includes the IP joint helps support the weight of the instrument, thereby decreasing stress on the MP joint UCL.

FIGURE 24–7 This playing orthosis supports both the thumb CMC and MP joints by restricting excessive radial deviation and hyperextension via the distal radial portion of the orthosis. In the way the orthosis is fabricated, it also provides a dorsal volar stabilization of the 1st CMC joint.

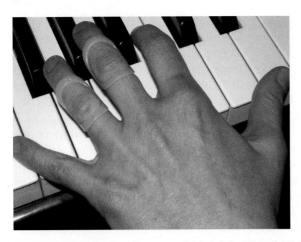

FIGURE 24–8 Oval-8 ring orthoses on pianist's left MF and RF PIP joints to prevent hyperextension and reduce pain while playing (3-Point Products, Stevensville, MD).

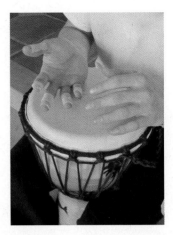

FIGURE 24–9 Steri-strip application to lessen repetitive stress on fingertips in drummer.

The finger IP joints may also sustain ligamentous injuries from repetitive playing, as seen in a right-handed pianist who injured her left middle finger (MF) and ring finger (RF) after she practiced for hours and days. She was trying to create a certain sound in a passage of a piano sonata using a forceful percussive technique that positioned her fingers straight down and coming in at an angle on the piano key (which was the technique demanded by her teacher). She presented with constant pain at the proximal interphalangeal (PIP) joints of her left MF and RF worsening with force into extension. These symptoms necessitated positioning the inflamed joints into slight flexion to restrict hyperextension with playing (Fig. 24–8). She used prefabricated Oval-8 ring orthoses, which fit her well and did not interfere with playing but rather assisted her movement by preventing hyperextension at the PIP joints. These orthoses blended in with her skin color and were not visible to the audience. All of these considerations are very important to the selection and design of a playing orthosis.

Soft tissue impact injuries are also seen in musicians. The palmar skin, fingertips, and sides of the fingers are areas that receive repetitive mechanical stresses from some instruments. They are subject to reactive injury, painful and inflamed soft tissues, or development of small masses. Reactive soft tissue problems on the finger or fingertips of players may be successfully protected with soft materials, such as Leuko tape or Steri-strips (Fig. 24–9). String players are subject to painful fingertip subcallus blisters, neuromas, or small glomus tumors on the finger pads of the left hand from the repeated blows struck against sharp metal strings. Callus injuries tend to resolve over a period of months if they are not irritated further (R. G. Eaton, personal communication, 1997). Many patients try taping the fingertip, but sharp strings quickly cut through the tape. Although the use of any material on the fingertip can be unacceptable to some players, in a concert, some musicians can often tolerate the use of a silicone-lined finger cap (Fig. 24–10) (Manske, 1999).

Orthotic Fabrication for Injuries Related to Handling Instruments

Many instruments must be held to the mouth or lifted in some way for playing, resulting in injuries related to lifting and positioning the instrument. Woodwind instruments are good examples; all must be supported and held near the body and mouth for playing. Lifting the weight of these instruments places stress on the whole upper extremity, especially the joints of the thumb. Playing orthoses can support the instrument by transferring part of the instrument weight to a more proximal joint and muscle group (Johnson, 1992a). Two types of custom-molded playing orthoses for the thumb can be fabricated to assist woodwind players in

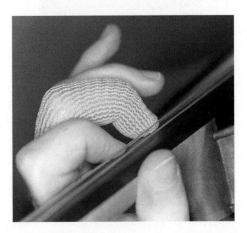

FIGURE 24–10 A Silipos Digital Cap used to protect a violinist who has an MF neuroma. The sleeve can be trimmed to the DIP or PIP crease to allow greater freedom of movement.

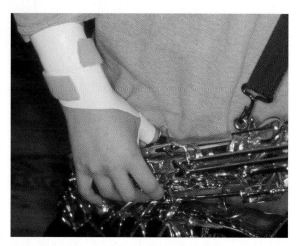

FIGURE 24–11 This spiral design of a wrist/thumb immobilization orthosis decreases the lateral stress on the thumb for this saxophonist.

supporting their instrument. A more supportive orthosis is a variant of a wrist/thumb immobilization orthosis that transfers part of the instrument's weight from the thumb to the dorsal ulnar wrist (Fig. 24–11). The other orthosis is a hand-based thumb MP immobilization orthosis wrapped from ulnar to radial and around the thumb as shown in Figures 24-3 and 24-6B.

Prefabricated orthoses can be challenging to fit perfectly for instrument support compared to the intimate fit achieved from a well-molded, custom-fabricated orthosis. In the absence of a custom option, a form-fitting, prefabricated thumb orthosis may give partial support to the MP and IP joints (Fig. 24–12). When choosing a prefabricated

orthosis, it is helpful to consider the same factors as when designing a custom-molded orthosis: Avoid any obstruction to the instrument or its moving parts and respect the player's customary hand and wrist position (see Chapter 11 for additional information). Custom-fabricated neoprene orthoses are an additional option and are described in Chapter 14.

Other commercially available adaptive devices used for instrument support include neck straps, the **FHRED** (Finger and Hand Retraining Ergonomic Device) **oboe or English horn support** (rests on the chair and supports the instrument on a rigid stem), and the post (holds the instrument out from the body braced against the player's abdomen). Refer to the listing at the end of this chapter for various instrument Web sites/catalogs that offer many solutions to this common problem. These Web sites also offer various straps, stands, supports for musical instruments, and other accessories that might be helpful for the musician to prevent injury.

Playing Orthoses for Age-Related Problems

Musicians do not stop playing their instrument at a certain age, and their ability to play can be affected by age-related problems, such as arthritis, as seen in the left MF distal interphalangeal (DIP) joint of this cellist. Her left MF DIP joint presents with osteoarthritis and deviates ulnarly and her PIP joint rotates radially, preventing her from placing her digit down on the string correctly, affecting the sound of the note. Also, she cannot maintain the space between her fingers, which affects her ability to reach the correct note. She was fitted with a dorsal PIP and DIP joint orthosis that was molded as she positioned her fingers on the cello strings (Fig. 24–13). The orthosis prevents her DIP joint from deviating, and it allows her fingers to maintain the correct spacing on the strings because of the improved alignment of her PIP and DIP joints.

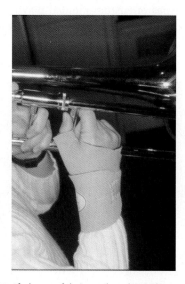

FIGURE 24–12 If the prefabricated orthosis has a wrist component, as shown, it will assist in CMC stability and may decrease wrist symptoms.

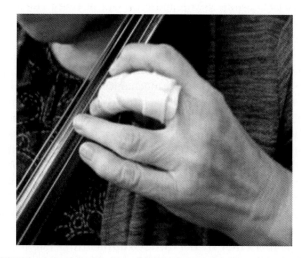

FIGURE 24–13 Lateral view of PIP and DIP orthosis to align joints with osteoarthritis into a better playing position.

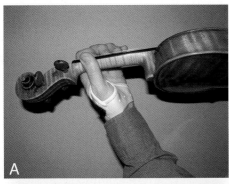

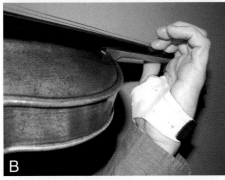

FIGURE 24–14 A and B, A thumb CMC joint immobilization orthosis to lessen CMC joint pain. Notice how this design does not restrict movement at the thumb MP joint.

If the musician has osteoarthritis and pain at the CMC joint, a custom-molded thumb CMC joint immobilization orthosis that does not include the MP joint (Colditz, 2000) has helped some musicians during practice sessions but was noted to be too restrictive during performance (Fig. 24–14A,B). The Push CMC orthosis is a new, more flexible design for the thumb CMC joint (Colditz & Koekebakker, 2010) that may be another option; however, the color of the thermoplastic polyurethane contrasts with the skin color, and the musician still may not want to wear the orthosis during a performance because it is noticeable.

Constructing a Playing Orthosis

Taking a thorough physical and musical history and completing a thorough initial evaluation (with and without the instrument) precede construction of a playing orthosis. If the patient has an acute or traumatic injury, he or she needs two orthoses: a resting or protective orthosis and, when the injury allows, a playing orthosis to assist the return to the instrument. If the patient has an inflammatory or chronic problem, observation of the musician playing his or her instrument should be included in the initial evaluation. This observation method is often referred to as a **functional movement analysis**. During this functional movement analysis with his or her instrument, the following information is collected:

- **Musician's posture**
- Head position

- Upper extremity balance and imbalances
- Joint positions during playing
- Body mechanics
- Excessive tension in muscle groups
- Increases in body or facial tension
- Playing endurance
- Correctness of functional movement
- Note any substitutions and/or compensatory movements (especially with repetitive use injuries; be sure to educate musician)

The therapist must determine the treatment plan and consider the use of a playing orthosis as soon as clinically possible. If a playing orthosis is appropriate, consulting with the physician about any restrictions or contraindications is important (Norris, 2002; Stephens & Leilich, 1998; Stotko, 1998). The patient should bring the instrument to the fabrication appointment, and the therapist should schedule a generous amount of time if possible. Table 24–1 outlines a step-by-step procedure for evaluation and fabrication of a playing orthosis. This information is specifically related to fabrication of an orthosis for a musician; more general fabrication guidelines can be found in Chapter 6.

Orthotic Fabrication

Material Selection

Thermoplastic materials with a prolonged setup time and little memory are usually preferred for playing orthoses. A high degree of conformability is necessary to ensure comfort and optimal fit (Fig. 24–15). A longer setup time allows for adjustments before the position of the orthosis is finalized. Thick ⅛″ thermoplastic materials, with some degree of conformability, such as TailorSplint or NCM Clinic, are best used for instrument-weight-bearing orthoses and orthoses that cross the wrist. Thicker materials are more suited for larger hands. Thinner thermoplastic materials, such as ¹⁄₁₆″ and ³⁄₃₂″ Aquaplast or Orfit, are best used for alignment orthoses on the fingers or thumb, Figure-8 orthoses for IP joints, and light thumb supports. Sometimes a thin thermoplastic material, such as ¹⁄₁₆″ perforated Orfit or Fabriplast, is used best for a **training orthosis**—not to provide rigidity but to serve as a gentle reminder (tactile biofeedback) of proper joint position.

The choice of perforated or nonperforated thermoplastics depends on the purpose and function of the orthosis and the amount of adjustment time needed for construction. Perforated materials tend to set up more quickly and may not allow for the multiple adjustments needed when making a playing orthosis comfortable. Whether to use coated or uncoated material depends on the design and any part of the orthosis that needs to be bonded to the base (Austin, 2003; Breger-Lee & Buford, 1992; Moberg, 1984).

TABLE 24–1

Evaluation and Fabrication of a Playing Orthosis

1. Observe the patient as he or she plays the instrument. Note the synergistic movement patterns of the bones, joints, and soft tissues in relation to the instrument.

2. Determine an appropriate orthosis pattern by taking into account the goals for the playing orthosis based on the diagnosis, stage of healing or symptoms, and the treatment plan.

3. Choose a suitable material based on the function and fit needed.

4. Measure to fabricate an orthosis pattern from a paper towel.

5. Again, observe the patient playing the instrument and review the rationale for the design. Try the pattern on the patient, and test for interference with instrument parts.

6. Cut and prepare the material. The patient should be ready to play the instrument for the fitting.

7. Mold the material on the patient's extremity while he or she maintains a playing position with the instrument; take great care when conforming the material to avoid the moving parts of the hand and instrument.

8. Apply straps or tape if needed, making sure they do not interfere with the hand or instrument; the material used should be the patient's choice.

9. Test the orthosis. Ask the patient to try playing with the orthosis firmly in place. Encourage him or her to identify any parts that are uncomfortable or hinder playing. Take time with this step; if the patient does not use the orthosis, it may slow down or hinder the healing process.

10. Test the orthosis while the patient plays in several musical contexts: a slow passage, a fast passage, and a technically demanding section. Note: Some players have to change instruments or costumes in the course of a performance; test the patient's ability to remove and apply the orthosis.

11. When the patient decides that the orthosis is comfortable and fits well and does not interfere with his or her ability to play his or her instrument, and the therapist determines that the design achieves its goals of support, assist, and/or restriction of movement, it is then necessary for the therapist to observe the effect of wearing an orthosis on the movement of the upper extremity as a whole. Does wearing the orthosis cause any abnormal muscle movements, compensations, and/or substitutions that may lead to other musculoskeletal problems? If noted, the cause of the movement problem needs to be identified and changed. Is it the effect of wearing an orthosis on tactile input or joint proprioception or is it the effect of the restriction of the orthosis on the movement? Or is it something else specific to the patient?

12. Plan a follow-up visit for the patient with his or her instrument to make any necessary alterations. Be sure the patient is able to play at his or her level of ability in the orthosis.

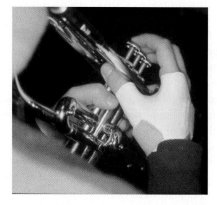

FIGURE 24–15 Note the precise fit achieved with the use of plastic material on this hand-based thumb immobilization orthosis.

Another consideration when choosing a material is that musicians who will be performing in public with their orthosis may prefer a material that is similar to skin color to minimize visibility.

Strapping Selection

Straps are best made of traditional hook and loop when firm stabilization is required. When soft tissues have to move beneath the straps, softer materials, such as elastic, neoprene, or foam, are a more appropriate choice. Finger orthoses that require stabilization can be applied with an elasticized wrap, such as Coban™ or elastic tape. Wrap these materials without applying too much tension to avoid compression of the neurovascular structures.

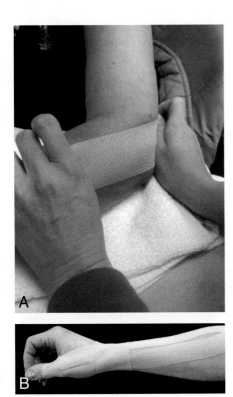

FIGURE 24–16 **A,** Kinesio taping being applied to musicians with lateral epicondylitis and **(B)** deQuervain's syndrome. Skin-colored tape is available and may be more acceptable for onstage performances.

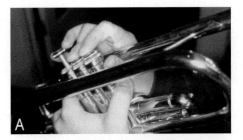

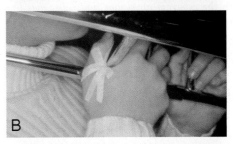

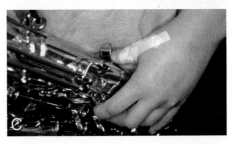

FIGURE 24–17 **A,** "X" taping to improve lateral stability of the right index finger PIP joint in a trumpet player. **B,** "X" taping with additional lateral strips to improve thumb MP joint stability in a trombone player. **C,** Basket-weave taping to support the thumb of a saxophone player.

Taping techniques, using Kinesio® tape or Leuko tape, are suitable as playing orthoses. Taping can often substitute for orthosis use (Fig. 24–16A,B). Taping gives the patient a chance to try playing with some degree of restriction. Taping may also be appropriate as a form of emergency immobilization if a player must perform with an injury and there is no time to fabricate a protective orthosis. Useful taping patterns for musicians include "X" taping to allow a joint to move while being supported laterally (Fig. 24–17A). The "X" pattern can be combined with lateral or longitudinal taping for firmer support (Fig. 24–17B). On the thumb, basket-weave taping can be used for partial stability and can be combined or reinforced with longitudinal strips to support areas of stress (Fig. 24–17C). Taping is not a long-term solution for musicians because it must be applied and removed frequently, which can be irritating to the skin (Reese, Burruss, & Patten, 1990).

Conclusion

Fabrication of orthoses is a vital and challenging component in the therapeutic treatment of the injured musician. To construct an orthosis that allows the musician to make an earlier and safe return to his or her instrument is rewarding for both the musician and the therapist (Meinke, 1998). Three-dimensional analysis of movement, understanding of tissue healing and timing, realistic goals and expectations, patient education, and suitable design and materials lead the way to the fabrication of a playing orthosis for the musician that is functional and self-actualizing.

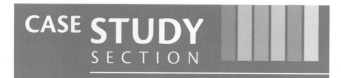

CASE STUDY SECTION

The case studies presented here are meant as a teaching guideline only. Treatment and orthosis protocols vary greatly from surgeon to surgeon and from therapist to therapist. The therapist should check with the referring physicians and colleagues to define the preferred treatment and appropriate orthotic intervention.

CASE STUDY 1: Violinist with Distal Radius Fracture

JP is a 42-year-old violinist who fell and sustained a nondisplaced fracture of the left distal radius. He was placed in a short arm plaster cast with the fingers and thumb free. The patient was started on a program of exercise to maintain range of motion (ROM), strength, and muscle balance of all uninvolved joints. At 1-month postinjury, x-rays showed good fracture alignment; the cast was removed, and a wrist immobilization orthosis was ordered to provide continued protection of the fracture site.

Eager to return to work, JP was fitted with an additional play-ing orthosis that allowed him to start practicing (Fig. 24–18). Based on left-hand use for violin playing, a radial wrist immobi-lization playing orthosis was constructed to protect and main-tain fracture alignment and to prevent disruption of the newly formed callus. With the orthosis in place, JP could start to regain finger strength and facility. After 2 weeks of using the transitional playing orthosis, he was able to return unencumbered to his instrument and to work.

CASE STUDY 2: Bass Player with Distal Phalanx Fracture

BRT is a 40-year-old double bass player who fractured the distal phalanx of his left MF when he was thrown off a horse. Radio-

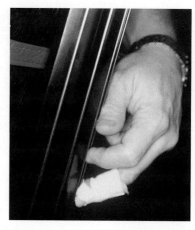

FIGURE 24–19 A dorsal DIP immobilization orthosis fabricated from ¹⁄₁₆″ thermoplastic material for the MF of a double bass player. Special considerations included acceptable protection of the fracture during impact on the string and soft but stable strapping that would not interfere with sensory input from the string.

graphs revealed a bony mallet injury that did not require sur-gical intervention. Because the DIP joint of the MF moves very little during string depression on the bass, it was safe to fabri-cate a playing orthosis without risking disruption of the healing tendon/bone interface.

A simple dorsal DIP immobilization orthosis allowed an early return to work (Fig. 24–19). The orthosis was conformed to the dorsum and lateral borders of the DIP joint. Elastic tape was directed diagonally to ensure maximum conformity with the finger pulp; DIP joint hyperextension was maintained, and the fracture was protected during instrument use. BRT was able to return to work 3 days after the injury; the fracture remained aligned and healed without incident.

CASE STUDY 3: Percussion Player with Proximal Interphalangeal Joint Sprain

FW is a 23-year-old percussion player who was injured in a basket-ball game when he jammed his right MF against another player, spraining the radial collateral ligament (RCL) of the PIP joint. After x-rays determined there was no fracture, he was referred for a PIP joint immobilization orthosis. An orthosis was molded dorsally over the proximal and middle phalanges with the PIP in maximum achievable extension to provide lateral support and complete immobilization. This orthosis was worn full time for 10 days.

FW expressed great concern over an upcoming audition that was scheduled in 3 weeks. To prepare for the audition, the patient needed to return to practicing. A PIP extension block orthosis was constructed to maintain lateral support while allowing a limited flexion/extension arc of motion (Fig. 24–20). FW was able to con-trol the stick while wearing the orthosis and return to practicing for the audition on a modified schedule. Before FW's treatment was complete, he had several playing orthoses constructed be-cause the joint edema fluctuated with increased use. The injured joint, maintained in alignment, progressed satisfactorily to well-aligned healing, and the patient was able to play at his audition.

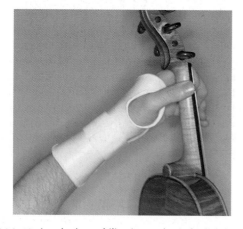

FIGURE 24–18 A wrist immobilization orthosis (radial design) for a violinist with a left distal radius fracture. The orthosis was cut away on the ulnar side, allowing motion into moderate ulnar deviation and full finger use in the first four positions.

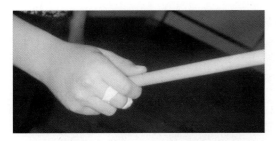

FIGURE 24–20 A PIP extension restriction orthosis for the MF PIP joint of a percussion player. After the material was molded to the PIP joint but before the material had hardened, the patient gripped a drumstick so the orthosis conformed to the stick.

CASE STUDY 4: **Guitarist with Wrist Tendonitis**

PCG is a 32-year-old guitar player who presented with complaints of burning and pain at the right elbow medial epicondyle that extended distally along the ulnar border of the forearm. The onset of his symptoms developed over the previous 3 ½ months, during which time his job schedule had increased from two to six nights a week. He was started on anti-inflammatory medication and fitted with a dorsal wrist immobilization orthosis that kept the wrist in 5 to 10° of flexion. Pain kept PCG from returning to his instrument for 2 weeks, at which time he believed it was imperative to start playing again.

At his instrument evaluation, PCG was observed to use extreme ulnar deviation in forceful repeated swipes for strumming. When questioned about this style of playing, he reported that his band had been working on a new strident style of playing and had asked him to slap the strings more and more forcefully. When he began to repeat this motion, he realized it was directly related to his pain. At 2 weeks into his treatment, PCG was fitted with a playing orthosis designed to provide a partial restriction of ulnar deviation (Fig. 24–21). He was able to play in the orthosis, and the restriction of extreme ulnar deviation helped him revise his right-hand technique. He used the orthosis for practicing and part of his performing hours until he accomplished the modification of technique. After 4 weeks of tapered use, the orthosis was discontinued.

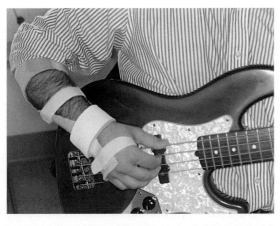

FIGURE 24–21 A wrist immobilization orthosis (ulnar design) for the right wrist of guitar player with flexor carpi ulnaris (FCU) tendonitis.

CASE STUDY 5: **Bassoonist with Thumb Instability**

SD is a 40-year-old bassoonist who was referred to therapy with a 4-month history of progressive pain in the left thumb. This problem had finally led her to take a leave of absence from her full-time orchestra job. Physical findings included pain along the thenar eminence, dorsally over the first metacarpal, and proximally into the CMC and radiocarpal joint with tenderness over the UCLs of the MP and IP joints. Passively, both the MP and IP joints could be moved 20° and 15°, respectively, into radial deviation, demonstrating a significant laxity at both joints compared to the other side. Bassoonists use the left thumb to depress many different keys (Fig. 24–22A).

SD's painful thumb was treated for 8 weeks, progressing from immobilization to partial immobilization and then to gradual strengthening. A playing orthosis was then designed to assist her thumb joint stability at the instrument (Fig. 24–22B). Owing to the progressive nature of this problem, SD continues to wear her playing orthosis, thus avoiding further acute episodes.

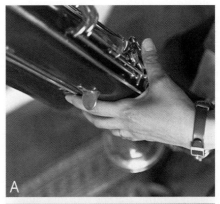
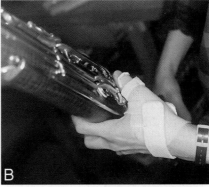

FIGURE 24–22 A, Note the stress to the left thumb of this bassoonist. **B,** A variation of a hand-based thumb immobilization orthosis constructed from ¹⁄₁₆″ perforated thermoplastic material with memory with lateral support to the MP and IP joints. The orthosis includes a slim volar opening to allow variable IP joint flexion and a protective palmar edge to block the first metacarpal from maximum adduction. Soft material was used for strapping, and the contact edges were bound with adhesive-backed ¹⁄₁₆″ liner to improve comfort.

CASE STUDY 6: **Woodwind Player with Thumb Pain and Lateral Epicondylitis**

LT is a 45-year-old professional musician who plays clarinet and saxophone. He was referred with two diagnoses: right thumb pain and right elbow lateral epicondylitis. Symptoms included diffuse pain along the thumb radially after 30 minutes of playing, pain on palpation at the CMC and MP joints, and pain on resisted active and isometric thumb extension and adduction. Provocative testing of resisted extensor carpi radialis longus (ECRL) and extensor carpi radialis brevis (ECRB) was also positive, with increased pain at the lateral epicondyle. LT was not tender over the first dorsal compartment, and the Finkelstein's test was negative, suggesting that he did not have deQuervain's tenosynovitis.

Both the clarinet and saxophone are constructed with a thumb support on the back of the instrument that rests on the ulnar border of the player's right thumb. Much of the instrument's weight transfers to the thumb, stressing the MP and CMC thumb joints. Although playing his instrument caused pain, LT was unwilling to take more than an occasional night off from his job playing on stage in a Broadway show. Taping (thumb basket-weave taping with vertical supports to the radial and UCLs) was used as a trial immobilization and was found to be somewhat helpful, providing partial support to the MP and IP joints (Fig. 24–17C). Therefore, a hand-based thumb immobilization orthosis was constructed to assist the thumb in supporting the instrument (Fig. 24–23). This orthosis requires exact molding to the instrument for the thumb support to be successful. No good skin match was available in splinting material of the required consistency, so the orthosis and straps were painted with acrylic paint, making it invisible to the audience.

LT was also placed on a program to reduce the inflammation, including anti-inflammatory medication, isometric strengthening exercises, and the use of a wrist/thumb immobilization orthosis when not playing. He progressively returned to the show while wearing the orthosis, starting with four shows a week and then making weekly increases. The orthosis was worn onstage for 3 months, and then wearing time was tapered over a period of

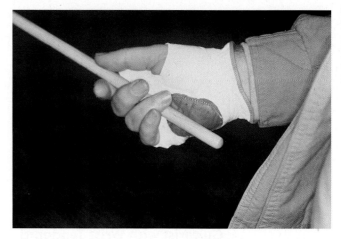

FIGURE 24–24 A protective glove for the right palm of a drummer.

4 weeks. LT keeps the orthosis in his dressing room so he can use it if his thumb becomes symptomatic.

CASE STUDY 7: **Drummer with Ulnar Neuritis**

TF is a 58-year-old drummer who presented with a painful palm 2 months after the excision of a reactive inflammatory mass over the digital ulnar nerve in the right palm. The drumstick hit the excision area with each stroke, repeating the original cause of injury. Unwilling to give up any more playing time, TF requested a mechanism for softening the stick's impact without interfering with touch and control. A light leather golf glove was chosen as the base for the playing orthosis (Fig. 24–24). A patch of thicker leather was used to cover a piece of ⅛" Styrofoam padding cut to align with the stick-striking area. TF was able to play while wearing the glove because it did not interfere with motion or sensation in the fingers or thumb.

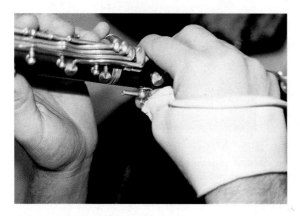

FIGURE 24–23 A hand-based thumb immobilization orthosis fabricated for the right hand of a clarinet player. By wrapping distally and radially around the thumb and crossing the thenar crease, this orthosis stabilizes the CMC and MP joints. In addition, part of the weight of the instrument is transferred to the ulnar border of the hand.

Chapter Review Questions

1. What are the main objectives of a playing orthosis in a musician?

2. Describe the considerations and orthotic intervention for a musician that has sustained a forearm repetitive trauma. Include what orthosis or taping techniques can be applied throughout the course of healing.

3. What injury to the thumb does the woodwind player often acquire? Why does this happen and how can this injury be managed?

4. What musicians may have soft tissue injuries? What are two examples of these injuries and what are the appropriate orthotic intervention choices for each?

5. During a functional movement analysis with the musician's instrument, what information should be collected in order to develop the most appropriate treatment plan that includes the orthosis?

25 Hand and Upper Extremity Transplantation

Marie Pace, OTR/L, CHT
Kimberly Zeske-Maguire, MS, OTR/L, CHT

Chapter Objectives

After study of this chapter, the reader should be able to:

- Describe the preoperative and postoperative role of the hand therapist in the care of the patient who underwent allotransplantation.
- Explain the relative indications and contraindications in allotransplantation versus replantation.
- Understand when allotransplantation is most appropriate and who is the ideal candidate for this procedure.
- Appreciate the overall rehabilitation of the transplanted limb, in particular, the role of orthosis management.
- Clearly describe the potential postoperative immediate and long-term complications in allotransplantation.

Key Terms

Carter™ pillows
Donor match
Graft-versus-host disease
Helmet orthosis
Host tissue

Neuromuscular electrical stimulation
Pittsburgh Protocol
Primary reconstruction
Prosthetic device
Replantation

Residual limb
Sensory innervation
Transplantation
Universal cuff

Introduction

Upper extremity allotransplantation is a relatively new technique in hand reconstruction. Allotransplantation is the transplantation of cells, tissues, or organs to a recipient from a genetically different donor of the same species (Lanzetta, Dubernard, & Petruzzo, 2007).

With significant loss of tissue due to injury or illness, there are few options to restore function and cosmesis. These options are limited to **primary reconstruction**, use of a **prosthetic device**, or **transplantation**. Reconstruction with **host tissue** can be a good option if enough sensate tissue is available for producing a functional result, such as an opposable pinch. A prosthetic can be fit to restore function with skilled training. Newer prosthetic devices are available that are not only functional but also cosmetically appealing. Conversely, there are well-documented limitations to a prosthetic in both overall quality of function and natural appearance.

Upper extremity allotransplantation is an option for reconstruction if the **residual limb** has healthy tissue, the recipient has stable health, and the recipient agrees to be compliant with antirejection medication and rehabilitation. Potential hand transplant recipients go through a battery of medical tests and assessments of functional skills and deficits. Once a **donor match** is found, a composite tissue allograft is harvested, the residual limb is prepared, and the limb is surgically attached (Lanzetta et al., 2007; Schuind, Abramowicz, & Schneeberger, 2007).

To date and to the authors' knowledge, private health insurance has not paid for the transplant procedure or follow-up visits. Funding has typically been provided from grants and institutional support (Amirlak, Gonzalez, Gorantla, Breidenbach, & Tobin, 2007; Chung, Oda, Saddawi-Konefka, & Shauver, 2010; Gordon & Siemionow, 2009).

The Transplanted Hand versus the Replanted Hand

Treating the transplanted upper extremity is unique from **replantation** for several reasons (Cendales & Breidenbach, 2001; Hartzell et al., 2011). After an injury that requires replantation, there is often a significant amount of tissue trauma that must be overcome in order to eventually have functional outcomes. Surgeons have to make use of the viable tissue that remains in order to create a working hand or limb. For example, if a patient has an amputation transcarpally and the surgeons are able to replant the hand, the carpus must be fused due to bone loss and ligament damage. Permanent loss of wrist motion would result, but it is likely that sensation and motor function to the fingers would be spared. The postsurgical orthosis would be the same as with a transplant, except wrist support would continue longer to ensure proper fusion. The goals for restoring tendon glide, functional use, and intrinsic muscle function would be the same. Compensatory strategies for loss of wrist motion would be addressed in therapy.

In the case of a hand transplant, the donated hand is chosen in part because it is not damaged. The optimal level of transplantation is carefully planned to closely restore normal anatomy. There is time to plan and enlist the cooperation of a full team of skilled surgeons to harvest the donor tissue and prepare the recipient's residual arm(s). The team carefully and securely attaches the allograft in order to maximize the eventual function of the reconstruction.

Transplantation

After the surgery, all transplant recipients take antirejection medications. In some transplant centers, the patient undergoes a bone marrow transplant and drug regimen that is referred to as the **Pittsburgh Protocol** to promote physiologic acceptance of the limb and minimize the amount of antirejection medication required (Gorantla et al., 2011).

The post–hand transplant rehabilitative process requires the following:

- Edema management
- Wound care and scar management
- Monitoring signs of rejection

- Protective orthoses
- Positioning devices
- Assistive equipment
- Range of motion (ROM) exercise
- Sensory retraining
- Patient and family education/training
- Social and vocational counseling

Each transplant recipient has individualized care based on the level of transplant attachment, residual abilities and skills, personal contexts, and the postsurgical function of the limb. The level of attachment has the most influence on postsurgical function; therefore, the postsurgical therapy protocol is unique to each level of attachment.

Rehabilitation of the transplanted limb can extend 2 to 5 years after the initial surgery (Breidenbach et al., 2008; Herzberg, Weppe, Masson, Gueffier, & Erhard, 2008; Schneeberger et al., 2006). Most of the transplant recipients have been in therapy 4 to 5 days per week for 4 to 6 hours a day. After approximately 6 months of living near the medical facility where the transplant is done, recipients are transferred to a therapist specializing in hand therapy near their home. Extensive therapy is needed to train the transplant recipient to use muscle–tendon units because they are reinnervated. Orthotic intervention is a crucial aspect of the rehabilitation in this unique patient population, and there are various designs that can be used throughout the months of healing. Table 25–1 summarizes the most common orthoses used with these patients.

Functional skills that are important to the recipient are broken down into smaller segments and relearned. For many of the recipients, they have not had a hand for many years; therefore, they must reintegrate the new hand into the brain's cortical mapping (Lee & Nguyen, 2005; Piza-Katzer & Estermann, 2007; Vargas et al., 2009; Washington et al., 2009).

Below Elbow Transplants

Immediate Postoperative Phase

The hand therapist is intimately involved with the surgical team for transplant positioning, minimizing edema, preventing pressure sores on the insensate skin, and patient/family education. Approximately 2 days postoperatively, an orthosis is fabricated in the intrinsic plus position, digits positioned at 50° of metacarpophalangeal (MCP) joint

TABLE 25–1

Transplant Orthoses

Time Frame	Orthosis	Level of Transplant	Comments
0–6 weeks	Dorsal-based MCP extension mobilization orthosis ("crane outrigger") Figure 25–2	Below elbow	Provides optimal balance to healing flexor and extensor tendons
0–6 weeks	Forearm-based hand and wrist immobilization orthosis ("safe position"—either dorsal or volar) Figure 25–1	Above and below elbow	Positions the hand in antideformity position and protects forearm bones during early healing stage
2 months to 1 year	Hand-based dorsal MCP extension restriction orthosis with thumb included Figure 25–8	Below elbow	When extrinsic finger muscles are functioning in the above elbow transplant
0–6 weeks	Volar elbow immobilization orthosis in 30–60° of flexion Figure 25–16	Above elbow	Optional dorsal frame to protect olecranon process from pressure
2 months to 1 year	Hand-based thumb immobilization orthosis with IP joint free Figure 25–9	Below elbow	For use with ADL and in clinic functional tasks

flexion, and interphalangeal (IP) joints extended (Hodges, Chesher, & Feranda, 2000; Scheker & Hodges, 2001) (Fig. 25–1A,B). The wrist and forearm are positioned in neutral and the thumb carpometacarpal (CMC) joint midway between palmar and radial abduction. The orthosis can be either volar or dorsal, depending on vascular integrity, surgeon preference, or to accommodate any other circumstances such as Doppler wires, wounds, drainage tubes, and skin fragility. An alternative to keeping the hand in proper

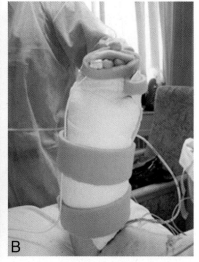

FIGURE 25–1 A and B, Postsurgical orthosis to allow for protective motions. Notice the thick postoperative padding and drains.

position is the MCP extension mobilization orthosis, also referred to as a "dynamic dorsal crane outrigger" (Chesher, Schwartz, & Kleinert, 1988) (Fig. 25–2A,B). Wounds are usually covered with nonadherent gauze and absorbent pads appropriate to the drainage. The dressings are changed daily to check skin for signs of rejection and monitor wound healing. Choosing a thermoplastic material that provides a general fit that can be remolded frequently is crucial. Soft, wide, contouring straps should be used to prevent excess pressure on the body part the strap traverses and prevent compromise of the vascular system (Fig. 25–1). Cotton stockinette over light fluff gauze can be used for edema management, and this will assist in wicking away moisture. Compressive bandages are not typically used due to concerns of the vascular structures' ability to withstand even the slightest external compression from applications such as Coban™ or Isotoner® gloves. Combinations of **Carter™ pillows**, foam wedges, and orthoses are used to promote safe positioning. Forearm placement and consistent elevation optimize vascular flow and edema control (Fig. 25–3). Precise orthosis fabrication with particular attention to joint angles is critical and must take into account minimizing any tension on the vascular system. For hand transplants, the wrist joint is normally positioned in neutral. In the patient with an above elbow transplant, the elbow is positioned in 30 to 60° of flexion.

The forearm position should be alternated from the end range of pronation to the end range of supination. Instruction should be given to the patient and/or involved family member on how to change safely into these forearm positions.

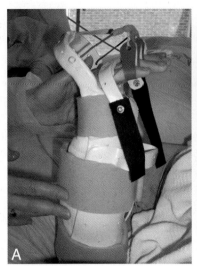
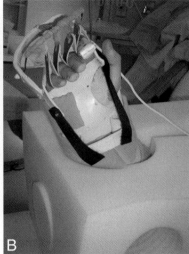

FIGURE 25–2 **A and B,** PIP extension mobilization orthosis allowing active digit flexion against tension on elastics with passive extension to neutral.

Shoulder and elbow active range of motion (AROM) should be done several times a day by the patient. The therapist should instruct the patient to move the extremity slowly with the orthosis on for proximal ROM exercises. The patient should also walk, at minimum, once daily for 10 to 20 minutes to prevent blood clots and enhance circulation to the transplanted limb. While walking, the arm should be elevated, which will contribute to edema reduction and facilitate proximal muscle activation/strengthening. A platform walker or a sling should be used if the patient is unable to hold the affected arm in an elevated position independently (Lee, Garcia, Lee, & Munin, 2011). The therapy schedule is approximately 1 to 2 hours a day, 6 to 7 days a week, focusing on proximal exercises, positioning, and assuring the appropriate fit of any or all orthoses.

10 Days Postoperative

Based on the patient's activities of daily living (ADLs) goals and when approved by the surgical team, functional tasks

and adaptive techniques should be initiated (e.g., pushing buttons on the cell phone with an extension to the orthosis, wrapping the affected hand to a brush with a bandage, applying lotion, using a tissue to wipe eyes) (Fig. 25–4). Only tasks that can be done safely (i.e., no resistance to healing structures such as bone, vessels, and tendons) with the newly transplanted arm/hand should be executed with the orthosis in place. An example is teaching how to use the orthosis as an assist against the noninjured hand in order to pick up light objects, such as a cup, towel, or TV remote control. If the transplant is bilateral, training with a **universal cuff** for eating, writing, and shaving is recommended (Fig. 25–5).

The therapist performs visual inspection of the skin at each session to monitor for signs of possible rejection (patient's body attacking the transplanted tissue). The

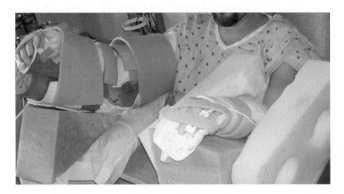

FIGURE 25–3 Positioning for vascular flow and edema control in this patient with bilateral transplantations. Notice the Carter™ pillow elevating his left upper extremity.

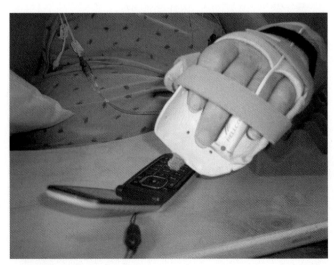

FIGURE 25–4 Adaptation at distal end of volar wrist and hand immobilization orthosis to increase independence.

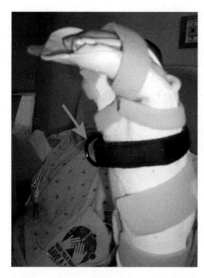

FIGURE 25–5 This is a volar orthosis for a forearm level transplant that has a universal cuff attached for function. The patient can eat and use a comb in the cuff. This provides functional exercise for the proximal muscles while the tissues are healing.

native skin is included in the inspection to monitor for **graft-versus-host disease (GVHD)**. GVHD occurs when the cells from the graft begin attacking the patient's native tissue. It is a complication that can develop after introduction of any transplanted tissue and can appear as a rash on the host tissue that does not blanch when touched (Gorantla et al., 2011; Schuind, 2010). Rejection episodes are easier to monitor in hand transplantation than with organ transplantation due to the ability to visibly inspect the skin. It is essential to notify the physicians and scientists who are on the decision-making teams about medication immediately if there is suspicion of a rejection or GVHD. There should be no delay in adjusting the patient's medication.

3 Weeks Postoperative

The therapy schedule is up to 6 hours a day, 5 days a week. Place/hold finger flexion exercises can begin. Functional tasks and adaptive techniques are adjusted to accommodate the patient's increasing endurance and abilities. By the third week, most of the therapy issues (orthosis fit, assignment of appropriate activities, and exercises) are settled, and a routine is established. The patient should be independent with the assigned self-ROM and activities. The patient has learned adaptive techniques with the appropriate precautions. Weeks 3 to 6 function as a waiting period for the tissues to heal enough to advance to the next level of exercise and function.

6 Weeks Postoperative

AROM is begun with the wrist and digits (Fig. 25–6). Passive finger ROM should continue, including flexion and extension in composite and isolation and finger abduction. Thumb abduction ROM exercises in palmar and radial abduction

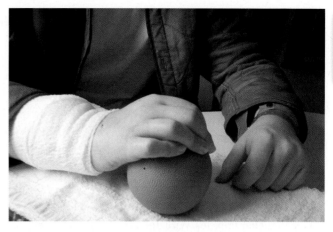

FIGURE 25–6 Gentle active wrist motion performed over a small therapy ball.

are continued because the intrinsics will not be fully innervated for many more months. Orthotic intervention at this stage will depend on need. The forearm-based wrist and hand immobilization orthosis (in the intrinsic plus position) will be used when the patient is not in therapy to prevent undesirable contractures and protect healing forearm bones (Fig. 25–1). Orthoses to increase function include a neutral position wrist orthosis (Fig. 25–7) and a "helmet" orthosis (a dorsal hand-based MCP flexion/IP extension with palmar/radial abduction of thumb) (Fig. 25–8). During controlled therapeutic activity, the wrist orthosis allows stability of the wrist in order to maximize distal motion in the fingers. Similarly, the **helmet orthosis** facilitates IP joint extension by blocking the extensor digitorum communis (EDC) effect on MCP extension. This position harnesses the power of EDC tendon excursion to extend the IP joints. Functional pinch is enhanced with the thumb supported dorsally substituting

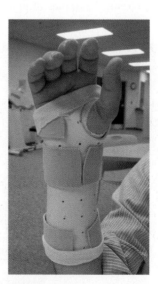

FIGURE 25–7 Wrist immobilization orthosis in neutral to allow for protection of healing tissue yet provide for safe ROM and function distal and proximal.

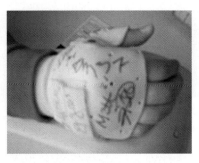

FIGURE 25–8 "Helmet" orthosis blocks extension of MCP joints but allows functional flexion for activities.

for weak thenar muscles. With dorsal support, the flexor pollicis longus (FPL) can be used for an efficient lateral pinch.

In order to minimize edema, the transplanted extremity continues to be elevated and supported in a sling, on a lap tray, or placed on a rolling platform. If the vascular system is functioning adequately, light compression with an elastic stockinette can be started for edema control and scar management.

Frequent execution of identical movement patterns has been shown to be vital in achieving motor recovery (Butefisch, Hummelsheim, Denzler, & Mauritz, 1994). Due to the length of time since the hand transplant recipient's amputation, the portion of the brain that activates the target hand muscles may be less active and will require repetition for cortical reintegration. Having the patient carefully execute repetitive motions (such as PIP flexion) with maximal concentration and effort will contribute to improving the quality of that motion (Butefisch et al., 1994). Tasks must be performed several times each day to encourage cortical integration, allowing the brain to regain control of motor movement patterns (Fig. 25–9). The set of tasks that the recipient performs each day are unique to his or her abilities and interests. For each of the recipients, the list of tasks can be in excess of 20 items. Examples of possible tasks could

include picking up cotton balls, stacking cones, turning a lever, clicking a pen, tapping a drum, or using a keyboard.

Care continues to be taken with functional activities as not to cause damage to reinnervating skin. Burns, friction blisters, and cuts can occur easily due to altered sensation. As functional activity increases, precautions to avoid friction, heat, and sharp edges are paramount. This is especially important with dorsally applied devices given the bony anatomy and fragility of the dorsal skin.

Protective measures include the following:

- Incorporating padding into the orthosis during fabrication (if added after fabrication, the padding may cause a focal area of pressure)
- Smoothing any rough border on the orthosis that may come in contact with skin
- Allowing full clearance of joint creases
- Using straps that are wide and soft versus traditional loop that may have stiff, nonconforming borders
- Considering the use of bicycle or edema gloves to protect the skin from tool handles such as the Baltimore Therapeutic Equipment (BTE) and the upper body ergometer (UBE)
- Educating patient on visual inspection of the skin and compensation for sensory loss

Recipients are excited to have a new hand(s) and will often attempt activities without realizing the inherent potential harm that activity may cause. For example, to avoid a possible burn, the recipients are repeatedly instructed to first use the nonaffected extremity to test the temperature of water before hand washing (Cendales & Breidenbach, 2001).

3 Months Postoperative

At this time, the orthoses serve several purposes:

- Preventing extension contractures at the MCP joints
- Facilitating active IP joint extension
- Improving overall function for life tasks

A hand-based dorsal MCP extension restriction orthosis (intrinsic plus position) will be appropriate for all three purposes (Fig. 25–10). It is worn during daily activity and

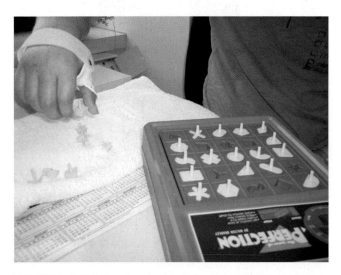

FIGURE 25–9 This thumb orthosis substitutes for the opposition muscles that are not fully innervated, allowing for functional prehension.

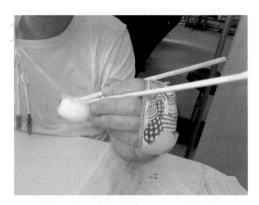

FIGURE 25–10 Fine motor control using chopsticks in combination with the "helmet" orthosis.

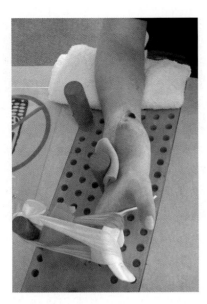

FIGURE 25–11 At 4 months postoperative, a hand-based digit orthosis was used in combination with the Hough™ Hand table and exercise bands to provide low-load, prolonged stretch to tight long flexors.

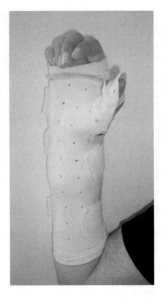

FIGURE 25–13 This wrist and thumb orthosis uses a serial static approach to stretch the thumb into radial abduction with the IP joint extended.

with all exercise. If there are limitations in passive motion, mobilization orthoses can be used therapeutically for daily sessions to improve motion (Fig. 25–11). A flexion glove can be used to improve fingertip-to-palm limitations. If thumb flexion is a problem, a hand-based composite thumb flexion orthosis can be initiated (Fig. 25–12). Limitations in pronation and supination can be managed with static progressive or dynamic mobilization devices, whether custom made or prefabricated (Hodges et al., 2000). Custom-made neoprene supination/pronation straps are an alternative for skin that is less tolerant to thermoplastic material or for those patients that may need a "less bulky" or "lower profile" design. Refer to Chapters 11 on Prefabricated Orthoses and 14 on Neoprene Orthoses for further information on alternative materials and devices. Any passive stretching of the transplanted forearm, wrist, and/or digits should be done with a low-load, prolonged stretch (Liebesman & Carfelli, 1994).

If persistent edema is a problem, the patient should be fitted with custom-made edema sleeve. The consistent low-grade pressure of the garment aids in minimizing edema and remodeling scar tissue. Elastic stockinette and "off-the-shelf" elasticized gloves may be considered as an alternative. Caution must be used when dispensing off-the-shelf garments because (1) circumferential pressure is not always uniform throughout the garment, (2) the garment may not be aesthetically pleasing to the patient, and (3) durability of the garment may be problematic.

6 Months Postoperative

At this time frame, it is not unusual to see a decrease in passive ROM (PROM) due to the increased muscle tone from emerging innervations. Mobilization orthoses can be applied to improve functional movement (Fig. 25–13) (Scheker, Chesher, Netscher, Julliard, & O'Neill, 1995). Mobilization orthoses should be used when the patient is not in therapy. Therapy should focus on strengthening muscles and improving motor skills (Fig. 25–14). It is

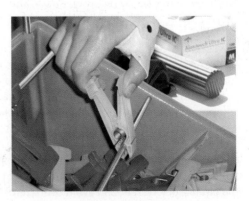

FIGURE 25–14 This hand-based thumb immobilization orthosis has the volar portion cut away to allow flexion.

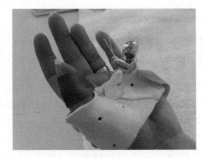

FIGURE 25–12 Hand-based thumb IP flexion mobilization orthosis.

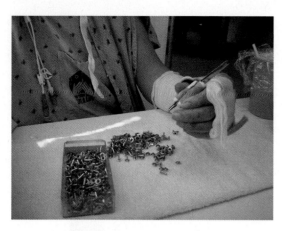

FIGURE 25–15 Built-up tweezers and use of the MCP flexion/thumb opposition orthosis.

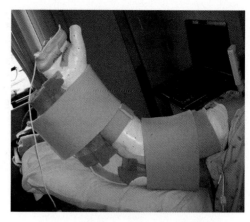

FIGURE 25–16 Arm-based volar immobilization orthosis with a dorsal "sled" with foam padding at the elbow.

imperative that fine motor training include activities such as (but not limited to) moving the fingers individually for writing, manipulating coins in the hand, using utensils, and performing keyboard work (Fig. 25–15). Training for writing should be in the hand that was dominant prior to the amputation. However, if the patient has a bilateral transplant and the dominant hand has a higher level of attachment or complications, retraining dominance may be necessary to facilitate increased independence. Sensory stimulation techniques including a mini–massage device, touch/tap/rubbing the area with various textures, and identifying objects with vision occluded should begin as sensation in the hand returns. The therapy schedule is 6 hours a day, 5 days a week. This schedule can taper off if return to work is possible and progress is acceptable. Higher levels of injury in the forearm will require a longer commitment to full-time therapy to achieve desired goals (Breidenbach et al., 2008; Cavadas, Landin, & Ibanez, 2009; Herzberg et al., 2008; Jablecki et al., 2010; Ravindra et al., 2008; Schneeberger et al., 2006).

Above Elbow Transplants

Immediate Postoperative Phase

As with the below elbow transplanted hand, the hand therapist is intimately involved with the surgical team for transplant positioning, minimizing edema, preventing pressure sores on the insensate skin, and patient/family education.

Orthosis application with the elbow in 30° of flexion will allow for stabilization in a protected position, prevent pressure on the circulatory vessels, and avoid overstretching the healing tendons (Fig. 25–16). The forearm and wrist are held in a neutral position, whereas the MCP joints are in 70° of flexion, the IP joints are extended, and the thumb CMC joint is positioned midway between radial and palmar abduction. Most often, the orthosis should be fabricated volarly incorporating a dorsal "sled" with foam padding to prevent pressure on the olecranon process.

Shoulder exercises consist of active assisted range of motion (AAROM) while wearing the volar portion of the orthosis to protect the elbow (Shores, Brandacher, Schneeberger, Gorantla, & Lee, 2010). Finger and wrist PROM can begin 3 to 5 days after transplantation. A rolling walker with arm rests will be required to support the extremity during daily walking (Lee et al., 2011). To compensate for hand and elbow use, training the patient in the use of a mouth stick can temporarily increase independence with environmental controls (e.g., telephone, TV remote, computer, lights, nurse call button).

3 Weeks Postoperative

The orthosis is adjusted to 60° of elbow flexion to allow scarring and tightening of the biceps. Gentle PROM of the elbow is performed from 0 to 90°. PROM continues distally to all joints (Dubernard et al., 2003; Scheker & Hodges, 2001; Shores et al., 2010). Light AAROM of the bicep and triceps muscles can begin when approved by the surgeons.

6 Weeks Postoperative

AAROM of the elbow(s) can begin, gradually progressing to AROM in gravity-reduced planes such as on a table with the arm on a skateboard or towel (Fig. 25–17). The elbow orthosis should be used when the patient is not in therapy. Because the shoulders obtain adequate strength, the patient (with assistance from the therapist as needed) can begin using a universal cuff to practice controlling utensils and combing hair (Fig. 25–5). This requires elbow control as well as focused concentration.

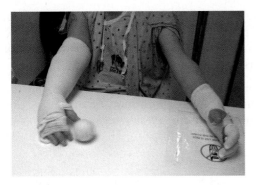

FIGURE 25–17 AROM in the gravity-eliminated plane.

8 Weeks Postoperative

The elbow orthosis is discontinued. The use of a sling and a forearm-based wrist orthosis is sufficient for protecting the involved extremity when out of bed. The sling can be discontinued when the muscles of the elbow are strong enough to move the arm against gravity. When distal muscles have a manual muscle test of $2-/5$ (the joint can move less than full ROM with gravity eliminated) or better, AAROM exercises can begin. **Neuromuscular electrical stimulation** can be used safely once the patient has adequate **sensory innervation** to feel the electrical stimulation. Combining the electrical stimulation with AAROM can help the patient concentrate on activating the newly innervated muscles.

Conclusion

The primary responsibility for therapy practitioners is to increase the independence of our patients. The occupational/physical therapist plays a vital role on the team that treats the patient with upper extremity transplantation. Positioning, orthotic intervention, cortical reintegration, therapeutic exercises, and training for ADLs are all means by which we must carefully and meticulously guide clients through the phases of rehabilitation. Brushing teeth, performing toilet hygiene, playing video games, holding a hand, and feeling the touch of a loved one's face are meaningful goals to these patients. Seemingly little things can be taken for granted, but in this patient population, they become therapy goals because they contribute to the sense of self and "feeling whole." Through commitment, hard work, communication, and dedication from the surgeon-therapist-patient-family team, the goal of functional independence can be achieved.

CASE STUDY SECTION

The case studies presented here are meant as a teaching guideline only. Treatment and orthosis protocols vary greatly from surgeon to surgeon and from therapist to therapist. The therapist should check with the referring physicians and colleagues to define the preferred treatment and appropriate orthotic intervention.

CASE STUDY 1: **Distal Forearm Transplant**

JM is a 26-year-old, right hand–dominant male who sustained a transcarpal amputation from a blast injury to the hand. He was not satisfied with the function of his hand while using a prosthetic. He was subsequently selected for the transplant recipient waiting list. When the appropriate donor was identified, JM was brought into the hospital and his residual limb was prepared. The team of surgeons attached all of the structures of the prepared donor limb to corresponding parts in JM's residual limb. Following surgery, the patient had a bulky gauze dressing with a protective plaster slab applied in the operating room.

Three days postoperative, the surgeons ordered a custom dorsal wrist/hand immobilization orthosis with the wrist in neutral, MCP joints flexed, and IP joints extended (Fig. 25–1). The hand therapist fabricated the orthosis over the bulky dressing. The thumb was positioned midway between palmar and radial abduction with the MP and IP joints extended. At 10 days postoperative, the bulky dressing was reduced, and the wound drains and monitoring wires were discontinued. The decision was made to apply the MCP extension mobilization orthosis to maximize digital mobilization and minimize tendon stress (Fig. 25–2).

At 3 weeks postoperative, for functional activities, a dorsal-based MCP extension restriction orthosis was fabricated to maintain the MCP joints in flexion and the thumb midway between palmar and radial abduction (Fig. 25–8). This orthosis was used during light functional activity and during wrist AROM. A lightweight material was used to minimize stress to the healing structures. During the fabrication process, padding was integrated into the orthosis to prevent potential tissue breakdown on very insensate skin.

After the postoperative week 6, the forearm-based mobilization orthosis was discontinued, and a hand-based orthosis was worn when not performing exercises for the digits. A forearm-based orthosis was used to protect the healing forearm bones during activities such as driving, using the arm bike, and performing proximal exercises with cuff weights. After 8 weeks, the patient used the hand-based orthosis to prevent PIP flexion contractures and make pinching stronger until intrinsic muscle function improved.

Additional case studies can be found on the companion web site on thePoint.

Chapter Review Questions

1. What is allotransplantation? Who are the candidates?

2. Explain the preoperative and postoperative role of the hand therapist in this patient population.

3. Explain the difference between the transplanted hand and the replanted hand.

4. How important is the level of attachment, how does this influence the postoperative protocol, and what are some of the postoperative complications that a therapist should be keenly aware of?

5. For a below elbow transplantation, describe the stages and time frames for orthotic intervention, along with the rationale during each stage.

Index

Page numbers followed by "*b*," "*f*," and "*t*" denotes boxes, figures, and tables respectively.